NUTRITIONAL AND METABOLIC DISORDERS

José Adán Amaya Duarte and
Kareling Alexandra Lopez Sandoval

ALLIED
HEALTH
PRESS

Nutritional and Metabolic Disorders

Author: **José Adán Amaya Duarte and Kareling Alexandra Lopez Sandoval**

Allied Health Press
4164 Lakeshore Road
Burlington ON L7L 1A4
Canada
www.alliedhealthpress.com
Email: orders@arclereducation.com

ISBN: 978-1-77956-798-7

ABOUT THE AUTHORS

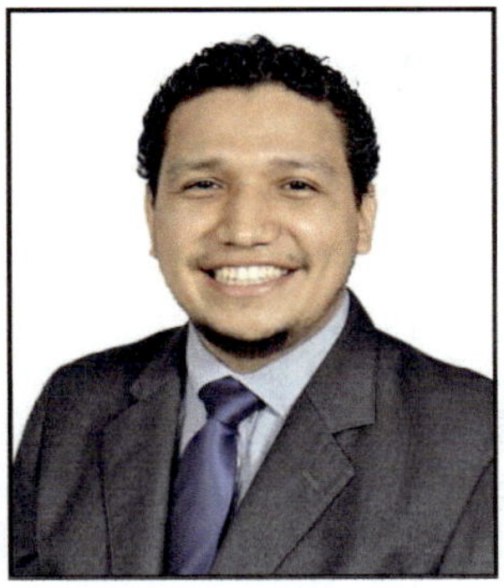

José Adán Amaya Duarte is a medical doctor, academic consultant, and entrepreneur with extensive experience in the industrial, educational, and public health sectors. He currently serves as General Manager (CEO) and co-founder of INVALA S.A., a manufacturing company in Nicaragua, where he has led operational and financial development since 2019.

With a medical degree from UNAN-León, where he also worked as a university professor and research assistant, his profile combines scientific rigor with advanced managerial skills. He also has worked as a medical academic content consultant on global platforms such as Upwork and as a technical advisor and instructional designer for the Pan American Health Organization (PAHO/WHO), participating in multiple virtual training projects, course design, and the updating of pedagogical health content.

In the academic field, he has served as an online tutor, academic coordinator, and designer of educational materials, including audiovisual media, for the Virtual Campus of Public Health. He has also conducted workshops and collaborated in international seminars on topics such as Biofabrication, anatomy, environmental toxicology, educational innovation, and human resource management.

Adán is fluent in English (advanced level) and has basic knowledge of German. In addition, he possesses strong skills in digital tools, ERP/CRM systems, data analysis (SPSS), audiovisual editing, and basic programming (AS3, Swift, Java). His multidisciplinary approach and leadership capacity position him as an influential figure at the intersection of medicine, virtual education, and business management.

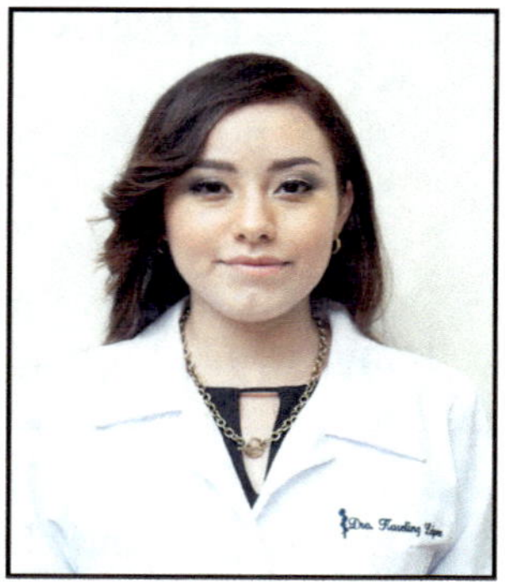

Kareling Alexandra López Sandoval is a medical doctor with experience in clinical care, healthcare operations supervision, and medical translation. She currently serves as Clinical Operations Supervisor at Oclinicals/GI Alliance, coordinating remote teams and maintaining direct communication with clinics in the United States to ensure high standards of patient care.

Graduated as a Doctor of Medicine and Surgery from the National Autonomous University of Nicaragua (UNAN-León), Kareling has worked across various medical areas, developing solid skills in patient assessment, diagnosis, and education. Her career includes roles in both hospital and remote settings, allowing her to adapt to diverse healthcare environments.

In the academic and scientific communication field, she has worked as a medical content reviewer for academic texts, medical article writer based on scientific evidence, and translator of medical documents (Spanish English) with technical accuracy. Her C2-level English proficiency has enabled her to collaborate on international projects, ensuring terminological precision and effective communication with global healthcare teams.

With a combination of clinical training, operational expertise, and medical communication skills, Kareling stands out for her commitment to quality, self-discipline, and continuous improvement in the healthcare sector.

Brief Table of Contents

1. Introduction to Nutritional and Metabolic Disorders 1
2. Macronutrient Metabolism 39
3. Micronutrient Metabolism 73
4. Nutritional Assessment 107
5. Protein-Energy Malnutrition (PEM) 143
6. Obesity and Overnutrition 175
7. Diabetes Mellitus 209
8. Metabolic Bone Disorders 243
9. Lipid Metabolism Disorders 277
10. Inborn Errors of Metabolism 313
11. Eating Disorders 347
12. Gastrointestinal and Liver Disorders 383
13. Nutritional Disorders in Special Populations 417
14. Nutrigenomics and Personalized Nutrition 449
15. Prevention and Public Health Strategies 483

Index 519

Detailed Table of Contents

List of Figures *xv*
Preface *xxiii*

CHAPTER 1

Introduction to Nutritional and Metabolic Disorders 1

Introduction **1**
1.1. Types of Nutritional Disorders **5**
1.1.1. Malnutrition and Its Effects 6
1.1.2. Micronutrient Deficiencies 7
1.1.3. Eating Disorders (e.g., Anorexia, Bulimia) 8
1.2. Types of Metabolic Disorders **9**
1.2.1. Inborn Errors of Metabolism 10
1.2.2. Diabetes Mellitus and Its Complications 11
1.2.3. Thyroid Disorders and Their Impact 12
1.3. Causes of Nutritional Disorders **14**
1.3.1. Socioeconomic Factors 15
1.3.2. Cultural Influences on Diet 16
1.3.3. Psychological Factors Affecting Eating Habits 17
1.4. Causes of Metabolic Disorders **18**
1.4.1. Genetic Predispositions 19
1.4.2. Environmental Triggers 20
1.4.3. Lifestyle Choices and Their Consequences 22
1.5. Diagnosis of Nutritional and Metabolic Disorders **23**
1.5.1. Clinical Assessments and History 25
1.5.2. Laboratory Tests and Imaging 26
1.5.3. Role of Dietary Evaluations 27
1.6. Treatment and Management Strategies **28**
1.6.1. Nutritional Interventions and Dietary Modifications 29
1.6.2. Pharmacological Treatments 31
1.6.3. Importance of Multidisciplinary Approaches 31
Summary **34**
References **36**

CHAPTER 2

Macronutrient Metabolism 39

Introduction **39**
2.1. Types of Macronutrients **43**
2.1.1. Carbohydrates 43
2.1.2. Proteins 44
2.1.3. Fats 45
2.2. Digestion of Macronutrients **46**
2.2.1. Process of Carbohydrate Digestion 47
2.2.2. Process of Protein Digestion 48
2.2.3. Process of Fat Digestion 49
2.3. Absorption of Macronutrients **50**
2.3.1. Mechanisms of Carbohydrate Absorption 51
2.3.2. Mechanisms of Protein Absorption 53
2.3.3. Mechanisms of Fat Absorption 54
2.4. Production of Energy from Macronutrients **55**

2.4.1. Glycolysis and Energy from Carbohydrates 56
2.4.2. Krebs Cycle and Energy from Proteins 57
2.4.3. Beta-Oxidation And Energy from Fats 58
2.5. Role of Hormones in Macronutrient Metabolism 58
2.5.1. Insulin and Carbohydrate Metabolism 60
2.5.2. Glucagon and Protein Metabolism 60
2.5.3. Cortisol and Fat Metabolism 62
2.6. Factors Affecting Macronutrient Metabolism 62
2.6.1. Age and Metabolism 64
2.6.2. Physical Activity and Metabolism 64
2.6.3. Dietary Composition and Metabolism 66
Summary 68
References 70

CHAPTER 3

Micronutrient Metabolism 73

Introduction 73
3.1. Types of Micronutrients 77
3.1.1. Vitamins: Water-Soluble and Fat-Soluble 78
3.1.2. Minerals: Major and Trace Elements 79
3.1.3. Role of Phytochemicals in Micronutrient Metabolism 80
3.2. Absorption of Micronutrients 81
3.2.1. Mechanisms of Absorption in the Gastrointestinal Tract 82
3.2.2. Factors Affecting Absorption Rates 83
3.2.3. Role of Dietary Components in Micronutrient Bioavailability 84
3.3. Transport of Micronutrients 85
3.3.1. Transport Mechanisms in Bloodstream 86
3.3.2. Role of Proteins in Micronutrient Transport 87
3.3.3. Impact of Transport on Cellular Uptake 88
3.4. Metabolism of Vitamins 89
3.4.1. Conversion of Vitamins to Active Forms 90
3.4.2. Role of Coenzymes in Metabolic Pathways 91
3.4.3. Effects of Deficiencies on Metabolic Processes 92
3.5. Metabolism of Minerals 93
3.5.1. Bioavailability and Utilization of Minerals 94
3.5.2. Interactions Between Different Minerals 96
3.5.3. Consequences of Mineral Imbalances 97
3.6. Health Implications of Micronutrient Metabolism 98
3.6.1. Contribution to Health Promotion and Disease Prevention 98
3.6.2. Impact of Deficiencies on Public Health 100
3.6.3. Importance of Micronutrient Supplementation 101
Summary 103
References 105

CHAPTER 4

Nutritional Assessment 107

Introduction 107
4.1. Types of Nutritional Assessment 111
4.1.1. Dietary Assessment Methods 112
4.1.2. Anthropometric Measurements 113
4.1.3. Biochemical Analysis 114
4.2. Dietary Assessment Methods 115
4.2.1. 24-Hour Dietary Recall 116
4.2.2. Food Frequency Questionnaires 117
4.2.3. Diet Diaries 118
4.3. Anthropometric Measurements 119
4.3.1. Body Mass Index (BMI) 120
4.3.2. Waist-to-Hip Ratio 122
4.3.3. Skinfold Thickness Measurements 123
4.4. Biochemical Analysis 123
4.4.1. Blood Tests for Nutrient Levels 125
4.4.2. Metabolic Marker Urine Tests 125
4.4.3. Tissue Biopsies for Nutrient Status 127
4.5. Factors Influencing Nutritional Status 128
4.5.1. Socioeconomic Status 128
4.5.2. Cultural Food Habits 129
4.5.3. Age and Gender Differences 130
4.6. Applications for Nutritional Assessment 131
4.6.1. Patient Care and Clinical Settings 132
4.6.2. Public Health Initiatives 133
4.6.3. Research and Policy Development 134
Summary 137
References 139

CHAPTER 5

Protein-Energy Malnutrition (PEM) 143

Introduction 143
5.1. Causes of Protein-Energy Malnutrition 146
5.1.1. Insufficient Dietary Intake 147
5.1.2. Socioeconomic Factors 148
5.1.3. Health Conditions Affecting Nutrient Absorption 149
5.2. Types of Protein-Energy Malnutrition 150
5.2.1. Kwashiorkor 151
5.2.2. Marasmus 152
5.2.3. Mixed Forms of PEM 153
5.3. Symptoms and Health Effects 154
5.3.1. Physical Symptoms 155
5.3.2. Psychological Effects 155
5.3.3. Long-Term Health Implications 157
5.4. Populations at Risk 157
5.4.1. Children and Infants 159
5.4.2. Elderly Individuals 159
5.4.3. Individuals in Low-Income Countries 160
5.5. Diagnosis of Protein-Energy Malnutrition 161
5.5.1. Clinical Assessment Methods 162
5.5.2. Laboratory Tests 163
5.5.3. Nutritional Screening Tools 164
5.6. Treatment and Management 165
5.6.1. Nutritional Rehabilitation 166
5.6.2. Medical Interventions 167
5.6.3. Community-Based Programs 168
Summary 171
References 173

CHAPTER 6

Obesity and Overnutrition 175

Introduction 175
6.1. Causes of Obesity 178
6.1.1. Genetic Factors 179
6.1.2. Environmental Influences 180
6.1.3. Behavioral Patterns 182
6.2. Health Consequences of Obesity 182
6.2.1. Physical Health Risks 183
6.2.2. Psychological Effects 184
6.2.3. Economic Implications 185
6.3. Nutritional Aspects of Overnutrition 186
6.3.1. Excess Caloric Intake 187
6.3.2. Nutrient Imbalance 188
6.3.3. Role of Processed Foods 189
6.4. Societal Impact of Obesity 190
6.4.1. Stigmatization and Discrimination 191
6.4.2. Impact on Healthcare Systems 192
6.4.3. Influence on Productivity and Workforce 193
6.5. Prevention Strategies 194
6.5.1. Public Health Initiatives 195
6.5.2. Educational Programs 196
6.5.3. Community-Based Interventions 197
6.6. Treatment Options 198
6.6.1. Lifestyle Modifications 199
6.6.2. Medical Interventions 200
6.6.3. Surgical Options 201
Summary 204
References 206

CHAPTER 7

Diabetes Mellitus 209

Introduction 209
7.1. Types of Diabetes Mellitus 212
7.1.1. Type 1 Diabetes 214
7.1.2. Type 2 Diabetes 214
7.1.3. Gestational Diabetes 216
7.2. Causes and Risk Factors 216
7.2.1. Genetic Predisposition 217
7.2.2. Lifestyle Factors 218
7.2.3. Environmental Influences 219
7.3. Symptoms and Diagnosis 220
7.3.1. Common Symptoms of Diabetes 221
7.3.2. Diagnostic Tests and Criteria 222

7.3.3. Importance of Early Detection 223
7.4. Complications of Diabetes 224
7.4.1. Short-Term Complications 225
7.4.2. Long-Term Health Risks 226
7.4.3. Impact on Quality of Life 227
7.5. Management and Treatment 228
7.5.1. Lifestyle Modifications 229
7.5.2. Medication and Insulin Treatment 230
7.5.3. Monitoring Blood Sugar Levels 231
7.6. Prevention Strategies 232
7.6.1. Healthy Eating Habits 233
7.6.2. Regular Physical Activity 234
7.6.3. Education and Awareness Programs 235
Summary 238
References 240

CHAPTER 8

Metabolic Bone Disorders 243

Introduction 243
8.1. Types of Metabolic Bone Disorders 246
8.1.1. Osteoporosis 248
8.1.2. Osteomalacia 248
8.1.3. Paget's Disease 250
8.2. Causes of Metabolic Bone Disorders 251
8.2.1. Nutritional Deficiencies 252
8.2.2. Hormonal Imbalances 253
8.2.3. Genetic Factors 254
8.3. Risk Factors 254
8.3.1. Age and Gender 256
8.3.2. Lifestyle Choices 256
8.3.3. Medical History 257
8.4. Symptoms and Diagnosis 258
8.4.1. Common Symptoms 259
8.4.2. Diagnostic Tests 260
8.4.3. Importance of Early Detection 261
8.5. Treatment Options 262
8.5.1. Medications 263
8.5.2. Lifestyle Modifications 264
8.5.3. Surgical Interventions 265
8.6. Prevention Strategies 266
8.6.1. Nutritional Guidelines 267
8.6.2. Exercise Recommendations 268
8.6.3. Regular Health Screenings 268
Summary 271
References 273

CHAPTER 9

Lipid Metabolism Disorders 277

Introduction 277
9.1. Types of Lipid Metabolism Disorders 281
9.1.1. Hyperlipidemia 282
9.1.2. Lipid Storage Diseases 283
9.1.3. Fatty Liver Disease 284
9.2. Causes of Lipid Metabolism Disorders 285
9.2.1. Genetic Factors 286
9.2.2. Dietary Influences 287
9.2.3. Lifestyle Choices 288
9.3. Symptoms and Diagnosis 289
9.3.1. Common Lipid Metabolism Disorder Symptoms 290
9.3.2. Diagnostic Tests and Procedures 291
9.3.3. Importance of Early Detection 293
9.4. Impact on Health 294
9.4.1. Cardiovascular Diseases 295
9.4.2. Pancreatitis 296
9.4.3. Liver Dysfunction 297
9.5. Treatment Alternatives 298
9.5.1. Dietary Modifications 299
9.5.2. Pharmacological Interventions 300
9.5.3. Lifestyle Changes 301
9.6. Research and Advances 302
9.6.1. Current Research Trends in Lipid Metabolism 303
9.6.2. Emerging Therapies and Treatments 304
9.6.3. Future Directions in Lipid Metabolism Research 305
Summary 308
References 310

CHAPTER 10

Inborn Errors of Metabolism 313

Introduction 313
10.1. Types of Inborn Errors of Metabolism 317
10.1.1. Carbohydrate Metabolism Disorders 318
10.1.2. Amino Acid Metabolism Disorders 319
10.1.3. Lipid Metabolism Disorders 320
10.2. Genetic Basis of Inborn Errors of Metabolism 321
10.2.1. Function of Genes in Metabolic Pathways 322
10.2.2. Inheritance Patterns (Autosomal Recessive, Dominant, etc.) 323
10.2.3. Genetic Mutations and Their Effects 324
10.3. Symptoms and Diagnosis 325
10.3.1. Common Clinical Manifestations 326
10.3.2. Diagnostic Tests and Procedures 327
10.3.3. Importance of Early Detection 328
10.4. Treatment Options 329
10.4.1. Dietary Management and Restrictions 330
10.4.2. Enzyme Replacement Therapy (ERT) 331
10.4.3. Gene Therapy Advancements 332
10.5. Case Studies 333
10.5.1. Phenylketonuria (PKU) 334
10.5.2. Maple Syrup Urine Disease (MSUD) 335
10.5.3. Galactosemia 336
10.6. Impact on Patients and Families 337
10.6.1. Psychological Effect on Patients 338
10.6.2. Financial Burden of Treatment 339
10.6.3. Support Systems and Resources Available 340
Summary 343
References 345

CHAPTER 11

Eating Disorders 347

Introduction 347
11.1. Types of Eating Disorders 351
11.1.1. Anorexia Nervosa 352
11.1.2. Bulimia Nervosa 353
11.1.3. Binge Eating Disorder 354
11.2. Causes of Eating Disorders 355
11.2.1. Genetic Factors 356
11.2.2. Psychological Influences 357
11.2.3. Societal and Cultural Pressures 358
11.3. Symptoms and Diagnosis 359
11.3.1. Physical Symptoms 360
11.3.2. Emotional and Behavioral Symptoms 361
11.3.3. Diagnostic Criteria and Assessment 362
11.4. Consequences of Eating Disorders 363
11.4.1. Physical Health Complications 364
11.4.2. Psychological Effects 365
11.4.3. Social and Relational Impacts 366
11.5. Treatment Options 367
11.5.1. Counseling and Therapy 368
11.5.2. Nutritional Rehabilitation 369
11.5.3. Medication and Medical Intervention 370
11.6. Prevention Strategies 371
11.6.1. Awareness and Education Campaigns 372
11.6.2. Promoting Healthy Body Image 373
11.6.3. Support Systems and Community Resources 374
Summary 377
References 379

CHAPTER 12

Gastrointestinal and Liver Disorders 383

Introduction 383
12.1. Anatomy and Physiology of the Gastrointestinal System 387
12.1.1. Structure of the Gastrointestinal Tract 388
12.1.2. Functions of the Gastrointestinal System 389
12.1.3. Interaction Between the Gastrointestinal System and Liver 390
12.2. Common Gastrointestinal Disorders 391
12.2.1. Gastroesophageal Reflux Disease (GERD) 392
12.2.2. Inflammatory Bowel Disease (IBD) 393
12.2.3. Irritable Bowel Syndrome (IBS) 394
12.3. Liver Disorders Overview 395
12.3.1. Types of Liver Disorders 396

12.3.2. Causes of Liver Disorders 397
12.3.3. Symptoms Associated with Liver Disorders 398
12.4. Diagnostic Strategies for Gastrointestinal and Hepatic Disorders 399
12.4.1. Imaging Techniques (e.g., Ultrasound, CT scan) 400
12.4.2. Endoscopic Procedures 401
12.4.3. Laboratory Tests (e.g., Liver Function Tests) 401
12.5. Treatment Options for Gastrointestinal Disorders 402
12.5.1. Dietary Modifications 403
12.5.2. Laboratory Tests (e.g., Liver Function Tests) 404
12.5.3. Treatment Options for Gastrointestinal Disorders 405
12.6. Pharmacological Treatments 406
12.6.1. Surgical Interventions 407
12.6.2. Treatment for Liver Disorders 408
12.6.3. Lifestyle Changes and Dietary Recommendations 409
Summary 411
References 413

CHAPTER 13

Nutritional Disorders in Special Populations 417

Introduction 417
13.1. Nutritional Disorders in Children 420
13.1.1. Common Disorders Affecting Children 422
13.1.2. Impact of Socioeconomic Status on Nutrition 422
13.1.3. Role of Schools in Promoting Healthy Eating 424
13.2. Nutritional Disorders in the Elderly 424
13.2.1. Age-Related Changes Affecting Nutrition 425
13.2.2. Common Deficiencies in Elderly Populations 426
13.2.3. Strategies for Improving Nutritional Intake 427
13.3. Nutritional Disorders in Pregnant Women 428
13.3.1. Importance of Nutrition During Pregnancy 429
13.3.2. Common Nutritional Deficiencies Among Pregnant Women 430
13.3.3. Effects of Maternal Nutrition on Fetal Development 431
13.4. Nutrition Disorders Among Athletes 432
13.4.1. Unique Nutritional Needs of Athletes 433
13.4.2. Risks of Disordered Eating in Sports 434
13.4.3. Importance of Hydration and Recovery Nutrition 435
13.5. Nutritional Disorders Among Persons with Disabilities 436
13.5.1. Challenges Faced by Individuals with Disabilities 437
13.5.2. Specific Nutritional Needs and Considerations 438
13.5.3. Role of Caregivers in Managing Nutrition 439
13.6. Cultural Influences on Nutritional Disorders 440
13.6.1. Impact of Cultural Beliefs on Dietary Practices 441
13.6.2. Nutritional Disorders Prevalent in Specific Cultures 442
13.6.3. Strategies for Culturally Sensitive Nutrition Education 443
Summary 445
References 447

CHAPTER 14

Nutrigenomics and Personalized Nutrition 449

Introduction 449
14.1. The Science of Nutrigenomics 452
14.1.1 Genetic Variations and Their Impact on Nutrition 453
14.1.2. Mechanisms of Gene-Nutrient Interactions 454
14.1.3. Role of Epigenetics in Dietary Responses 455
14.2. Historical Context 457
14.2.1. Evolution of Nutritional Science 457
14.2.2. Key Milestones in Nutrigenomics Research 458

14.2.3. Development of Personalized Nutrition Concepts 459
14.3. Applications for Nutrigenomics 460
14.3.1. Tailored Dietary Recommendations 461
14.3.2. Nutrigenomic Assessment and Testing 462
14.3.3. Case Studies of Successful Personalized Nutrition Plans 463
14.4. Benefits of Personalized Nutrition 464
14.4.1. Improved Health Outcomes 465
14.4.2. Enhanced Weight Management Measures 466
14.4.3. Prevention of Diet-Related Diseases 467
14.5. Challenges and Limitations 468
14.5.1. Ethical Considerations of Nutrigenomics 469
14.5.2. Accessibility and Affordability of Testing 470
14.5.3. Variability in Individual Response to Diets 471
14.6. Future Directions in Nutrigenomics 472
14.6.1. Advances in Genomic Technologies 473
14.6.2. Integration of Nutrigenomics into Healthcare 474
14.6.3. Potential for Public Health Initiatives 475
Summary 478
References 480

CHAPTER 15

Prevention and Public Health Strategies 483

Introduction 483
15.1. Historical Context of Public Health 487
15.1.1. Evolution of Public Health Practices 489
15.1.2. Significant Public Health Achievements 490
15.1.3. Impact of Historical Pandemics on Health Strategies 491
15.2. Epidemiology and Disease Prevention 492
15.2.1. Role of Epidemiology in Public Health 493
15.2.2. Disease Surveillance and Monitoring 494
15.2.3. Strategies for Outbreak Control 495
15.3. Health Education and Promotion 496
15.3.1. Importance of Health Literacy 497
15.3.2. Community Outreach and Engagement 498
15.3.3. Use of Social Media in Health Promotion 499
15.4. Vaccination Programs 500
15.4.1. Overview of Vaccination Strategies 501
15.4.2. Impact of Vaccines on Public Health 502
15.4.3. Challenges in Vaccine Distribution and Acceptance 503
15.5. Policy and Legislation 504
15.5.1. Role of Government in Public Health 505
15.5.2. Key Public Health Policies and Legislation 506
15.5.3. Advocacy for Health-Related Legislation 507
15.6. Global Health Initiatives 508
15.6.1. International Organizations and Their Roles 509
15.6.2. Global Strategies for Disease Prevention 510
15.6.3. Collaboration Between Countries for Health Improvement 511
Summary 514
References 516

Index 519

LIST OF FIGURES

Figure 1.1. Child eating fresh raspberries, promoting healthy early nutrition
Figure 1.2. Children with rickets showing bone deformities due to vitamin D deficiency
Figure 1.3. Overview of common metabolic disorders and associated conditions
Figure 1.4. Types of nutritional disorders
Figure 1.5. Clinical effects of malnutrition across major body systems
Figure 1.6. Whole foods as natural sources of nutrients
Figure 1.7. Key symptoms associated with major eating disorders: AN, BN, and BED
Figure 1.8. Types of metabolic disorders affecting human health
Figure 1.9. Inborn errors of metabolism
Figure 1.10. Major complications associated with diabetes
Figure 1.11. Types of thyroid diseases compared to healthy thyroid gland
Figure 1.12. Medical examination of a bruised and swollen knee
Figure 1.13. Illustration of traditional foods from around the world
Figure 1.14. Key emotional, social, and economic factors affecting eating habits
Figure 1.15. Main causes contributing to metabolic syndrome
Figure 1.16. DNA visualization highlighting genetic predisposition to disease
Figure 1.17. Factors contributing to inflammatory bowel disease (IBD)
Figure 1.18: Healthy vs. unhealthy lifestyle habits
Figure 1.19. Dietary impact on inflammation and metabolic disease risk
Figure 1.20. Methods for assessing physician clinical competency
Figure 1.21. A scientist performing laboratory research with modern equipment
Figure 1.22. A nutritionist preparing a healthy diet and lifestyle plan
Figure 1.23. Therapeutic strategies for managing obesity
Figure 1.24. Impact of dietary modification on type 2 diabetes and its complications
Figure 1.25. Caregiver assisting with daily medication management
Figure 2.1. Comparison of essential macronutrients and micronutrients
Figure 2.2. Sources of macronutrients essential for metabolism
Figure 2.3. Types of macronutrients: Carbohydrates, proteins, and fats
Figure 2.4. Common dietary sources of carbohydrates
Figure 2.5. Labeled diagram of digestive organs involved in nutrient processing

Figure 2.6. Steps and organs involved in carbohydrate digestion
Figure 2.7. Enzymatic breakdown of proteins into amino acids
Figure 2.8. Process of fat digestion and absorption in the body
Figure 2.9. Peptide and amino acid absorption in the small intestine
Figure 2.10. Mechanisms of carbohydrate absorption in the intestine
Figure 2.11. Digestion and absorption pathway of dietary proteins
Figure 2.12. Sources of essential dietary macronutrients
Figure 2.13. Inputs and outputs of the Krebs (citric acid) cycle
Figure 2.14. ATP production from macronutrient metabolism pathways
Figure 2.15. Glucagon signaling pathway promoting catabolic activity in hepatic cells
Figure 2.16. Age, gender, and body composition impact metabolic rate
Figure 2.17. Overview of metabolic inputs and outputs in the human body
Figure 3.1. Food sources rich in essential vitamins and minerals
Figure 3.2. Colorful fruits, vegetables, and seeds as sources of essential micronutrients
Figure 3.3. Assorted nutrient-dense foods rich in vitamins, minerals, healthy fats, and proteins for a balanced diet
Figure 3.4. Types of micronutrients: fat- and water-soluble vitamins, macrominerals, and microminerals
Figure 3.5. Classification of minerals into major minerals (e.g., calcium, magnesium) and trace elements (e.g., iodine, zinc)
Figure 3.6. An assortment of legumes and seeds highlights common dietary sources of essential micronutrients, vital for metabolism, immunity, and overall health
Figure 3.7. Structure and regional divisions of the gastrointestinal tract, including the foregut, midgut, and hindgut
Figure 3.8. Route-specific factors influencing drug absorption into systemic circulation
Figure 3.9. Micronutrient transport by MEC from maternal blood to milk
Figure 3.10. Types of membrane transport proteins: Pumps, ion channels, and transporters
Figure 3.11. Pathway of vitamin B12 absorption and metabolism from dietary sources to intestinal uptake
Figure 3.12. Structure of Coenzyme A showing its key components: Amino ethanethiol, pantothenic acid, and phosphorylated ADP
Figure 3.13. Carbohydrate deficiency and its link to related diseases
Figure 3.14. Diagram of mineral metabolism and dietary sources of essential minerals
Figure 3.15. Key factors affecting mineral bioavailability in the body
Figure 3.16. Common forms of mineral and vitamin supplements
Figure 3.17. Promoting disease prevention through healthy lifestyle habits
Figure 3.18. Nutrition's impact on brain health and mental well-being
Figure 4.1. Clinical nutrition assessment and dietary counseling

Figure 4.2. Nutritional planning with fresh vegetables
Figure 4.3. Digital nutrition tracking and calorie assessment
Figure 4.4. A nutritionist guiding healthy eating and meal planning
Figure 4.5. Different methods of anthropometric measurement
Figure 4.6. Nutritional assessment through balanced dietary choices
Figure 4.7. Variety of fresh, nutritious ingredients for a balanced diet
Figure 4.9. Meal planning with fruits and a structured diet chart
Figure 4.10. Measuring waist circumference for nutritional assessment
Figure 4.11. BMI chart categorizing weight status by body mass index ranges
Figure 4.12. Waist-to-hip ratio chart linking body shape to health risk
Figure 4.13. Biochemical analysis conducted in a laboratory setting
Figure 4.14. Doctor preparing patient for blood sample collection
Figure 4.15. Various personal and cultural factors affecting nutrition
Figure 4.16. Cultural influences on food choices and seasoning preferences
Figure 4.18. Demographic factors like sex, age, and cultural differences
Figure 4.19. The medical team performing bedside patient evaluation
Figure 4.20. Healthcare workers supporting public health initiatives
Figure 5.1. Comparison of Kwashiorkor and Marasmus in protein-energy malnutrition
Figure 5.2. Clinical presentation of Kwashiorkor and Marasmus
Figure 5.3. Factors leading to and resulting from protein energy malnutrition
Figure 5.4. Key socio-economic factors influencing well-being
Figure 5.5. Types of protein energy malnutrition: Kwashiorkor, Marasmus, and Marasmic Kwashiorkor
Figure 5.6. Key signs and symptoms of Marasmus in children
Figure 5.7. Infant showing signs of protein-energy malnutrition
Figure 5.8. Illustration of brain activity and neural connections
Figure 5.9. Populations at higher risk for health and nutritional challenges
Figure 5.10. Elderly people enjoying social interaction in the park
Figure 5.11. Diagnostic steps for identifying protein-energy malnutrition
Figure 5.12. Nutritional consultation between the patient and the healthcare provider
Figure 5.13. Women participating in a community nutrition education session
Figure 5.14. Surgeons performing a medical procedure in an operating room
Figure 6.1. Foods high in sugar and fat contribute to overnutrition
Figure 6.2. Causes and health consequences associated with obesity
Figure 6.3. Illustration of genetic modification through DNA editing techniques
Figure 6.4. Environmental factors influencing human development
Figure 6.5. Health complications arising from obesity

Figure 6.6. Psychological effects of workplace bullying include anxiety, depression, panic attacks, and difficulty concentrating
Figure 6.7. Types of malnutrition: Undernutrition, overnutrition, and micronutrient deficiency
Figure 6.8. Nursing diagnosis chart for imbalanced nutrition less than body requirements
Figure 6.9. Impact of food environment on dietary choices and obesity
Figure 6.10. VR and AI integration in advanced medical diagnostics
Figure 6.11. Three levels of disease prevention: Primary, secondary, and tertiary
Figure 6.12. Participants attending an in-person training or educational seminar
Figure 6.13. Treatment options for prostate cancer
Figure 6.14. Core elements of a healthy lifestyle
Figure 6.15. Types of medical interventions and tools
Figure 7.1. Overview of diabetes mellitus diagnosis and management
Figure 7.2. Insulin and glucose function in healthy, Type 1, and Type 2 diabetes
Figure 7.3. Types of diabetes mellitus and their classification
Figure 7.4. Glucose and insulin activity in normal vs. Type 2 diabetes
Figure 7.5. Common causes of hypertension
Figure 7.6. Major lifestyle factors influencing health
Figure 7.7. Key symptoms associated with diabetes
Figure 7.8. Key methods and limitations in diagnosing ADHD
Figure 7.9. Common health complications caused by diabetes
Figure 7.10. Viral infection affecting the human respiratory system
Figure 7.11. Doctor guiding patients on medication and care plan
Figure 7.12. Common treatment methods for diabetes management
Figure 7.13. A healthcare professional checking a patient's blood glucose level using a glucometer
Figure 7.14. Choosing between unhealthy fast food and healthy nutrition
Figure 7.15. Different types of physical exercises for teens
Figure 8.1. Visual representation of osteoporotic bone structure
Figure 8.2. Metabolic bone disorders affecting bone strength and structure
Figure 8.3. Bone remodeling cycle showing key cellular processes
Figure 8.4. Bone density comparison: normal vs. Osteomalacia
Figure 8.5. Common signs and symptoms of Paget's disease
Figure 8.6. Effects of nutritional deficiency on energy and health
Figure 8.7. Common symptoms of hormonal imbalance
Figure 8.8. Healthy bone vs. osteoporotic bone comparison
Figure 8.9. Healthy lifestyle habits for overall well-being
Figure 8.10. Bone disorders linked to systemic conditions

Figure 8.11. Blood samples prepared for laboratory testing
Figure 8.12. A nurse supporting a young cancer patient during recovery
Figure 8.13. Healthy lifestyle tools for fitness and wellness
Figure 8.14. Balanced diet plate illustrating key food groups
Figure 8.15. Routine health check-up for early disease detection
Figure 9.1. Overview of lipid metabolism and tissue distribution
Figure 9.2. Neuron affected by lipid metabolism disorder
Figure 9.3. Arterial plaque buildup due to hyperlipidemia
Figure 9.4. Healthy liver versus cirrhotic liver comparison
Figure 9.5. DNA double helix structure illustrating genetic material
Figure 9.6. Balanced diet and regular exercise support heart health and overall well-being
Figure 9.7. Impact of smoking and high-fat diet on lungs, liver, and gut health contributing to chronic inflammation and metabolic disorders
Figure 9.8. Genetic testing through blood analysis in a clinical laboratory setting
Figure 9.9. Blood pressure check for early detection of hypertension
Figure 9.10. Illustration of the human cardiovascular system showing the heart, arteries, and veins
Figure 9.11. Acute inflammation of the pancreas and nearby digestive structures
Figure 9.12. Essential medical tools and medications used in patient treatment and care
Figure 9.13. Various prescription medications used in chronic disease management
Figure 9.14. Medical researcher working with a microscope and a computer in a laboratory setting
Figure 9.15. Advanced laboratory research exploring the human microbiome and genetic science
Figure 10.1. Illustration of gene editing showing targeted modification within a DNA strand
Figure 10.2. Complications associated with metabolic syndrome
Figure 10.3. Visualization of carbohydrate metabolism with enzymes active in the bloodstream
Figure 10.4. Overview of insulin resistance cascade: from liver disease and dyslipidemia to adiposity and systemic complications
Figure 10.5. Conversion of food into ATP and heat through metabolic processes in the human body
Figure 10.6. Autosomal recessive inheritance showing carrier parents and risk distribution in offspring
Figure 10.6. Monitoring blood pressure to manage and diagnose hypertension
Figure 10.7. Plant researchers analyzing tissue culture samples in a laboratory setting
Figure 10.8. Laboratory technician handling blood samples for diagnostic testing and analysis
Figure 10.9. Overview of leukemia treatment options including chemotherapy, targeted therapy, stem cell transplant, radiation therapy, and immunotherapy
Figure 10.10. Illustration of i-ERT formulation using lipid nanoparticles and polymers to deliver encapsulated mRNA
Figure 10.11. Infant undergoing routine clinical examination for early health assessment

Figure 10.12. Newborn receive specialized monitoring and support in a clinical environment
Figure 10.13. Symptoms of galactosemia in an infant, highlighting organ and neurological complications
Figure 10.14. Chemotherapy patients sharing support during treatment
Figure 10.15. Support systems play a vital role in the care and recovery of cancer patients
Figure 11.1. Individuals exhibiting signs of restrictive eating behavior, commonly associated with eating disorders
Figure 11.2. Group dining fostering connection and mindful eating
Figure 11.3. Key warning signs of anorexia nervosa
Figure 11.4. Binge eating episode with excessive intake of high-calorie foods
Figure 11.5. Venn diagram showing common psychological and environmental causes of anorexia, bulimia, and binge-eating disorders
Figure 11.6. Mother comforting her daughter during an emotional moment
Figure 11.7. Sharing a joyful moment over a hearty meal
Figure 11.8. Signs of an eating disorder including behavioral and physical indicators
Figure 11.9. Binge eating behavior involving excessive consumption of high-calorie foods
Figure 11.10. Doctor discussing digestive health symptoms with a patient during consultation
Figure 11.11. Craving high-calorie foods while restricting intake—an illustration of disordered eating behavior
Figure 11.12. Therapeutic approaches commonly used in the treatment of eating disorders
Figure 11.13. A dietitian offering personalized nutritional counseling during a client consultation
Figure 11.14. Eating Disorder Awareness: Promoting healthy eating habits for all ages
Figure 11.15. Distracted eating: A young girl focused on her phone during mealtimes
Figure 12.1. Visual representation of digestive discomfort in the stomach and intestines
Figure 12.2. Visual representation of the liver's location within the human digestive system
Figure 12.3. Digestive system diagram showing key organs from the oral cavity to the anus
Figure 12.4. The gastrointestinal system showing digestion, absorption, and excretion functions
Figure 12.5. Healthy guts supported by beneficial microbes and probiotic-rich foods
Figure 12.6. Ulcerative colitis and Crohn's disease shown as types of inflammatory bowel disease (IBD)
Figure 12.7. Irritable bowel syndrome (IBS) showing abdominal pain and colon inflammation
Figure 12.8. The human liver is shown in anatomical position within the abdominal cavity
Figure 12.9. Liver pain indicating potential inflammation or liver-related disorder
Figure 12.10. Gastroenterology concept image showing abdominal discomfort and the digestive tract
Figure 12.11. Upper endoscopy showing the scope inserted to examine the upper digestive tract
Figure 12.12. Gastrointestinal disorders treatment targeting digestive tract issues
Figure 12.13. Liver function test sample used to evaluate liver health markers
Figure 12.14. Medications used for treating injuries or medical conditions

Figure 12.15. Treatment options for fatty liver include L-carnitine, glutathione, vitamins C and E, and Myers' protocol
Figure 13.1. Nutritional deficiencies can lead to diet-related diseases and poor health
Figure 13.2. Balanced nutrition and physical activity tailored to special populations for optimal health
Figure 13.3. Child enjoying a nutritious meal, promoting healthy eating habits from a young age
Figure 13.4. Mother and daughter cook together, promoting healthy eating and bonding
Figure 13.5. Elderly woman refusing food, highlighting nutritional challenges in aging populations
Figure 13.6. Older adults managing medications for common age-related health issues
Figure 13.7. Pregnancy nutrition choices affecting fetal growth and maternal health
Figure 13.8. Balanced nutrition during pregnancy supports the mother and baby's health
Figure 13.9. Couple refueling with bananas and water after playing basketball
Figure 13.10. Cycle showing how low self-esteem and stress contribute to eating disorders in athletes
Figure 13.11. Caregiver assisting elderly woman at mealtime, encouraging nutrition and care
Figure 13.12. Healthy meal prep highlighting the nutrition needs of working men and women
Figure 13.13. Families enjoying traditional meals, highlighting culture's role in healthy eating
Figure 13.14. Social media influence on food choices and eating behaviors
Figure 14.1. Nutrigenomics links diet, lifestyle, genetics, and health
Figure 14.2. Nutrigenomics connects nutrition and genes for personalized health
Figure 14.3. Fruits and vegetables forming a DNA strand to represent nutrition–gene connection
Figure 14.4. Diet influences health and disease risk through epigenetic and transgenerational effects
Figure 14.5. Personalized nutrition shaped by genetics, lifestyle, and metabolic factors
Figure 14.6. Applications of nutrigenomics in personalized diet and gene interaction
Figure 14.7. Nutrition influences gene expression and overall health
Figure 14.8. Benefits of personalized nutrition for health, diet, and disease prevention
Figure 14.9. Balanced diet and exercise support effective weight management
Figure 14.10. Nutrition guidance supports disease prevention and healthy living
Figure 14.11. Nutrigenetics and nutrigenomics influence metabolism and disease risk through gene–diet interactions
Figure 14.12. Fresh vegetable salads rich in nutrients, promoting a healthy and balanced diet
Figure 14.13. Tools like CRISPR and sequencing enhance fruit and vegetable genetics
Figure 14.14. Gut microbiota and nutrients affect gene expression and cardiovascular risk
Figure 15.1. A healthcare professional providing nutrition and lifestyle counseling to older adults
Figure 15.2. Doctor providing health advice to support public health awareness
Figure 15.3. Historic scene of childhood vaccination in early public health care
Figure 15.4. Health workers providing community care during Ebola response efforts

Figure 15.5. Healthy diet and active lifestyle support disease prevention

Figure 15.6. Global epidemiological surveillance through research and data analysis

Figure 15.7. Core components of health education: promotion, empowerment, lifelong learning, and information spread

Figure 15.8. Masked community members participate in an interactive public health education session

Figure 15.9. Child receiving vaccination with parental support to promote immunization and public health

Figure 15.10. Close-up of vaccine preparation by a masked healthcare worker, emphasizing immunization safety

Figure 15.11. Digital interface illustrating legal policies and regulatory frameworks

Figure 15.12. Symbolic representation of healthcare policy and governmental reform initiatives

Figure 15.13. Hands of diverse colors encircling the globe, symbolizing global cooperation and equity in health

Figure 15.14. Key components of NCD prevention depicted through lifestyle and health management icons

PREFACE

The study of nutritional and metabolic disorders encompasses a vast spectrum of conditions arising from the complex interplay between dietary intake, biochemical processes, and genetic predispositions. Over the lifespan, macronutrient and micronutrient imbalances lead to states of deficiency, excess, or dysfunction that impair growth, development, and health. From cellular mechanisms that govern energy generation to the systemic effects of hormonal regulation, understanding how nutrients are processed, stored, and utilized is essential to preventing and treating disease. In addition, altering food availability patterns and lifestyle behaviors in modern societies have reshaped the epidemiology of these disorders, presenting new challenges to clinicians, researchers, and public health practitioners.

Metabolic pathways are context-dependent; their function is regulated by factors as diverse as age, sex, environmental exposure, and culture. Advances in molecular biology and omics technologies have begun to define how single-gene mutation variation in inherited metabolic diseases builds through to polygenic risk in common conditions such as obesity and type 2 diabetes, impacts nutritional requirement and disease susceptibility. As knowledge increases, so does the potential of targeted intervention, by way of dietary modification, drug treatment, or gene-directed therapy. The convergence of clinical experience, laboratory research, and epidemiologic data offers a special potential to enhance our techniques for diagnosis, treatment, and prevention of disorders depending on nutritional and metabolic deviation.

To meet the need for a comprehensive resource, *Nutritional and Metabolic Disorders* integrate basic principles, clinical practice, and recent research in a single easy-to-use volume. The text can be utilized as a resource for practitioners and as a teaching text for trainees and students. By presenting new evidence together with practical guidance, the book aims to attempt to bridge the gap between theory and practice, equipping the reader with the skills to address the entire range of nutritional and metabolic challenges in contemporary healthcare settings.

Chapter 1 sets the stage for our historical and epidemiological background and trends that brought us to our present perception of nutritional and metabolic diseases and sets the stage for a more detailed exploration of metabolic processes and clinical syndromes. Chapter 2 describes the digestion, absorption, transport, and utilization of carbohydrates, proteins, and fats with a focus on the enzymatic reactions and regulatory hormones that govern macronutrient metabolism. Chapter 3 explains vitamins and trace elements and their roles as cofactors, antioxidants, and signaling molecules, and also deficiency and toxicity status. Chapter 4 discusses assessment tools, from anthropometry and food surveys to biochemical markers and function tests, and how to choose the right ones for populations.

Chapter 5 reviews the spectrum of protein-energy malnutrition, ranging from kwashiorkor and marasmus to mixed, with emphasis on pathophysiology, clinical presentation, and therapeutic considerations. Chapter 6 reviews the global epidemic of obesity and overnutrition, including pathogenesis, comorbidities, and multi-specialty management strategies. Chapter 7 covers pathologic and physiologic processes of diabetes mellitus separately for type 1, type 2, and other selected types and surveys contemporary pharmacologic and lifestyle treatments. Chapter 8 surveys metabolic bone disease, including osteoporosis, osteomalacia, and Paget's disease and emphasizes interaction among vitamin D, calcium homeostasis, and bone integrity.

Chapter 9 summarizes lipid metabolism disorders, such as dyslipidemias, atherosclerosis risk factors, and inherited metabolic disorders like familial hypercholesterolemia, in addition to lipid-lowering treatment and dietary and lifestyle changes. Chapter 10 covers inborn errors of metabolism, offering a classification system and summarizing leading examples, such as phenylketonuria, maple syrup urine disease, and urea cycle defects, and also newborn screening, testing and diet therapy. Chapter 11 examines eating disorders, including anorexia nervosa, bulimia nervosa, and binge-eating disorder, focusing on psychological factors, medical complications, and multidisciplinary treatment paradigms. Chapter 12 addresses gastrointestinal and liver disorders with associated nutritional factors, including celiac disease, inflammatory bowel disease, and hepatic steatosis, as well as nutritional support and therapeutic diets.

Chapter 13 discusses special population nutritional disorders—e.g., lactating and pregnant women, infants and children, old age, and chronic disease, and considers unique nutrient requirements and risk factors. Chapter 14 introduces nutrigenomics and personalized nutrition to the forefront, discussing the role of genetic variation in nutrient metabolism and how dietary manipulation may be tailored to an individual's genomic profile. Chapter 15 concludes on prevention and public health practice, summarizing policy development, community intervention, and global activities to reduce the burden of nutritional and metabolic disease.

This book is for medical students, dietitians, nutritionists, physicians, and allied health practitioners who desire a comprehensive but applicable overview of nutritional and metabolic disorders. Researchers and policy analysts alike will also gain from the blending of clinical acumen and public health knowledge. As a textbook in courses taught by health professionals or as a bench reference in clinical settings, *Nutritional and Metabolic Disorders* aims to promote evidence-based decision making and stimulate ongoing exploration of the complex intersections of nutrition, metabolism, and health.

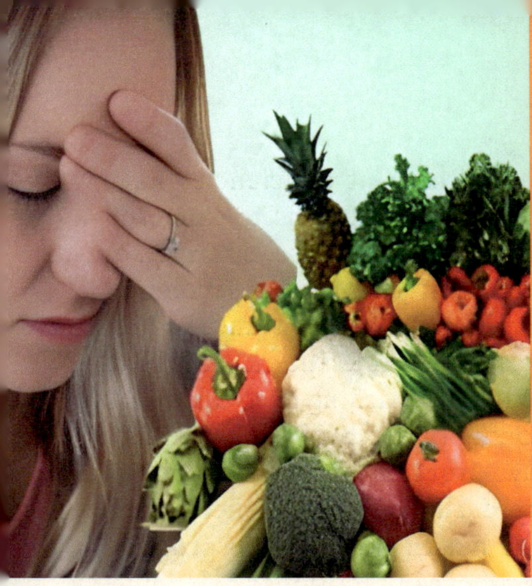

Chapter 1

INTRODUCTION TO NUTRITIONAL AND METABOLIC DISORDERS

Contents

Introduction 1
1.1. Types of Nutritional Disorders 5
1.2. Types of Metabolic Disorders 9
1.3. Causes of Nutritional Disorders 14
1.4. Causes of Metabolic Disorders 18
1.5. Diagnosis of Nutritional and Metabolic Disorders 23
1.6. Treatment and Management Strategies 28
Summary 34
References 36

Introduction

The category nutritional and metabolic disorders encompasses a broad spectrum of ailments that arise because of an imbalance in the intake, assimilation, and processing of nutrients. The term nutritional disorders is restricted to describing those issues that result from an excess or deficiency or relative deficiency of primary nutrients such as vitamins, minerals, and macronutrients. Scurvy and rickets are disorders caused by a deficiency of vitamin C and vitamin D, respectively. In contrast, metabolic disorders are due to disturbances of biochemical processes that lie behind the metabolic functions, for example, the breakdown of food to energy through metabolism. Metabolic disturbances like such are either congenital, e.g., phenylketonuria, or acquired, typically due to lifestyle factors like nutrition and lack of exercise. This duality underscores the complex interrelation of nutrition and metabolism, implying the necessity of an integrated understanding of both to prevent and manage these disorders. Nutritional and metabolic disorders have far-reaching impacts that can significantly influence the health of individuals as well as public health systems. Nutrient deficiencies have the potential to produce a range of complications, ranging from immune weakness to impaired cognitive growth and metabolic illnesses such as diabetes and cardiovascular disease. Overload of certain nutrients, such as sodium or sugar, triggers hypertension and obesity, leading to secondary metabolic disorders. According to Murray et al. (2022), the load of antimicrobial resistance, which is likely to emerge due to poor nutrition and associated health problems, sets the nexus of the relationship between dietary patterns and general well-being. Awareness regarding such disorders is not only crucial for their clinical management but also for developing public health measures to check diet quality and the availability of nutrition education. Effective prevention and management of nutritional and metabolic diseases need a multi-component approach that engages healthcare practitioners, policymakers, and communities. It can include public health measures to promote nutritional literacy, the availability of health food and exercise. Healthcare practitioners also play a significant role in early detection and intervention, particularly among high-risk populations such as children and the elderly. The effects of neglecting nutritional health are palpable, such as increased healthcare spending and compromised quality of life. An integrated, community-oriented approach in managing the disorders, as seen in evidence in Livingston et al. (2020), is crucial in achieving long-term gains to health and constructing resilience against the growing incidence of these diseases in our society (Figure 1.1).

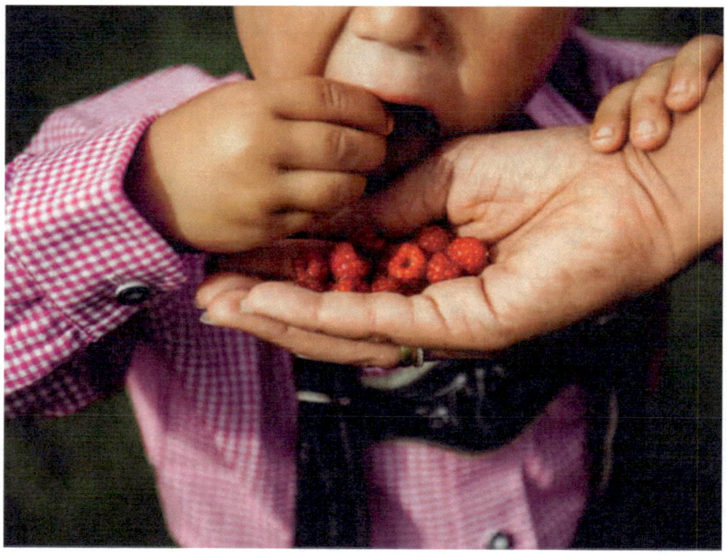

Figure 1.1. Child eating fresh raspberries, promoting healthy early nutrition.

Source: https://media.post.rvohealth.io/wp-content/uploads/2021/12/child-eating-raspberries-732x549-thumbnail-732x549.jpg.

Overview of Nutritional Disorders

Nutritional disorders are a category of conditions resulting from an imbalance in the intake of nutrients that can be presented as deficiency or excess. Nutritional disorders include, but are not limited to, malnutrition, obesity, micronutrient deficiencies, and eating disorders. Malnutrition, a poor intake of necessary nutrients, usually leads to serious health complications, particularly among risk groups such as children and the elderly. Conversely, conditions like obesity are caused by excess caloric intake and unwholesome eating habits combined with physically sedentary lifestyles. Both ends of nutrition contribute negatively to physical health and can precipitate the development of chronic diseases like diabetes, cardiovascular disease, and osteoporosis. Appreciating the intricacy of such diseases renders adequate and balanced nutrition imperative for good health and well-being. The relationship between dietary components and mental health is increasingly known, particularly regarding obesity and its psychological correlations. Interestingly, research indicates that obese individuals have higher rates of depression and anxiety, an association due to multiple metabolic derangements and inflammatory pathways of excess fat. These diets involving saturated fats and sugars are thought to make this connection worse, leading to neuroinflammation, responsible for affecting mood regulation and emotional balance. In addition, having metabolic syndrome, or a cluster of factors like high blood pressure, high blood sugar, and abnormal cholesterol levels, increases the likelihood of developing these psychiatric diseases. This growing awareness of the interlinkages between nutrition and mental health reiterates the importance of integrated strategies to include both dietetics and psychotherapy in the treatment of obesity disorders (Fulton et al., 2021). Prevention and control of nutritional disorders require an integrated and multidisciplinary process that brings together public health interventions, educational interventions, and clinical interventions. Public health strategies promoting diet and exercise have been encouraging in arresting the prevalence of obesity and its comorbidities of obesity. Practitioners of health also play an important part in identifying at-risk populations and providing personalized nutrition counseling, which can be extremely helpful in low-resource settings. Addressing root causes such as socioeconomic status, food environment, and cultural beliefs is essential in forging long-term solutions for nutritional disorders. Ultimately, a shift towards preventive measures, such as an enhancement of focus towards evidence-based dietary principles, is the key to successful management and improved outcomes in the context of nutritional and metabolic disorders (Murray et al., 2022) (Figure 1.2).

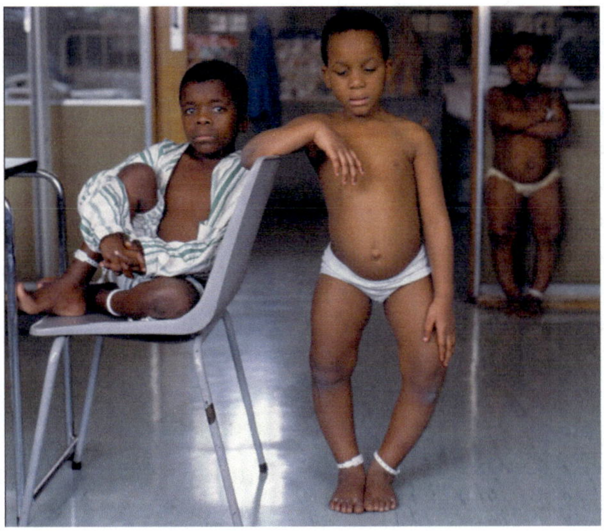

Figure 1.2. Children with rickets showing bone deformities due to vitamin D deficiency.

Source: https://cdn.britannica.com/01/148701-050-02F947BF/Children-rickets-disease-bone-deformities-bowlegs-Rickets.jpg.

Overview of Metabolic Disorders

Metabolic disorders are a broad group of diseases that disrupt normal metabolic processes within the body, affecting the function of converting food to energy. Metabolic disorders are the result of genetic problems, lack of nutrients, or environmental factors. They may present in numerous symptoms that influence body functions, including the creation of energy, the utilization of nutrients, and the excretion of waste. Diabetes, metabolic syndrome, and obesity are the most prevalent metabolic diseases and have a significant impact on public health worldwide. The rise in the prevalence of these conditions is typically blamed on lifestyles such as unhealthy dieting and lack of physical activity, thus making preventive measures and health education play a pivotal role in managing risk factors for these conditions. The classification of metabolic disorders may be complex, with heterogeneous groups according to their pathogenetic mechanisms. Some disorders are due to isolated enzymatic defects, which are directed against specific biochemical pathways, but others may be due to systemic issues, such as insulin resistance in type 2 diabetes. Genetic metabolic disorders, such as phenylketonuria and galactosemia, illustrate how atypical enzymatic deficiencies can cause serious health effects if undetected. Moreover, secondary metabolic disorders can occur as a complication of other illnesses, e.g., liver or endocrine disorders. Recognizing these categories is central to developing targeted treatment programs and improving patient outcomes among diverse populations. Lastly, the link between nutrient intake and metabolic disorders underlines the central position that diet takes in managing these illnesses. Nutritional therapy is generally a central element of the treatment and prevention of metabolic disorders, with therapy being directed towards satisfying individual nutritional needs. For instance, low-carbohydrate diets are very helpful in diabetics by improving glycemic control. Dietary fiber is encouraged to promote metabolic health as well as reduce cholesterol levels. Understanding the biochemical pathogenesis of these disorders can inform lifestyle modification and dietary interventions, culminating in better health outcomes. In harmony with public health reactions to rising metabolic disorder incidence, the incorporation of evidence-based nutritional advice into prevention programs is central to creating healthier populations and reducing healthcare expenditures associated with these disorders (Figure 1.3).

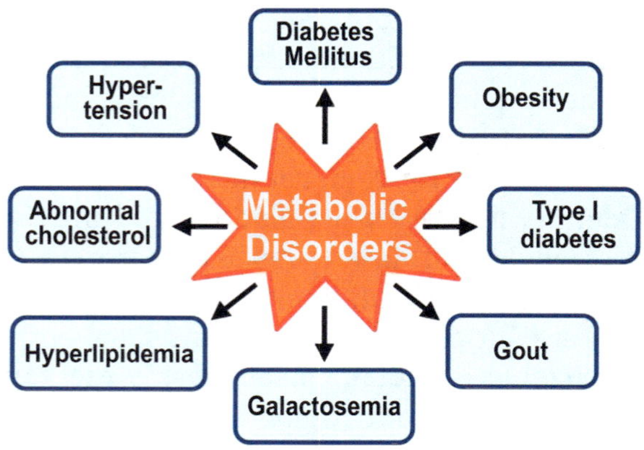

Figure 1.3. Overview of common metabolic disorders and associated conditions.

Source: Dama A, Shpati K, Daliu P, Dumur S, Gorica E, Santini A. Targeting Metabolic Diseases: The Role of Nutraceuticals in Modulating Oxidative Stress and Inflammation. *Nutrients*. 2024; 16(4):507. https://doi.org/10.3390/nu16040507

Importance of Understanding These Disorders

Understanding nutritional and metabolic disorders is crucial in the maintenance of human health complexity. These disorders, which may be caused by genetic dispositions, environmental factors, or eating habits, have extremely serious impacts on the overall health of an individual. Disbalances in metabolism, for instance, lead to conditions such as diabetes or obesity, which are increasingly common in modern society. By understanding these conditions and the mechanisms involved, practitioners of health can design targeted interventions and prevention regimens and, consequently, improve health outcomes. Moreover, education and awareness of such conditions allow people to make appropriate dietary decisions, which call for an active role in health care and prevention. The complex relationship between diet, gut microbiota, and metabolic health highlights the importance of nutrition in handling such conditions. Recent research indicates that the human gut harbors trillions of microbes that have a critical function in shaping nutritional status through the degradation of nutrients into bioactive molecules (Vernocchi et al., 2020). Microbial metabolites can have an effect on various biochemical pathways and therefore have an important role in the maintenance of homeostasis. Disruptions in gut microbiota composition have been linked to a range of metabolic and inflammatory diseases. This is essential as it is made possible to design precise nutrition and treatment interventions based on individual microbiota composition, which in the long run makes treatment plans more effective and improves patient adherence. Finally, the rising incidence of non-communicable diseases and their impact on healthcare systems worldwide emphasize the need for intensive research and education regarding these diseases (de Vos et al., 2017). Increased life expectancy has presented populations with an increasing pattern of years lived with metabolic and nutritional complications. This calls for early intervention in healthcare through lifestyle modifications and dietary counseling. From critical analysis of the implications of such disorders, the health system can prioritize resource allocation, enhance therapeutic approaches, and create community awareness, leading to better health outcomes and reduced healthcare spending. Thus, studying nutritional and metabolic disorders is a matter beyond intellectual pursuit but a necessary undertaking to move forward in public health.

1.1. Types of Nutritional Disorders

The scope of nutritional disorders is broad and encompasses ailments caused by both insufficiencies and excesses of the necessary nutrients. Deficiency diseases such as pellagra and scurvy occur when the body lacks certain indispensable vitamins or minerals, and this causes serious health issues. Pellagra, whose symptoms include dermatitis, diarrhea, and dementia, occur due to a deficiency in niacin (vitamin B3), normally found in most food sources. Concurrently, scurvy, induced by improper ingestion of vitamin C, yields symptoms involving fatigue, bleeding gums, and impaired healing of wounds. Both conditions underscore the utmost importance of a good diet that supplies the necessary vitamins and minerals needed to maintain physiological wellness. At the other end of the spectrum, the field of excessive consumption of diet can also cause nutritional disorders. Overconsumption of some nutrients can lead to illnesses such as hypervitaminosis, in which the overloading of vitamins, particularly fat-soluble vitamins A, D, E, and K, is detrimental to the body. Disease is another major example and is found to trigger numerous diseases, i.e., diabetes, cardiovascular diseases, and joint disorders. It is essential to realize the balance between nutritional intake and body needs because abnormal increments of dietary content can drastically deplete health and wellbeing. It is for this reason that there must be training in nutrition among the population to be able to create awareness and preventive strategies against deficiency and overconsumption. The above conditions highlight a critical interface between nutrition and metabolism where it is clear that nutritional health is not solely an issue of adequate food intake but, rather, optimal composition and organization of the diet. For example, in equine populations, there is a significant knowledge gap regarding nutrition management in relation to disease, as indicated by research into veterinary practice in horse populations of differing health status, including metabolic disease (Garber et al., 2018). Horse owner surveys also demonstrate an alarming trend: the majority of respondents were unaware of nutrition disorders, and this lack of awareness can have devastating consequences for animal health (Murray et al., 2015). This information lacuna not only mirrors the complexity of nutritional diseases in different species but also marks the universal implications of deficiency in adequate education and information in achieving optimal gains in health (Figure 1.4).

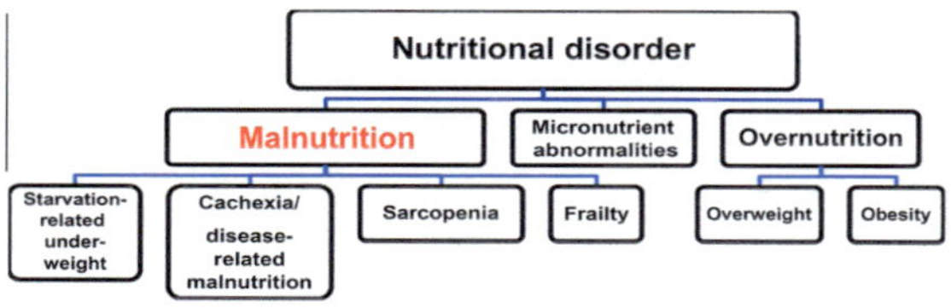

Figure 1.4. Types of nutritional disorders.

Source: https://www.researchgate.net/profile/Alison-Jesus/publication/308040914/figure/fig2/AS:1108565947351041@1641314126382/A-conceptual-tree-of-nutritional-disorders.png.

1.1.1. Malnutrition and Its Effects

Malnutrition is a significant public health problem, with significant consequences for individual and population health outcomes. Malnutrition encompasses both undernutrition, symbolized by poor calorie or essential nutrient intake, and overnutrition, signified by high calorie and food energy intake culminating in obesity and its accompanying chronic illnesses. Malnutrition has extensive and complex effects extending across physical, cognitive, and psychological health. Malnourished individuals tend to have an increased risk of infections since their immune function becomes compromised, and the body cannot produce proper immune responses since the proper nutrients for proper immune functions are not present. In addition, malnutrition was associated with higher death rates and longer hospitalizations, hence contributing to greater healthcare burdens and reduced economic productivity in affected populations. Improved nutrition appears to be essential for maximizing overall health and reducing the incidence of many diseases associated closely with malnutrition. The relationship between malnutrition and some health complications cannot be underestimated, particularly among high-risk individuals such as chronic disease patients. For instance, malnutrition is among the leading causes of the onset of frailty and sarcopenia, particularly among older patients and patients with diseases such as cirrhosis. Malnutrition among cirrhotic patients represents an imbalance of nutrients that adversely affects the function and health status of the body. Scarily, malnutrition was reported to exacerbate liver disease, creating a vicious loop of deteriorating disease and quality of life. Specifically, muscle atrophy and strength loss from malnutrition lead to increased levels of disability and hospitalization, further complicating treatment regimens and recovery processes. Hence, the treatment of such malnutrition in these patient groups demands an integrated, coordinated approach to enable effective management and improved health outcomes, highlighting the urgency for awareness and intervention. Also, the socio-economic factors contributing to malnutrition increase the prevalence and severity of malnutrition in different populations. Factors causing reduced nutrition are food insecurity, limited healthcare access, and educational inequalities. Undernutrition as well as increased obesity are more prevalent in the majority of low-resource settings; individuals have not had proper access to high-quality foods. The American Association for the Study of Liver

Diseases emphasizes that the key to overcoming malnutrition is also in tackling its root causes, including social determinants of health and systemic inequalities affecting access to resources. By maximizing access to healthy food and healthcare services, communities can stem the effects of malnutrition and enhance overall well-being. The determination of these linkages is significant in developing effective public health strategies that will assist in curbing malnutrition and its long-term implications, hence establishing a healthier and more productive nation in the long term (Figure 1.5).

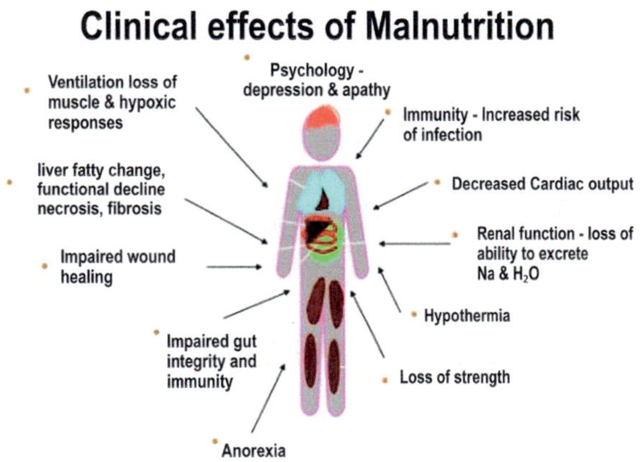

Figure 1.5. Clinical effects of malnutrition across major body systems.

Source: https://beyoungstore.com/Content/images/Blog/Clinical.png.

1.1.2. Micronutrient Deficiencies

Micronutrient deficiencies remain a pressing concern even in a calorie-surplus world. The paradox arises from unbalanced diets that result in inadequate amounts of essential vitamins and minerals for healthy living. These micronutrients have pivotal biochemical roles and are involved in homeostatic mechanisms that allow control of body processes. Causes of deficiencies can include socioeconomic status, inability to access a diverse source of foods, or comorbid illnesses that interfere with nutrient absorption. Diagnosis of deficiencies is typically complex, reliant on many tests, including dietary assessment, biochemical testing, and functional testing. It is essential to understand the intricacies of micronutrient deficiency as it has far-reaching implications for the health of a person in terms of developing conditions such as anemia, weakened immunity, and poor cognitive ability (Combet & Buckton, 2014). Deficiencies of micronutrients are not only of personal health significance but also have public health implications. Populations with a high prevalence of deficiency have an increased risk of disease and decreased overall productivity, which can place a strain on health systems and slow economic growth. Vitamins and minerals, for instance, are important in avoiding chronic diseases such as type 2 diabetes and some cancers, further emphasizing the importance of nutritional sufficiency for long-term health status. As the world market continues to promote vitamins as a means of enhancing health, it should be noted that supplements alone will not do in having a healthy diet. Multivitamins have been suggested to fail in offering benefits that have been touted and, in certain situations, can be detrimental to the point of promoting mortality among certain groups (Combet & Buckton, 2014). Therefore, focusing on whole foods as the foundation of nutrition is of paramount importance for public health. The risk of micronutrient deficiency can become higher in special populations, e.g., those set to undergo bariatric surgery, due to altered digestive physiology and reduced food intake. Postoperative patients require personalized nutritional treatment to prevent deficiency due to the influence of surgery on nutrient absorption. After weight-loss treatment, patients typically have particular medical needs, and special training in nutrition, co-morbidity management, and psychological assistance is necessary to deliver comprehensive care. Clinical practice guideline implementation and awareness are crucial to address these complexities adequately. Healthcare providers need to closely monitor micronutrient status in these patients since deficiency is common for iron, vitamin B12, and folate and can cause vast health issues in the long run. In understanding the nuances involved in addressing micronutrient deficiencies, health care providers are better able to safeguard the long-term health of post-bariatric patients while continuing to foster a comprehensive model of nutrition care (Figure 1.6).

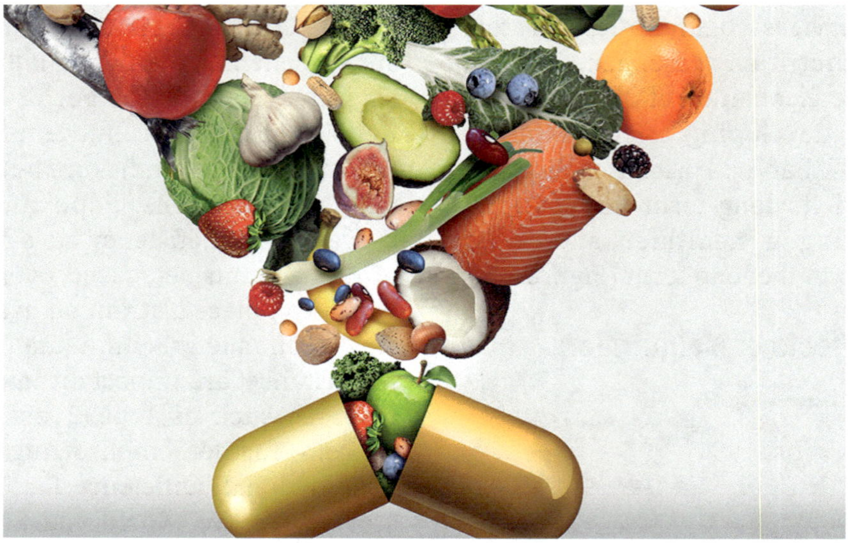

Figure 1.6. Whole foods as natural sources of nutrients.

Source: https://ds982gbwnvyso.cloudfront.net/Pictures/380x253/7/0/4/704_nutraceuticals_742289.jpeg

1.1.3. Eating Disorders (e.g., Anorexia, Bulimia)

The prevalence of eating disorders, such as anorexia nervosa and bulimia nervosa, has become a significant concern within the discipline of nutritional and metabolic disorders. Eating disorders are not simple food intake or body image issues; they are serious psychiatric illnesses with profound biochemical, psychological, and sociocultural components. The incidences of the disorders have experienced increases globally, sounding an alarm, particularly with evidence suggesting an increased surge in cases driven by stressors such as the COVID-19 pandemic. The DSM-5-TR explains that anorexia and bulimia manifest through various patterns of behavior and body physiological symptoms but share similar underlying characteristics, such as fear of weight gain and disturbances in perceptions regarding their body shape. Therefore, the complex interplay of environmental and neurological forces mandates a multi-dimensional model of prevention, treatment, and comprehension of eating disorders (Yu and Muehleman, 2023). Comorbidities of eating disorders also make them difficult to treat. Patients with anorexia and bulimia often present with other psychiatric disorders, including anxiety and depression, which complicate medical therapy and significantly impair the quality of life. In addition, there exist ominous correlations between the existence of eating disorders and the development of metabolic diseases like obesity, diabetes, and other cardiovascular ailments. Patients tend to have high rates of metabolic syndrome, getting stuck in a cycle that impacts mental and physical health negatively. The complex interaction between food consumption and emotional well-being reflects the need for treatment protocols that address all these issues at once. Early treatment and detection are most critical in order to prevent the long-term effects of these disorders on physical and psychological health (Murray et al., 2022). The treatment of eating disorders is typically a multidisciplinary intervention that includes psychotherapy, dietary instruction, and medication in some cases. Psychotherapy, particularly therapies such as cognitive-behavioral therapy (CBT), has proven effective in the treatment of eating disorders' cognitive distortions. Concurrently, nutrition education targets reversing normal eating patterns and normalizing food-related behavior. Treatment programs need to target the individual's own specific needs, emphasizing individual responsibility in recovery. The combination of both types of therapies has been shown to improve treatment outcomes, but further research is required on effective interventions as well as prevention programs. Emphasizing early detection and complete treatment can potentially provide improved prognoses for those afflicted with these incapacitating diseases (Yu et al., 2023).

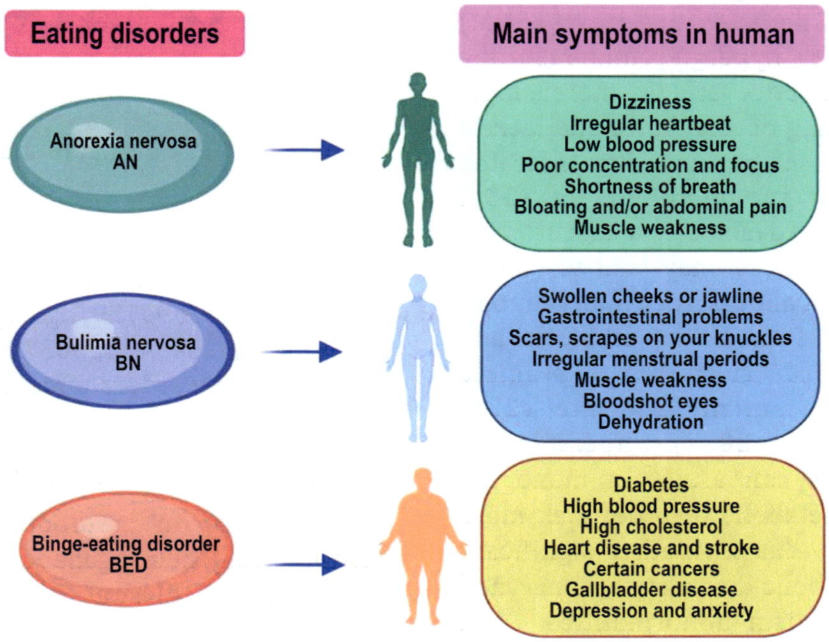

Figure 1.7. Key symptoms associated with major eating disorders: AN, BN, and BED.

Source: Feng B, Harms J, Chen E, Gao P, Xu P, He Y. Current Discoveries and Future Implications of Eating Disorders. *International Journal of Environmental Research and Public Health*. 2023; 20(14):6325. https://doi.org/10.3390/ijerph20146325

1.2. Types of Metabolic Disorders

Metabolic disorders consist of a range of conditions that disrupt normal metabolic processes, resulting in severe health conditions. Metabolic disorders are typically classified into two large categories: inherited and acquired. Inherited metabolic disorders are often genetic in nature and affect the body's ability to metabolize certain substances, which is typically due to a deficiency of enzymes. Examples include phenylketonuria (PKU) and galactosemia, disorders leading to toxic substance buildup when the diet is not controlled. Acquired metabolic disorders, on the other hand, e.g., type 2 diabetes mellitus (T2DM), are more likely to develop due to habits and environmental influences, primarily diet and sedentary lifestyle. Management of such conditions requires an understanding of the metabolic pathways involved and the influence of dietary intervention and modification. Among the range of metabolic disorders, carbohydrate metabolism disorders are particularly noteworthy. Diabetes mellitus, both type 1 and type 2, is a significant public health problem. Type 2 diabetes mellitus (T2DM) is characterized by hyperglycemia resulting from insulin resistance and is increasingly prevalent with rising obesity rates and lack of exercise. More recent research has indicated the importance of gut microbiota in T2DM progression, where dysbiosis, a disturbance in gut microbial balance, may lead to insulin resistance and metabolic disorder. Interventions, such as dietary adjustment using prebiotics and probiotics, have been suggested to promote gut health and potentially alleviate T2DM effects (Basista et al., 2022). Understanding these connections can assist in managing and preventing metabolic disorder risk more effectively in individuals. Another significant clustering in metabolic disorders is concerned with lipid metabolism abnormalities. Such disorders as hyperlipidemia, in which blood has excess lipids, can result in serious cardiovascular disease and more. Genetic susceptibility is often involved in such conditions, but lifestyle factors like diet, physical activity, and obesity also have important roles to play in their manifestation. High LDL cholesterol and low HDL cholesterol are potent risk predictors for atherosclerosis and coronary heart disease. More significantly, current research links chronic inflammation and oxidative stress to lipid metabolic disturbances, leading investigators to explore new treatment approaches that are capable of interfering with these pathways. A synthesized appreciation of the lipid metabolic disorders' multifactorial etiology has a significant potential to enhance public health measures to prevent their incidence and associated morbidity (Murray et al., 2022) (Figure 1.8).

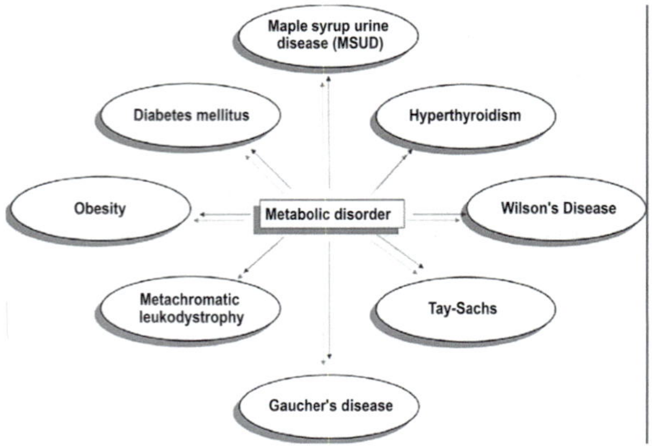

Figure 1.8. Types of metabolic disorders affect human health.

Source: https://www.researchgate.net/profile/Saravanan-Ramachandran-2/publication/330899929/figure/fig5/AS:723157241569281@1549425530378/Different-types-of-metabolic-disorders-affecting-humans.png.

1.2.1. Inborn Errors of Metabolism

Inborn errors in metabolism (IEM) are a phenotypically heterogeneous group of genetic disorders that disrupt metabolic pathways, leading to the generation of pathogenic compounds or lack of essential metabolites. They are caused by mutations of genes encoding enzymes for biochemical reactions such as carbohydrate, protein, and lipid metabolism. Early recognition and treatment of IEM are crucial to avoid severe health outcomes that can occur in the case of untreated illness. Different signs and symptoms are presented by patients, including neurological dysfunction, failure to grow, and organ dysfunction. An active therapeutic and diagnostic strategy, such as newborn screening programs, plays a key role in effective management of these complicated disorders and in improving outcomes for patients. Nutritional care is a central component of the treatment of IEM, with an emphasis on dietary adjustment to limit toxic metabolites and deliver essential nutrients. Treatment with specially prepared diets permits clinicians to forestall toxic buildup in individuals. For example, in the treatment of phenylketonuria (PKU), patients require a diet low in protein but supplemented with tyrosine to control phenylalanine levels. Innovations in dietetic care, such as those researched in recent work, demonstrate the improvements in IEM adult inpatients' treatment by means of individualized intervention. The innovations include instituting clinical alerts to facilitate timely dietary assessments, which offer nutritionally proper care to 100% of the patients.

Such interventions, as noted, form a critical component in optimizing nutritional therapy in high-risk individuals, highlighting the significance of dietary measures in the management of such metabolic conditions (McGill et al., 2019). Formulation of PN protocol is another critical component in the care of patients with IEM who cannot be tolerated orally. Protein catabolism must be minimized while supporting anabolic activity through the use of targeted amino acid (AA) supplementation. Ordinary AA solutions are generally sufficient, but in severe metabolic derangement, proprietary products might be necessary. For the normally healthy patient, an AA intake of approximately 0.8 g/kg/day is standard, but for patients with inborn errors in amino acid metabolism, the intake can be raised to avoid complications. Furthermore, a satisfactory nitrogen-to-calorie ratio has to be provided to make the best use of the nutrients. Utilizing precise nutritional therapy is thus essential in facilitating optimal recovery and growth in IEM patients, demonstrating the complex association between diet and metabolic health (Blumenstein et al., 2009) (Figure 1.9).

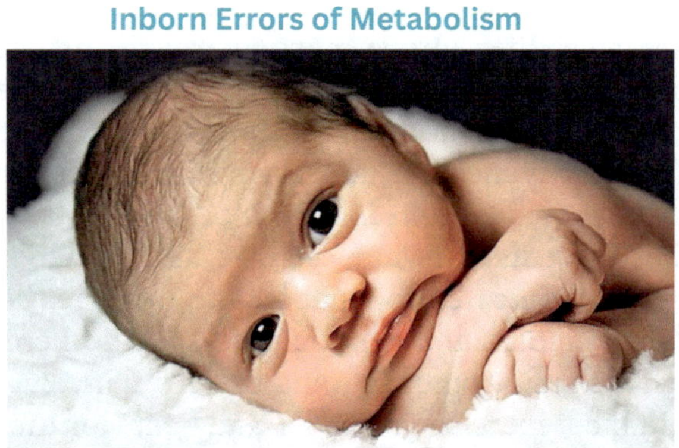

Figure 1.9. Inborn errors of metabolism.

Source: https://www.diagnopein.com/img/BlogImages/Inborn%20Errors%20of%20Metabolism.jpg.

1.2.2. Diabetes Mellitus and Its Complications

Diabetes mellitus is a metabolic disorder that is multifactorial and consists of chronic hyperglycemia caused by defects in insulin secretion, insulin action, and both. The two primary forms of the disease are Type 1 diabetes, which is an autoimmune beta-cell destruction, and Type 2 diabetes, which typically involves insulin resistance. Diabetes is highly associated with lifestyle, with physical inactivity and diet playing the biggest role. Poor eating patterns, i.e., excessive caloric consumption and low fiber intake, are key in the etiology of diabetes and its complications. Its complications most frequently include cardiovascular disease, neuropathy, and retinopathy, which contribute importantly to quality of life and morbidity in those who have diabetes mellitus. Diabetes mellitus treatment should be multidisciplinary and include nutritional therapy and lifestyle modification. Dietary changes, particularly the inclusion of macronutrients with a focus on fiber, are protective of the gut and glucose metabolism. For instance, a high-fiber diet may stabilize gut barrier functions and lower systemic inflammation, which are both vital in metabolic disorder patients , such as diabetes patients. Nevertheless, it should be observed that excessive fiber intake, particularly in instances of pancreatic insufficiency, is proven to lead to complications , such as increased fecal elimination of fat, supporting the need for personalized dietary interventions. The interventions should preferably be evidence-based to preclude any possibility of ineffectiveness in addressing diabetes complexities (Badiali et al., 2019). In addition, obesity and diabetes is causes for concern since excess body fat is a top contributor to insulin resistance. Obesity in itself is now viewed as a metabolic disease that is challenging to treat and makes it more complicated for diabetes to manage. Contributory factors , such as physical inactivity, poor dietary habits, and genetic predisposition create a challenging situation for effective intervention. Holistic management should therefore involve a multi-disciplinary approach, integrating nutritional guidance, exercise protocols, and behavior therapy. It fosters sustained weight loss, generally aiming to combat the risks of diabetes-related complications. By understanding the multi-faceted nature of such diseases, medical practitioners can set more effective, individually adjusted treatment protocols that contribute to better health outcomes for diabetic individuals (Busetto et al., 2015) (Figure 1.10).

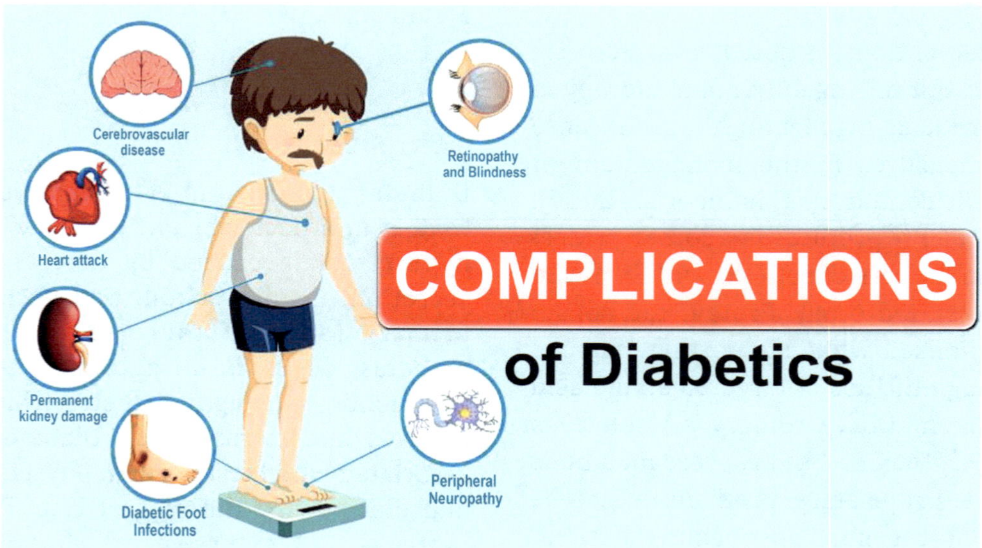

Figure 1.10. Major complications associated with diabetes.

Source: https://webcdn.freedomfromdiabetes.org/storage/blog/394/0c504cf6-4721-466e-86ad-99b2b4e04a1b.jpg

1.2.3. Thyroid Disorders and Their Impact

Thyroid conditions represent a complex interface of nutritional and metabolic determinants with significant effects on human health. The thyroid gland plays a crucial role in regulating metabolism by producing the hormones thyroxine (T4) and triiodothyronine (T3). These hormones play significant roles in metabolic homeostasis, and abnormalities in their production have varied clinical presentations. Hypothyroidism and hyperthyroidism are an imbalance of hormonal output that can result in weight gain or weight loss, fatigue, and cognitive impairment. Understanding the biochemical pathways in thyroid hormone regulation emphasizes the need for proper nutritional strategies for the gland to perform optimally and diet becomes a necessary part of the management of thyroid function and prevention of associated disorders, as favored by current research studies on metabolic derangements due to diet (Sarmidi et al., 2012). Iodine deficiency is well recognized across thyroid diseases and contributes significantly to public health policy everywhere in the world. In Belgium and other countries, mild iodine deficiency has been linked to increased prevalence of thyroid nodular diseases and metabolic disorders. The anticipatory intervention by the governments in the form of the iodization programs has been effective in highlighting the economic burden of uncontrolled iodine deficiency.

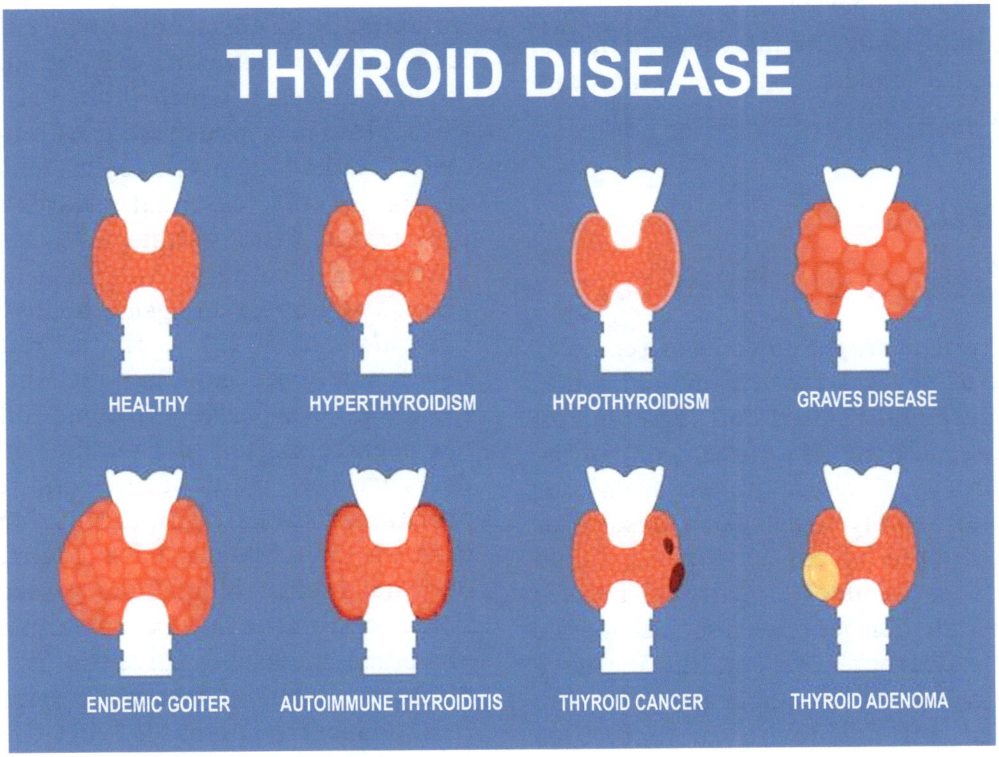

Figure 1.11. Types of thyroid diseases compared to healthy thyroid gland.

Source: https://www.sparshhospital.com/wp-content/uploads/2024/10/thyroidimg3.jpeg.

The economic costs of thyroid nodular diseases in Belgium, for instance, are significant, approximating 38 million euros annually, primarily among adults (Annemans et al., 2010). Implementation of diet-based measures that enhance iodine supplementation not only improves such health challenges but also heightens overall social benefits. Therefore, detection and intervention of such nutritional deficiency are significant to maximizing overall health outcomes, reflecting the significant nexus between nutrition and metabolic disorder. Furthermore, the implications of untreated thyroid disorders branch out beyond immediate impact on health, influencing quality of life and economic effectiveness. Thyroid dysfunction patients usually report diminished physical and emotional status, equating to increased healthcare costs and decreased labor force participation. Given that thyroid hormones control a broad spectrum of physiological events, subnormal levels may initiate a cascade of metabolic derangement ranging from energy homeostasis to brain activity. Hypothyroidism and hyperthyroidism are serious concerns among the general population of affected individuals, justifying the use of beneficial nutritional measures. By raising awareness and advocating for comprehensive nutritional programs, policymakers can respond well to the extensive reach of thyroid diseases, opening the doors for improved public health programs including personal as well as social well-being, implied by the interdependence of food, metabolism, and health in recent literature (Sarmidi et al., 2012) (Figure 1.11).

1.3. Causes of Nutritional Disorders

Nutrition disorders are the outcome of a complex interaction of several factors involving diet habits, socioeconomic status, and psychological factors. Inadequate intake of food is one of the prime reasons, which typically stems from poor availability of healthy foods. Food deserts or areas with limited access to affordable and healthy food cause poor nutritional intakes and thus malnutrition. Moreover, socioeconomic status can exacerbate the condition, where poor people are more concerned with the quantity and not the quality of food, thus producing imbalances that enhance nutritional disorders. Poor nutritional education also exacerbates the condition, as most individuals are unaware of what they require in terms of dietary recommendations. Resolution of these basic issues is essential not only to improve the health status of individuals but also nutritional consciousness at a community level and equity and thus decrease the social cost of nutritional disorders. Psychological factors are also significant in the etiology of nutritional disorders. Stress, depression, and anxiety can cause eating disorders in terms of excessive or inadequate food consumption. General stress has been linked to metabolic dysregulation that results in poor diets due to tendencies to consume high-calorie foods for comfort under stressful situations. Metabolic stress and inflammation are consequences of poor diets, creating a loop of deteriorating health status. For instance, the term obesity-inflammation describes how excess body fat results in metabolic disruption, , such as Type II diabetes, which often has associated physiological processes. Consequently, understanding the psychological underpinnings of food habits is essential towards developing effective intervention strategies that will prevent nutritional disorders while also maintaining mental well-being alongside bodily well-being (Delgado et al., 2022). Finally, the role played by inflammatory processes in nutritional disorders cannot be exaggerated. Chronic inflammation has been connected to a number of metabolic dysfunctions, which are found to impact nutritional status significantly. For instance, cachexia and obesity have been associated with heightened inflammatory reactions that introduce negative impacts on normal metabolic processes, increasing susceptibility to various diseases, , such as metabolic syndrome and cardiovascular diseases. In this regard, biomarkers like albumin and C-reactive protein are employed to measure the inflammatory status of individuals and provide valuable information regarding their nutrition. Understanding these correlations better explains how inflammation causes or leads to nutritional disorders through which mechanisms. The implication is clear: fighting inflammation through diet and way of life potentially plays a central role in the prevention and management of nutritional disorders, highlighting the need for holistic approaches to healthcare practice as well as policy (Daghigh et al., 2014) (Figure 1.12).

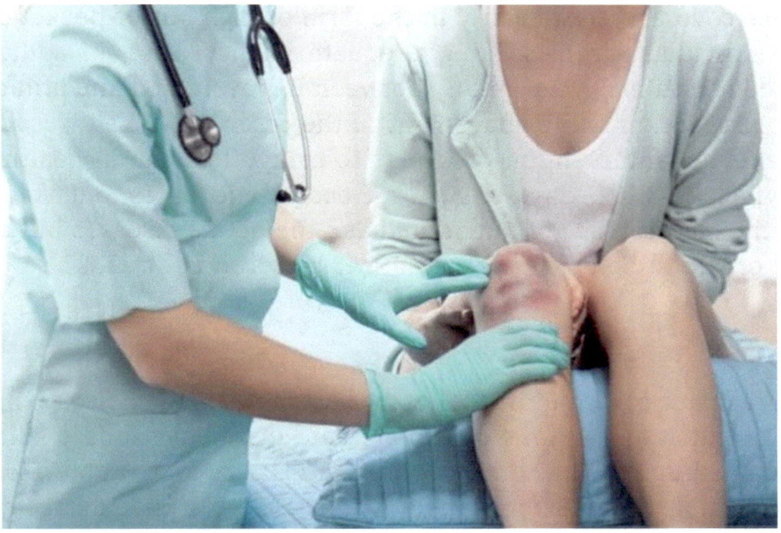

Figure 1.12. Medical examination of a bruised and swollen knee.

Source: https://cms.patrika.com/wp-content/uploads/2019/07/04/amb.png?w=450&q=90

1.3.1. Socioeconomic Factors

The socioeconomic determinants of nutritional and metabolic disease are profound in that they influence an individual's access to the resources necessary for nourishment and maintenance of health. Individuals with poor socioeconomic status often suffer from food insecurity, which may lead to a diet lacking essential primary nutrients and cause obesity, malnutrition, or other types of nutritional disease. Food deserts, areas with limited access to healthy, affordable food, only perpetuate the issue by putting pressure on citizens to spend their time and finances in convenience stores and fast-food chains, where unhealthy options rule. Education also plays a vital part; health illiteracy can render people incapable of making knowledgeable food choices and thereby perpetuating cycles of poor health and nutritional status. Thus, these socioeconomic problems yield a complex set of factors with significant effects on physical well-being and render metabolic disorders more common among vulnerable populations. In addition to that, socioeconomic determinants influence the ability to regularly exercise, further exacerbating the likelihood of metabolic disorders , such as diabetes and obesity. Poorer communities are deprived of access to clean recreational spaces and organized sports or exercise facilities, thereby experiencing barriers to adopting an active lifestyle. Time restrictions like extended working hours and working multiple jobs also undermine time for physical activity. Furthermore, health and fitness attitudes within society impact lifestyle choice negatively within communities indirectly. Therefore, physical inactivity may be the reason for an inactive lifestyle, which also contributes to health risks. This vicious cycle of inactivity coupled with poor nutritional consumption on the basis of socioeconomic status pinpoints the importance of managing these broader determinants in public health interventions that seek to reduce nutritional and metabolic diseases in at-risk populations. Besides, the socioeconomic determinants' interaction continues to the extent and availability of health care that an individual experiences. Members of lower socioeconomic communities will experience significant barriers to receiving adequate health care, resulting delays in diagnosis and treatment of nutritional and metabolic conditions. Exclusion from health insurance coverage, particularly in the form of high out-of-pocket costs and transport barriers, dissuades individuals from seeking adequate medical care. In addition, the quality of healthcare services delivered may vary greatly between impoverished and affluent communities to reveal disparities in prevention and management of the disorders. The discovery of these gaps is crucial in devising effective intervention programs to bridge this gap in health equity. Healthcare providers and policymakers must consider such socioeconomic forces to develop holistic solutions addressing not just the medical face of nutritional and metabolic diseases but also the supporting social determinants of health below (Lai et al., 2021; Visseren et al., 2021).

1.3.2. Cultural Influences on Diet

Cultural influences are major contributors to dietary habits and food choices, which have a dramatic impact on health and nutrition. Various cultures create distinctive food traditions that not only determine what one eats but also how one prepares and shares food. In Mediterranean traditional diets, for example, vegetables, legumes, and healthy fats , such as olive oil are given due attention, as they are highly recommended for heart health. Conversely, the diet typically found in certain Asian populations would be rice and fish, which is an expression of regional agricultural trends and religious beliefs. This food and nutritional belief then follow cultural influences, such that dietary guidelines are followed.

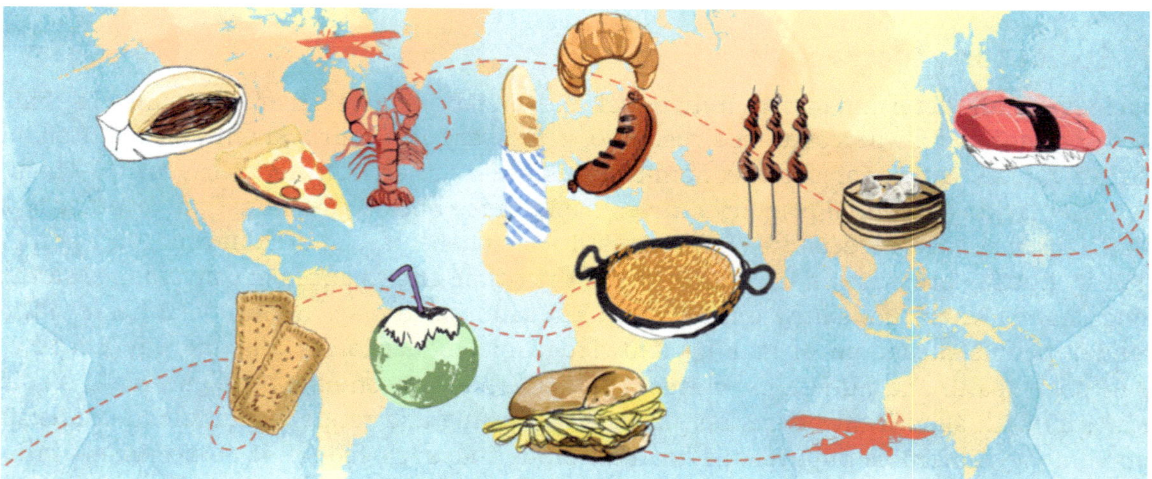

Figure 1.13. Illustration of traditional foods from around the world.

Source: https://media.licdn.com/dms/image/v2/C5612AQEnRLVUoBJBhQ/article-cover_image-shrink_720_1280/article-cover_image-shrink_720_1280/0/1532173823809?e=2147483647&v=beta&t=QeNgs1Wex3lmpMRJ0pbc51ixiBzCD6ZA0dkNvWv3dUA.

By appreciating these facets of culture, nutritionists can design specific interventions that more closely appeal across diverse populations and, in the end, have improved dietary compliance and clinical outcomes. Moreover, understanding cultural food is often inextricably linked with social identity and family culture and, as such, influences individual choice and practice concerning food. Commensality is a fundamental aspect of social life in most societies, producing behavioral and cultural continuity as well as familial bonds. Commensality occasionally conflicts with modern dietary guidelines, particularly those intended to prevent nutritional and metabolic disease. For instance, patients who are on a low-phenylalanine diet that is required to manage diseases like phenylketonuria may find it useful but difficult to negotiate social eating situations without drawing attention to their restriction. The sense of belonging derived from shared eating can unwittingly undermine adherence to prescribed dietary therapies, highlighting the need for culturally sensitive dietary advice. The psychosocial environment of diet may encourage or hinder healthy eating habits, and due attention is required in dietary education and care (Bensi et al., 2018). Also, the intersection of psychosocial determinants and culture affects dietary adherence, particularly among populations with metabolic disorders. A study of Italian adults with phenylketonuria showed that the majority of individuals did not consider their disease a health issue, and this had an effect on diet restriction compliance (Bensi et al., 2018). This is a case of how cultural perceptions directly affect an individual's belief and mastery over a health issue. Moreover, social pressures around food, e.g., the stigma of certain dietary supplements, can complicate compliance further. Heightened cultural factors, , such as education sensitive to local beliefs and practices, are necessary for clinicians who want to enhance compliance in their patients. By matching these cultural and psychological subtleties, health professionals can develop better dietary interventions that appeal to their patients lived lives and cultural environment (Figure 1.13).

1.3.3. Psychological Factors Affecting Eating Habits

Psychological processes play an important role in controlling individuals' eating habits, food intake, portion sizes, and overall dietary style. Emotions, e.g., stress and anxiety, can lead to abnormal eating habits, e.g., binge eating or food avoidance. These psychological conditions typically stem from underlying emotional disturbances, thus forming a vicious cycle of abnormal eating behaviors. Research shows that individuals with emotional problems can find it challenging to maintain healthy eating habits, as the effort to cope with the distress of feeling ill at ease tends to lead to using food as a source of comfort or escape. Such reliance has the potential to make individuals oppose adherence to dietary guidelines necessary for metabolic disorder control, be it obesity or diabetes, thereby complicating the issue of disordered eating. Aside from emotional distress, cognitive determinants , such as consciousness and knowledge of nutritional needs also exert a huge influence on diet. In a survey of Italian adult patients with phenylketonuria (PKU), the majority of subjects did not consider PKU as a disease and therefore were not compliant with dietary restrictions needed to control their illness (Bensi et al., 2018). This shift in perception brought an increase in the consumption of natural protein sources, threatening the efficacy of the low-phenylalanine diet. These results demonstrate the necessity of intervention within education that not only educates dietary knowledge but also introduces a better comprehension of the psychological effects of their illnesses. Increasing patients' awareness and adjusting their cognitive frameworks might be shown to improve their diet compliance and outcomes. Social pressures are another significant psychological factor that can affect eating habits. The desire to fit socially with how one eats has the potential to cause them to prioritize peers' acceptance over adherence to healthy diet patterns. Social pressure concerning food consumption was emphasized in the PKU study as the main factor influencing patients' adherence to their medical requirements (Bensi et al., 2018). This underscores the interplay between individual psychology and the broader social forces, suggesting that the interventions aimed at modifying food habits must consider the social world in which individuals operate. By establishing support systems that enhance good eating rather than sabotaging it, clinicians can help to buffer these social forces and promote healthier lifestyle decisions. Finally, addressing the interconnected psychological factors affecting food intake is essential to effectively treat nutritional and metabolic disorders (Figure 1.14).

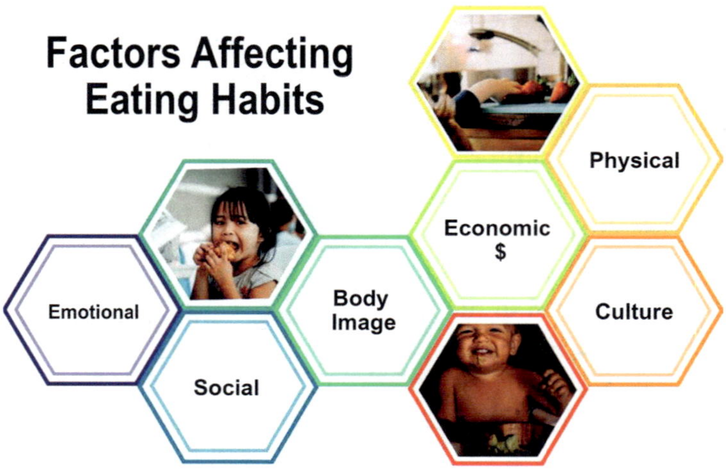

Figure 1.14. Key emotional, social, and economic factors affecting eating habits.

Source: https://external-content.duckduckgo.com/iu/?u=https%3A%2F%2Fpressbooks.saskpolytech.ca%2Fapp%2Fuploads%2Fsites%2F30%2F2021%2F11%2FMuted-Rainbow-Hexagon-Thinking-Graphic-Organizer-1024x730.png&f=1&nofb=1&ipt=df05bb9281cedbe985a7a367b1e39cb4400e9ec6abec05a9345fa7d725d2d0b5.

1.4. Causes of Metabolic Disorders

Metabolic disorders are caused by multifactorial interaction between genetics, environment, and lifestyle. Genetic susceptibility has a direct influence on one's susceptibility to these diseases. For instance, inherited diseases like phenylketonuria and cystic fibrosis demonstrate the role of genetics in metabolic dysfunction. In addition, genetic polymorphisms , such as in the genes PNPLA3 and TM6SF2 have also been associated with non-alcoholic fatty liver disease (NAFLD), emphasizing the role of genetic variants in fat metabolism and liver function. Lastly, revelations in gene-environmental interactions explain the ways by which some dieting habits lead to genetic vulnerabilities, resulting in metabolic disorders. This complex relationship highlights that even though genetic predisposition is extremely significant, it could take environmental influences to manifest as clinical conditions. Environmental influences, particularly nutrition and lifestyle, have a critical role in the onset of metabolic disorders. Poor eating habits like high calorie intake, high sugar and fat content, and saturated fats are strongly linked with obesity, type 2 diabetes, and cardiovascular complications. Overnutrition can lead to insulin resistance and later metabolic syndrome, marking the initiation of metabolic disorder from health (Chalasani et al., 2017). Sedentary lifestyle also worsens these conditions because, without exercise, metabolic processes become difficult and body fat deposition is made easy. The rising prevalence of these disorders can thus be attributed directly to modern lifestyle patterns, where convenience foods and a lack of physical activity have become the new norm. They should be addressed in order to counteract the rising trend of metabolic disorders and achieve maximum public health outcomes. In addition to environmental and hereditary factors, clinical disorders like endocrine disturbances may be significant etiologic forerunners to metabolic disorders. Polycystic ovary syndrome (PCOS) and hypothyroidism, for example, show how hormonal deregulation can lead to insulin resistance and deranged metabolic pathways (Chalasani et al., 2017).

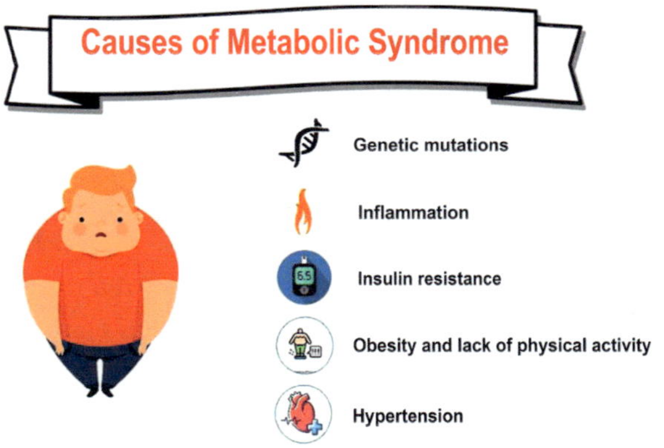

Figure 1.15. Main causes contributing to metabolic syndrome.

Source: https://www.researchgate.net/profile/Shimaa-Emam/publication/371951530/figure/fig1/AS:11431281171170090@1688066210818/Causes-of-metabolic-syndrome-MetS.jpg

For instance, patients of PCOS tend to have a greater tendency towards type 2 diabetes due to insulin resistance. The relationship between stress and metabolic condition cannot be overlooked either; chronic stress can actually disrupt hormonal pathways, leading to inflammation and consequent metabolic derangement. This nexus of hormonal and metabolic activity creates fertile ground for the onset of diseases, emphasizing their complexity of origin. It becomes significant in the process of formulating prevention and treatment modalities in nutritional and metabolic medicine to recognize the multifactorial pathogenesis of these conditions (Figure 1.15).

1.4.1. Genetic Predispositions

Genetic predispositions play a pivotal role in the etiology and progression of nutritional and metabolic disorders, determining how individuals respond to eating habits and lifestyle. Genetic predispositions would enhance the vulnerability for developing disorders , such as obesity, diabetes, and NAFLD, among others. For instance, genetic differences in genes involved in fat storage and metabolism, e.g., FTO and MC4R, have been associated with increased body weight and altered control of appetite. Similarly, single nucleotide polymorphisms (SNPs) of the PNPLA3 gene have been linked with the severity of hepatic steatosis, meaning that patients with certain genetic backgrounds would be more susceptible to fat deposition in the liver and subsequent development of NAFLD. Awareness of these genetic factors is important for clinicians to properly individualize preventive measures and therapeutic interventions. The interaction between predispositions that are genetic and predispositions that are environmental is particularly important when it comes to metabolic syndromes. Overnutrition, together with genetic predispositions, can lead to insulin resistance and, in turn, to chronic diseases , such as type 2 diabetes and cardiovascular disease. Individuals may have genetic polymorphisms predisposing them to poorer lipid metabolism or elevated glucose levels, combined with a diet rich in fat and sugar (Golubnitschaja et al., 2021). Besides, the frequency of specific genotypes associated with metabolic syndrome also differs across populations, hence is a reason why a personalized diet is needed. The integration of genetics into dietary advising is all part of a broader view of health, which goes beyond the philosophy one-size-fits-all, and the high emphasis it places on the requirement for personalized nutrition according to individual genetic composition. Moreover, genetic predispositions are increasingly valued as central elements influencing the reaction to interventions in metabolic and nutritional diseases. For example, individuals with specific genetic markers may react differently to weight-reducing diets or medication treatment for obesity and diabetes (Wong et al., 2017). The discovery of such genetic factors can influence clinical practice to enable more precise and effective management strategies for at-risk or currently experiencing metabolic dysfunction patients. Accordingly, continued investigation into nutrigenomics, diet interacting with genes, can lead to new ways of preventing and treating metabolic disease based on a person's genetic makeup. This trend toward personalized medicine underscores the potential to not only enhance patient outcomes, but also to address the rising prevalence of metabolic disease among populations around the world (Figure 1.16).

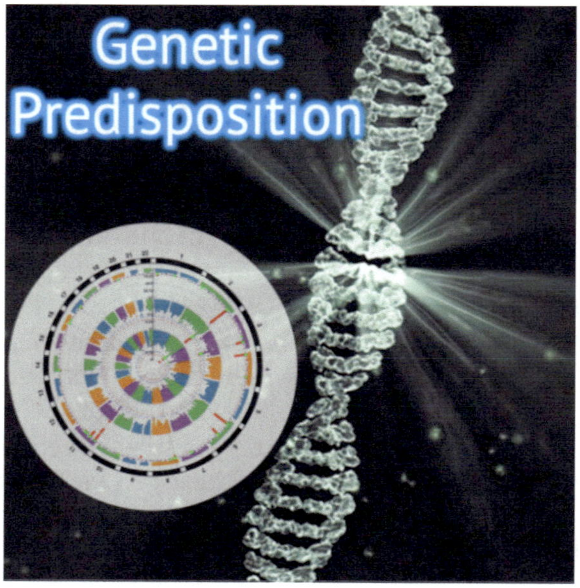

Figure 1.16. DNA visualization highlights genetic predisposition to disease.

Source: https://external-content.duckduckgo.com/iu/?u=https%3A%2F%2Fdiskinlab.org%2Fwp-content%2Fuploads%2F2019%2F08%2FResearch-headings_Predis_v3.png&f=1&nofb=1&ipt=ee60b21cdd58ac71cf4a21534b75a3ad90803eb20d8d6199054e168e8f4fc919.

1.4.2. Environmental Triggers

Environmental stimuli are the core initiating and propagating factors for the majority of nutritional and metabolic disorders, acting as agents catalyzing inherited genetic predispositions. The modern world has opened up an infinite number of lifestyle alternatives and environmental stimuli that can have a deep influence on metabolism. All three elements, i.e., diet, exercise, and stress levels, are closely related to environmental conditions. For instance, high-calorie, nutrient-poor foods that are common in modern diets have been linked to the rising instances of obesity, which make individuals vulnerable to depression and anxiety disorders (Fulton et al., 2021). Moreover, overloads of fast foods and processed foods, with accompanying inflammation and metabolic dysfunction, further make individuals' health dynamics more complicated. It is imperative to get to the bottom of these environmental stimuli to be able to develop effective preventive interventions and therapeutic interventions that will reverse the impact of metabolic disorders on mental health. Environmental stressors aside from diet are also key factors in worsening nutrition as well as metabolic disorders. Chronic stress due to several sources , such as profession, interpersonal relationships, and manner of life pressures, has been revealed to disrupt endocrine equilibrium and lead to metabolic syndrome. The interface between stress and dietary habits generally results in a vicious circle where increased cortisol levels stimulate desires for high-fat and high-sugar foods, which further improve obesity as well as the resulting linked health complications (Roszkiewicz et al., 2019). Also, recent research indicates the critical influence of psychosocial stressors on mental health, suggesting that long-term exposure to such environmental stimuli could increase the occurrence of mood disorders. By recognizing the complex interaction of environmental signals and metabolic well-being, researchers are better equipped to encourage public health interventions that can address healthier behavior and reduce the public health impact of these disorders. An environmental stimulus demands a multi-faceted approach that includes education, policy change, and behavior modification. Public health interventions like enhancing nutrition awareness and promoting physical activity play a pivotal role in restricting the influence of obesogenic environments. In addition, the incorporation of mental health services in nutrition programs will put them in a position to provide holistic support to individuals experiencing both metabolic and psychological problems. There should also be an emphasis on the system-level determinants generating unfavorable food environments, , such as socioeconomic disparities and limited access to healthy foods. By encouraging community-level interventions and implementing specially tailored interventions, we can create supportive environments that are able to foster metabolic health maintenance and prevent associated disorders. Understanding the environmental stimuli of nutritional and metabolic derangements plays an important role in supporting long-term health and wellbeing (Figure 1.17).

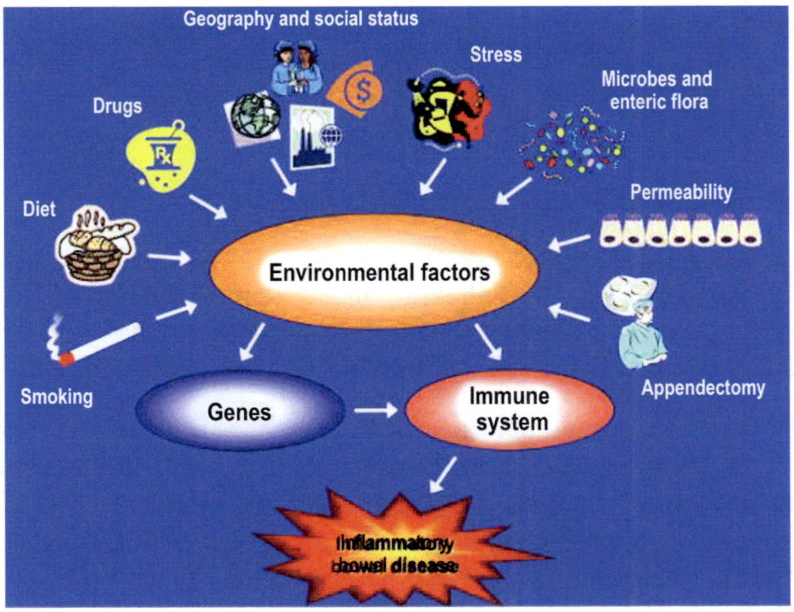

Figure 1.17. Factors contributing to inflammatory bowel disease (IBD).

Source: https://ars.els-cdn.com/content/image/1-s2.0-S1568997204000400-gr1.jpg

1.4.3. Lifestyle Choices and Their Consequences

Lifestyle choices have a strong influence on overall health and may have a major impact on the prevalence and management of nutritional and metabolic diseases. Individual diet, exercise, and sleep choices all influence metabolic function and refine or hinder energy homeostasis. Unhealthy diet with a focus on processed foods rather than whole foods, for instance, can lead to obesity, a major risk factor for type 2 diabetes and cardiovascular disease. Furthermore, sedentary living conditions add to these risks, as physical inactivity is associated with decreased insulin sensitivity and increased blood glucose.

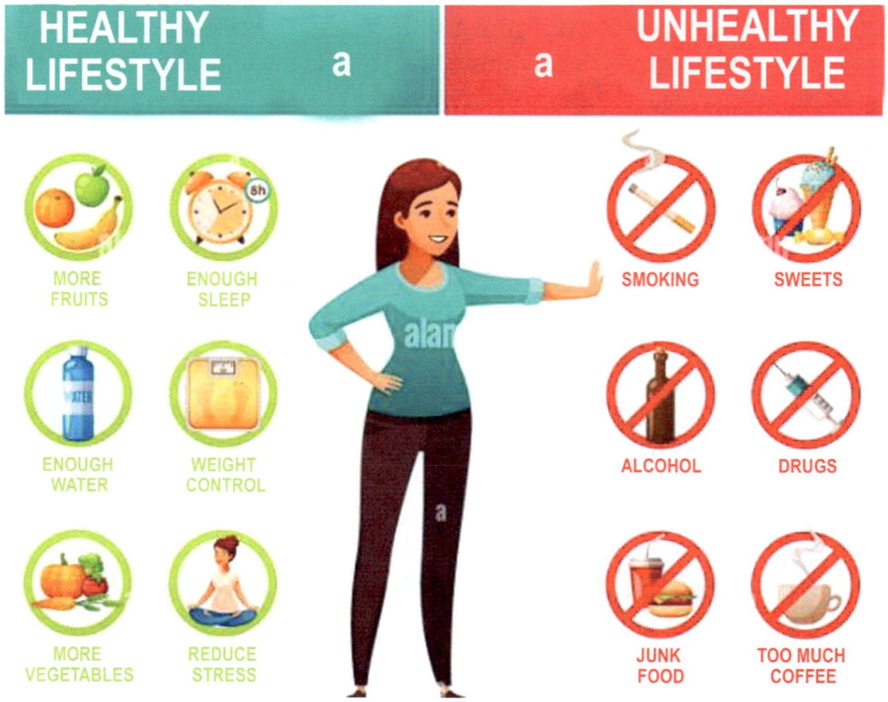
HEALTHY LIFESTYLE
UNHEALTHY LIFESTYLE
MORE FRUITS
ENOUGH SLEEP
ENOUGH WATER
WEIGHT CONTROL
MORE VEGETABLES
REDUCE STRESS
SMOKING
SWEETS
ALCOHOL
DRUGS
JUNK FOOD
TOO MUCH COFFEE

Figure 1.18: Healthy vs. unhealthy lifestyle habits.

Source: https://external-content.duckduckgo.com/iu/?u=https%3A%2F%2Fc8.alamy.com%2Fcomp%2F2G760YT%2Fhealthy-unhealthy-lifestyle-infographic-cartoon-poster-with-fruit-vegetable-diet-vs-smoking-drugs-caffeine-consumption-vector-illustration-2G760YT.jpg&f=1&nofb=1&ipt=1cada7448eada4a35892aa1a290b4eb7b26f6b4991b29244fd85fd42eb68351c.

Regular exercise can enhance metabolic health and decrease the risk of developing such chronic diseases. Thus, lifestyle consequences becomes paramount for individuals who wish to optimize their well-being and minimize their risk of nutritional and metabolic diseases. The impact of lifestyle decisions is not only experienced at an individual level but also ultimately affects public health trends and healthcare spending.

Over the past several decades, rising obesity and related metabolic disorder patterns have been severely burdening healthcare systems all over the world. Evidence points towards lifestyle control as a key intervention to reduce the escalating epidemic. For instance, intense lifestyle interventions focusing on diet and exercise have been observed to prevent diabetes and manage overweight and obesity. Health agencies' latest recommendations emphasize that targeted weight loss interventions and education in healthy living have the potential to induce positive health outcomes. In addition, social determinants of health , such as access to healthy food and access to ways of participating in physical activity significantly influence these lifestyle habits, and therefore public health interventions addressing these barriers are required (Davies et al., 2018).

Therefore, the application of preventive intervention focusing on more desirable lifestyle behaviors can alleviate health disparities and reduce healthcare costs associated with metabolic disorders.

The interplay between lifestyle and metabolic disorders is further exacerbated by the correlation among mental health, diet, and general well-being. Chronic stress and poor mental health can lead to unhealthy diets and less motivation to exercise, creating a vicious cycle of self-abuse that sustains metabolic dysfunction.

Moreover, research identifies the significance of mental stimulation and sensory stimulation in determining mental well-being, particularly among older adults where conditions like dementia are prevalent (Livingston et al., 2020). Maintaining balanced lifestyles with a healthy diet, physical activity, and mental well-being habits can prevent the occurrence of not only metabolic disorders but also cognitive decline. Therefore, interventions that target comprehensive lifestyle choices must be highlighted to enhance healthier physical and psychological well-being, ultimately contributing to improved quality of life and functional independence in the affected individuals with nutritional and metabolic disorders (Figure 1.18).

1.5. Diagnosis of Nutritional and Metabolic Disorders

The nutrition and metabolic disease diagnosis is a multidisciplinary process that relies on the utilization of several diagnostic modalities and tests to establish an accurate representation of the health status of a patient. The initial examinations are typically a thorough medical history and physical examination, which allow clinicians to screen for potential nutritional deficiency or metabolic derangement. Laboratory tests play a central part in this effort, measuring some biomarkers , such as blood sugar, lipid content, and hormone concentrations. Analysis of diet, perhaps through the use of food frequency questionnaires or 24-hour recall methods, also provides additional richness to the clinical presentation by explaining the patient's dietary pattern and habits. This association of clinical data and laboratory results enables healthcare professionals to establish the etiology of disorders, guiding targeted interventions and individualized treatment plans for both nutritional intake and metabolic processes. Diagnosis of nutritional and metabolic disorders is compounded by the inter-relatedness of genetics, environment, and lifestyle. Metabolic disorders like obesity, diabetes, and cardiovascular disease usually have similar symptoms as well as risk factors, making diagnosis more challenging. In some instances of inherited metabolic disorders, specialized genetic testing is required to gain insights into certain gene mutations that influence nutrient metabolism. With the incorporation of technology, including metabolic profiling and advanced imaging, one can gain a better understanding of the metabolic status and nutritional condition of an individual. Through the application of a comprehensive diagnostic model, physicians can make precise diagnoses of diseases like metabolic syndrome or nutritional deficiencies, setting the foundation for effective functional management schemes that result in enhanced health outcomes for patients. Healthcare providers are faced with significant challenges when making timely and precise diagnoses of metabolic as well as nutritional diseases, particularly in populations with low access to diagnostic services.

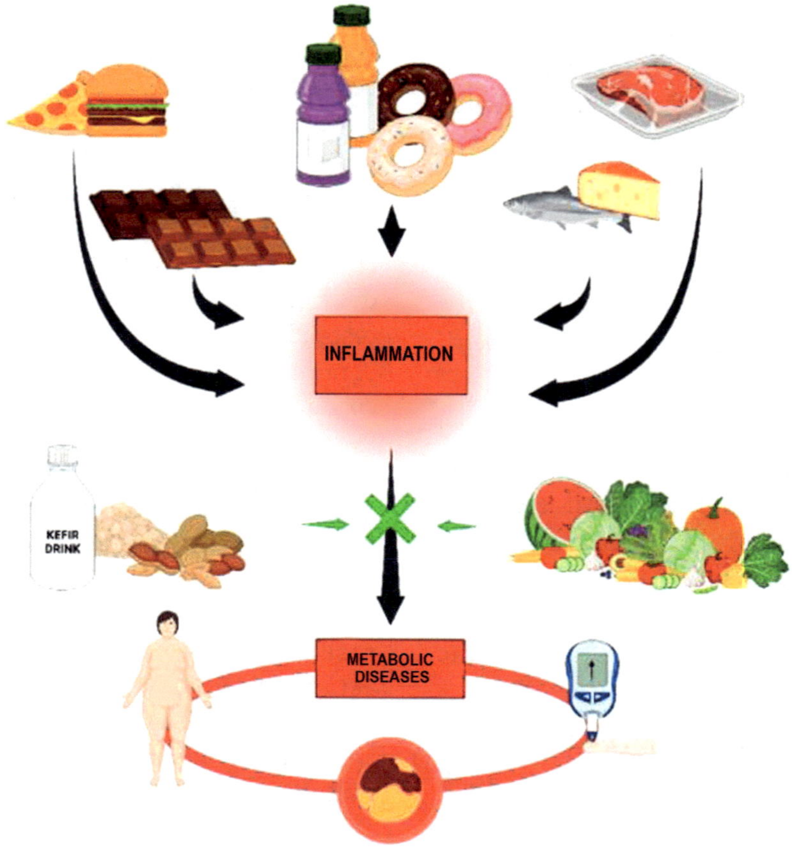

Figure 1.19. Dietary impact on inflammation and metabolic disease risk.

Source: https://www.researchgate.net/publication/371929619/figure/fig4/AS:11431281388459495@1745177571499/Description-of-the-types-of-diet-that-can-cause-inflammatory-processes-including-animal.tif

The variations in laboratory facilities in different health institutions may lead to variations in the efficiency of diagnosis and treatment. Besides, health professionals are advised to keep themselves updated on the latest advancements and guidelines, e.g., as available in Visseren et al. (2021), to facilitate evidence-based decision-making regarding diagnostics and treatments. Social determinants of health care are also necessary, as socioeconomic factors might highly affect nutritional status and access to care. Lastly, an interdisciplinary approach combining clinical knowledge, technological innovation, and patient-specific education is crucial to optimizing the diagnosis and treatment of nutritional and metabolic diseases and public health outcomes in general (Figure 1.19).

1.5.1. Clinical Assessments and History

In metabolic and nutritional diseases, patient history and clinical assessment systematically are essential for accurate diagnosis and appropriate treatment. These assessments consist of a range of methods involving a range of in-depth interviews and structured questionnaires for assessing diet intake, activities, and signs of metabolic health. These broad-based evaluations not only form the basis for the diagnosis of some conditions like non-alcoholic fatty liver disease (NAFLD), but also for identifying risk factors associated with other metabolic disorders. By employing methods like anthropometry and biochemical analysis, clinicians are able to represent a patient's health profile in a multiple-dimensional format, ultimately determining interventions aimed at addressing immediate as well as long-term problems of health. This combined approach highlights the importance of keeping clinical assessments in the broader nutritional health perspective. Adequate attention to the patient's dietary history will enlighten us about essential aspects of their health trajectory, particularly concerning derangement of metabolism. For instance, studies have demonstrated that deficiencies in essential vitamins will aggravate psychiatric disorder accompanying deranged metabolism, rendering nutritional assessment a critical diagnostic part. In a patient population with severe mental illnesses, deficiencies in vitamins , such as D, B9, and B12 were correlated with adverse psychiatric outcomes and increased metabolic syndrome rates (Faugère et al., 2025).

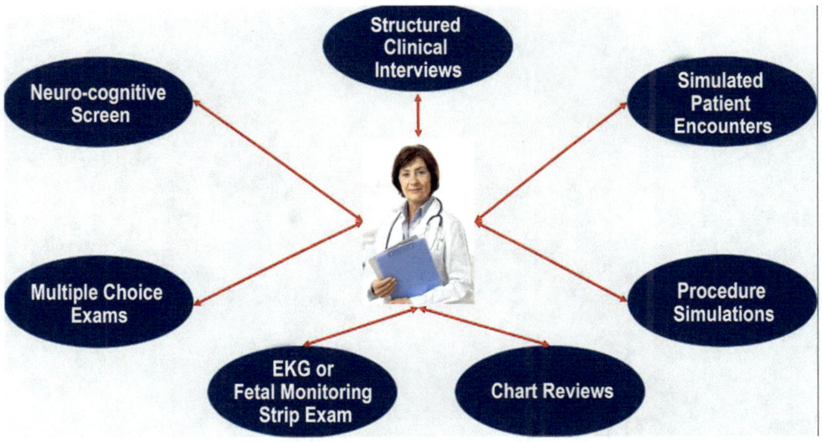

Figure 1.20. Methods for assessing physician clinical competency.

Source: https://external-content.duckduckgo.com/iu/?u=https%3A%2F%2Fwww.cpepdoc.org%2Fwp-content%2Fuploads%2F2018%2F05%2FRevised-Assessment-Flowchart-1.png&f=1&nofb=1&ipt=1ab305e56ab4f051cff050e5b900762ac05717e4935d95d31ae10e240597373d.

This correlation highlights clinicians' need to address not just the patient's physical, but also psychological, component of nutrition. An in-depth clinical history, therefore, becomes an absolute necessity, assisting health professionals in devising detailed treatment strategies including both psychological well-being and metabolic management. Furthermore, the multifactorial etiology of nutritional and metabolic disorders demands personalized clinical assessment acknowledging heterogeneity in risk factors and disease process. For instance, research explains that NAFLD patients have diverse risk profiles according to BMI and hormonal markers, owing to the necessity of tailored evaluation (Znakharenko et al., 2024). Perception of the differential implication of dietary habits, lifestyles, and metabolic factors offers clinicians the wisdom to carry out targeted interventions. Thus, careful examinations of clinical history and assessments allow for early treatment and diagnosis, perhaps halting the development of diseases like NAFLD. Lastly, a rigorous and responsive approach to clinical assessments can significantly affect the efficacy of treatment as well as patient outcomes overall for patients with metabolic and nutritional problems (Figure 1.20).

1.5.2. Laboratory Tests and Imaging

Knowledge of the function of imaging and laboratory tests in the diagnosis of nutritional and metabolic disorders is essential for proper management and treatment. Laboratory tests may be able to reveal biochemical imbalances characteristically found in these disorders. An example is that serum biomarkers are necessary in assessing liver function and detecting conditions , such as nonalcoholic fatty liver disease (NAFLD). Patients with suspected NAFLD typically receive a sequence of tests to establish the presence of hepatic steatosis, inflammation, and fibrosis. In this instance, it is important to differentiate between various disease phases using accurate biomarkers because the accuracy of diagnosis has a significant effect on the outcome of the patients and thus makes effective laboratory techniques extremely vital. Imaging modalities like ultrasound, computed tomography (CT), and magnetic resonance imaging (MRI) play as important role in the evaluation of patients presenting with suspected metabolic disease.

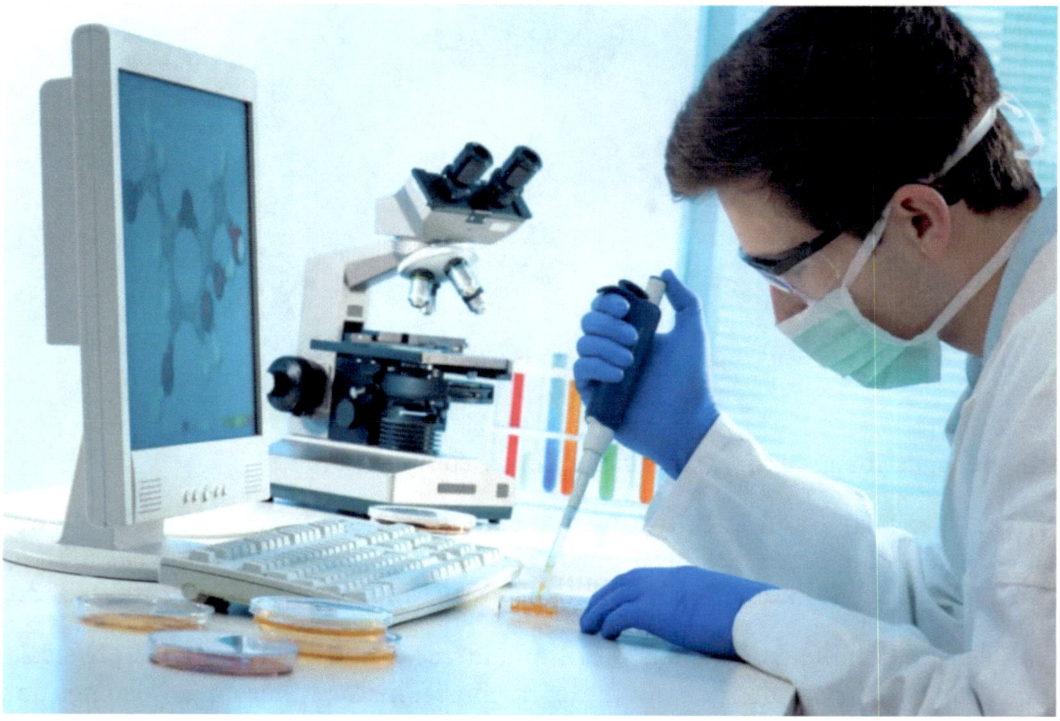

Figure 1.21. A scientist performing laboratory research with modern equipment.

Source:

While traditional imaging modalities like ultrasound can identify hepatic steatosis, they are not sensitive enough for the detection of early disease in most cases. Specialized imaging techniques like MRI spectroscopy have, however, come into use and offer increased sensitivity as well as quantitative assessment of hepatic fat. These advances not only help in the diagnosis but also monitor the development of disorders over time. Thus, integration of newer imaging modalities with routine clinical practice would significantly enhance our capability to understand and manage metabolic derangements (Cryan et al., 2019). Interaction between imaging and laboratory tests offers the best approach for diagnosing and monitoring nutritional and metabolic disorders. New research on the gut microbiota supports the necessity for robust diagnostic mechanisms. This association of the microbiota with metabolic health underscores other pathways through which laboratory tests and imaging can provide critical insights. As non-invasive techniques further evolve, particularly in unraveling the microbiota-gut-brain axis, they may reveal novel avenues for intervention for metabolic disease. Briefly put, ongoing innovation in laboratory and imaging modalities is essential to maximize diagnostic precision and propel directed therapies for this fast-evolving disease (Cryan et al., 2019) (Figure 1.21).

1.5.3. Role of Dietary Evaluations

During the assessment of metabolic and nutritional disorders, dietary evaluations are pivotal to establishing the connection between nutrition and health outcomes. These evaluations provide critical data on an individual's diet, nutrient intake, and lifestyle, which can play a major role in metabolic health. By the systematic analysis of foods taken, clinicians are able to identify possible excesses or deficits that could contribute to the causation or progression of metabolic disorders. The relationship, for instance, between food consumption and conditions , such as diabetes or obesity underscores the requirement for an overall assessment, which can inform targeted interventions in maximizing health.

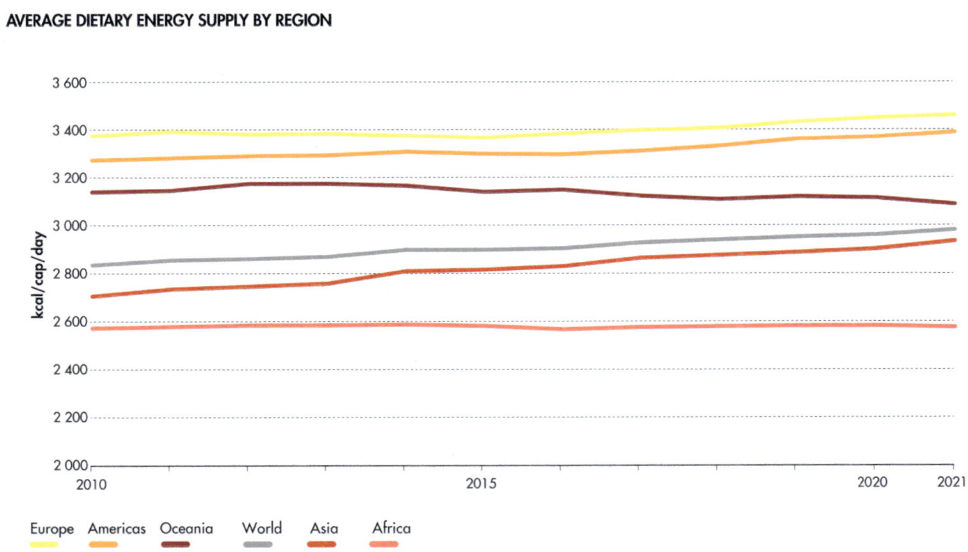

Figure 1.22. A nutritionist preparing a healthy diet and lifestyle plan.

Source: By FAO - https://www.fao.org/documents/card/en/c/cc8166en , File:World Food and Agriculture - Statistical Yearbook 2023.pdf, CC BY -SA 3.0 igo, https://commons.wikimedia.org/w/index.php?curid=142154565

Besides, nutritional evaluations are also useful for monitoring response to nutritional therapies with provisions for changes based on patient response and variable health status. Further, the inclusion of nutritional evaluation in clinical practice allows for the development of patient-tailored dietary plans. The realization that each person has unique nutritional needs defined by genetics, lifestyle, and health status is essential in the management of metabolic disorders. By using techniques , such as food frequency questionnaires or recall diets, practitioners are able to have a clear picture of a patient's dietary behavior and nutrient intake patterns. This facilitates the identification of specific food components that are likely to be altered, thus enhancing patient compliance with guidelines for treatment. For example, dietary evaluations can recognize excessive intake of processed foods, trans fats, or sugars, which are linked with undesirable health outcomes (Ceulemans et al., 2017). Thus, by making clear evident the dietary components of metabolic diseases, physicians can better help patients bring about a change in behavior and become healthier in general. Moreover, nutrition evaluations are also helpful in providing information regarding the potential impact of certain nutritional supplements on the treatment of a range of ailments. Recent studies, for instance, have explored the efficacy of antioxidant and immunomodulatory nutrients in attention-deficit hyperactivity disorder (ADHD) treatment, suggesting a link between food insufficiency and behavior (Ceulemans et al., 2017).

This then makes it pertinent to evaluate eating patterns not only to supplement present deficiencies but also to investigate the far-reaching implications of nutrition on mental well-being. Additionally, as recent studies point to the relationship between diet, immune response, and metabolic health, dietary assessments could disclose patterns that may trigger preventative measures against metabolic diseases. Therefore, the function of dietary assessments goes beyond simple measurement; it involves a proactive stance on health management, highlighting the need for individuals to pay attention to their dietary habits alongside clinical advice (Figure 1.22).

1.6. Treatment and Management Strategies

Successful treatment and management of metabolic and nutritional disorders, however, involve an interdisciplinary strategy that integrates diet changes, way of life changes, and, where required, drugs. One such condition is polycystic ovary syndrome (PCOS), which occurs in a significant percentage of women and leads to various metabolic as well as reproductive problems. Extensive management of PCOS includes personalized diet therapy to improve insulin sensitivity and weight control, which may also affect the course of the disease. Treatments include the adoption of a low-calorie diet with the view of reducing intake of simple carbohydrates and foods with high calorie value. Furthermore, diet regimens should comprise monitoring saturated and trans fatty acids intake and could comprise prebiotic food with regard to potential deficiencies, especially in vitamin D and omega-3 fatty acids, as these are essential to metabolic health (Jain et al., 2025). A further innovative method in obesity management and related metabolic disorders is the application of very low-energy ketogenic diets (VLEKT). This approach has been a promising weight-loss and metabolic intervention in people who are suffering from obesity-related comorbidities. VLEKT is found to promote ketosis efficiently, favoring fat oxidation and metabolic control, with potential benefits for important organ systems like the liver and adipose tissue. However, maintaining such a regimen strictly can prove challenging, which requires strict oversight and customized programming by professionals to offset deficits and avoid long-term failure. Such a diet regimen not only focuses on enhancing weight control but also works toward enhancing complications , such as metabolic syndrome and resultant cardiovascular diseases (Balestra et al., 2025). Furthermore, successful management programs must incorporate diet therapies with other lifestyle adjustments, , such as exercise and behavior modification. Some advantages of regular exercise include significantly enhancing the efficacy of dietary therapy by promoting metabolic function and a healthy weight. By adopting a healthier lifestyle, as patients become physically more active, synergistic interactions of physical activity and diet adjustment can lead to improved insulin sensitivity and complications reduction of metabolic disorders. Besides, the incorporation of digital health technology , such as mobile health applications to track diet and exercise, will further increase the effectiveness of a comprehensive management plan. Therefore, treatment of nutritional and metabolic disorders demands an integrated and individualized approach whereby ongoing research continues to inform optimum practices and strategies for enduring health outcomes through maximal dietary and lifestyle modification (Figure 1.23).

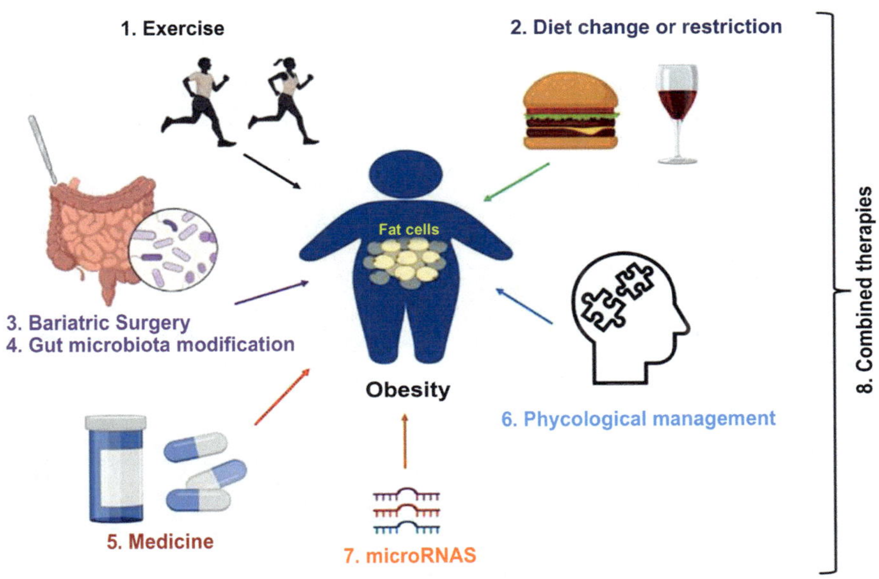

Figure 1.23. Therapeutic strategies for managing obesity.

Source: Yang M, Liu S, Zhang C. Related Metabolic Diseases and Treatments of Obesity. *Healthcare*. 2022; 10(9):1616. https://doi.org/10.3390/healthcare10091616

1.6.1. Nutritional Interventions and Dietary Modifications

Nutritional modification and dietary intervention are of vital importance in the control of many metabolic syndromes, with the efficacy established in the prevention and management of diseases , such as obesity and type 2 diabetes. These interventions are usually comprehensive strategies that seek to reduce caloric intake and alter food habits to enhance health. For instance, a comprehensive program consisting of behavioral therapy, exercise, and drug treatment has been reported to achieve significant weight loss. Data indicates that individuals participating in multicomponent lifestyle modification programs can achieve a 5% to 10% weight loss that is associated with substantial improvements in glucose metabolism and blood pressure in people with diabetes and hypertension. Effective dietary approaches can be modified to suit an individual's predilections, thereby enhancing adherence and long-term success in achieving metabolic homeostasis (Elmaleh-Sachs et al., 2023). Moreover, early-life nutrition has a strong influence on metabolic health across life. It is pointed out through research that maternal overnutrition and undernutrition, respectively, can make the offspring susceptible to metabolic disease, pointing towards the vital role played by nutrition during crucial periods of development. Most notably, fetal programming theory suggests that nutritional intake during pregnancy could have long-lasting effects on energy metabolism in children during growth. This interaction is mediated by epigenetic mechanisms, , such as DNA methylation and histone modification, by which nutritional exposure acts. By interrupting early-life imbalances of nutrients through dietary intervention, disease courses are susceptible to being altered and preventive measures against subsequent metabolic disease can be instituted. This proactive approach to dietary intervention may ultimately reverse the tide of diseases like type 2 diabetes and obesity (Zhou et al., 2020).

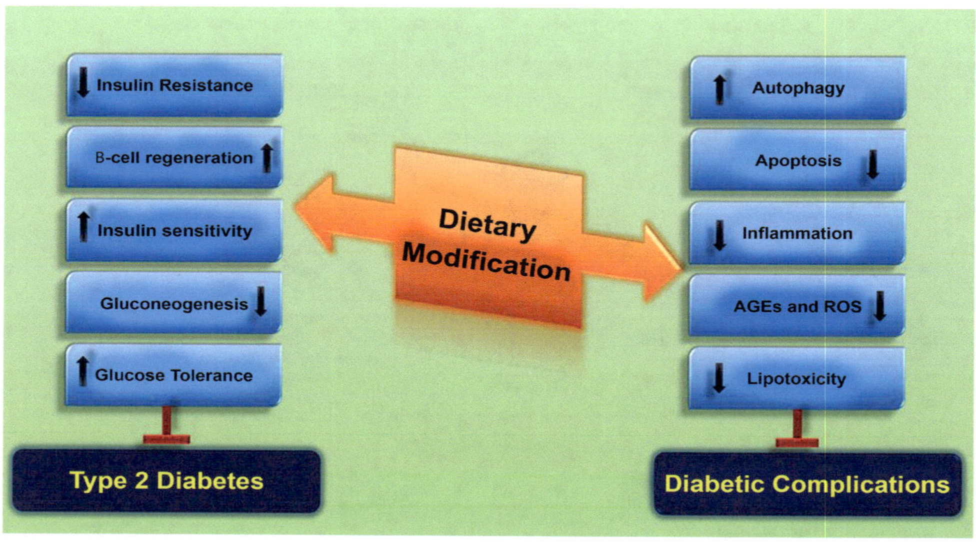

Figure 1.24. Impact of dietary modification on type 2 diabetes and its complications.

Source: https://ars.els-cdn.com/content/image/1-s2.0-S1043661821001869-ga1_lrg.jpg.

Additionally, the integration of pharmacotherapy with diet modification validates the effectiveness of weight loss programs. The past decade has seen remarkable advancements in anti-obesity medications that offer new forms of therapy for individuals with treatment-resistant weight loss, particularly when lifestyle modifications are insufficient. For instance, medications , such as glucagon-like peptide 1 (GLP-1) agonists have revealed significant value in promoting weight loss with a simultaneous improvement of concomitant metabolic factors. Clinical practice guidelines today recommend the use of a multi-component treatment protocol that includes dietary modification, individualized lifestyle interventions, and, where necessary, pharmacologic therapy. Such a wide-ranging approach not only facilitates significant and sustained weight loss but also assists in the management, in general, of obesity-related comorbidities, and emphasizing the value of individualizing treatment plans based on the patient's specific needs and challenges (Elmaleh-Sachs et al., 2023) (Figure 1.24).

1.6.2. Pharmacological Treatments

Pharmacologic treatments have emerged as a key component of the control of nutrition and metabolic disorders, particularly obesity. Obesity management demands treatment for this multifactorial disease. in addition to the added complexities of biological, behavioral, environmental, and social factors. Medications can assist patients in achieving realistic weight loss and compliance with lifestyle interventions. For example, pharmacotherapy can mitigate obesity-associated health risks by supplementing 'dieting' and exercise. Although diet therapy, for example, hypocaloric diets, continues to be a pillar of weight loss, pharmacological agents can provide supplementary assistance to obese individuals, ultimately enhancing the overall quality of life and reducing obesity-associated co-morbidities (Busetto et al., 2015). In the pharmacotherapeutic field, some medications have been created to affect appetite and the absorption of fat. Medications , such as orlistat inhibit the absorption of fat in the digestive system, while others , such as liraglutide, decrease appetite and promote feelings of fullness. These drugs may also prove extremely beneficial when diet and exercise alone cannot trigger dramatic weight loss. However, the proper utilization of these pharmacologic treatments can be greatly reliant on a well-coordinated coordination among healthcare professionals, including dietitians and behavioral therapists, to monitor the treatment process and adjust treatment plans in response. Significantly, the pharmacodynamic and pharmacokinetic profiles of the drugs should be comprehended to prevent potential side effects and ensure patient safety during the treatment period (Busetto et al., 2015). Besides, the co-administration of pharmacological therapies should be approached with caution, particularly among patients with compromised health histories, , such as disabled veterans. As has been observed, poor lifestyle and dietary patterns complicate the pharmacological treatment process. Even in medication-drug interactions, interactions with food supplements or herbal remedies are a concern. The veterans can be served with individual nutrition plans suiting their specific needs, avoiding the risk of drug interactions. Also, integrative medicine principles like dietary changes like the Mediterranean diet can be used in conjunction with pharmacotherapy to encourage a healthier lifestyle and treat the patients as a whole. Thus, the wise application of pharmacologic therapy as a component of an appropriate health care regimen is important in order to achieve maximal benefits for patients with nutritional and metabolic disorders (Figure 1.25).

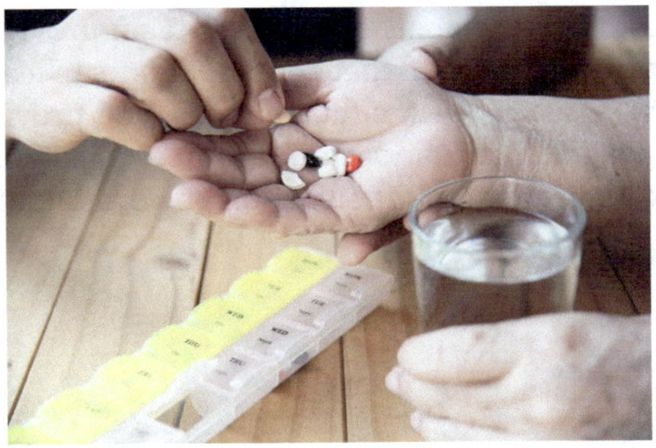

Figure 1.25. Caregiver assisting with daily medication management.

Source: https://nirvanhospital.com/wp-content/uploads/2023/12/Integrating-Medication-Management.png.

1.6.3. Importance of Multidisciplinary Approaches

Metabolic and nutritional disorders demand multidisciplinary management to offer comprehensive patient care. Several health professionals, including dietitians, physicians, and metabolic disorder specialists, offer varying perspectives essential to addressing the diverse needs of patients with metabolic and nutritional disorders. Such collaboration can readily enhance the accuracy of diagnosis and therapeutic interventions, since each professional offers specialist knowledge that informs better clinical decisions. For example, a dietitian will identify some deficiencies in diet, while a metabolic specialist can identify biochemical abnormalities underlying the disorder. Overall, such a collective combination of expertise constructs an integrated understanding of the patient's status, ultimately resulting in improved health status and quality of life. The multidisciplinary team not only enhances clinical management but also addresses psychosocial aspects of nutritional and metabolic disorders. Patients are often forced to encounter psychological problems, including depression and anxiety, as a result of chronic illness and dietary restrictions. Including mental health professionals on the care team provides timely intervention that allows patients to learn how to cope. Team educators can also provide important information and resources to patients and their families, allowing empowerment and engagement in their own plans of care. This common environment is particularly valuable in the management of the multi-faceted nature of such disorders, as it synthesizes medical treatment with emotional support and education into a more integrated healthcare experience. With the ongoing development in nutritional and metabolic sciences, active dialogue among members of multidisciplinary teams remains vital. The introduction of new therapies and interventions, particularly for patients with complex needs, necessitates active dialogue to tailor care plans accordingly. For instance, the case of spinal muscular atrophy type 1 (SMA1) illustrates this point because advancements in precision medicine require thorough nutritional and metabolic monitoring for optimal patient outcomes (Corsello et al., 2021). This calls into question not only the necessity of having a multidisciplinary team but also having them work as an integrated unit. Finally, stimulating cooperation among various specialists can lead to groundbreaking solutions having a significant influence on the prevention and treatment of patients with nutritional and metabolic disorders, emphasizing the significance of a multidisciplinary model in contemporary healthcare.

CLOSER LOOK

MALNUTRITION

Malnutrition is a serious global health issue that occurs when a person's diet lacks the necessary nutrients for proper growth, development, and overall health. In children, malnutrition can manifest as undernutrition, including wasting (low weight for height), stunting (low height for age), and underweight (low weight for age), or as overnutrition, such as obesity and nutrient imbalances caused by unhealthy diets. The most common causes of malnutrition in children include poverty, food insecurity, poor feeding practices, recurrent infections, and lack of access to clean water and healthcare. In developing countries, undernutrition remains a major concern, often leading to weakened immune systems, increased risk of infections, delayed development, and even death in severe cases. In contrast, overnutrition and micronutrient deficiencies (such as lack of iron, vitamin A, or iodine) are also rising concerns, even in wealthier nations, due to increased consumption of processed, nutrient-poor foods. The signs of malnutrition can include fatigue, slow growth, swollen belly, dry skin, hair loss, and frequent illness. Diagnosis involves assessing a child's weight, height, and nutritional intake, often supported by blood tests to identify deficiencies. Treatment depends on the type and severity of malnutrition but may include therapeutic feeding programs, vitamin and mineral supplementation, and addressing underlying medical or social issues. Prevention is key and involves promoting breastfeeding, providing education on balanced diets, improving sanitation, and ensuring food security. A closer look at malnutrition reveals that it is not merely a lack of food but a complex issue influenced by social, economic, and environmental factors. Addressing malnutrition requires a coordinated effort between healthcare providers, governments, communities, and families to ensure every child has the opportunity to grow up healthy and reach their full potential.

SUMMARY

The research on nutritional and metabolic disease reveals a profound understanding of their increasing prevalence and wide-ranging implications on global health. The increase in the prevalence of conditions , such as metabolic syndrome (MetS) suggests the intersection of lifestyle choices and health outcomes, particularly in developing nations where industrialization has transformed dietary patterns. As documented, the syndrome of metabolic burden has not only cardiovascular but also polyphyletic neurological risks, posing immediate public health challenges. This complex relationship between diet, physical inactivity, and chronic disease development reflects an urgent need for a meticulous understanding of these disorders, considering their relevance not only to their individual impact on health but also to society as a whole, calling for urgent attention from clinicians and policymakers (Busetto et al., 2017). Moreover, the findings of the Global Burden of Diseases study highlight that while years lived with disability (YLDs) on an age-standardized basis slightly improved, the overall burden of non-fatal disease from nutritional and metabolic disorders has risen significantly. The trend resonates with the fact that progress in mortality has to be complemented by strategies focusing on the quality of life of people suffering from the disorders. The differences observed in illnesses , such as depressive disorders in conjunction with metabolic syndrome, justify the necessity for an integrated therapy and prevention plan. As populations age and have high-risk health profiles, the necessity to deal with the constellation of causative factors of YLDs needs to be met so that the impact of metabolic and diet-related diseases on people and the healthcare system can be curtailed (James et al., 2018). Lastly, the complex interaction between nutrition, metabolism, and health outcome necessitates interdisciplinary and multidisciplinary action from lifestyle modifications to novel pharmacologic therapies. In the face of the increasing prevalence of such conditions as metabolic syndrome constitutes a severe public health challenge, prevention-based and management-based specific interventions are absolutely essential. By taking on an integrated strategy that addresses both environmental determinants and individual health behaviors, not only can risk for these disorders be lowered, but quality of life for individuals with these disorders may also be improved. As nutritional and metabolic ailments continue to increase in complexity, continued research and progressive action will be necessary to meet these complexities and create healthier populations overall (Etchegoyen et al., 2018).

Understanding the complex relationship of nutrition with metabolic diseases is key to addressing the public health problems of the modern era. Nutritional deficiencies have the potential to lead to metabolic abnormalities and, in a way, create a cycle of bad health. To cite, some micronutrient deficiencies are linked with type 2 diabetes and obesity. Such metabolic diseases not only worsen one's health but also exert significant economic burdens on healthcare systems. Moreover, recent research has highlighted the role of gut microbiota in regulating the metabolism of the host. Dysfunctions within the gut microbiome can have a profound impact on the metabolic processes of the body, which result in various disorders. Thus, the study of , such associations provide new directions for therapeutic approaches targeting nutritional intake and microbiome composition as therapeutic interventions for the management and prevention of metabolic disorders (de Vos et al., 2022). In addition to exploring the interface of nutritional disorders, more general consequences of antimicrobial resistance (AMR) need to be addressed for nutritional status. Antimicrobial resistance is a threat to global health now, and research has indicated that malnutrition may hasten the effects of AMR, leading to enhanced infection-related mortality. The effect of infectious illnesses compounded by AMR particularly affects vulnerable populations, making it an imperative problem within low-income settings. What has been discovered through research is that malnutrition would compromise immune function and, consequently, increase susceptibility to drug-resistant infections. It is therefore essential to understand the interface of nutrition, metabolism, and AMR to devise effective health interventions. Decision-makers must prioritize nutritional interventions as a key component of wider public health programs to mitigate the impact of both nutritional deficiencies and the rising tide of AMR in the population (Murray et al., 2022). Finally, elucidating the interactions between metabolic disorders, nutrition, and AMR underlines an integrated strategy for enhancing health and avoiding disease. With the inclusion of nutritional assessment in practice, clinicians can determine susceptible individuals and provide them with certain dietary suggestions for improving the metabolic health outcome. Public health initiatives also need to emphasize the contribution of balanced nutrition towards avoiding metabolic disorders as well as infection. Multisectoral cooperation between sectors, including health care, agriculture, and education, is imperative in formulating effective policies that guarantee nutritional health. Eventually, these problems are addressed through an eclectic method that will enhance the efficacy of interventions aimed at reducing the occurrences of nutritional and metabolic diseases while simultaneously fighting against the emergence of AMR. Interactions of these elements point to the importance of an integrated understanding of health with respect to nutritional aspects and microbial interactions within the human body (Ciccotti et al., 2018).

References

1. Ciccotti, M., Raguzzini, A., Sciarra, T., Catasta, G., Aiello, P., Buccolieri, C., Reggi, R., Palmery, M., Lista, F., & Peluso, I. (2018). Nutraceutical-based Integrative Medicine: Adopting a Mediterranean Diet Pyramid for Attaining Healthy Ageing in Veterans with Disabilities. Current pharmaceutical design, 24(35), 4186–4196. https://doi.org/10.2174/1381612824666181003113444 (accessed on 13th June 2025).

2. Annemans, L., Moreno-Reyes, R., Tafforeau, J., et al. (2010). Projected reduction in healthcare costs in Belgium after optimization of iodine intake: Impact on costs related to thyroid nodular disease. https://core.ac.uk/download/55842999.pdf (accessed on 13th June 2025).

3. Busetto, L., Dicker, D., Azran, C., Batterham, R. L., Farpour-Lambert, N., Fried, M., Hjelmesæth, J., Kinzl, J., Leitner, D. R., Makaronidis, J. M., Schindler, K., Toplak, H., & Yumuk, V. (2017). Practical Recommendations of the Obesity Management Task Force of the European Association for the Study of Obesity for Post-Bariatric Surgery Medical Management. Obesity facts, 10(6), 597–632. https://doi.org/10.1159/000481825 (accessed on 13th June 2025).

4. Badiali, D., Bruno, G., Ribichini, E., et al. (2019). Role of fiber in nutritional management of pancreatic diseases. https://core.ac.uk/download/231748461.pdf (accessed on 13th June 2025).

5. Basista, R. S., Jaiswal, S., & Veeranna, R. P. (2022). Modulation of gut microbiota by bioactive compounds for prevention and management of type 2 diabetes. Biomedicine & Pharmacotherapy, 152, 113148–113148. https://doi.org/10.1016/j.biopha.2022.113148 (accessed on 13th June 2025).

6. Blumenstein, I. U., Böhles, H., Goeters, C., et al. (2009). Aminosäuren–Leitlinie Parenterale Ernährung, Kapitel 4. https://core.ac.uk/download/14527635.pdf (accessed on 13th June 2025).

7. Combet, Emilie and Buckton, Christina (2014) Micronutrient deficiencies, vitamin pills and nutritional supplements. Medicine, 14(2), pp. 66-72. (doi: 10.1016/j.mpmed.2014.11.002) (accessed on 13th June 2025).

8. Chalasani, N., Younossi, Z. M., Lavine, J. E., Charlton, M., Cusi, K., Rinella, M. E., Harrison, S. A., et al. (2017). The diagnosis and management of nonalcoholic fatty liver disease: Practice guidance from the American Association for the Study of Liver Diseases. Hepatology, 67, 328–357. https://doi.org/10.1002/hep.29367 (accessed on 13th June 2025).

9. Cryan, J. F., O'Riordan, K. J., Cowan, C. S. M., Sandhu, K. V., Bastiaanssen, T. F. S., Boehme, M., Codagnone, M. G., et al. (2019). The microbiota-gut-brain axis. Physiological Reviews, 99, 1877–2013. https://doi.org/10.1152/physrev.00018.2018 (accessed on 13th June 2025).

10. Daghigh, F., Harris, J. E., King, J., et al. (2014). Nutri One-on-One: Improving patients' metabolic profile with one-on-one nutritional coaching. https://core.ac.uk/download/234124880.pdf (accessed on 13th June 2025).

11. de Vos, W. M., Tilg, H., Van Hul, M., & Cani, P. D. (2022). Gut microbiome and health: Mechanistic insights. Gut, 71, 1020–1032. https://doi.org/10.1136/gutjnl-2021-326789 (accessed on 13th June 2025).

12. Delgado, A. F. (2022). Resposta inflamatória e alterações nutricionais: Biomarcadores. https://core.ac.uk/download/492971549.pdf (accessed on 13th June 2025).

13. Etchegoyen, M., Nobile, M. H., Báez, F., Posesorski, B., González, J., Lago, N., Milei, J., et al. (2018). Metabolic syndrome and neuroprotection. Frontiers in Neuroscience, 12. https://doi.org/10.3389/fnins.2018.00196 (accessed on 13th June 2025).

14. Fulton, S., Décarie-Spain, L., Fioramonti, X., Guiard, B. P., & Nakajima, S. (2021). The menace of obesity to depression and anxiety prevalence. Trends in Endocrinology and Metabolism, 33, 18–35. https://doi.org/10.1016/j.tem.2021.10.005 (accessed on 13th June 2025).

15. Garber, A., Hastie, P., Kaya Karasu, G., et al. (2018). Equine nutrition: A preliminary investigation of feeding practices in equine veterinary hospitals in the USA. https://core.ac.uk/download/157812853.pdf (accessed on 13th June 2025).

16. Gigliotti, S., Maio, R., Perticone, F., et al. (2019). Ketogenic diet-induced weight loss is associated with an increase in vitamin D levels in obese adults. https://core.ac.uk/download/231747945.pdf (accessed on 13th June 2025).

17. Murray, C. J. L., Ikuta, K. S., Sharara, F., Swetschinski, L. R., Robles Aguilar, G., Gray, A. P., Han, C., et al. (2022). Global burden of bacterial antimicrobial resistance in 2019: A systematic analysis. The Lancet, 399, 629–655. https://doi.org/10.1016/s0140-6736(21)02724-0 (accessed on 13th June 2025).

18. Murray, J. A. M. D., Bloxham, C., Kulifay, J., Stevenson, A., & Roberts, J. (2015). Equine nutrition: A survey of perceptions and practices of horse owners undertaking a massive open online course in equine nutrition. Journal of Equine Veterinary Science, 35(6), 510–517. https://core.ac.uk/download/30638562.pdf (accessed on 13th June 2025).

19. Vernocchi, P., Del Chierico, F., & Putignani, L. (2020). Gut microbiota metabolism and interaction with food components. International Journal of Molecular Sciences, 21, 3688–3688. https://doi.org/10.3390/ijms21103688 (accessed on 13th June 2025).

20. Visseren, F. L. J., Mach, F., Smulders, Y. M., Carballo, D., Koskinas, K. C., Bäck, M., Bénétos, A., et al. (2021). 2021 ESC guidelines on cardiovascular disease prevention in clinical practice. European Heart Journal, 42, 3227–3337. https://doi.org/10.1093/eurheartj/ehab484 (accessed on 13th June 2025).

21. Wong, V. W. S., Chan, W. K., Chitturi, S., Chawla, Y., Dan, Y. Y., Duseja, A., Fan, J. G., et al. (2017). Asia–Pacific Working Party on Non-alcoholic Fatty Liver Disease guidelines 2017—Part 1: Definition, risk factors and assessment. Journal of Gastroenterology and Hepatology, 33, 70–85. https://doi.org/10.1111/jgh.13857 (accessed on 13th June 2025).

22. Yu, Z., & Muehleman, V. (2023). Eating disorders and metabolic diseases. International Journal of Environmental Research and Public Health, 20, 2446–2446. https://doi.org/10.3390/ijerph20032446 (accessed on 13th June 2025).

23. Zhou, L., Deng, M., Zhang, Q., & Xiao, X. (2020). Early-life nutrition and metabolic disorders in later life: A new perspective on energy metabolism. Chinese Medical Journal, 133, 1961–1970. https://doi.org/10.1097/cm9.0000000000000976 (accessed on 13th June 2025).

24. Znakharenko E.A., Gerasimenko O.N., Maximov V.N., Gorbunova A.M. Clinical-nutritional and metabolic disorders in the formation of non-alcoholic fatty liver disease. Experimental and Clinical Gastroenterology. 2024;(9):55-62. (In Russ.) https://doi.org/10.31146/1682-8658-ecg-229-9-55-62(accessed on 13th June 2025).

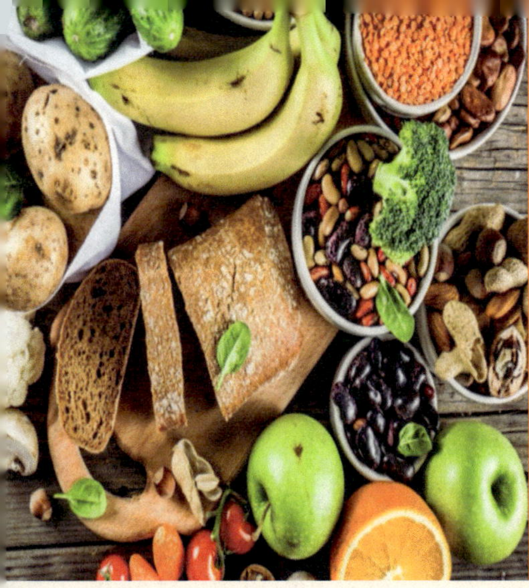

Chapter 2

MACRONUTRIENT METABOLISM

Contents

Introduction....39
2.1. Types of Macronutrients....43
2.2. Digestion of Macronutrients....46
2.3. Absorption of Macronutrients....50
2.4. Production of Energy from Macronutrients....55
2.5. Role of Hormones in Macronutrient Metabolism....58
2.6. Factors Affecting Macronutrient Metabolism....62
Summary....68
References....70

Introduction

Macronutrient metabolism is the term that describes the biochemical processes through which the body extracts energy from macronutrients: fats, carbohydrates, and proteins. These nutrients are of paramount significance for the maintenance of physiological functions and homeostasis. The ability of the body to metabolize these macronutrients efficiently is of paramount significance for energy formation as well as for health in general. As it is with changing modern dietary patterns, particularly with increased intake of ultra-processed foods, an understanding of the importance of macronutrient metabolism has never been so important. The variations in digestion and absorption that come with each macronutrient demand a detailed appreciation of nutritional science, where the interconnectedness of diet and metabolic function comes into focus. More and more research points to the importance of diet quality as a determinant of health outcomes, particularly for chronic disease. It has been shown that high-fiber diets that are generally low in processed foods play a significant role in gut health and metabolic function. Fiber, predominantly from plant foods, not only aids digestion but is also essential for maintaining processes , such as insulin sensitivity and regulation of appetite. The history of a poor fiber diet among Western populations is alarming because such changes can potentially destabilize homeostasis as well as exacerbate several diseases. The intestinal microbiome is an essential part of this balance, tasked with mediating the beneficial properties of fiber in the diet as well as structuring the overall metabolic environment (Barber et al., 2020). Further investigation into the role of short-chain fatty acids (SCFAs) produced by the fermentation of fiber demonstrates their complex interplay with metabolic health. SCFAs not only serve as a source of cellular energy in the colon but also regulate systemic inflammation and immune response, connecting gut health to more general metabolic pathways. A lack of SCFAs has been associated with a myriad of disorders, ranging from inflammatory bowel conditions and cardiovascular illness (Fusco et al., 2023). As researchers delve further into the intersection of gut microbiota, diet, and metabolic health, it also becomes increasingly evident that balancing macronutrient intake, particularly fiber, contributes significantly toward better well-being. Therefore, an understanding of macronutrient metabolism supports the construction of public health interventions for the prevention of the unwanted effects of modern lifestyles and the promotion of well-being.

Definition of Macronutrients

The three broad categories of nutrients necessary for human health are referred to by the term macronutrient: proteins, carbohydrates, and fats. There is a particular but complementary function of all three macronutrients in metabolism and overall physiological processes. Proteins are necessary for tissue repair, growth, hormones and enzyme production. They provide amino acids that contain some that are nonessential but necessary to be provided through food. Carbohydrates are the body's main energy source, quickly metabolized into glucose to meet the energy demands of the moment, particularly for brain function and physical activity. Lastly, fats composed of triglycerides, fatty acids, and cholesterol facilitate nutrient assimilation and compact energy reservoir, essential for metabolic functions and brain functions. Thus, understanding the definition and roles of macronutrients is fundamental to understanding their metabolism and health and disease implications. The relationship between macronutrient intake and health status is particularly accentuated in specific populations, e.g., children and the elderly. For instance, adequate protein intake is imperative for growth and development in children since it is responsible for the maintenance of linear growth and muscle growth. Here, nutritional recommendations like the Acceptable Macronutrient Distribution Range (AMDR) are used to guide the ideal proportion of macronutrients in a child's diet. However, in the elderly, with the development of changes with aging in muscle mass and function impacting metabolism, the role of macronutrients becomes complicated. The aging process itself predisposes to insulin resistance and reduced energy expenditure, thereby altering the use of these macronutrients in the body. Imitation of such dynamics stresses the need for age-related dietary guidelines (Cameron et al., 2020). Additionally, the interaction between macronutrients and other diseases stresses their definition and metabolic significance. For instance, in Type 1 diabetes, regulation of carbohydrates is critical due to the correlation between carbohydrate consumption and blood sugar management. Yet, the contribution of proteins and fats in diets is also crucial, specifically in alleviating complications of the condition. Freeling (2024) point out that as carbohydrates contribute mostly to energy, proteins have a dual function in growth as well as energy supply, thus are specifically beneficial in managing growth patterns in children. Research has shown potential relationships between macronutrient distribution and health status, emphasizing the need for further research into the impact that eating habits have on metabolic efficiency. There is a requirement for a comprehensive understanding of macronutrients and macronutrient metabolism to develop proper nutritional regimes that foster health along the life cycle (Figure 2.1).

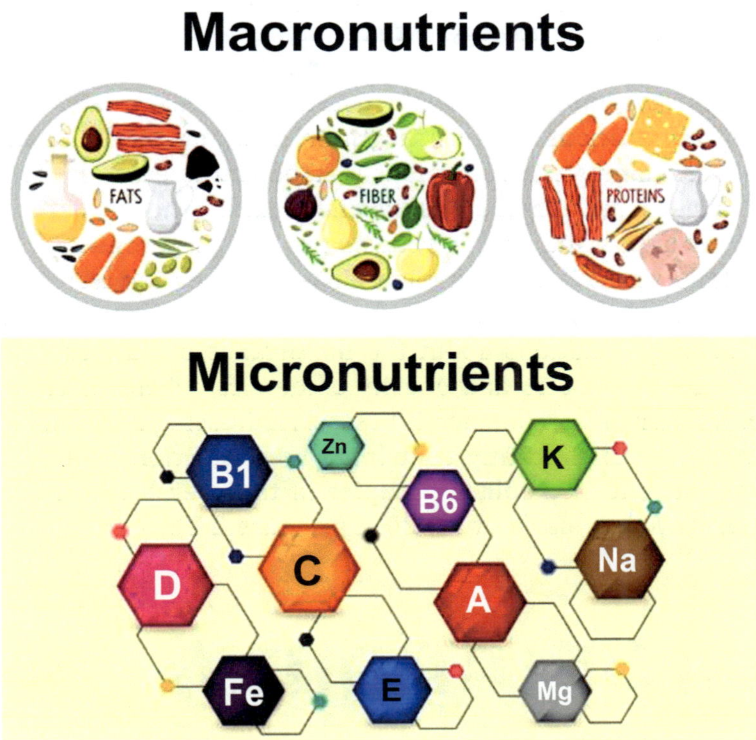

Figure 2.1. Comparison of essential macronutrients and micronutrients.

Source: https://external-Content.duckduckgo.com/iu/?u=https%3A%2F%2Fi.pinimg.com%2F736x%2F27%2F25%2F9e%2F27259edec59e56821321483794d5ae9e.jpg&f=1&nofb=1&ipt=1aedcece3e2307fe6a542d04cba836a4b63adece450f4d458ec1529cf4718fdd.

Importance of Macronutrient Metabolism

Understanding macronutrient metabolism is key to appreciating how the human body utilizes and processes essential nutrients into energy and building materials for cellular processes. Macronutrients are significant energy sources that provide the energy needed for different physiological processes, including growth, repair, and maintenance of tissues. Each of these macronutrients plays a specific role; carbohydrates merely provide quick energy, fats offer compact energy, and proteins are involved in cellular architecture and enzyme function. The interdependence of these metabolic processes indicates how the body relies on balanced assimilation to perform at optimal levels. Dysregulation or deficiency in the metabolism of any of these macronutrients can lead to a range of health issues; thus, the need for an all-around understanding of how these nutrients influence overall metabolic health and disease prevention, particularly in the backdrop of growing obesity and related diseases in the population (María et al., 2021). Furthermore, macronutrient metabolism is not a singular occurrence but is interwoven with a number of biological systems, including hormonal regulation and gut bacteria. Insulin and glucagon are hormones that regulate the balance between nutrient use and storage and their regulation impacts how the body will react to varying caloric consumption and exercise levels. Moreover, recent studies suggest the role of gut microbiota in dietary fiber and other complex carbohydrate metabolism to yield short-chain fatty acids that contribute to energy metabolism and gut health. Such interaction also shows the complex networks within human physiology, with the ability to promote or impair metabolic health. Accurate macronutrient metabolism is thus essential not just to energy production but also to the control of metabolic pathways important to homeostasis maintenance and prevention of metabolic disorders, with strong implications for nutritional science and public health (Lai et al., 2021). Last but not least, understanding macronutrient metabolism is essential for formulating dietary advice and therapeutic measures aimed at maximizing health benefits. Through comprehension of the distinct metabolic pathways and energy returns for every macronutrient, health professionals can more accurately tailor dietary recommendations—whether for weight, sports performance, or disease recovery. With the world trend moving toward processed food, there is a concerted effort required to educate populations about the importance of nutrient quality and balance. It is particularly in the case of diabetes and obesity epidemics, where macronutrient imbalance in food intake is the central driver behind such illnesses. Addressing such dietary problems through evidence-based methods can significantly contribute to population well-being, underscoring the critical position macronutrient metabolism occupies in the overall framework of nutritional and health promotion interventions (María et al., 2021) (Figure 2.2).

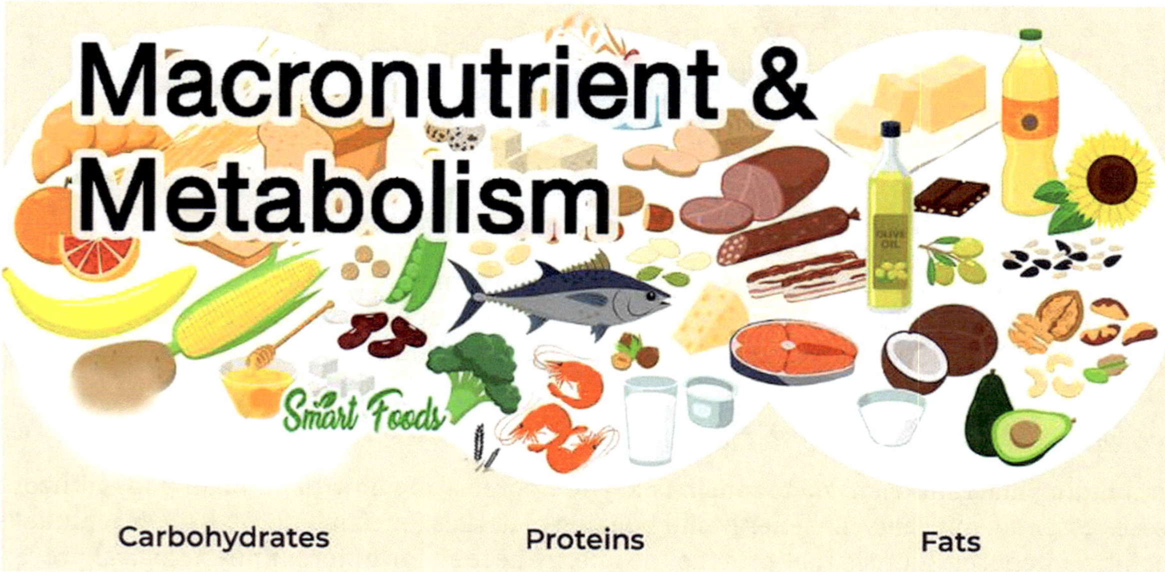

Figure 2.2. Sources of macronutrients are essential for metabolism.

Source: https://external-content.duckduckgo.com/iu/?u=https%3A%2F%2Fstatic.wixstatic.com%2Fmedia%2F25f9a1_7895cdb8d00e4e0c95de0e7b887068be~mv2.jpg%2Fv1%2Ffill%2Fw_1000%2Ch_500%2Cal_c%2Cq_85%2Cusm_0.66_1.00_0.01%2F25f9a1_7895cdb8d00e4e0c95de0e7b887068be~mv2.jpg&f=1&nofb=1&ipt=97ce9e838af7ce46bd3feaa3c0e556d72fc286e8b889823e278ad88eaac413ae.

2.1. Types of Macronutrients

Understanding the types of macronutrients is critical for their function in health and metabolic disease. Macronutrients are classified into three categories: carbohydrates, proteins, and fats, all playing different physiological functions. The body uses carbohydrates as the primary source of energy, readily broken down to glucose through metabolic processes. Rapid breakdown provides instant energy, most beneficial in exercising, to provide immediate energy. However, the type and quantity of carbohydrates consumed can also profoundly influence metabolic processes, as overconsumption, particularly of simple carbohydrates like fructose, can lead to pathological conditions , such as insulin resistance and fatty liver disease. This kind of metabolic disturbance raises the issue of carbohydrate control in diets, as an understanding of macronutrient composition is required for optimizing health. Proteins, consisting of amino acids, play numerous essential roles beyond the provision of energy, including cell repair, immune function, and hormone production. Consuming quality protein sources can enhance satiety and preserve muscle synthesis, thereby contributing to the regulation of body composition. Postprandial responses, , such as gastrointestinal hormone secretion following protein intake, may modulate metabolism through the control of hunger and satiety (Klementov et al., 2019). The relative amino acid intake also comes into play; certain of the essential amino acids were discovered to be particularly beneficial to muscle accretion and metabolic well-being. With the growing popularity of plant-based diets, it is important to contrast different sources of protein, as bioavailability and biological value can dramatically affect metabolic impact. Fats, commonly assumed to be unhealthy, are a part of a healthy diet, essential for hormone production, nutrient absorption, and the construction of cells. Saturated, unsaturated, and trans fats need to be distinguished because each has differing effects on health. Unsaturated fats, found in foods like avocados and nuts, are positive for cardiovascular health, while trans fats are associated with an increased risk of chronic illness (Gutierrez et al., 2021). Metabolism of fat also involves a complex interplay with carbohydrate metabolism, particularly in energy storage and equilibrium. Recent evidence has clarified the role of macronutrient content, including fat amount and type, in the control of metabolic markers like insulin sensitivity and liver fat content. Such evidence supports the necessity of composite evaluation of diet with a focus on macronutrient types to ensure optimal health outcomes (Figure 2.3).

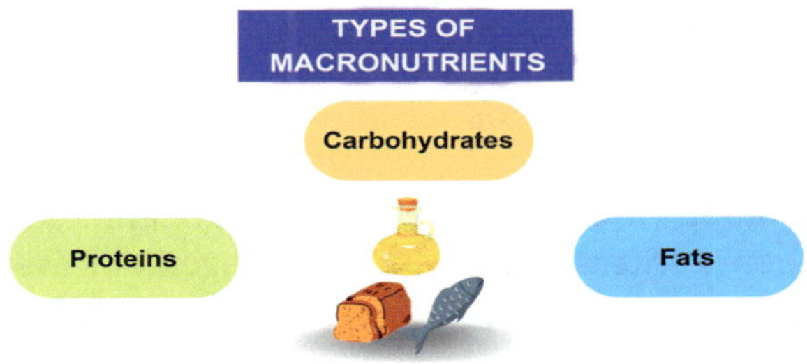

Figure 2.3. Types of macronutrients: Carbohydrates, proteins, and fats.

Source: https://external-content.duckduckgo.com/iu/?u=https%3A%2F%2Fimages.examples.com%2Fwp-content%2Fuploads%2F2024%2F04%2FTypes-of-Macronutrients.png&f=1&nofb=1&ipt=b1fecaa795f8d35b8158a2daba4581f4eac6cd9a682d9feff367625ff434c96f.

2.1.1. Carbohydrates

Carbohydrates are a macronutrient of great importance with a primary role in energy metabolism and overall body processes. Made up of simple sugars, complex carbohydrates, and fiber, the molecules are primarily utilized by the body as a source of fuel to power cellular functions and maintain metabolic homeostasis.

Carbohydrates are broken down by the digestive system to convert to glucose, which is absorbed in the bloodstream and distributed to cells. This is a process that highlights the significance of carbohydrates as energy sources and regulators of blood sugar levels. Excess, and particularly in the form of processed sugars, carbohydrates lead to metabolic derangements like insulin resistance and obesity. This leads to the significance of carbohydrate discrimination in dietary counseling in order to optimize health and avoid unwanted metabolic consequences. The metabolic consequences of carbohydrate consumption have been a focus of great interest, particularly with growing concerns over the impact of fluctuation. The emerging evidence is that excessive consumption of fructose is linked with insulin resistance, DNL, and hepatic steatosis, which may further result in severe health outcomes , such as type 2 diabetes and non-alcoholic fatty liver disease. Specifically, studies with a ketohexokinase (KHK) inhibitor have demonstrated that disruption of fructose metabolism can repress hyperinsulinemia and other markers of metabolic derangement even when subjects are fed diets comparable to typical American diets. These findings point to the potentially pathogenic nature of fructose metabolism, not simply due to excess calories, but due to the metabolic activation inherent in fructose per se. Hence, the new evidence proves that there is a need to reassess carbohydrate sources in diet advice. Furthermore, the collaboration of micronutrients and carbohydrate metabolism is one area of increasing relevance. While macronutrient research will most often overshadow research on micronutrients, new research indicates that minerals and vitamins are also important in optimizing metabolic processes related to carbohydrates. For instance, certain B-vitamins have been shown to influence gene and epigenetic control of lipid metabolism, which overlaps with carbohydrate metabolism via shared metabolic pathways. When consumed in conjunction with plant diets, appropriate quantities of these micronutrients can maximize metabolic function, perhaps preventing some ill effects of excessive carbohydrate intake. Such a practice that harmonizes macronutrients and micronutrients may therefore help address the issues associated with modern dietary practices and their influence on metabolic health (Saito et al., 2020; Gutierrez et al., 2021) (Figure 2.4).

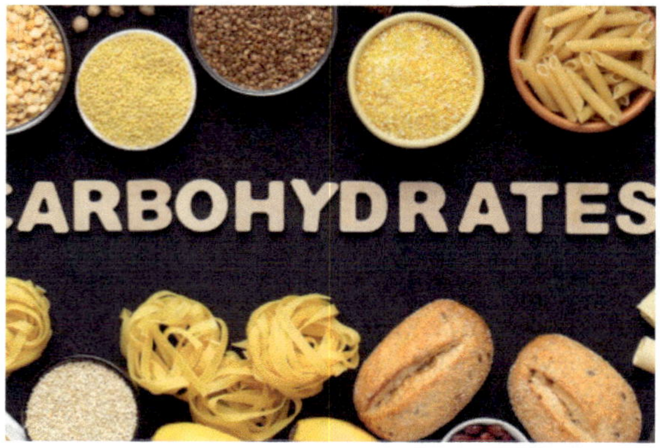

Figure 2.4. Common dietary sources of carbohydrates.

Source: https://external-content.duckduckgo.com/iu/?u=https%3A%2F%2Fwww.kaizo-health.com%2Fwp-content%2Fuploads%2F2020%2F09%2FCarbohydrate-Blog-scaled.jpeg&f=1&nofb=1&ipt=ce0ed26f8ab2c5367524ddefc441f2164b3d098912113d8333e8684ab016104d.

2.1.2. Proteins

Proteins are essential macromolecules with essential roles in cell structure, function, and signaling. Composed of amino acids, proteins are involved in numerous biological processes , such as catalyzing metabolic reactions such as enzymes, immune response, and molecular transport. Proteins contribute to muscle mass, tissue repair, and the synthesis of hormones and enzymes utilized in the regulation of metabolism. The variability in proteins makes them participate in specialized functions based on the needs of different tissues and organs, indicating their importance in achieving homeostasis in the body. Moreover, variation in protein intake can influence metabolic processes, hence further emphasize the role of such macronutrients in overall health and nutrition. As far as macronutrient metabolism is concerned, the role of autophagy is particularly important when autophagy is considered with reference to protein degradation and turnover. Autophagy is a cellular mechanism that ensures the removal of faulty proteins and organelles, utilizing their contents for energy or as precursors necessary for new protein synthesis. In nutrient starvation, such a role is indispensable, where the body utilizes autophagic breakdown to sustain metabolism by mobilizing intracellular resources to provide the necessary energy. For instance, studies indicate that autophagy significantly contributes to metabolic processes, pointing out protein metabolism-autophagy interdependency.

The interdependency points to the necessity of equilibrium in protein intake to realize balance between synthesis and breakdown, thereby achieving overall efficiency of the metabolic process and cellular health (Magen et al., 2022). Further, protein metabolism is known to cover the malnutrition effects on muscle growth, particularly among individuals suffering from conditions , such as cirrhosis. In such a case, protein malnutrition can lead to complications like frailty and sarcopenia, where the muscle strength and mass are depleted by the body, and its health is jeopardized. Research describes complex interplays between various proteins, essential amino acids, and the body's ability to sustain muscle function, particularly when it has a chronic illness. Healthy consumption of protein is critical for these individuals to recover from muscle loss and provide the substrates needed for energy metabolism and tissue repair. Because protein metabolism incorporates both dietary intake as well as protein turnover dynamics, deficiencies need to be corrected for optimal health benefits in population groups with the metabolic effects of various diseases (Lai et al., 2021).

2.1.3. Fats

The function of fats in macronutrient metabolism cannot be overstated because they play very important roles in the supply of energy, nutrient absorption, and cell development. Fats are largely composed of triglycerides, and these are the body's most concentrated source of energy, with over nine calories per gram compared to carbohydrates and proteins that provide four calories per gram. Besides, fats enable the incorporation of fat-soluble vitamins (A, D, E, and K) essential to many physiological functions, including vision, bone development, and immunity. In spite of this, the balance of fats in the diet is crucial as excessive consumption, particularly saturated and trans fats, can lead to undesirable health conditions, including hypertriglyceridemia and cardiovascular diseases. Thus, identifying the role of dietary fats in metabolic processes is important to achieve optimal health and prevent chronic illnesses (Luna-Castillo et al., 2022). Metabolic processes involved in fat include several procedures, including lipolysis, β-oxidation, and ketogenesis, which play a key role in ensuring energy homeostasis. Lipolysis involves the hydrolysis of triglycerides into glycerol and free fatty acids, which then proceed into the Krebs cycle to generate ATP. In states of low carbohydrate availability, , such as fasting or endurance exercise, fatty acids are shunted into ketone bodies through ketogenesis to serve as a fuel for other tissues, including the brain. Surprisingly, dietary lifestyle has been discovered to have a significant impact on these metabolic processes. The Mediterranean diet, with emphasis on the healthy fats of olive oil and nuts, has been associated with improved lipid profiles and reduced metabolic syndrome risk. This kind of diet emphasizes the effect of fat quantity and quality on metabolic status in general (Smith and Betts, 2022). Current research has also suggested that macronutrient timing plays a crucial role in fat metabolism. The period of fat intake might influence metabolic adaptation and subsequent energy expenditure throughout the day. For instance, the consumption of higher-fat meals in the morning can enhance the body's ability to oxidize fat in the latter part of the day and thereby improve the body's energy balance. Conversely, late-night consumption of fats has been implicated in metabolic process of dysregulation and obesity, showing that food synchronization with the circadian rhythms is critical for optimal metabolic function. Thus, dietary advice must consider not only the amount and quality of macronutrients but also the timing of their consumption. Last but not least, this multifaceted strategy of macronutrient metabolism can enable more effective approaches to weight management and prevention of related diseases (Smith and Betts, 2022).

2.2. Digestion of Macronutrients

Macronutrient digestion, carbohydrate, proteins, and fat, commences within the oral cavity and is carried on by a sequence of processes in the gastrointestinal tract. Salivary enzymes like amylase begin the breakdown of carbohydrates, and food mechanical processing is offered by mastication. Upon the attainment of acidic conditions in the stomach, pepsin activation is achieved, an enzyme that is essential for protein digestion. The environment also acts as a significant contributor to triggering lipid emulsification, enhancing lipid and enzyme contact. It is finished in the small intestine, where the majority of macronutrient digestion and absorption occur. Pancreatic enzymes there continue to hydrolyze carbohydrates into monosaccharides, proteins into amino acids, and fats into fatty acids and glycerol, mirroring the complex interaction between mechanical and chemical digestion as food is transported through the digestive tract. The microbial population of the gastrointestinal tract contributes substantially to macronutrient digestion and absorption, particularly in the small intestine.

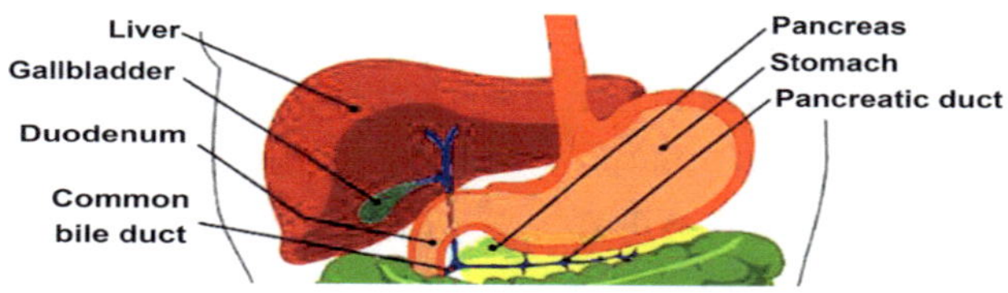

Figure 2.5. Labeled diagram of digestive organs involved in nutrient processing.

Source: https://external-content.duckduckgo.com/iu/?u=https%3A%2F%2Fopen.oregonstate.education%2Fapp%2Fuploads%2Fsites%2F51%2F2019%2F08%2F3_413.png&f=1&nofb=1&ipt=683e559974d26a761e51e95a8dca2a25e5622dcf3ab5d3733877c892a0afccef.

The activity and presence of some gut bacteria enable carbohydrate fermentation and facilitate the metabolism of lipid and protein substrates. The interactions enhance the bioavailability of nutrients by breaking down complex structures that human enzymes would otherwise be incapable of processing. Of special note is the *Lachnospiraceae* family of colonic microbes that has been shown to play a major role in the production of short-chain fatty acids (SCFAs) from fibers in the diet through fermentation, which serve not only as substrates for energy for colon cells but also control many hosts' metabolic functions (Vacca et al., 2020). Dynamic composition and function of the gut microbiota thus emphasize microbial inputs to efficient macronutrient metabolism. Further, the metabolism of macronutrients has a significant effect on health conditions. Furthermore, fat digestion is another clear example of how macronutrient metabolism affects health. Lipid emulsification in the duodenum by bile salts increases the action of pancreatic lipase, with effective hydrolysis of fats to fatty acids and monoglycerides (Kastl et al., 2019). The molecules then come together to create micelles that help them be transported through the intestinal epithelium to the lymphatic system prior to circulation in the blood. Whereas they are utilized for energy generation or storage when they arrive at tissues. Gut dysbiosis, which is a disruption in gut microbiota, can impair lipid metabolism and lead to systemic disorders , such as obesity and metabolic syndrome. Therefore, it is necessary to know the complex mechanisms related to macronutrient digestion in nutrition and health promotion (Figure 2.5).

2.2.1. Process of Carbohydrate Digestion

Carbohydrate digestion starts in the mouth, where the enzymatic breakdown begins to break down polysaccharides begin. Saliva has the enzyme amylase, which breaks starch to maltose and dextrin. This is the first step, and it is important because it not only gets carbohydrates ready for the rest of their digestion in the gastrointestinal tract but also makes the energy release more efficient. As the bolus of food is propelled by peristalsis down the esophagus into the stomach, the acidic pH inhibits the activity of amylase, suspending carbohydrate digestion.

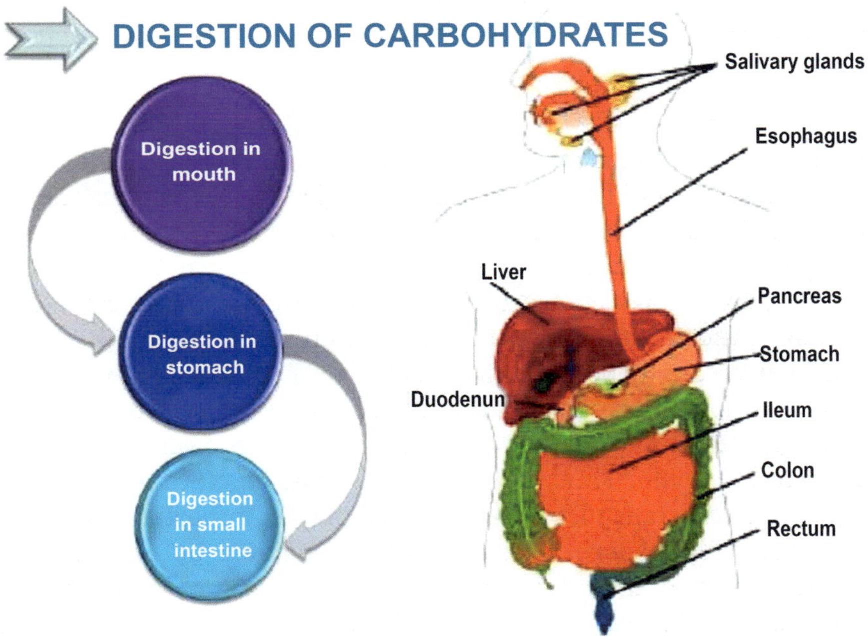

Figure 2.6. Steps and organs are involved in carbohydrate digestion.

Source: https://external-content.duckduckgo.com/iu/?u=https%3A%2F%2F2.bp.blogspot.com%2F-C_PD14gh1gA%2FVhxBkFbsJDI%2FAAAAAAAAjuw%2FNU2KQAJrllk%2Fs1600%2Fdigestion-absorption-of-carbohydrates.jpg&f=1&nofb=1&ipt=61f557d34896d1ecf884636b2f4f0a9c376b758886ddd59d8057cde2f4aba1c4.

This dynamic interplay between mechanical and enzymatic activity mirrors the exquisite choreography of carbohydrate digestion, the necessity for which emphasizes both the salivary enzymes and the digestive secretions in successful carbohydrate assimilation as macronutrients. On arriving in the small intestine, the pieces of the complex carbohydrate are acted upon by further enzymatic digestion. The pancreas also releases other enzymes , such as pancreatic amylase, which further split the polysaccharides to form disaccharides. Brush border enzymes present on the microvilli of the intestinal lining, , such as maltase, sucrase, and lactase, complete the process by converting the disaccharides to monosaccharides. This process enables glucose, galactose, and fructose to be pumped efficiently into the bloodstream via specific transporters. The rapid absorption of such small sugars is important because they are the principal energy fuel for cellular metabolism, thereby underscoring the importance of effective carbohydrate digestion in overall metabolic health. Following absorption, the monosaccharides join the hepatic portal circulation, directing them to the liver for further metabolism. The liver also plays a regulatory role where it converts fructose and galactose to glucose, and this is important in maintaining the level of blood glucose constantly. This glucose may be stored as glycogen or released into the bloodstream for the use of energy directly or stored in the adipose tissues and muscles. In addition, their impact on the gut microbiota, e.g., the *Lachnospiraceae* family, has been reported as a consequence of their production of short-chain fatty acids, which can influence host physiology and disease. Consequently, it logically follows that the complexity of carbohydrate digestion is not merely significant in relation to individual nutrient absorption but also pertains to large-scale metabolic impact, extending to include the interconnectedness of dietary components and overall well-being, as suggested in Vacca et al. (2020) (Figure 2.6).

2.2.2. Process of Protein Digestion

Protein digestion begins in the stomach, where an acidic pH facilitates the denaturation of protein structures and the exposure of peptide bonds to enzymatic cleavage. Pepsin, an acid-activated enzyme, plays a key role in cleaving large protein molecules into smaller peptide fragments. Digestion is required because it generates substrates that are further degradable in the small intestine. Once the chyme passes into the duodenum, it is buffered by pancreatic bicarbonate, which creates optimal conditions for the pancreatic enzymes, trypsin and chymotrypsin, to continue protein breakdown. The sequence of enzymes breaks up peptides into smaller forms, which are predominantly dipeptides and tripeptides, available for uptake in the enterocytes lining the intestinal wall. While digestion of proteins goes on, the resulting peptides are broken down into amino acids by brush border enzymes on enterocyte microvilli. Transport of these smaller molecules into the bloodstream is facilitated by many amino acid transport systems, which play an important role in the overall amino acid homeostasis in the body. Absorption efficiency is promoted by short-chain fatty acids, the products of carbohydrate fermentation by the gut microbiome, highlighting the inter-relationship of macronutrient metabolism. Further, the gut microflora composition, particularly *Lachnospiraceae* members, could influence protein digestion processes by regulating the intestinal environment and allowing beneficial metabolites and nutrients for absorption that can enhance protein utilization and well-being overall (Vacca et al., 2020). The interaction between protein digestion and gut microbiota illustrates the complex relationship between health and diet. Microbiome breaks down unabsorbed proteins and creates metabolites , such as ammonia and branched-chain fatty acids that have both beneficial and potentially deleterious impacts, which change with their concentration and environment in the gastrointestinal tract (Oliphant et al., 2019). Such interactive association underscores the need for a balanced diet in order to promote a healthy microbiome, which also regulates various metabolic functions. Understanding these processes reveals fundamental insights into how protein metabolism affects human health, particularly in the setting of various disease states related to protein malabsorption or abnormal gut microbiota composition. This knowledge is essential in the design of dietary strategies aimed at optimizing macronutrient metabolism and enhancing well-being (Figure 2.7).

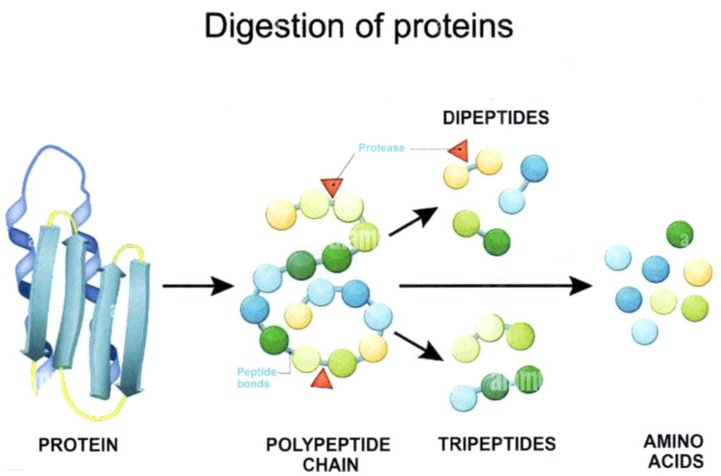

Figure 2.7. Enzymatic breakdown of proteins into amino acids.

Source: https://external-content.duckduckgo.com/iu/?u=https%3A%2F%2Fc8.alamy.com%2Fcomp%2F2GD6J2H%2Fprotein-digestion-enzymes-proteases-and-peptidases-are-digestion-breaks-the-protein-into-smaller-peptide-chains-and-into-single-amino-acids-2GD6J2H.jpg&f=1&nofb=1&ipt=62b129c8fa85bffc4b7adfe3ef377b2aa785af13e8f6a9571150ae87a5ab095a.

2.2.3. Process of Fat Digestion

The breakdown of fat, or lipids, is far more complex than carbohydrates or protein. The process initially starts in the stomach and mouth with the mechanical breakdown, and enzymes , such as lingual lipase, begin to degrade the triglycerides. This early stage, however, is short-lived, and the majority of the breakdown of fat takes place in the small intestine. Emulsification by the bile salts secreted by the liver here breaks big fat globules into small droplets and augments the surface for enzymatic action. Pancreatic lipase then hydrolyzes emulsified fats to monoglycerides and free fatty acids that become absorbable via the mucosa of the intestine. The process is a demonstration of how complex lipid metabolism is, which provides not only energy but also essential functions for cell structure and signaling. When monoglycerides and fatty acids are absorbed, they are reformed as triglycerides within enterocytes, which are intestinal lining cells. It plays a key role in the formation of chylomicrons, which are lipoprotein particles that transport dietary lipids from the intestines to other organs. By entering lymphatic circulation before entering the circulation, chylomicrons very effectively deliver fats into the body, where they can be utilized as energy, stored in adipose tissue, or utilized in various metabolic activities. Fat absorption can be influenced by a variety of dietary factors and physiological conditions, , such as the age of the subject, initiating the need to adjust diet to optimize lipid utilization. As is demonstrated through research, the young birds have fat utilization limits, demonstrating the specific dietary strategies necessary for lipid digestion and absorption improvement, in particular, the potential benefits of emulsifiers (Oketch et al., 2023). The outcomes of fat digestion extend beyond simple energy provision; they also play a critical role in gut health regulation and modulation of the population of microbiota. Short-chain fatty acids (SCFAs), produced by the fermentation of unabsorbed lipids by bacteria in the gut, have been shown to have a significant impact on host physiology. As an example, *Lachnospiraceae* family bacteria are major producers of SCFAs, influencing improved gut health and other physiological functions. Not surprisingly, microbiota welfare can be influenced by dietary fat consumed, a finding that underscores the interaction between macronutrient metabolism and optimal health. The lipid consumption vs. gut microbial equilibrium encourages enhanced understanding and potential food-based changes aiming to leverage these correlations to encourage enhanced health outcomes (Vacca et al., 2020) (Figure 2.8).

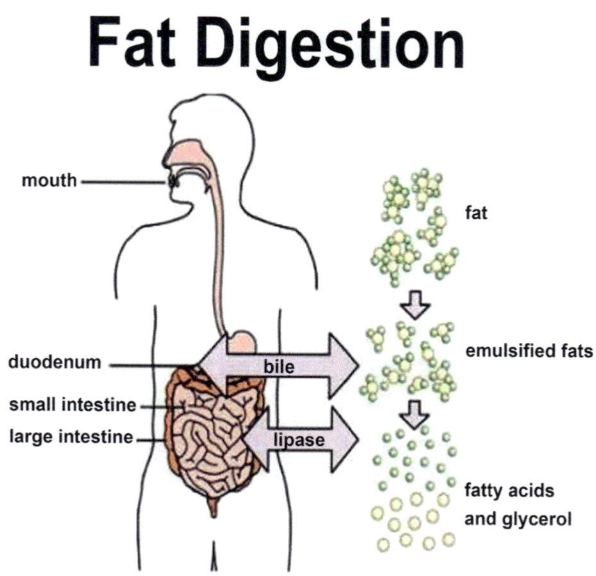

Figure 2.8. The process of fat digestion and absorption in the body.

Source: https://external-content.duckduckgo.com/iu/?u=https%3A%2F%2Fimage1.slideserve.com%2F2271785%2Ffat-digestion-l.jpg&f=1&nofb=1&ipt=27246e45f116b59847bf509acfdb4f955b3adcef31b1af4e244cb3179a18b83e.

2.3. Absorption of Macronutrients

The process of absorption of macronutrients is a key part of macronutrient metabolism, and it has important considerations for overall health and function. Macronutrients like carbohydrates, proteins, and lipids are digested before they get absorbed into the bloodstream. Carbohydrates are broken down to simple sugars, proteins to amino acids, and lipids to fatty acids and glycerol in the gastrointestinal tract. The efficiency of such an absorption process relies on several factors varying from food matrix to enzyme availability as well as the presence of co-factors , such as bile salts. Dysfunction in these processes of absorption leads to deficiencies and metabolic conditions and, accordingly, the importance of understanding macronutrient absorption within a bigger perspective of metabolic health (Gonzalez, 2022). Discoveries about mechanisms of absorption reveal pathways that are potentially targeted to maximize nutrient bioavailability with the ultimate aim of designing dietary strategies for enhancing health benefits and performance. Timing of nutrient intake has also emerged as an element of importance in macronutrient absorption, with research suggesting that metabolic responses may differ significantly depending on the time of consuming food. Glucose and triacylglycerol profiles, for example, show higher postprandial increases in the evening after rather than at morning intake. This phenomenon is likely a result of dynamic changes in hormone secretion throughout the day, like insulin release and sensitivity (Gonzalez, 2022). Appreciation of these circadian fluctuations in metabolism is necessary to optimally apply dietary strategies, particularly in individuals interested in weight management or improved sport performance. New findings on nutrient timing show that the manipulation of the timing of macronutrient intake enhances metabolic efficiency and appetite regulation, and these subsequently can contribute to better health and the prevention of diet-associated chronic diseases. Moreover, the role of some foods in influencing macronutrient uptake cannot be ruled out. For instance, the macronutrient content of a meal, , such as the ratio of fats, proteins, and carbohydrates, affects the secretion of gastrointestinal hormones, which in turn regulate the process of absorption. Some patterns of dietary intake, , such as those that emphasize better quality carbohydrates and healthful fats, have been reported to support enhanced nutrient uptake and utilization, and thus better metabolic well-being. In addition, components of diet , such as fiber content, can influence the macronutrient absorption dynamics. High-fiber diets have been found to be associated with retarded rates of absorption and digestion, resulting in more stable postprandial glycemia. These findings emphasize the crucial role of macronutrient quality and food composition in regulating effective absorption channels, ultimately leading to the optimization of global nutrition status and health (Figure 2.9).

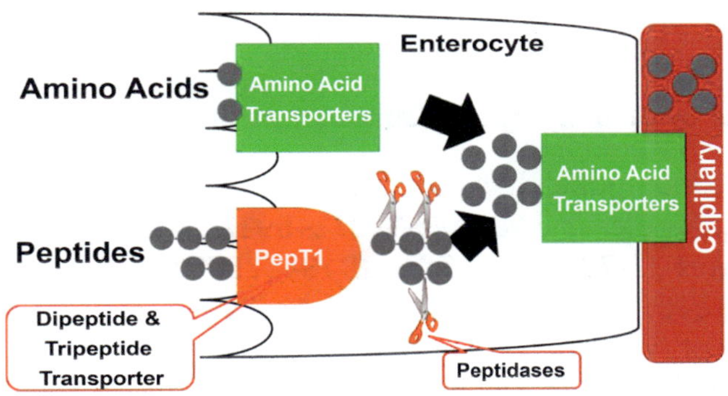

Figure 2.9. Peptide and amino acid absorption in the small intestine.

Source: Source: https://s3-us-west-2.amazonaws.com/courses-images/wp-content/uploads/sites/2569/2017/10/23201915/100000000000046F000002693CA157FD.png

2.3.1. Mechanisms of Carbohydrate Absorption

Absorption of carbohydrates plays a significant role in macronutrient metabolism since it determines the rate at which sugars and glucose are absorbed into the bloodstream. Carbohydrate digestion first occurs in the mouth, where salivary amylase starts digesting the polysaccharides into digested sugars. The site of primary carbohydrate absorption, however, is in the small intestine. Here, enzymes , such as maltase, isomaltose, and sucrase finish disaccharide digestion to monosaccharides, primarily glucose, fructose, and galactose. These monosaccharides are transported across the intestinal epithelium into the bloodstream actively. The regulation of the numerous transport systems indicates the complexity of the process; sodium-glucose co-transporters are utilized for glucose absorption, while fructose is absorbed by facilitated diffusion. This is done by the GLUT5 transporter.

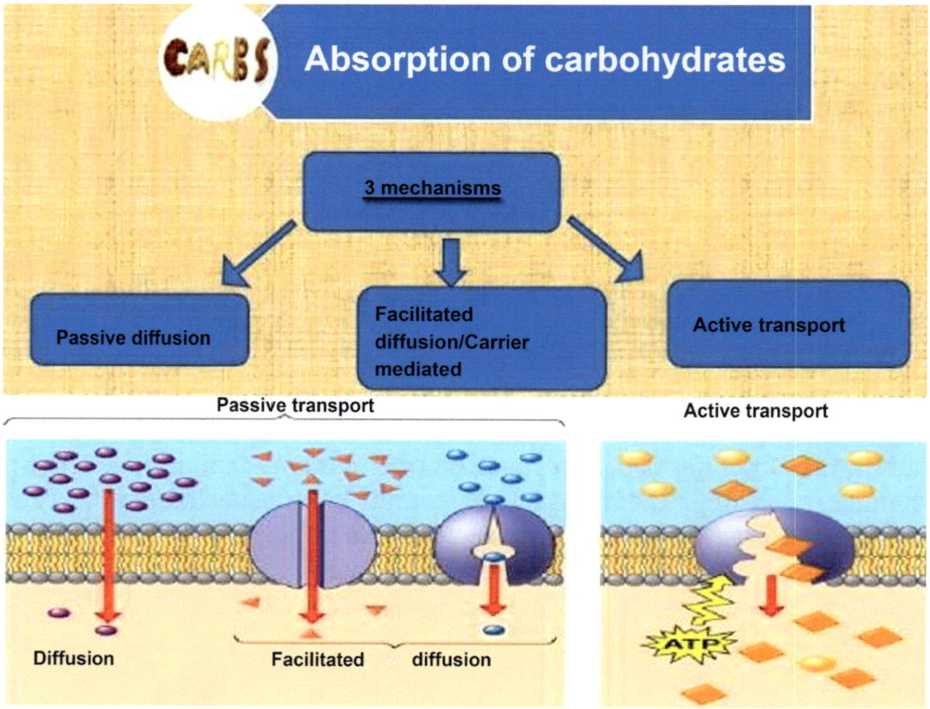

Figure 2.10. Mechanisms of carbohydrate absorption in the intestine.

Source: https://external-content.duckduckgo.com/iu/?u=http%3A%2F%2Fimage.slidesharecdn.com%2Fdigestionandabsorptionofcarbohydrates-120714091201-phpapp01%2F95%2Fdigestion-and-absorption-of-carbohydrates-32-728.jpg%3Fcb%3D1342257320&f=1&nofb=1&ipt=cf286d17414a9f64861d37c05a0f115fe84e408ac3c67118df5043c2fd1ce363.

Control of these transporters is of paramount importance since they can adapt to dietary changes and regulate overall glucose homeostasis. Monosaccharides, upon absorption, undergo a series of metabolic processes necessary for energy production and homeostasis. The liver is the site where fructose and galactose are converted into glucose via gluconeogenesis or glycogen synthesis. In addition, glucose can be utilized for immediate energy needs, being stored within muscle and liver glycogen, or transported into the circulatory system to maintain the level of glucose. The correlation between the digestion of carbohydrates and metabolism in general is also bolstered by the function played by microbiota to reinforce such processes. The gut microbiota members, , such as those of the *Lachnospiraceae* family, have been reported to produce short-chain fatty acids (SCFAs) as a result of the fermentation of dietary fiber, further influencing the physiology and metabolism of the host by regulating carbohydrate absorption and metabolism (Vacca et al.,

2020). The complex relationship between gut microbiota and carbohydrate absorption also displays how food composition is essential in ensuring metabolic health. Evidence brings to light that the presence of certain fibers can enhance microbial richness and enable the production of health-beneficial SCFAs, which have been associated with several impacts on health, including enhanced insulin sensitivity and reduced inflammation (Silva et al., 2020). Such metabolic interactions indicate how food choice may directly affect carbohydrate absorption efficacy and overall well-being. Therefore, understanding the mechanisms of carbohydrate absorption is paramount to the development of nutritional strategies that optimize metabolic health. As science continues to uncover the many ways diet and gut microbiota interface, it is becoming ever more evident that facilitating a well-balanced microbiome can be essential in managing carbohydrate metabolism in an optimal manner (Figure 2.10).

2.3.2. Mechanisms of Protein Absorption

The physiological mechanisms of protein absorption lie at the heart of macronutrient metabolism and are crucially important in human health. The basis of protein absorption lies in the mechanism of digestion that begins in the stomach, where proteins are denatured by gastric juices and broken down into smaller polypeptides. These polypeptides are then transported to the small intestine, where they are further hydrolyzed by pancreatic enzymes , such as chymotrypsin and trypsin into free amino acids and smaller peptides.

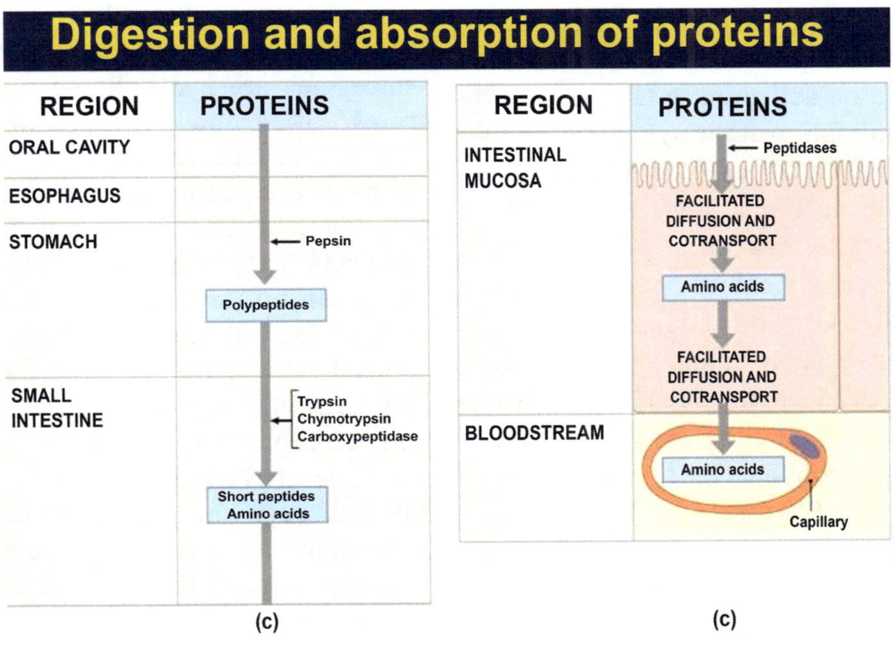

Figure 2.11. Digestion and absorption of dietary proteins.

Source: https://external-content.duckduckgo.com/iu/?u=https%3A%2F%2Fcf.ppt-online.org%2Ffiles%2Fslide%2Fw%2FwDr7OMEvlS3oyjcpH2zqhtR94JgGLaUsN6idTC%2Fslide-51.jpg&f=1&nofb=1&ipt=2426623d76b6c84b9d4bbe45e00e82c9f324f3d2bf13175cd37538f60d377bf0.

Specific transport mechanisms in the intestinal epithelial cells absorb these amino acids and small peptides. Notably, absorption occurs by both facilitated diffusion and active transport, the latter of which typically relies on sodium gradients to help shuttle amino acids across the cell membrane. This alteration is important, as it not only supplies protein-synthesizing building blocks but also influences overall metabolic pathways within the body. Following the initial absorption into the enterocytes, amino acids and peptides meet with an intracellular medium, on which their fate is determined. In the enterocytes, amino acids can be used for cellular functions, for instance, energy production or synthesis of new proteins for cellular repair and development. The majority, however, are moved still deeper into the bloodstream by a second transporter set that translocate the amino acids out of the enterocytes across the basolateral membrane. Their transport throughout the body is necessary so that they will be delivered to tissues where they are needed for protein synthesis or as precursors to other such necessary compounds. It is pertinent to note that some conditions, , such as cystic fibrosis, break these processes due to impaired pancreatic enzyme secretion, and this leads to malabsorption and insufficiency of nutrients that are capable of improving existing health status (Bass et al., 2021). Moreover, various factors can modulate the effectiveness and processes of protein uptake, , such as diet nature, state of health, and age. For instance, the presence of some amino acids may influence transport activity, enhancing the efficiency of absorption. The role of gut microbiota also takes center stage as a relevant factor, particularly in how it influences dietary protein metabolism, with a likely leaning towards differences in efficacy of absorption. These intricacies are highlighted in certain states of health , such as liver disease, wherein altered metabolism can disrupt efficient utilization and absorption of nutrients (Lai et al., 2021). Understanding these sophisticated mechanisms is critical in developing strategies to treat malnutrition and achieve the highest possible health outcomes, particularly in individuals whose absorption ability is compromised or have elevated protein needs (Figure 2.11).

2.3.3. Mechanisms of Fat Absorption

Absorption of fat is a critical process in macronutrient metabolism, which occurs mainly in the small intestine. When dietary fat is emulsified by bile salts in the duodenum, it is broken down into micelles, enabling the lipids to be moved over to the intestinal mucosa. The process is crucial because it increases the surface area of fat, making it vulnerable to enzymatic action. Pancreatic lipase then hydrolyzes triglycerides into monoglycerides and free fatty acids, which are more capable of passing through the enterocyte membranes since they are hydrophobic. Triglycerides are re-esterified and packaged in chylomicrons, lipoprotein particles that transport dietary lipids through the lymphatic vessels before entering the bloodstream. The complex process of fat absorption aptly illustrates how well the human body can utilize lipids from diet as energy, as well as for cell functions. Chylomicrons play a crucial role in transporting absorbed fats to the body. Lipoproteins are synthesized within the endoplasmic reticulum of enterocytes and are afterwards secreted into the lymph fluid through the process of exocytosis. Once chylomicrons enter the bloodstream after passing through the thoracic duct, they enter various tissues like muscle and adipose tissues. Here, the enzyme lipoprotein lipase, which is stimulated by apolipoprotein C-II, is used for the hydrolysis of triglycerides. During this process, free fatty acids are released. Free fatty acids may be oxidized to generate energy or stored for future purposes. The roles of these complexes underscore the complex interaction of metabolism, as they not only deliver essential nutrients but also regulate energy homeostasis in the body. Interruptions of chylomicron metabolism or fat absorption thus result in various metabolic disorders, underscoring the significance of these processes in health. Gut microbiota and dietary fat interaction also significantly contribute to fat absorption and metabolism. Recent studies have demonstrated that the composition of intestinal microbiota can affect the efficiency of fat digestion and absorption, which is critical in maintaining energy balance. Some bacterial populations can enhance the metabolism of dietary fats and, therefore, impact the bioavailability of fatty acids and enterocyte uptake. Moreover, a well-balanced gut microbiome will have an impact on fat-soluble vitamin absorption, an important function in many physiological processes. These interactions need to be viewed within the framework of the eating patterns of various populations, as lifestyle elements have the potential to influence microbial activity and diversity. Understanding these mechanisms and their impact on metabolic well-being, particularly relating to conditions , such as obesity and insulin resistance, is crucial for guiding effective nutritional intervention that can enable optimized fat absorption (Lai et al., 2021; Gonzalez et al., 2023).

2.4. Production of Energy from Macronutrients

Macronutrients-carbohydrates, fats, and proteins, are the major sources of energy for human metabolism. On consumption, these macronutrients undergo several biochemical transformations to be converted into adenosine triphosphate (ATP), the currency of energy for the cell. Carbohydrates are particularly efficient at this because they can be catabolized easily to glucose, which is funneled into glycolysis, a metabolic pathway that produces ATP by oxidation. The by-products of glycolysis lead to further ATP synthesis in the citric acid cycle and oxidative phosphorylation, illustrating how carbohydrates are utilized mainly for short-term energy demands. This high-speed and efficient conversion is necessary for physical exercise as well as to maintain basic bodily functions, illustrating the significance of carbohydrates for generating energy from macronutrients. Fats are a secondary but significant storehouse of energy. Triglycerides are hydrolyzed into glycerol and free fatty acids by a mechanism called lipolysis, which can be further oxidized for energy. This metabolism is most critical in the case of prolonged physical activity and fasting conditions, when fat stores are utilized for long-term energy. Beta-oxidation is the mechanism of cleaving free fatty acids into acetyl-CoA, which is channeled into the citric acid cycle, thereby contributing to the generation of ATP. Also, fats provide more energy per gram compared to carbohydrates, and their importance as a dense caloric source for caloric metabolism and roles in hormone production and cell structure are emphasized. Proteins, though primarily employed for growth and repair, can also be utilized as an energy source, although not primarily. Under conditions of low carbohydrate and lipid stores, the body can deaminate proteins to yield intermediates that can be diverted into metabolic pathways , such as gluconeogenesis or the citric acid cycle. Macronutrient metabolism and energy capture are also significantly influenced by the gut microbiota. Short-chain fatty acids (SCFAs), the bacterial fermentation end-products of dietary fibers, are essential for energy control and gastrointestinal well-being, enhancing host metabolism. In this regard, understanding the interface between macronutrient metabolism and microbial activity provides a broad framework of energy production within the human organism, a field that must be developed and studied widely (Kastl et al., 2019; Silva et al., 2020) (Figure 2.12).

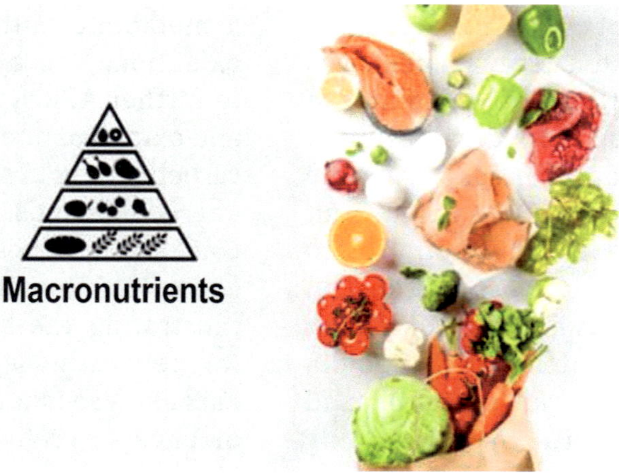

Figure 2.12. Sources of essential dietary macronutrients.

Source: https://external-content.duckduckgo.com/iu/?u=https%3A%2F%2Ftse1.mm.bing.net%2Fth%3Fid%3DOIP.FweyW7V_oAsUpMlZmiN0jQHaEn%26pid%3DApi&f=1&ipt=663999df7a3c336811210b77d3517a877966ced3a5c253f62ad29daf7e751a9f.

2.4.1. Glycolysis and Energy from Carbohydrates

Glycolysis is a critical metabolic pathway for the extraction of carbohydrate energy, one of the most important pathways of macronutrient metabolism. It is a ten-step pathway that occurs in the cytoplasm and converts glucose to pyruvate with a net production of two molecules of ATP and two molecules of NADH for every molecule of glucose metabolized. The energy liberated during glycolysis is critical, particularly during anaerobic conditions where cells rely on glycolysis as their primary means of ATP production. Such reliance is especially crucial in muscle cells during extreme exercise, where oxygen supply may be impaired. Additionally, glycolysis serves as a central metabolic hub, providing intermediates that feed into other metabolic pathways, thereby supporting its function in cell metabolism. Integration of these observations emphasizes the pivotal position of glycolysis in the promotion of energy production from carbohydrate consumed, together with the maintenance of metabolic flexibility. Glycolysis is a strongly regulated process by a myriad of factors, including substrate availability, energy status, and hormone signals. Regulation of enzymes is primarily attained through major regulatory enzymes hexokinase, phosphofructokinase-1, and pyruvate kinase, which catalyze glycolytic irreversible reactions. Phosphofructokinase-1, in particular, is considered the key regulatory location, responsive to levels of ATP and AMP to transmit the cellular energy status. Under conditions of high energy demand, under strenuous exercise or an abundance of nutrients, glycolytic flux is enhanced to meet energy demands. Under conditions of low energy, under fasting or starvation, glycolysis is lowered to conserve glucose for essential processes. This fine balance underscores the crucial role of glycolysis in controlling cell energy production based on the organism's metabolic requirements. Further, the integration of glycolysis into other biochemical pathways proves its importance in broader metabolic processes. Glycolytic intermediates are diverted to the citric acid cycle and oxidative phosphorylation so that efficient production of ATP through aerobic respiration can be achieved. In addition, interaction of glycolysis with fermentation allows for the generation of ATP during low oxygen availability, as in most tissues, like the retina. The unique energy requirements of various cell types can also guide their reliance on glycolytic metabolism. For instance, studies have indicated that photoreceptors are primarily found on oxidative phosphorylation but are supplemented by glycolytic mechanisms under certain conditions, and the different types of photoreceptors exhibit varying degrees of dependency on these metabolic processes (Chen et al., 2024). Similarly, cancer cell reprogramming of energy metabolism is also an expression of the universality of glycolysis, in which the energy production of cancer cells is often diverted towards increased glycolytic processes, a phenomenon known as the Warburg effect (Wang et al., 2024). This interplay between glycolysis and overall energy metabolism speaks volumes about its role in normal physiology as well as disease processes.

2.4.2. Krebs Cycle and Energy from Proteins

The Krebs cycle, or tricarboxylic acid cycle or citric acid cycle, is at the hub of the metabolic breakdown of macronutrients , such as proteins. It occurs primarily in mitochondria and entails the cyclic oxidation and degradation of acetyl-CoA from a variety of sources , such as carbohydrates, fats, and proteins. When proteins are undergoing breakdown, they undergo deamination, in which the amino group is removed from the amino acids to give ammonia and a corresponding keto acid.

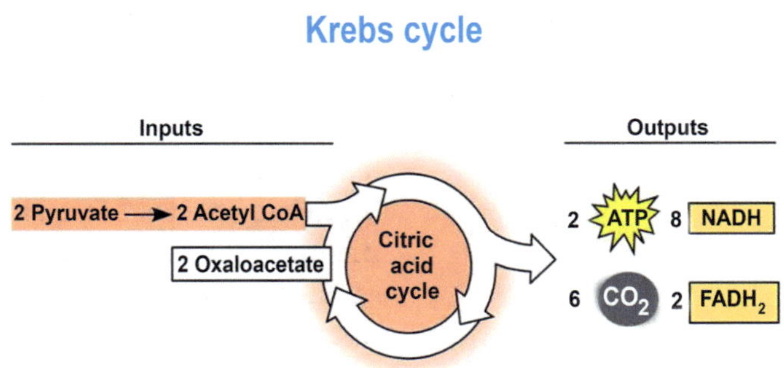

Figure 2.13. Inputs and outputs of the Krebs (citric acid) cycle.

Source: https://external-content.duckduckgo.com/iu/?u=https%3A%2F%2Fcf.ppt-online.org%2Ffiles1%2Fslide%2Fb%2FBVGgMrEbKADuN34HO20vTzjaCy71mpXIiJYRslZckf%2Fslide-17.jpg&f=1&nofb=1&ipt=5f56bd5664373da0f4ec6a037c95f38c59c7229c33dcbe7b98262eb9463cd233.

The resulting keto acid can be processed further into acetyl-CoA or fed into the Krebs cycle at numerous different entry points so that the organism can optimally utilize energy. This energy is essential for various cellular functions, homeostasis maintenance, and the support of body functions, hence underlining the importance of protein metabolism in the larger context of macronutrient metabolism. Apart from being involved in energy production, the Krebs cycle has an important function of bringing together different metabolic pathways. For example, under carbohydrate shortage, the organism can make up for it by increasing protein catabolism, thereby powering the Krebs cycle using amino derivative molecules. Such metabolic flexibility is crucial, particularly under starvation or metabolic stress conditions, when reliance on protein sources of energy becomes augmented. By its incorporation of carbohydrate, fat, and protein metabolism, the Krebs cycle facilitates efficient production of energy regardless of macronutrient composition in the diet. Moreover, disruptions in this cycle hold serious consequences for overall metabolism and energy balance, highlighting its importance in maintaining metabolic health and efficiency, as evidenced by research examining the interaction between environmental determinants and nutrient intake (Allgood, 2009). Continued examination of the Krebs cycle illustrates its crucial function in regulating energy return from proteins and influencing varying physiological responses. Because the Krebs cycle catabolizes acetyl-CoA, it generates significant byproducts , such as NADH and FADH2 that contribute to the electron transport chain for ATP synthesis. This energy-generation mechanism becomes more relevant under conditions of impaired glucose metabolism, , such as in diabetes. During such a condition, the nutritional shift towards greater protein intake can facilitate energy generation from the Krebs cycle regardless of carbohydrate (Bando et al., 2020). Also, energy equilibrium is regulated by energy intake and expenditure, with metabolic rates dictated by the Krebs cycle, and it highlights the significance of protein metabolism in the more general context of macronutrient metabolism and disease and health management implications (Figure 2.13).

2.4.3. Beta-Oxidation And Energy from Fats

Beta-oxidation is a major metabolic pathway for the catabolism of fatty acids that helps convert fat reserves into energy. The process is catabolic and occurs in the mitochondria where long-chain fatty acids are cut by enzymes to produce acetyl-CoA, a major metabolite that enters the citric acid cycle. As the beta-oxidation of fatty acids proceeds, the process also produces reducing equivalents, NADH and FADH2, which themselves are utilized in the electron transport chain to produce ATP. Given that fats are much more energy-concentrated molecules than carbohydrates, their correct metabolism by beta-oxidation becomes of specific interest during prolonged fasting or extreme exercise, highlighting the body's capacity to adapt to varying energy demands and substrates. Significantly, beta-oxidation is not only vital in the production of energy but also a significant component of overall metabolic regulation. Fat availability to undergo oxidation is regulated by hormonal signals, dietary availability, as well as the physiological status of the subject. For instance, during caloric deprivation or carbohydrate low status, , such as in ketogenic diets, beta-oxidation is enhanced to supply energy, reflecting a preference away from glucose metabolism. Research indicates that this elevation in fat oxidation is associated with increased metabolic flexibility, hence the body's capacity to utilize various macronutrients. This metabolic flexibility is of special importance in diseases like nonalcoholic fatty liver disease, where the improved utilization of fatty acids can reduce hepatic fat accumulation and enhance liver function overall (Watanabe et al., 2020). Aside from that, the connection between beta-oxidation and metabolic illnesses further underscores the importance of understanding fat metabolism in the clinical context. PCOS is a prime example that can be used to highlight the role of fat intake on insulin sensitivity as well as on general health outcomes. Given that PCOS patients often exhibit a higher rate of obesity and insulin resistance, dietary intervention is crucial. A diet of low saturated and high unsaturated fats, complemented with balanced carbohydrates and proteins, can provide effective metabolism and symptom control of the disorder (Ghazeeri et al., 2021). This indicates that macronutrient composition and pathways of their metabolism are inherently mixed up in metabolic health and disease management. Thus, identification of beta-oxidation function is not only important for energy production but also has overall health implications in metabolic control.

2.5. Role of Hormones in Macronutrient Metabolism

Hormones play a key role in macronutrient metabolism through the regulation of carbohydrate, fat, and protein use, storage, and absorption within the body. Insulin, released from the pancreas in response to elevated blood glucose levels, drives glucose uptake by cells and glycogen storage in the liver and muscle. It further inhibits gluconeogenesis, thus maintaining blood glucose in a narrow range. Furthermore, insulin promotes lipogenesis through the mobilization of excess glucose into fatty acids. On the other hand, during fasting, another pancreatic hormone, glucagon, triggers glycogenolysis and gluconeogenesis, allowing mobilization of fats and glucose to sustain energy.

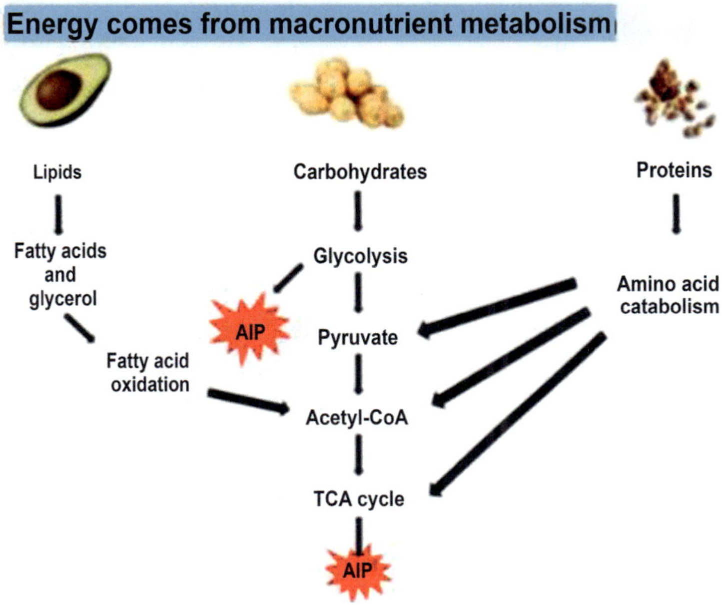

Figure 2.14. ATP production from macronutrient metabolism pathways.

Source: https://external-content.duckduckgo.com/iu/?u=https%3A%2F%2Fo.quizlet.com%2FRDVuPqPr3f6EzWYTa4NC8A.png&f=1&nofb=1&ipt=e2ee51d54fd33c6d5fdf4c16ef1412c6cff7937504ea3681f52ebbfa68d89216.

These dynamic interactions among hormones mirror the highly regulated balance required for maintenance of metabolic homeostasis, and they illustrate how the hormonal signaling pathways can facilitate or impair the efficient usage of macronutrients in the body (Tao and Cheng, 2023). Estrogen also plays a critical role in controlling macronutrient metabolism, particularly in women. Research has shown that estrogen signaling can influence numerous aspects of metabolism, ranging from fat distribution to insulin sensitivity. Estrogen enhances tissue glucose use through the upregulation of glucose transporters and also enhances the use of fatty acids as a fuel source. Estrogen signaling also cross-talks with other metabolic hormones , such as insulin, to modulate protein turnover and mitochondrial metabolism. For instance, estrogen receptors can regulate PGC-1α, which is a major coactivator of mitochondrial biogenesis and function, thereby maximally generating energy (Tao and Cheng, 2023). Estrogen signal dysregulation has also been linked to metabolic disease, further highlighting the significance of the hormone in well-regulated metabolism and energy homeostasis in the framework of macronutrient dynamics.

Coordination with the biological rhythms of the day, as regulated by circadian clocks, further highlights the complexity of macronutrient metabolism. The effect of hormones , such as insulin, glucagon, and cortisol on each other may be under circadian control, changing the body's response to nutrient intake at different times of the day. It is proposed that variations in hormone levels across the circadian cycle may significantly influence glucose tolerance and lipid metabolism and that timing of food might change metabolic responses by leveraging such hormonal controls. Robust evidence shows that circadian disruption can lead to metabolic disorders, , such as obesity and diabetes, by altering the normal hormone secretory patterns and response to dietary macronutrients. Such integration of ideas regarding the function of hormones in macronutrient metabolism and circadian biology could provide novel strategies to control metabolic well-being (Figure 2.14).

2.5.1. Insulin and Carbohydrate Metabolism

Insulin plays a key function in carbohydrate metabolism, primarily by facilitating the entry of glucose into cells for energy production or storage. After carbohydrate digestion, blood glucose levels elevate, stimulating pancreatic β-cells to secrete insulin. The hormone acts on a number of tissues, including muscle and fat tissues, to cause glucose transport by glucose transporter proteins. Additionally, insulin regulates the conversion of glucose to glycogen in the liver, or glycogenesis, in order to enable the body to store surplus glucose for later use. Imbalances in insulin signaling are also recognized to lead to metabolic disease, , such as insulin resistance, which is very prevalent in conditions , such as obesity and polycystic ovary syndrome (PCOS; Ghazeeri et al., 2021). Therefore, understanding the role of insulin in carbohydrate metabolism is of utmost significance in designing dietary regimens that will control metabolic disturbances associated with impaired glucose homeostasis. The interconnection between insulin and carbohydrate metabolism is again emphasized by the impact of food choices on insulin sensitivity. Diets that are high in carbohydrates and sugars can lead to blood glucose elevations that stimulate the pancreas to release more insulin. In the long run, excessive secretion of insulin has been proven to cause insulin resistance, a state in which cells become less responsive to insulin and thus tend to have elevated blood glucose. The condition is threatening since it can predispose to type 2 diabetes and other cardiovascular diseases. There has been evidence to show that modifying carbohydrate intake, most critically reducing levels of high GI food, can increase insulin sensitivity (Ghazeeri et al., 2021). Therefore, embracing dietary changes that emphasize complex carbohydrates and balanced macronutrient profiles is able to speed overall metabolic well-being and reverse the deleterious consequences of insulin resistance. New studies have provided insight into novel mechanisms whereby insulin controls carbohydrate metabolism and influences body weight regulation. For instance, neurosecretory protein GL (NPGL) has emerged as a critical modulator working together with insulin signaling for food intake adjustment and fat accumulation. NPGL increases food intake and stimulates the storage of energy in white adipose tissue, particularly under the influence of high-calorie intake. In addition, NPGL activity is associated with insulin levels, indicating a feedback loop that may affect metabolic pathways controlling hunger and energy storage. Dysregulation of these neuropeptides, along with insulin, could enhance obesity and metabolic syndrome conditions. This emphasizes the need for an integrative perspective in the study of macronutrient metabolism, where both foodways and endocrine responses are included in attaining metabolic health.

2.5.2. Glucagon and Protein Metabolism

Its role in protein metabolism is central to its broader importance in macronutrient metabolism. Glucagon is a pancreatic hormone that, in its major role, is responsible for elevating blood glucose. Its effects also involve significant roles in amino acid metabolism. In times of low energy supply, say fasting, glucagon functions to trigger the liver to increase gluconeogenesis, a process that constructs glucose from non-carbohydrate materials, like amino acids obtained in the process of breaking down proteins.

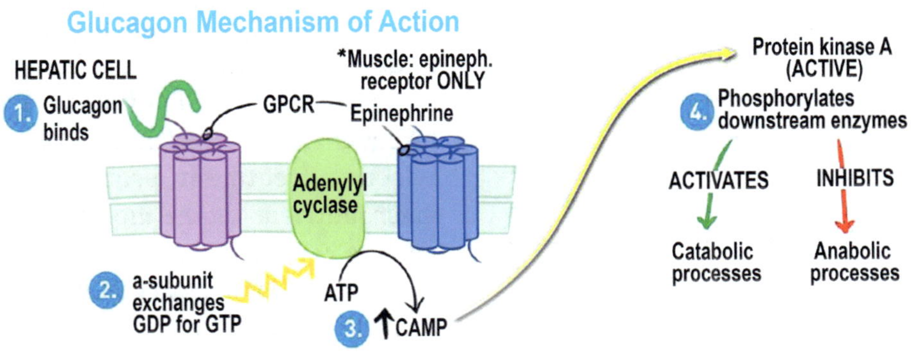

Figure 2.15. Glucagon signaling pathway promotes catabolic activity in hepatic cells.

Source:

Consequently, glucagon stimulates the release of amino acids from muscles so that, whenever caloric deprivation is present, the body has a ready source of energy and thereby recognizing the paramount interaction between glucagon and protein metabolism in achieving homeostasis in metabolic stress. In addition to its gluconeogenic effect, glucagon has an equally imperative function to perform in the control of protein synthesis and breakdown. Under increasing levels of glucagon, the body demonstrates several metabolic changes that enhance catabolism over anabolism, particularly in muscle tissue. The state of catabolism is characterized by increased proteolysis, releasing amino acids for energy production and gluconeogenesis. While this serves a purpose under prolonged fasting or exercise, it has connotations of muscle breakdown and protein balance. Understanding the way glucagon directs these metabolic pathways highlights the importance of balanced macronutrient intake, as chronically elevated glucagon without sufficient dietary protein has been demonstrated to lead to significant muscle loss. It is important to examine these interactions for developing nutritional strategies to optimize protein metabolism while moderating glucagon's catabolic action. Furthermore, glucagon's interaction with gut microbiota also must be considered in relation to protein metabolism. Recent studies suggest that gut microbiota can indirectly influence the concentration of glucagon and metabolic processes by altering protein breakdown and fermentation. For instance, certain gut microbial populations participate in the production of short-chain fatty acids (SCFAs) during protein fermentation. SCFAs can modulate host metabolic processes and influence glucose and protein homeostasis (Silva et al., 2020; Vacca et al., 2020). Furthermore, varying gut microbiota populations may also determine the individual's response to glucagon, and therefore, personalized nutrition may be of key importance. Since the interaction between dietary protein, hormonal homeostasis, and microbial function is so complex, an integrated nutrition strategy incorporating these may optimize protein metabolic effects and overall metabolic health (Figure 2.15).

2.5.3. Cortisol and Fat Metabolism

Cortisol is a glucocorticoid hormone produced by the adrenal cortex, and it plays a significant role in the regulation of numerous metabolic processes, including fat metabolism. Elevated levels of cortisol, typically caused by chronic stress or adrenal disease, are associated with enhanced lipolysis and redistribution of fat storage, with visceral fat being a favorite site. Redistribution is problematic because visceral fat is associated with numerous metabolic syndromes, including insulin resistance and type 2 diabetes. The action of cortisol on metabolic pathways gives it its pivotal position in the grand design of macronutrient metabolism and serves to illustrate that hormonal regulation can have an impact upon the body's handling of fats, carbohydrates, and proteins simultaneously. This information, then, becomes essential not only to the study of fat metabolism but also to the capacity to cope with broader endocrine regulation of metabolic health. It has been demonstrated by evidence that cortisol levels are interrelated with macronutrient intake, particularly under patterns of changing diets. It is revealed through research that some diets, for instance, low-carbohydrate diets, can decrease cortisol's metabolic effects, particularly on adipose tissues where fat is stored. Such diets appear to modulate tissue-specific glucocorticoid levels, perhaps by the mediation of 11β-hydroxysteroid dehydrogenase type 1 (11β-HSD1) activity, which is a crucial factor in the activation of glucocorticoids in the body. Observational studies indicate that reduced carbohydrate intake may reduce hepatic 11β-HSD1 expression, thus altering glucocorticoid metabolism and its effect on fat distribution. Dietary interventions thus could provide an avenue to reverse the dysregulation of the metabolic process commonly seen with elevated cortisol levels, linking the relationship between nutrition and hormonal homeostasis in macronutrient metabolism. Besides, an understanding of the interaction between cortisol and fat metabolism can provide insight into potential therapeutic interventions for metabolic disorders.

By modulating the regulatory pathways under the control of cortisol, especially in bariatric and other types of weight loss interventions, clinicians can devise more effective treatment protocols. For example, macronutrient intake modification of food can positively manage cortisol actions and improve metabolic responses. Secondly, the recognition of the role played by stress management therapies in cortisol regulation can lead to integrative treatments that include lifestyle changes to combat obesity and related comorbidities. As research continues to uncover the complexities of cortisol's effect on fat metabolism, more and more, it seems that a multi-faceted approach, including dietary modifications and counseling, can significantly enhance the management of metabolic health in individuals predisposed towards weight gain and its consequences.

2.6. Factors Affecting Macronutrient Metabolism

Macronutrient metabolism is controlled by a complex of physiological, environmental, and genetic factors that dictate how our bodies metabolize carbohydrates, fats, and proteins. Among these physiological factors, hormonal control is of specific significance. Hormones , such as insulin, glucagon, and cortisol significantly regulate metabolic pathways based on nutritional and energy requirements. For instance, insulin facilitates glucose and fatty acid storage and uptake, providing an anabolic state upon mealtimes. Glucagon, conversely, induces mobilization of stored energy upon fasting or extreme physical exertion. Genetic factors can further affect enzymic efficiency in macronutrient metabolism.

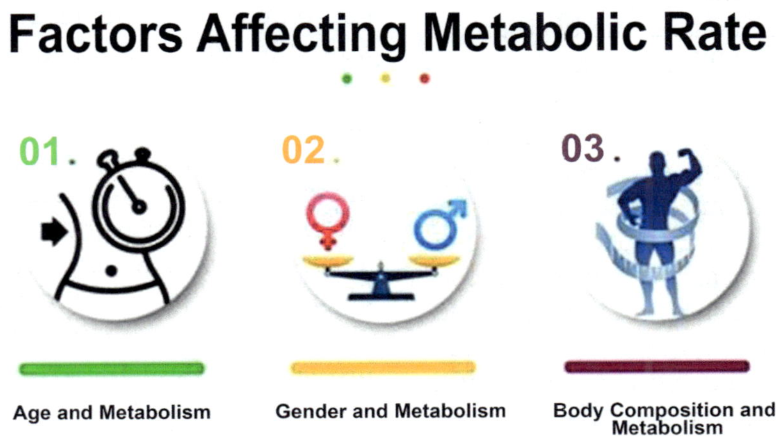

Figure 2.16. Age, gender, and body composition impact metabolic rate.

Source: https://external-content.duckduckgo.com/iu/?u=https%3A%2F%2Ftse2.mm.bing.net%2Fth%3Fid%3DOIP.SNtmWpk_GOHo0pTFkQ6FAAHaEK%26cb%3Diwp2%26pid%3DApi&f=1&ipt=de4303deab9c7fba5b bfab1a67e342acd67fcee92423a084076155822196 4f0e.

Variations in genes coding for metabolic enzymes account for variability in metabolism between people, demonstrating how genetics can influence complex metabolic function. In addition to physiological determinants, dietary composition also plays a pivotal role in the metabolism of macronutrients. The ratio of macronutrients in the diet can redirect metabolic pathways into catabolism or anabolism. High-carbohydrate diets, for instance, promote enhanced glucose oxidation, while increased fat consumption redirects energy metabolism into fatty acid oxidation. The effects of dietary fiber on carbohydrate metabolism are examples of how macromolecules of food can direct metabolic processes. Fiber slows the absorption of glucose and leads to more level insulin levels, which potentially can be beneficial for overall metabolic health. Therefore, understanding how various patterns of eating influence macronutrient metabolism is essential in creating effective interventions for metabolic disease and maximizing the health outcome. Moreover, environmental factors like physical activity and stress also have very important roles in macronutrient metabolism. Regular exercise improves the body's efficiency in using various macronutrients for energy, as physical activity enhances insulin sensitivity and consequently glucose uptake into the muscle. Moreover, stress can cause hormonal disturbances that affect metabolism, particularly through elevated cortisol production, which can result in disturbed fat and carbohydrate metabolism. Stress-related eating patterns can disrupt nutrient balance and interfere with metabolic homeostasis. Thus, an understanding of the multifaceted influence of both lifestyle and environmental factors is most crucial for a realistic comprehension of macronutrient metabolism. With further research into both areas continuing to develop, it will continue to reveal more about how best to maximize metabolic health and treat resulting disorders accordingly (Figure 2.16).

2.6.1. Age and Metabolism

As one grows older, the metabolic processes alter significantly and may play a critical role in macronutrient metabolism. The decrease in basal metabolic rate (BMR), resulting from loss of lean body mass and changes in hormones, affects the older population's carbohydrate, protein, and fat metabolism. A decreased ability to utilize glucose and an increased risk for insulin resistance and type 2 diabetes have been associated with aging. In addition, decreased protein metabolism brings about lowered rates of muscle protein synthesis, which may enhance sarcopenia. This further reduces not only functional mobility but also affects overall health outcomes. It is significant to understand these metabolic alterations in designing diet interventions based on the consumption of protein and the best macronutrient distribution to aid in health and vitality in aging adults. This focus on individualized nutrition will be able to mitigate some of the risk of metabolic decline with aging (ElSayed et al., 2022). Also, the interaction of age with macronutrient metabolism will extend to the way older individuals respond to different sources of dietary energy. From published studies, aging alters the way the body oxidizes fats relative to carbohydrates, the result of which may lead to fat oxidation becoming the priority. This shift allows for dietary planning modifications as it may call for shifting macronutrient composition to optimize metabolic health among older persons. For instance, higher fat intake may be desirable for energy status but must be matched by adequate carbohydrate intake to avoid undermining glucose metabolism. There are also nutrient intake regulation and absorption changes in older people that make nutritional interventions for the maximization of metabolic management more challenging. Therefore, understanding these dynamics is needed for physicians to organize age-related dietary measures to enable metabolic function and prevent associated diseases (Lai et al., 2021). Another critical area of aging and metabolism is how hormonal changes impact macronutrient processing. As individuals get older, hormone levels, insulin, growth hormone, and sex hormones, decline, which negatively affects macronutrient metabolism. Insulin sensitivity also reduces with age, which makes carbohydrate metabolism harder and increases the risk of metabolic disorder. Also, the reduction in estrogen and testosterone also affects muscle and fat, giving one more layer of imbalance in nutrient consumption. These alterations in hormonal levels highlight the inclusion of both lifestyle modifications and diet modifications based on the nutritional needs of the elderly. For instance, increased intake of micronutrients with a role in hormonal health, including vitamin D and omega-3 fatty acids, can enhance metabolic function. By paying attention to these interventions, one can promote healthier aging, simplifying the regulation of macronutrient metabolism over an individual's lifespan (ElSayed et al., 2022).

2.6.2. Physical Activity and Metabolism

Physical exercise plays a significant role in the development of metabolism, particularly with regard to macronutrient metabolism. Chronic exercise supplements the body's ability to metabolize carbohydrates, fats, and proteins better. During exercise, the skeletal muscle demands more energy, and this is initially made available through glycogen breakdown and later shifts to fat oxidation as the exercise continues. Increased exercise likewise leads to adaptations of muscle tissue, optimizing the functions of enzymes involved in energy production. In addition to providing short-term energy support, these metabolic adaptations contribute to long-term benefits in health by improving insulin sensitivity, lipid profiles, and overall metabolic health. Of most significance are the type and intensity of physical activity, which have a critical effect on how the body utilizes macronutrients. Aerobic exercise, or running and cycling, utilizes fatty acids as the predominant fuel during more extensive exercise bouts.

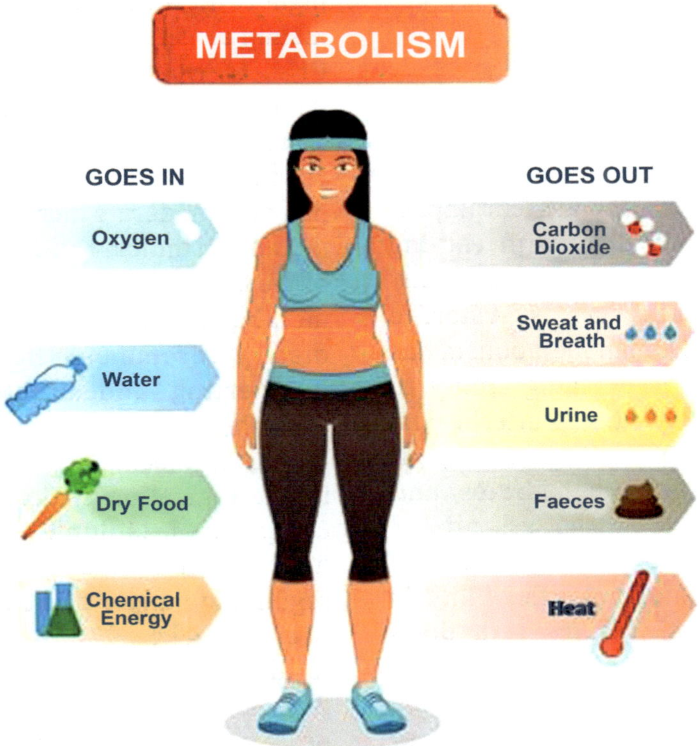
METABOLISM
GOES IN
Oxygen
Water
Dry Food
Chemical Energy
GOES OUT
Carbon Dioxide
Sweat and Breath
Urine
Faeces
Heat

Figure 2.17. Overview of metabolic inputs and outputs in the human body.

Source: https://external-content.duckduckgo.com/iu/?u=https%3A%2F%2Ftse4.mm.bing.net%2Fth%3Fid%3DOIP.GEhNBfHZsjkXZ4qP1yV01QHaH1%26pid%3DApi&f=1&ipt=ca54ff841047db8af9f60b2def0dc76b5ff1737e686d11d7a40b7c34ffd3de78.

Anaerobic exercise, , such as high-intensity interval training and weightlifting, utilizes glycogen stores as an energy source. These distinctions in substrate utilization would have some influence on dietary recommendations and when to take in nutrients in an effort to maximize performance and recovery. Understanding the role played by various forms of physical activity in affecting metabolic processes enables people to tailor their exercise program to achieve certain health benefits, whether fat loss, muscle gain, or improved sporting performance. The interrelationship between physical activity, metabolism, and nutrition reinforces the importance of a holistic approach to managing one's own health. Exercise not just enhances metabolic rate but also is an integral component of exercise, having a positive impact on the gut microbiota, which in turn has an indirect influence on the overall metabolic health. Recent evidence highlights the role of short-chain fatty acids (SCFAs), produced by fermentation of dietary fibers by gut microbes, in neuro-immunoendocrine control, demonstrating complex interactions among exercise, diet, and metabolic health. By pairing physical activity with a macronutrient-rich diet, the metabolic efficiency of an individual can be significantly optimized and chronic disease risk lowered. Ultimately, the key to maximizing macronutrient metabolism and long-term well-being is to create an active lifestyle that reconciles both exercise and macronutrient-rich foods (Figure 2.17).

2.6.3. Dietary Composition and Metabolism

The interaction between diet and metabolism is key to the recognition of macronutrient impact on overall health. Various diets with varying compositions of macronutrients can dramatically impact metabolic processes , such as fat storage and energy acquisition. Human metabolism has been found to possess an amazing ability to adapt to diverse dietary inputs by altering the fuel selection. Such flexibility allows adjustment of the utilization of fats, carbohydrates, and proteins as energy sources, which is essential to maintain homeostasis under varying conditions of the diet. While the metabolic flexibility is impressive, tremendous variations in diets may overburden such capacity and lead to harmful effects, showing the importance of macronutrient-balanced compositions in avoiding obesity and under-nutrition diets. This supports the need for dietary guidelines to take into consideration the diverse metabolic adaptation of human beings according to macronutrient consumption (Prentice et al., 2005). The glycemic index (GI) of carbohydrates is also a factor that can greatly affect metabolic health and body composition. High-GI diets have been associated with unfavorable changes in body fat mass and markers of metabolic well-being, particularly among young adults. Studies have established that young-adult animals on high-GI diets had larger fat stores and reduced insulin sensitivity compared to animals on low-GI diets. Notably, this relationship appears to be moderated by age, with older individuals or animals responding differently to high-GI diets. For instance, older participants on high-GI diets had only moderate increases in body weight and metabolic indices, as reflecting the intricacies of how age can exacerbate diet impacts on metabolism. This suggests that age-specific dietary recommendations can be beneficial in averting undesirable metabolic effects of high-GI diets (Abdelrahman et al., 2009). Moreover, mechanisms of appetite and energy intake regulation critically depend on dietary composition. Multiple macronutrient profiles may impact the hormones and neural signals regulating hunger and satiety and thus overall energy intake. Fatty diets have the potential to alter the secretion of centrally influential hormones, leptin and ghrelin. In contrast, protein diets tend to promote higher sensations of satiety and perhaps lower overall caloric intake. The relationships between macronutrient content and control of appetite underscore the need for personalized dietary advice based on individual metabolic responses and preferences. Personalized approaches to nutrition emphasize how a one-size-fits-all strategy may not be effective, particularly against the subtle ways in which food composition affects metabolism and energy expenditure in various groups (Prentice et al., 2005).

CLOSER LOOK

MACRONUTRIENTS

Macronutrients are the essential nutrients that the body requires in large amounts to provide energy and support growth, development, and overall health. They include carbohydrates, proteins, and fats, each playing a unique and vital role in the body's function. Carbohydrates are the body's primary source of energy, especially for the brain and muscles during physical activity. They are found in foods such as grains, fruits, vegetables, and dairy products. Complex carbohydrates, like whole grains and legumes, provide sustained energy and dietary fiber, while simple sugars offer quick energy but little nutritional value. Proteins are crucial for building and repairing tissues, producing enzymes and hormones, and supporting immune function. Sources of protein include meat, poultry, fish, eggs, dairy, legumes, and nuts. For children, adequate protein intake is particularly important for proper growth and development. Fats are often misunderstood but are essential for energy storage, hormone production, brain development, and absorption of fat-soluble vitamins (A, D, E, and K). Healthy fats—such as those found in avocados, nuts, seeds, and oily fish—should be prioritized, while trans fats and excessive saturated fats should be limited. Balancing macronutrients is key to maintaining a healthy diet. An imbalance—such as excessive intake of refined carbohydrates or unhealthy fats—can contribute to obesity, diabetes, and cardiovascular disease, while insufficient intake can lead to fatigue, poor growth, and nutrient deficiencies. A closer look at macronutrients highlights the importance of not only meeting energy needs but also choosing nutrient-dense foods that support long-term health. For growing children, athletes, and individuals with medical conditions, macronutrient needs may vary and should be adjusted accordingly. Understanding the role of macronutrients empowers individuals and families to make informed food choices that promote lifelong wellness.

SUMMARY

The complex interaction between macronutrient metabolism and many different physiological processes suggests that the time is ripe to understand how dietary factors influence health outcomes. Consistent with recent evidence, body composition and tissue-specific insulin sensitivity, both of which play central roles in the etiology of cardiometabolic disorders, are strongly influenced by diet. For instance, in the high-monounsaturated fatty acid (HMUFA) and low-fat, high-protein, high-fiber (LFHP) diet study, it was discovered that even though both diets improved body fat indicators, the LFHP diet by itself was associated with improved insulin sensitivity. These findings suggest that not every pattern of dietary intake is as effective at promoting metabolic health, and the need for selective nutritional interventions in weight regulation and disease prevention is therefore urgent (Trouwborst et al., 2024). Furthermore, insulin resistance has far-reaching implications extending far beyond metabolic disease, revealing concerning links with cognition. Research has shown that metabolic alterations exert large influences on brain glucose metabolism. During fasting states, insulin-resistant individuals have reduced glucose metabolism in the brain, which may cause cognitive impairments. However, under conditions of insulin stimulation, such individuals can exhibit heightened brain activity. These findings enlighten us on the complicated relationship between metabolic health and the functioning of the brain as a timely reminder of the broader health implications attendant to macronutrient intake in our diets (Jensen et al., 2024). Such relationships need to be comprehended in the development of dietary recommendations that will ensure both metabolic and cognitive health. With the growing body of evidence for macronutrient metabolism, it is increasingly clear that individualized nutritional management may prove to be essential for achieving maximum health outcomes. With the diversity of metabolic consequences of various diets and individual variability, nutrition cannot remain a one-size-fits-all endeavor. Future studies should attempt to continue refining diet guidelines by specific health profiles and disease states, not just weight control, but also optimization of overall metabolic health and cognitive function. With continued study of the complex impacts of macronutrient intake, we can better align public health initiatives for minimizing metabolic disease incidence with maximizing health in different populations (Iwakoshi-Ukena et al., 2017.

Understanding the subtleties of macronutrient metabolism is essential to understanding how foods impact human health and disease. Central to this process is the digestion and absorption of carbohydrates, proteins, and fats that provide essential energy and substrates for cellular function. Epidemiological studies and current research place emphasis on the role of gut microbiota in this metabolic environment, and evidence suggests its potential role in regulating not just metabolic functions but also immune and endocrine functions. The metagenesis between dietary fibers and gut microbiota generates short-chain fatty acids (SCFAs) through fermentation, which are assumed to play an essential role in health by modulating neuro-immunoendocrine systems. These findings into the metabolism of macronutrients emphasize the importance of bringing gut health into the broader story of metabolism and nutrition, paving the way for future therapeutic strategies that can treat numerous metabolic disorders and diseases linked with dietary imbalances and gut microbiome (Silva et al., 2020). Furthermore, the evolution of omics technologies has vastly transformed our understanding of macronutrient metabolism. By permitting scientists to think about genetic, transcriptomic, proteomic, and metabolomic data simultaneously, these platforms allow for a more comprehensive insight into the metabolic pathways engaged. The commingling of multi-omics facilitates the possibility of understanding how different macronutrients impact not only metabolic pathways but also the interactions among these pathways and greater physiological reactions. This integral strategy optimizes our ability to identify specific mechanisms through which macronutrients consumed as food affect health and provide potential avenues for personalized nutrition and targeted therapies. Therefore, ongoing optimization of research methods continues to expand the subject area of macronutrient metabolism, illuminating the complex interaction among diet, metabolism, and overall health (Hasin-Brumshtein et al., 2017). Finally, the implications of macronutrient metabolism extend far beyond basic nutrition. The findings from studies into the gut microbiota and their metabolites, specifically SCFAs, provide fresh hope for the discovery of new therapeutics for the treatment of a variety of illnesses, including central nervous system disease. Although scientists continue to explore deeper into the microbiota-gut-brain axis and its role in orchestrating neuro-immune interactions, it becomes evident that dietary options and the health of the gut are two interconnected enablers of health. These discoveries provide key potential for public health policy, directed toward the promotion of dietary patterns in support of a healthy microbiome and, conversely, enhanced metabolic health. As the debate surrounding nutrition becomes increasingly transmuted, the understanding of the key fields of macronutrient metabolism will remain imperative, not only for scientific investigation but also for practical applications toward health promotion (Silva et al., 2020).

References

1. Allgood, E. L. (2009). The effect of diet and polybrominated diphenyl ether (PBDE) exposure on adipocyte and whole-body metabolism in male Wistar rats. https://core.ac.uk/download/215515724.pdf (accessed on 13th June 2025).
2. Barber, T. M., Kabisch, S., Pfeiffer, A., & Weickert, M. O. (2020). The health benefits of dietary fiber. *Nutrients, 12,* 3209–3209. https://doi.org/10.3390/nu12103209 (accessed on 13th June 2025).
3. Watanabe, M., Tozzi, R., Risi, R., Tuccinardi, D., Mariani, S., Basciani, S., Spera, G., Lubrano, C., & Gnessi, L. (2020). Beneficial effects of the ketogenic diet on nonalcoholic fatty liver disease: A comprehensive review of the literature. *Obesity reviews: an official journal of the International Association for the Study of Obesity, 21*(8), e13024. https://doi.org/10.1111/obr.13024 (accessed on 13th June 2025).
4. Bass, R., Brownell, J. N., & Stallings, V. A. (2021). The impact of highly effective CFTR modulators on growth and nutrition status. *Nutrients, 13,* 2907–2907. https://doi.org/10.3390/nu13092907 (accessed on 13th June 2025).
5. Iwakoshi-Ukena, E., Shikano, K., Kondo, K., Taniuchi, S., Furumitsu, M., Ochi, Y., Sasaki, T., Okamoto, S., Bentley, G. E., Kriegsfeld, L. J., Minokoshi, Y., & Ukena, K. (2017). Neurosecretory protein GL stimulates food intake, de novo lipogenesis, and onset of obesity. *eLife, 6,* e28527. https://doi.org/10.7554/eLife.28527 (accessed on 13th June 2025).
6. Cameron, D., Hayhoe, R., & Welch, A. (2020). The relationships between sarcopenic skeletal muscle loss during ageing and macronutrient metabolism, obesity and onset of diabetes. https://core.ac.uk/download/237699394.pdf (accessed on 13th June 2025).
7. Freeling, Jessica L., "The Relationship of Macronutrient Intake with Growth in Children with Type 1 Diabetes Mellitus" (2024). *Electronic Theses and Dissertations.* 986. https://openprairie.sdstate.edu/etd2/986(accessed on 13th June 2025).
8. Fusco, W. G., Bernabeu, M., Cintoni, M., Porcari, S., Rinninella, E., Kaitsas, F., Lener, E., et al. (2023). Short-chain fatty-acid-producing bacteria: Key components of the human gut microbiota. *Nutrients, 15,* 2211–2211. https://doi.org/10.3390/nu15092211 (accessed on 13th June 2025).
9. Gonzalez, J. (2022). Novel dietary approaches to appetite regulation, health and performance. *The Journal of Physiology, 600.* https://www.semanticscholar.org/paper/6ce49da356cf0ca5462a8d481ab956bdd1df3419 (accessed on 13th June 2025).
10. Gutierrez, J. A., Liu, W., Perez, S., Xing, G., Sonnenberg, G. E., Kou, Blatnik, M., et al. (2021). Pharmacologic inhibition of ketohexokinase prevents fructose-induced metabolic dysfunction. *Molecular Metabolism, 48,* 101196–101196. https://doi.org/10.1016/j.molmet.2021.101196 (accessed on 13th June 2025).
11. Hasin-Brumshtein, Y., Seldin, M. M., & Lusis, A. J. (2017). Multi-omics approaches to disease. *Genome Biology, 18.* https://doi.org/10.1186/s13059-017-1215-1 (accessed on 13th June 2025).
12. Ijaz, H. (2025). An overview of bioavailability and bioequivalence study in human subjects. *Int. Jour. of Pharma Medix India.* https://www.semanticscholar.org/paper/1a554982fe378bf4c17a73a8a3d334a2e771f50d (accessed on 13th June 2025).

13. Magen, S., Seybold, H., Laloum, D., & Avin-Wittenberg, T. (2022). Metabolism and autophagy in plants—a perfect match. *FEBS Letters, 596*, 2133–2151. https://doi.org/10.1002/1873-3468.14359 (accessed on 13th June 2025).

14. Manungkalit, M. (M.), & Sari, N. P. (N.) (2019). Predictors of post prandial glucose level in diabetic elderly. https://media.neliti.com/media/publications/300706-predictors-of-post-prandial-glucose-leve-3dbe36d0.pdf (accessed on 13th June 2025).

15. Meng, Q., Boldt, J., & Runkle, E. (2020). Blue radiation interacts with green radiation to influence growth and predominantly controls quality attributes of lettuce. *Journal of the American Society for Horticultural Science, 145*, 75–87. https://www.semanticscholar.org/paper/0e51b5d56468e1ab50b3db4d16890a932a485425 (accessed on 13th June 2025).

16. Sato, T., & Sassone–Corsi, P. (2022). Nutrition, metabolism, and epigenetics: Pathways of circadian reprogramming. *EMBO Reports, 23.* https://doi.org/10.15252/embr.202152412 (accessed on 13th June 2025).

17. Smith, H., & Betts, J. A. (2022). Nutrient timing and metabolic regulation. *The Journal of Physiology, 600*, 1299–1312. https://doi.org/10.1113/jp280756 (accessed on 13th June 2025).

18. Sugioka, K., Nishida, T., Murakami, J., Itahashi, M., Yunoki, M., & Kusaka, S. (2024). Substance P promotes TGF-β-induced collagen synthesis in human corneal fibroblasts. *American Journal of Physiology. Cell Physiology.* https://www.semanticscholar.org/paper/f1268a229f9458e7c3a6317714058e9f48e0adda (accessed on 13th June 2025).

19. Tao, Z., & Cheng, Z. (2023). Hormonal regulation of metabolism—Recent lessons learned from insulin and estrogen. *Clinical Science, 137*, 415–434. https://doi.org/10.1042/cs20210519 (accessed on 13th June 2025).

20. Torres-Gonzalez, M., & Rice Bradley, B. H. (2023). Whole-milk dairy foods: Biological mechanisms underlying beneficial effects on risk markers for cardiometabolic health. *Advances in Nutrition, 14*, 1523–1537. https://doi.org/10.1016/j.advnut.2023.09.001 (accessed on 13th June 2025).

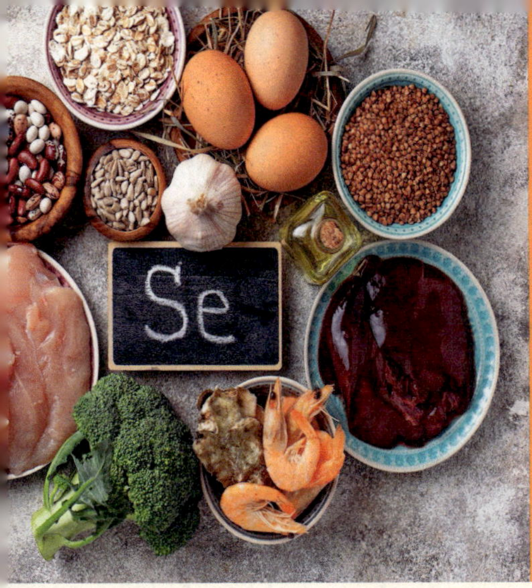

Chapter 3
MICRONUTRIENT METABOLISM

Contents

Introduction....73
3.1. Types of Micronutrients....77
3.2. Absorption of Micronutrients....81
3.3. Transport of Micronutrients....85
3.4. Metabolism of Vitamins....89
3.5. Metabolism of Minerals....93
3.6. Health Implications of Micronutrient Metabolism....98
Summary....103
References....105

Introduction

Micronutrients, i.e., minerals and vitamins, are essential components of human diets and play major roles in metabolic functions, immune function, and general health. Although they are of paramount importance, hundreds of millions of individuals globally have micronutrient deficiencies with serious health consequences. Of particular importance is that the relationship between micronutrient intake and chronic diseases underscores the importance of understanding micronutrient metabolism. Research has indicated that inadequacies, particularly at an initial phase, can have a lifetime impact, changing the body composition, glucose metabolism, and even potentially risking later-life disorders. Specifically, the World Health Organization estimates that about 2 billion people are micronutrient-insecure, and children below the age of five years are particularly vulnerable (Yousefi et al., 2025). This highlights a critical need for integrated nutrition strategies to improve micronutrient intake, particularly among populations at risk. The dynamics between some micronutrients and disease mechanisms is an area of escalating interest in nutritional science. For instance, iron, a very significant micronutrient, is well known for its role in oxygen transport and energy metabolism. In spite of this, its dual function as an essential nutrient and potential pro-oxidant raises significant questions regarding how it is metabolized in the context of disease , such as colorectal cancer (CRC). There is evidence to suggest that both iron deficiency and excess have roles in CRC pathogenesis through effects on cellular processes , such as proliferation and apoptosis (Yousefi et al., 2025). This necessitates an advanced comprehension of iron metabolism and its relevance to disease risk. By studying the impact of various dietary sources of iron, e.g., heme and non-heme, on health outcomes, researchers can enhance evidence for dietary guidelines and interventions aimed at reducing the incidence of iron-related disease. The theory of micronutrient metabolism is in continuous evolution, particularly with the Developmental Origins of Health and Disease (DOHaD) hypothesis in mind. This model proposes that deficiencies in nutrients during specific stages of development can lead to permanent changes in metabolism and disease risk later in life (Littlejohn et al., 2023). Recent evidence has highlighted co-occurring deficiency states , such as diminished zinc, folate, and vitamin levels that impact not only individual-pathway health outcomes but also reshape the gut microbiome, which underpins global metabolic health. The implications of such a discovery are far-reaching and suggest that broad strategies for micronutrient supplementation and dietary intervention could preempt long-term consequences of deficiency-related health issues. Situating the study of micronutrient metabolism in the broader context of public health, this research has the potential to contribute importantly to the mitigation and understanding of the pervasive issue of micronutrient deficiencies throughout the world.

Definition of Micronutrients

Micronutrients play a crucial role in human health as a diverse range of vitamins and minerals required in small amounts for sustaining distinct physiological functions. Unlike macronutrients like carbohydrates, proteins, and fats, micronutrients are characterized by their low dietary requirements but a critical role in metabolic functions. Such molecules encompass enzymatic reactions, influence gene expression, enable immune function, and provide overall cellular integrity. The deficiency of any required micronutrient has the potential to cause serious health consequences, ranging from stunted growth and developmental issues to greater vulnerability to disease. Therefore, the nuances of micronutrient classification, such as,, such as fat-soluble vitamins A, D, E, K and water-soluble vitamins, and the critical minerals like calcium, iron, and zinc, highlight their unique physiological functions and provide a foundation upon which to explore their metabolism within the body. The complexity of micronutrient metabolism only adds to their significance in disease and diet. Every micronutrient possesses its own distinct process of absorption that may be influenced by factors , such as food matrix, capacity for digestion by the individual, and health status. Certain vitamins, for instance, possess specific transport needs, while minerals , such as zinc, often depend on the presence of other food constituents to maximize utilization. These interactions show how the bioavailability of micronutrients can vary widely, which determines their efficacy in maintaining body processes. Research indicates that even when one has an apparently sufficient diet, he or she may still have deficiencies due to numerous factors like bioavailability and dietary selection. Deep scrutiny of food habits, food sources, and nutrient-nutrient interactions is thus needed to elucidate the mechanisms by which micronutrients act to affect health and metabolism (Combet & Buckton, 2014). Current developing research continues to analyze the impact of micronutrient supplementation in addressing public health demands. While the multivitamin and supplement industry often equate improved health and performance to its products, findings provide variable results regarding their efficacy. Surprisingly, though, there are some studies suggesting that unsupervised supplementation actually increases health risk, as seen in some subgroups where multivitamin intake is associated with heightened all-cause mortality rates and certain cancers. Thus, although supplementation may be tempting, nutritionally sufficient food consumption is the safest way to achieve micronutrient adequacy. Observing the interaction between intake of diet and serum levels of specific micronutrients, , such as zinc, illustrates the complexity of achieving optimal micronutrient status in groups. Systematic reviews point to gross heterogeneity in response to supplementation as justification for continued research in the development of evidence-based recommendations that reflect the complex nature of micronutrient metabolism (Ashwell et al., 2013) (Figure 3.1).

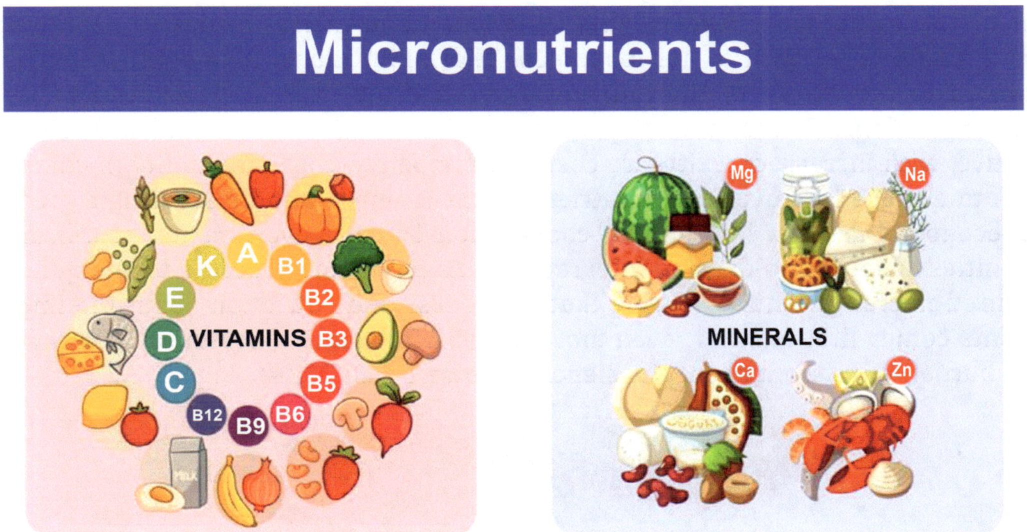

Figure 3.1. Food sources are rich in essential vitamins and minerals.

Source: https://external-content.duckduckgo.com/iu/?u=https%3A%2F%2Fimages.examples.com%2Fwp-content%2Fuploads%2F2024%2F04%2FMicronutrients-1.png&f=1&nofb=1&ipt=82f627215b7da49cd8ed00ea7c136fea5e2e2999e96411f96108d17e88eb043f.

Importance of Micronutrients in Human Health

The function of micronutrients in human health cannot be overstated, as they are instrumental in many processes within the body, including immunity, cell metabolism, and overall development and growth. Among such micronutrients, zinc has been recognized as a particularly significant entity for maintaining health throughout the human lifetime. Its varied functions range from being a catalyst of child development and infection resistance to the regulation of glucose metabolism. New findings indicate that zinc deficiency is highly linked to increased risks of diabetes and other cardiometabolic conditions, proving that zinc's inadequate nourishment can greatly impact public health. While crucial, zinc deficiency is still one of the most prevalent types of micronutrient malnutrition globally, and therefore, special interventions like supplementation, fortification of food, and agricultural interventions like biofortification are needed to increase dietary intake of zinc and tackle this highly prevalent problem (Lowe et al., 2024). The relationship between DNA integrity and micronutrient consumption also identifies another essential role of micronutrients in the enhancement of overall human health. Accumulation of DNA damage is implicated in many developmental and degenerative diseases and aging. Optimization of intake of some micronutrients, i.e., vitamins and minerals , such as vitamin C, vitamin E, folate, and zinc, can neutralize the effect of DNA damage. Research has proven that some micronutrients offer protective functions against oxidative injury by being involved in essential cellular processes regarding DNA metabolism and repair. For example, the supplementation with micronutrients have been proven to reduce biomarkers for DNA damage, thereby improving cellular health and genomic integrity. These associations improve individuals' and healthcare providers' ability to take adequate micronutrient consumption as a disease and age-related decline preventive action (Fenech et al., 2023). Furthermore, the realization of the combined effects of micronutrient deficiencies on public health accelerates the necessity to fill these nutritional loopholes. The implications of poor micronutrient intake are not limited to the health of the individual because they are likely to lead to far-reaching socioeconomic problems. To illustrate, populations with micronutrient malnutrition are likely to be less productive, with increased healthcare costs, and impaired cognitive ability in children. Hence, intervention to achieve improved micronutrient status is important for securing a greater quality of life and economic growth. Interagency cooperation among governments, healthcare systems, and communities is needed to develop integrated plans for ensuring access to an equilibrated diet rich in required micronutrients. Ensuring that awareness and education about the importance of micronutrients comes first makes it even more possible to create a healthier society and prevent the world's burden of micronutrient deficiencies (Lowe et al., 2024) (Figure 3.2).

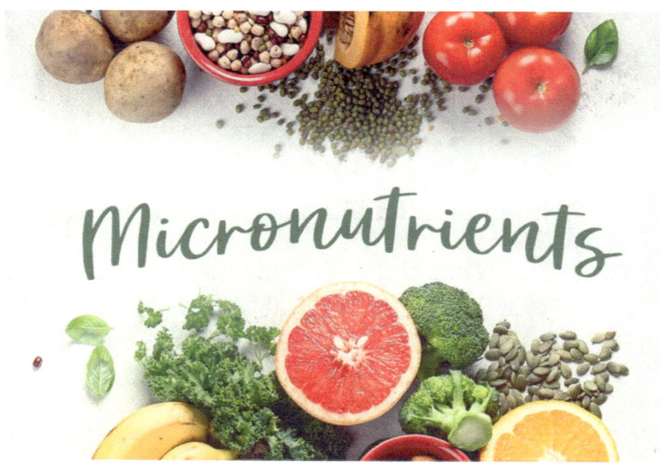

Figure 3.2. Colorful fruits, vegetables, and seeds as sources of essential micronutrients.

Source: https://miro.medium.com/v2/resize:fit:1000/1*W6zVR8rNqyJiVLKycAUeBQ.jpeg.

Overview of Micronutrient Metabolism

Micronutrient metabolism is a term for the biochemical processes by which our bodies metabolize required vitamins and minerals, ultimately leading to various physiological processes. Although micronutrients are required in small amounts, they are crucial in the management of cellular processes, metabolic processes, and overall health. Micronutrient metabolism consists of their uptake, transport, and utilization within cells, where they act as cofactors or precursors for enzyme reactions for the most part. For instance, bioactive polyphenol compounds are increasingly better known for their antioxidative properties, and their impact is seen in the prevention and treatment of metabolic syndrome. Recent studies highlight the therapeutic value of polyphenols in the mitigation of metabolic aberrations, indicating their ability to resist oxidative stress and to normalize carbohydrate and lipid metabolism, as is seen in the presented studies on their impact on non-communicable chronic diseases (Niewiadomska et al., 2022). An essential component of micronutrient metabolism is the complex relationship between various substances, which usually determines how the body is able to utilize these nutrients. One such trace mineral is selenium, which is an excellent example. Predominantly found in protein-bound form as selenocysteine, selenium has multifunctional roles that are critical to redox reactions and cell homeostasis. Research has offered insight into the evolutionary function and metabolic activities of selenium in prokaryotes and eukaryotes, underscoring its role in antioxidant defense and immune system processes (Zhang et al., 2022). Describing the dynamics of selenium metabolism and how it interacts with other micronutrients may shed more light on its utility in human health, particularly in the context of inflammatory and metabolic diseases. The complex interaction between micronutrient status and metabolic health underscores the relevance of well-balanced dietary nutrition. In addition, the function of micronutrient metabolism extends beyond single-function concepts to its integration into broader metabolic paradigms with relevance to systemic disease and disease prevention. In keeping with the trend towards modern diets, valuing whole, nutrient-rich foods supplemented by vitamins and minerals is important. The ongoing exploration of the bioactive effects of various micronutrients offers potential for the development of new dietary strategies or functional foods for the prevention of chronic diseases. Polyphenol plant source-supplemented diets, for instance, have been found to have beneficial effects on metabolic syndrome, further substantiating the need to understand the link between micronutrient consumption and metabolic health (Niewiadomska et al., 2022). Appreciation and use of micronutrient metabolism not only illuminate pathways to improved health but also inform nutrition policy and public health intervention for the avoidance of diet-related disease (Figure 3.3).

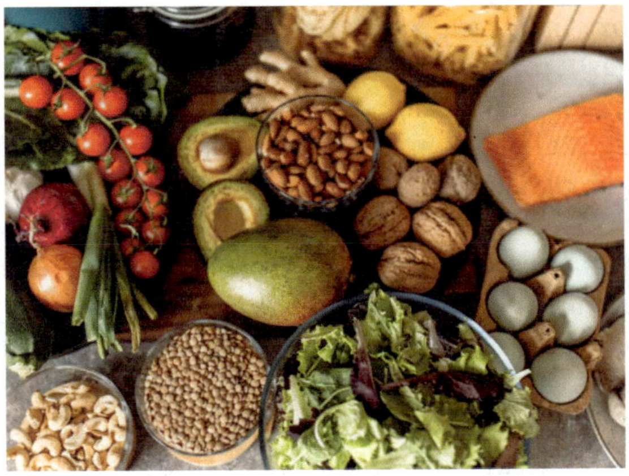

Figure 3.3. Assorted nutrient-dense foods rich in vitamins, minerals, healthy fats, and proteins for a balanced diet.

Source: https://media.post.rvohealth.io/wp-content/uploads/2024/10/overhead-nutritious-foods-on-counter-top-732x549-thumbnail.jpg.

3.1. Types of Micronutrients

Micronutrients, which include vitamins and minerals, have significant roles to play in the maintenance of metabolic processes within the human body. Vitamins are organic compounds required by the body for all biochemical reactions. Vitamins are found in two main classes: water-soluble and fat-soluble vitamins. Water-soluble vitamins, i.e., Vitamin C and B-vitamins, are required as coenzymes for metabolic reactions to help metabolize food into energy. Contrarily, fat-soluble vitamins (A, D, E, and K) are used in vision, bone, and clotting functions. Even though they are needed in small amounts, deficiencies of these vitamins lead to serious health issues, and thus their necessity in the diet as well as optimal intake through dietary sources (Mochulska et al., 2021; Wilson et al., 2024). Minerals are another form of micronutrients that serve vital functions in various physiological reactions. Minerals are inorganic compounds that play a variety of roles, from the development of robust bones to nerve conduction and muscle contraction. The essential major minerals are calcium, potassium, and magnesium, and the trace minerals are iron, zinc, and selenium, though needed in minute proportions, but equally critical. For instance, iron is not just vital in oxygen transport through the blood, and deficiency will result in anemia, which undermines energy levels and overall health. Intake and balance of such minerals are central to metabolic homeostasis and prevention of deficiencies that contribute to serious health complications (Mochulska et al., 2021; Wilson et al., 2024). The interactions between vitamins and minerals are central to optimal health and metabolism. Some vitamins depend on minerals to be effective; some of the B-vitamins, for example, require magnesium for their activation and utilization in the metabolic process. Likewise, vitamins have the potential to enhance the absorptivity and bioavailability of some minerals. Vitamin D, for example, enhances calcium absorption in the gut with a major influence on bone formation. It is also noteworthy that current dietary patterns have the tendency to lead to imbalances or deficiencies in such micronutrients, particularly in populations that consume highly processed diets. For this reason, identification and promotion of a diverse and high-density diet, both regarding vitamins and minerals, is indispensable in the maintenance of micronutrient metabolism as well as overall health (Mochulska et al., 2021; Wilson et al., 2024) (Figure 3.4).

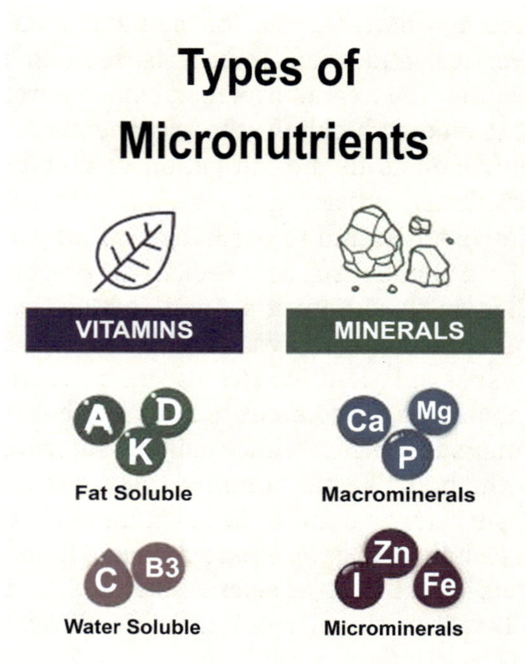

Figure 3.4. Types of micronutrients: fat- and water-soluble vitamins, macrominerals, and microminerals.

Source: https://external-content.duckduckgo.com/iu/?u=https%3A%2F%2Fkaynutrition.com%2Fwp-content%2Fuploads%2F2021%2F06%2Ftypes-of-micronutrients.jpg&f=1&nofb=1&ipt=9e7734c72347652bb7fbd07659a5e7c00ad0189578ee8c280d8a8abc85912a9c.

3.1.1. Vitamins: Water-Soluble and Fat-Soluble

The classification of the vitamins into water-soluble and fat-soluble is important in characterizing their metabolism as well as action within the body. Water-soluble vitamins like the B vitamins and vitamin C are readily absorbed in the blood and utilized in the metabolic functions. These types of vitamins are not stored in appreciable amounts; thus, they must be supplied continuously through diet to maintain correct levels. Their role in energy production and cellular metabolism is essential, as indicated by the influence of water-soluble vitamins on mental processes. Multivitamin/mineral complex supplementation has been found, using recent studies, to enhance cognitive function with prolonged task performances, highlighting the influence of these vitamins on efficient metabolic processes (Dodd et al., 2020). Therefore, understanding the action of water-soluble vitamins enables one to appreciate their role in general health and cognitive processes. Conversely, fat-soluble vitamins like vitamins A, D, E, and K possess different metabolic properties depending on whether they dissolve in fats or water. Fatty tissues and the liver store them, where the danger of toxicity through over-accumulation is potential. Their metabolic functions are diverse and critical, like vitamin D regulating calcium homeostasis, an integral function in bone condition, and vitamin A being critical for vision and immune function. The relationship between the fat-soluble vitamins and chronic disease has been of interest, where studies demonstrated a protective relationship between certain of the fat-soluble vitamins and the risk of disease for diabetic nephropathy. Findings show that increased observance of fat-soluble vitamin tendencies can significantly lower the rates of acquiring such disorders (Abaj et al., 2023). This points towards the necessity of equal intakes of nutrition to enhance metabolic health through effective utilization of both water-soluble and fat-soluble vitamins. The interrelation of water-soluble and fat-soluble vitamins must be grasped in order to develop overall nutrition strategies geared toward overall health and individual health outcomes. Each of these categories of vitamins plays a significant role in vital biological processes that form the basis of metabolic functions, but the specialized mechanism of intake, storage, and usage of each group influences different nutritional factors. For instance, generous amounts of vegetables and fruits provide ample water-soluble vitamins, while the use of healthy fat provides maximum utilization of fat-soluble vitamins. In addition, appreciation of the differential impact on health of these vitamins, , such as the role of multivitamin/mineral supplementation, can direct diet recommendations according to individual status and health needs. As subsequent studies elucidate the roles of these micronutrients, their use in dietary guidelines becomes increasingly important to promote health and to prevent disease, so that both water-soluble and fat-soluble vitamins are well controlled in the context of micronutrient metabolism.

3.1.2. Minerals: Major and Trace Elements

The function of major and trace elements as minerals in micronutrient metabolism cannot be overstressed. Major minerals , such as calcium, potassium, magnesium, and phosphorus, are crucial for many physiological processes, ranging from cell signaling, activation of enzymes, to structural protein and cell membrane integrity. Trace elements, though required in minute quantities, also play similarly basic roles in metabolic functions. For instance, iron is necessary for oxygen transport and electron transfer in metabolism, while zinc serves as a cofactor for numerous enzymes involved in DNA synthesis and the metabolism of proteins. There has to be an equilibrium of these minerals; deficiencies lead to metabolic aberration, growth retardation, and vulnerability to environmental toxins. Moreover, the interaction between these minerals governs plant productivity and health, which highlights the complex interaction between mineral nutrition and total micronutrient metabolism (Tariq et al., 2023). The availability of these minerals in the soil is greatly influenced by the environment, which can influence a plant's micronutrient uptake efficiency. Soil structure, pH level, and availability of competing ions may enhance or lower the uptake of essential minerals. For example, high levels of competing cations can lead to deficiencies in certain trace elements, e.g., copper or manganese, thus impacting plant metabolic functions. Furthermore, microbe action in the rhizosphere tends to modify the bioavailability of minerals, which can transform inorganic forms into more available forms for root uptake. With rising environmental pollution with heavy metals and pesticides, as illustrated by recent studies, the processes of mineral uptake and utilization by plants become even more complicated.

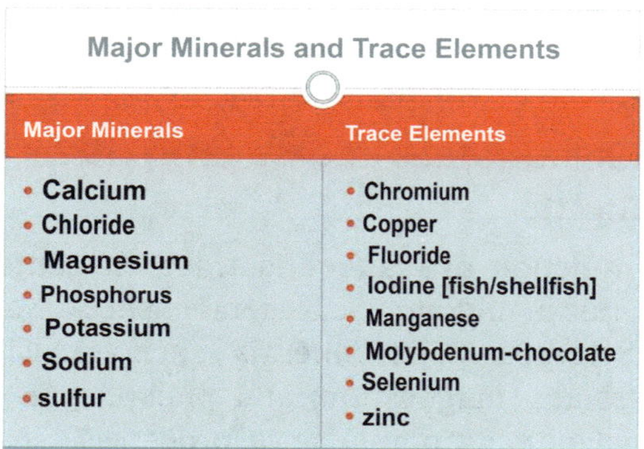

Figure 3.5. Classification of minerals into major minerals (e.g., calcium, magnesium) and trace elements (e.g., iodine, zinc).

Source: https://external-content.duckduckgo.com/iu/?u=https%3A%2F%2Fimage3.slideserve.com%2F6160231%2Fmajor-minerals-and-trace-elements-l.jpg&f=1&nofb=1&ipt=45f387c4e771de6d7f4b04bc018ef52f15e856aa332dee5425f3e2c587ea849b.

Understanding these facets is most important for proper agriculture tactics to optimize mineral availability in conjunction with limiting toxicant accumulation in plants (Alengebawy et al., 2021). Mineral nutrition management is very important in agricultural use for improving crop yield and quality. Soil amendments , such as compost or some balanced fertilizers with major and trace elements, can rectify nutrient deficiencies. More recent approaches , such as biofortified crops or microbial inoculants, may increase the bioavailability of the major minerals and hence the improve growth and metabolism. Not only do micronutrient deficiencies affect plant health, but they also have significant implications for human nutrition, particularly in staple crop-based countries that may be low in essential micronutrients. It is therefore critical to have a comprehensive understanding of micronutrient metabolism, ranging from the roles of major and trace minerals, to drive the discipline of agricultural sustainability and food security in an increasing global demand (Tariq et al., 2023) (Figure 3.5).

3.1.3. Role of Phytochemicals in Micronutrient Metabolism

Phytochemicals, or bioactive chemicals, are also significant in micronutrient metabolism and in influencing their absorption and bioavailability in the human organism. These compounds, , such as flavonoids, carotenoids, and polyphenols, possess various beneficial roles to health that can enhance the utilization of required micronutrients. For example, certain phytochemicals are able to enhance the uptake of minerals zinc and iron by improving gastrointestinal function or by optimally modulating gut flora. This interaction implies that phytochemical-rich foods may, theoretically, slow down deficiencies that are prevalent in people with suboptimal micronutrient intake. Such ingestion of varied plant foods, thus, not only provides necessary vitamins and minerals but also facilitates the processes by which these micronutrients are metabolized effectively in the body. The association between phytochemicals and the metabolism of micronutrients goes beyond absorption; these compounds also participate in cellular signaling processes that regulate vitamin and mineral metabolism. For instance, phytochemicals have been shown to act as antioxidants, protecting cells from oxidative stress and thereby increasing the longevity of micronutrients in the body. Research indicates that the gut microbiome, whose functioning is significantly influenced by dietary phytochemicals, can regulate the bioavailability of micronutrients, improving their metabolism and overall efficiency in impacting health. This engagement serves to emphasize the primary role phytochemicals can play not only in gut health but to influencing the systemic bioavailability of essential micronutrients, in keeping with mounting recognition of integrative nutritional approaches for prevention and management of micronutrient deficiency in various populations (Beane et al., 2021). Second, the enhancement of traditional and non-traditional food crops rich in phytochemicals is a very feasible solution for the control of global micronutrient malnutrition. Evidence shows that such crops, , such as millet, can be converted to nutrient-enriched foods that have a synergistic effect, where the micronutrients get the optimal absorption and utilization without the risk of antagonistic interaction (ILO & Famakinwa, 2022). With the promise of these neglected crops, regions afflicted with micronutrient deficiencies can now turn into home and sustainable sources of food that provide essential vitamins and minerals and a plethora of phytochemicals. Thus, encouraging the production and intake of several phytochemically dense plant foods can be an important determinant of enhanced micronutrient metabolism and overall health in populations of multiracial composition with dietary issues.

3.2. Absorption of Micronutrients

Micronutrient uptake is a complex process with inherently different relationships to various physiological functions of the human body. Micronutrients , such as vitamins and minerals, play critical roles in various biochemical processes and physiological functions. Micronutrient uptake begins primarily in the gastrointestinal system, where bioavailability is contingent on the nature of the food, intestinal health, and metabolic status. Factors like the presence of dietary fat have been found to enhance the absorption of fat-soluble vitamins, while others, like phytates and oxalates found in foods, will inhibit the absorption of elements like iron and calcium. This fine line has to be familiar for the sake of dealing with potential deficiencies, given that it is related to the Western diet common today, which specializes in convenience over nutrient density (Combet & Buckton, 2014). The role of the gut microbiome has emerged to become a crucial factor in the determination of micronutrient bioavailability and absorption. Recent studies indicate that the resident gut commensal microorganisms are potent modulators of micronutrient levels by regulating their absorption mechanisms and synthesis. For instance, some gut bacteria can facilitate the digestion of complex carbohydrates by releasing nutrients that allow vitamins B and K to be absorbed. This interdependent relationship underscores the promise of customized nutritional care with emphasis on optimizing gut microbiome content for enhanced micronutrient availability. Furthermore, an optimal microbiome also has implications on the overall metabolic well-being of an individual, underscoring the need for more awareness regarding the impact of diet on gut flora and subsequently, micronutrient absorption (Barone et al., 2022). Healing micronutrient deficiencies needs to be a complete process that recognizes the multifaceted nature of absorption and metabolism. Adequate nutrition is necessary, as deficiencies may not only be caused by low consumption but also by impaired absorption with other diseases or digestive disorders. Second, the premise that multivitamin tablets are a blanket solution to nutrient deficiency is being challenged more and more. There has been some evidence from studies that, instead of encouraging protection or health enhancement, such supplements will be detrimental, e.g., all-cause mortality in certain groups (Combet & Buckton, 2014). Therefore, encouraging the consumption of whole high-micronutrient foods and concurrently trying to enhance gut health is an essential approach in preventing and resolving micronutrient metabolism deficiencies (Figure 3.6).

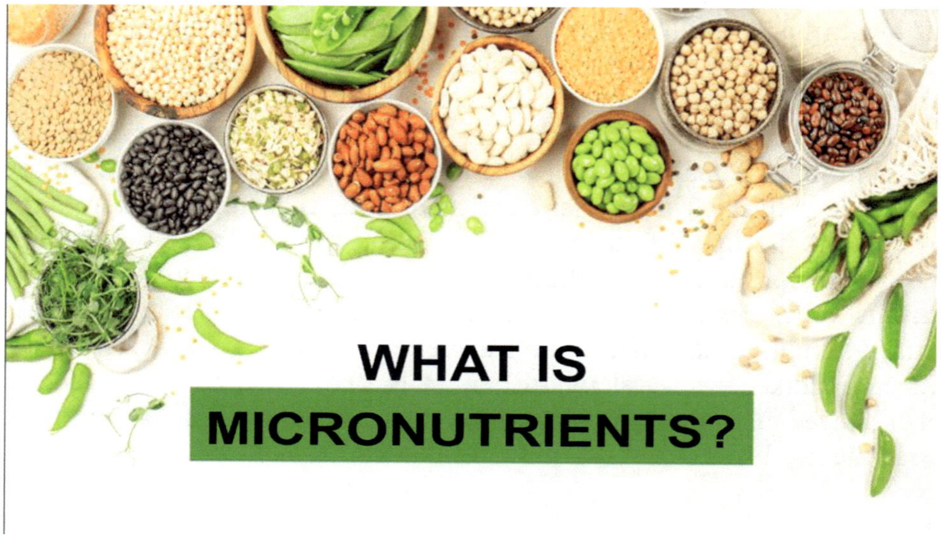

Figure 3.6. An assortment of legumes and seeds highlights common dietary sources of essential micronutrients, vital for metabolism, immunity, and overall health.

Source: https://external-content.duckduckgo.com/iu/?u=https%3A%2F%2Fthefitnessfalcon.com%2Fwp-content%2Fuploads%2F2024%2F01%2FWhat-is-Micronutrients.png&f=1&nofb=1&ipt=3ed90744fd2d4848406c55c007b09f9c94c7d5773feebbaa3b8a5cd594473606.

3.2.1. Mechanisms of Absorption in the Gastrointestinal Tract

Absorption mechanisms in the gastrointestinal tract are crucial for the efficient absorption of micronutrients, which participate in a number of critical biological processes. Micronutrients like vitamins and minerals are taken up by specific transport processes that vary across the various compartments of the gastrointestinal tract. For instance, the absorption of trace elements , such as zinc, is primarily the responsibility of the small intestine, facilitated by specialized intestinal epithelial transporters and channels. In recent times, research has increasingly resorted to the use of in vitro cell culture models, particularly the Caco-2 cell line, for studying these transport systems in detail. These models allow for the controlled examination of how food constituents influence micronutrient bioavailability and optimize best absorption, enabling explanation of zinc homeostasis and its systemic impact on health (Liu et al., 2020). The intestinal environment, including the presence of food constituents and inherent luminal circumstances, is also vital to micronutrient absorption. For example, food ligands can enhance or reduce the absorption and bio accessibility of trace elements in the intestinal lumen. Interaction between such food constituents and transport mechanisms plays a pivotal role in ascertaining micronutrient acquisition efficiency. An understanding of such processes can also shed light on potential deficiencies among populations with limited dietary diversity because inadequate essential constituents may hinder effective uptake. Studies on how particular conditions, , such as infections, impact these mechanisms can further reveal the complex nature of micronutrient metabolism in the gastrointestinal tract (Akubugwo and Ugwuja, 2010). Apart from food, physiological conditions of inflammation and infection can disrupt micronutrient absorption mechanisms to lead to adverse health effects. *Helicobacter pylori* infection, for instance, has been associated with aberrant trace element metabolism in pregnancy. Studies show that *H. pylori* decrease serum levels of prominent trace elements like copper, iron, and zinc substantially, with increased maternal morbidity and pregnancy complications. This is evidence of the importance of healthy gastrointestinal function for effective micronutrient absorption as well as general metabolic health. Awareness of the effects of such infections can guide dietary management and treatment plans, pointing to the need for vigilance and upkeep of gastrointestinal health so that normal micronutrient status in the body is not lost (Akubugwo and Ugwuja, 2010) (Figure 3.7).

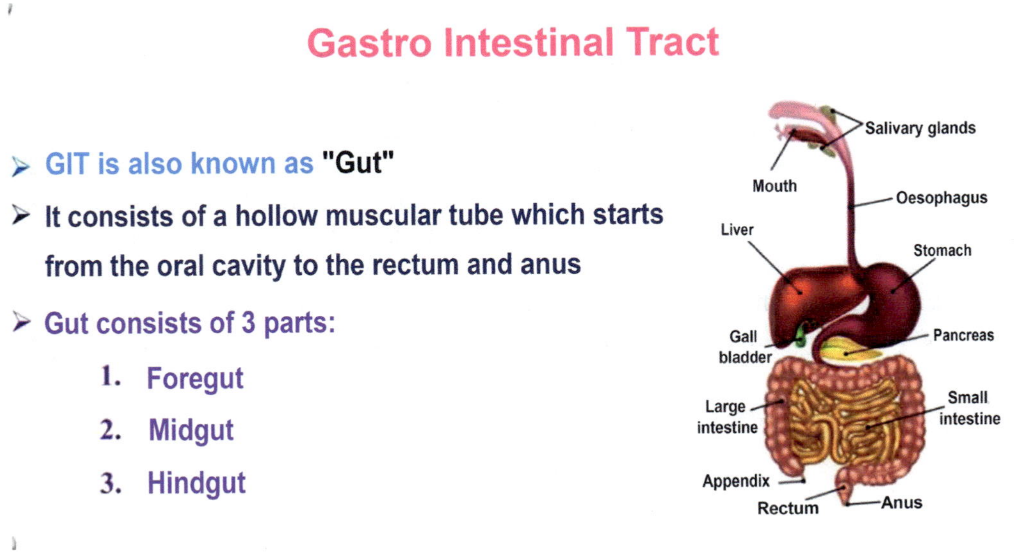

Figure 3.7. Structure and regional divisions of the gastrointestinal tract, including the foregut, midgut, and hindgut.

Source: https://external-content.duckduckgo.com/iu/?u=https%3A%2F%2Fimage.slidesharecdn.com%2Fgastrointestinaltractandmechanismofdrugabsorption-210730162359%2F75%2FGastrointestinal-tract-and-mechanism-of-drug-absorption-3-2048.jpg&f=1&nofb=1&ipt=f784ba3c4a66a73157312ae257ecae056c18d76e942ecfa26aeecf46b57afe6e.

3.2.2. Factors Affecting Absorption Rates

The bioavailability of micronutrients is influenced by a range of factors, including the nutrient content of the diet, competing nutrients' availability, and the physiological status of the subject. A diverse diet containing more fruits, vegetables, whole grains, and protein can enhance the bioavailability of essential micronutrients. Conversely, a few food constituents, like phytates in grains and legumes, can inhibit the uptake of minerals like zinc and iron. These inhibitory effects underscore the importance of understanding food sources and food combinations that facilitate or inhibit nutrient absorption, especially of concern in populations subjected to specific dietary limitations. Additionally, the environment of the gut is also very important as factors like pH levels, digestive enzymes, and intestinal lining status are bound to influence the degree of efficiency of nutrient absorption. In addition, intrinsic physiological factors like age, gender, and hormonal status are bound to have a significant impact on levels of micronutrient absorption. For instance,, during pregnancy and lactation, increased physiological needs necessitate a demand for more nutrients like zinc, requiring changes in rates of absorption to meet elevated rates of need. Evidence indicates that pregnant women can exhibit higher zinc absorption and decreased loss, a process that attempts to compensate for deficiency that may jeopardize fetal development and maternal health (Donangelo and King, 2012). The body employs complex homeostatic mechanisms in modulating the utilization of nutrients based on existing demands, demonstrating the way that metabolic status may influence the absorption of micronutrients. This reciprocal interaction between specific physiological states and nutritional demand serves to highlight the relevance of personalized nutritional protocols to achieve optimal rates of absorption as well as maximize health outcomes. Lastly, the contribution of gut microbiota to the modulation of nutrient absorption is a new focus of research within micronutrient metabolism. Gut bacteria are vital for the digestion of food and the release of nutrients, and certain strains of bacteria can enhance the bioavailability of certain micronutrients. For instance, the activity of favorable bacteria can facilitate the breakdown of phytate, thereby enhancing zinc absorption (Liu et al., 2020). In addition, gut microbiota balance can be modulated by diet, antibiotics, and general GI health status, further making the absorption landscape complex. As research continues to shed light on this complex relationship, elucidation of specific mechanisms by which microbiota modulate micronutrient absorption may enhance dietary advice and intervention to optimize general health and nutrient status in diverse groups (Figure 3.8).

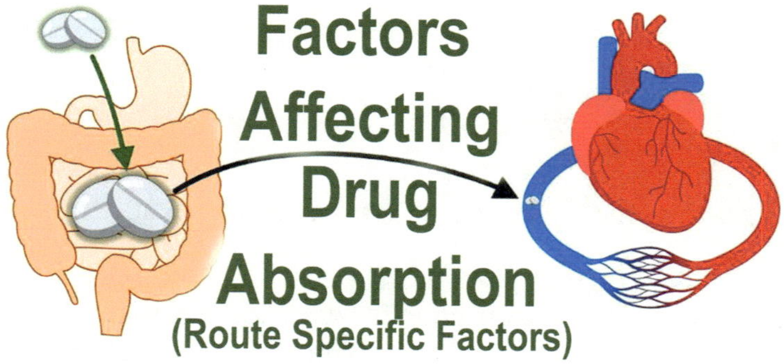

Figure 3.8. Route-specific factors influencing drug absorption into systemic circulation.

Source: https://external-content.duckduckgo.com/iu/?u=https%3A%2F%2Fi.ytimg.com%2Fvi%2FbTGIMoUiAS0%2Fmaxresdefault.jpg&f=1&nofb=1&ipt=7ca6ea972e50ee055b4735dcb356503afeee5ec25e9b775967d9675d19ab5b0a.

3.2.3. Role of Dietary Components in Micronutrient Bioavailability

Micronutrient bioavailability is greatly influenced by various dietary factors, which can either enhance or inhibit their absorption. For instance, certain phytochemicals in fruits and vegetables, flavonoids, and polyphenols, are known to increase minerals like iron and zinc's bioavailability.

Conversely, phytates found in whole grains and legumes can chelate essential minerals and decrease their effectiveness in absorption. This micronutrient bioavailability modulation is a critical consideration for ensuring adequate nutrient consumption, particularly among populations that rely on plant food consumption. Discovery of these interactions is critical to dietary recommendation development that ensures avoidance of deficiencies. More and more researchers are employing the use of in vitro cellular models, as cited in Liu et al. (2020), to discover the mechanisms of these complex interactions between food components and micronutrient uptake. Secondly, food fortification has emerged as a powerful instrument to enhance micronutrient intake and healthy public health outcomes. Fortification is a method of intentional addition of essential vitamins and minerals to food products, tailored to rectify specific deficiencies in populations.

The historic methods, , such as iodization of salt to suppress goiter and iron fortification of flour to avert anemia, attest to the efficacy of this intervention. As set out in Dwyer et al. (2015), fortification has now moved beyond the promotion of simply deficiency disease treatment to aiming at the upgrading of overall nutrient profiles in levels of dietary intake. This involves sensitive thought regarding the bioavailability of the added nutrients compared to other foods in the diet, in a way to optimize the potential benefits of such interventions to the population with as few harmful interactions as possible. Lastly, it is important to recognize the role of dietary fats in enhancing the absorption of fat-soluble vitamins A, D, E, and K. The latter relies on the presence of dietary lipids to be solubilized in the intestine and hence absorbed in the mucosal cells. Also, the proportion of dietary fats, the ratio of saturated to unsaturated fats, is able to affect the permeability of the intestinal membrane and vitamin absorption efficiency. Thus, healthy fat diets, , such as fish, nuts, and avocado fats, supply essential fatty acids but also boost the bioavailability of key micronutrients. These findings point out the connectedness of nutrients in maintaining effective micronutrient metabolism, and they highlight the importance of an appropriately balanced diet in sustaining health.

3.3. Transport of Micronutrients

Micronutrient transport is an essential process in micronutrient metabolism that defines plant health as well as human nutrition. Micronutrients like trace elements and vitamins are transported in plant systems by specialized mechanisms. These mechanisms rely on heterogeneous proteins that facilitate the entry and mobility of micronutrients into cell membranes. For example, transport proteins, , such as metal transport proteins, play a central role in the acquisition and redistribution of micronutrients within a plant tissue. Understanding these transport mechanisms enables the optimization of bioavailability and creates plants to fulfill not only their own nutritional needs but also those of the organisms that ingest them. In addition, the defects in such critical elements' transport have been proven to contribute to growth retardation, lower yields, and ultimately lead to human malnutrition, which signifies the imperative nature of ongoing research in this area of micronutrient metabolism. In addition to transport proteins, soil characteristics and environmental conditions play a major role in influencing the availability of micronutrients to plants. Soil water content, pH, and organic matter availability may all affect the solubility and mobility of micronutrients. High soil pH will precipitate certain micronutrients out of solution and render them unavailable to plant root systems. Furthermore, interactions among nutrients can complicate their transport dynamics, e.g., excessive levels of one nutrient can inhibit the uptake of another, leading to imbalance issues that harm plants. Thus, the interaction dynamics of nutrients and transport pathways are vital in developing effective agricultural strategies. Options , such as biofortification have subsequently emerged to overcome these challenges in efforts to enhance levels of micronutrients in crops to reduce the risk of deficiency among populations that rely on staple food that would otherwise lack these nutrients. Investing in the best transport of micronutrients in farming can be highly rewarding in combating malnutrition. Advances in genetic modification and biotechnology have also been promising in the enhancement of the uptake and assimilation of essential micronutrients by plants. For instance, breeding approaches that focus on the development of varieties with increased abilities for the transport of nutrients can lead to the harvesting of crops with higher levels of critical micronutrients , such as iron and zinc. All these research activities are highly relevant given the shocking statistics of "hidden hunger" affecting over two billion people globally due to improper intake of basic vitamins and minerals (Ballou et al., 2014). Also, with research continuing to unveil the complex machinery of micronutrient transport, it is evident that there is an urgent need for holistic knowledge of plant metabolism to power innovation in agriculture. By strategically improving micronutrient delivery, agricultural systems have the capacity to significantly contribute to public health and nutritional well-being worldwide (Ballou et al., 2014) (Figure 3.9).

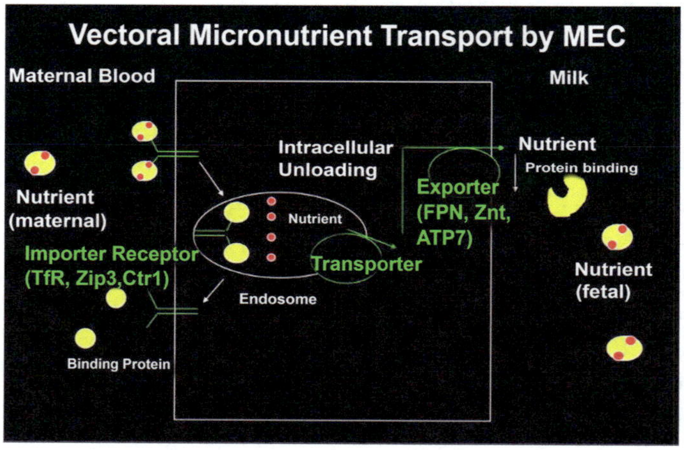

Figure 3.9. Micronutrient transport by MEC from maternal blood to milk.

Source: https://external-content.duckduckgo.com/iu/?u=https%3A%2F%2Fimage2.slideserve.com%2F4648590%2Fvectoral-micronutrient-transport-by-mec-l.jpg&f=1&nofb=1&ipt=a7be56affac595bd7ec10fb1116267c15108e253631fa5e2c61a773cf125aa77.

3.3.1. Transport Mechanisms in Bloodstream

The circulatory system serves as a vital vehicle for micronutrient transportation so that they can be delivered throughout the body for normal cellular function. This is reliant primarily on various transport mechanisms that can be divided into passive and active transport. Passive transport mechanisms like diffusion and facilitated diffusion allow micronutrients to cross endothelial cell membranes based on concentration gradients. This is an energy-requiring process and is crucial in the transport of water-soluble vitamins , such as vitamin C and B vitamins, which diffuse into the bloodstream through capillaries found in the intestines and find their target tissues. Active transport mechanisms, however, must use energy, usually in the form of ATP, to move micronutrients against the direction of their concentration gradient, as demonstrated by the sodium-transport-dependent mobilization of certain minerals , such as iron and calcium. Other than chemical gradients, the regulation of transport mechanisms within the blood is controlled by other factors, including nutritional requirements, hormonal levels, and the body's overall metabolic demands. For instance, during deficiency, there will be an augmentation in transport proteins that facilitate the uptake of needed micronutrients. Conversely, excess levels of certain vitamins and minerals have the effect of inducing competitive inhibition in which transport systems become saturated, ultimately inhibiting the uptake of other essential nutrients. Such interactive dynamics help to bring home the imperative of having a balanced intake of micronutrients to ensure the maximum transport and assimilation in the blood. Research underscores the importance of proper micronutrient transport for metabolic processes and overall health, as deficiencies result in a variety of diseases, , such as anemia due to improper iron transport. Furthermore, specific transport proteins often play a decisive role in the bloodstream's ability to transport micronutrients where and to what extent they are needed most. These proteins include some carriers and channels that regulate the transport of vitamins and minerals, , such as metallothionein's for zinc or transporters like vitamin D-binding protein for the transport of the lipid-soluble vitamin D. The presence of such transport proteins suggests not only their role in enabling micronutrients to access target tissues but also their role in regulating systemic levels of these essential compounds. For instance, genetic variation in transport proteins may impact sensitivity to nutrient intake at the individual level, further highlighting the complex interaction between genetic factors and micronutrient metabolism. Research into these transport processes continues to be warranted by immense research funding support, as illustrated in studies, exemplifying growing appreciation of their roles in nutrition and metabolism (Ballou et al., 2014; 2016).

3.3.2. Role of Proteins in Micronutrient Transport

Proteins play a vital role in the transport of micronutrients, enabling them to be absorbed, distributed, and converted to bioavailability in the body. Micronutrients, or vitamins and minerals, are utilized to facilitate numerous metabolic functions as well as overall health. Transport proteins, including members of the solute carrier (SLC) family and the ATP-binding cassette (ABC) transporters, play an important role in the healthy uptake of water-soluble vitamins , such as B-complex and vitamin C. These proteins operate by mechanisms that allow the selective absorption of micronutrients from the gastrointestinal tract into the systemic circulation, thereby enhancing their delivery to target tissues. Malfunction in the transport function of these transport proteins may lead to deficiencies or imbalances in micronutrient levels, which underscores the importance of ensuring metabolic homeostasis and preventing various medical conditions, as clarified from recent studies on dysfunctions of vitamin transporters and their implications for metabolism (Yuan et al., 2025). Furthermore, fat-soluble vitamins A, D, E, and K require specialized transport mechanisms due to their solubility. These vitamins are regulated via proteins , such as scavenger receptor class B type I (SR-BI) and Niemann-Pick C1-like 1 (NPC1L1), which synchronize lipid metabolism with vitamin absorption. Lipid interaction with fat-soluble vitamins has significant implications for micronutrient transport because lipid absorption influences the availability of these nutrients. Protein deficiencies of the transporters have been linked to varied pathologies, which extend to cardiovascular and skeletal diseases. Consistently, information on how the transport proteins work through mechanisms contains valuable insights into knowing the metabolism of micronutrients, as well as the therapeutic potential in overcoming deficiencies or associated disease conditions in practice (Yuan et al., 2025). Besides traditional mechanisms of transport, current studies highlight the role of extracellular vesicles, particularly exosomes, in micronutrient delivery and communication in the body. The nano-vesicles can encapsulate and transport a variety of biological molecules, , such as proteins and non-coding RNAs, which contribute to intercellular communication and influence metabolic processes like adipogenesis and lipid metabolism. This would mean that exosomes could be novel vectors for micronutrient transfer and expand our knowledge about the body's delivery of micronutrients. In addition, their therapeutic application to restore deficiencies in obesity and other metabolic diseases is starting to become apparent, as exosomes could transfer specific amounts of specific micronutrients or signaling molecules to enhance metabolism. Thus, the complex interplay of proteins and novel transport modes is a tangled web at the heart of micronutrient metabolism (Figure 3.10).

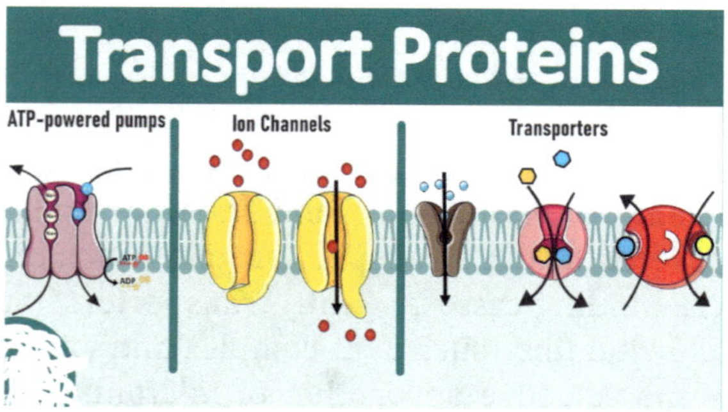

Figure 3.10. Types of membrane transport proteins: Pumps, ion channels, and transporters.

Source: https://external-content.duckduckgo.com/iu/?u=https%3A%2F%2Fi.ytimg.com%2Fvi%2FO8oMWHh2MIQ%2Fmaxresdefault.jpg&f=1&nofb=1&ipt=7c2796081e5b17e80ff2d5379b10418b418354c4d6c0ccd953b218f70e09f048.

3.3.3. Impact of Transport on Cellular Uptake

Micronutrient transport across cell membranes is a major factor governing the acquisition and overall metabolism of nutrients and plays a significant role in plant development and health. Micronutrients , such as iron, manganese, and zinc, are usually present in soils in the insoluble state, hence becoming inaccessible for plant assimilation. For their absorption, plants have employed various transport mechanisms , such as passive transport and active transport via specific transporters and channels. For instance, Strategy I and Strategy II systems are independent mechanisms adopted by various plant families to enhance iron bioavailability in the rhizosphere. Both systems are responsible for the solubilization of ferric iron into ferrous iron or phytosiderophore-mediated iron chelation, thereby enhancing cell uptake. Further, the efficiency of these transport processes can be regulated by environmental stressors, hence affecting the metabolic processes that are reliant on such essential micronutrients, and indicating the complex dependency between transport and uptake in microparticle metabolism. Extensive studies have shown the sophisticated dynamics of the interface between micronutrient transport and pathogen interaction in plants. Iron, for example, not only functions as a crucial cofactor in enzymatic activities but also plays a significant role in eliciting plant immune responses. Pathogen-associated molecular patterns (PAMPs) recognition sets off an extremely sophisticated defense-related signal transduction pathway that utilizes reactive oxygen species (ROS) generated via iron-dependent mechanisms. This generation of ROŠ is one integral part of immune activation and cellular signaling, showing the influence of transport and cellular uptake of micronutrients on plant defense strategies. Additionally, the iron transport gene dynamics can be altered with infection by pathogens, illustrating the feasibility of iron metabolism variation to modulate a plant's pathogen susceptibility or resistance strategy. These interactions bring forth the significance of understanding transport processes within the broader context of micronutrient metabolism and plant well-being. Furthermore, transport-mediated alterations in micronutrient metabolism have consequences extending beyond plant well-being to the environment and human health as well. Heavy metals, being in their typical association with soil contamination as a result of human activities, can potentially hinder the transport processes of vital micronutrients, leading to bioaccumulation and toxicity in plant tissues. High concentrations of metals , such as cadmium, lead, and mercury will disrupt normal cellular transport processes and highlight the importance of monitoring metal bioaccumulation in plants. With the potential incorporation of contaminated plants into the food chain, the determination of the transport and uptake processes of micronutrients in a polluted environment is important to assess food safety and public health risks. Transport process coordination in regular micronutrient metabolism, along with sensitization to current pollutants, marks significant areas of research in Agri-practices and environmental management.

3.4. Metabolism of Vitamins

Vitamin metabolism is a fundamental process of micronutrient metabolism since vitamins play vital roles in most biochemical reactions within the body. Vitamins are classified into two main categories depending on solubility: fat-soluble and water-soluble. Water-soluble vitamins like vitamin C and B-complex vitamins are all engaged in energy metabolism, amino acid, and antioxidant activity. On the contrary, fat-soluble vitamins , such as vitamins A, D, E, and K, are needed for uses , such as vision, bone growth, and blood coagulation. Health condition is important in the metabolism of these vitamins since deficiency can lead to some health disorders. Understanding the metabolic pathways of vitamins can be beneficial in comprehending nutritional needs and shaping food choices in order to achieve certain health outcomes. In addition, pharmacological therapy interactss with vitamin metabolism, requiring attention, that is, how certain drugs affect nutrient intake and metabolism. An example is medications like proton pump inhibitors (PPIs) and non-steroidal anti-inflammatory drugs (NSAIDs), which have the potential to interfere with the metabolism of critical nutrients, causing deficiencies. Evidence indicates that long-term use of such drugs is responsible for low blood levels of vital vitamins , such as B12 and calcium, which are crucial in various bodily processes (Geetha et al., 2025). This relationship emphasizes the significance of having medical personnel monitor patients for potential vitamin deficiency, especially when they are on drugs that can adversely affect nutrient metabolism. Both healthcare providers and pharmacists play a key role in advising patients regarding supplementation of nutrients and diet modifications to prevent such risks. Vitamin complexity in metabolism is also applied to its interaction with physical and mental well-being and linking deficiency with asthenia. Asthenia, or fatigue, along with diminished energy levels, can result from inadequate vitamins, particularly in chronic diseases or those with long-term medication intake. These kinds of conditions can also further enhance micronutrient imbalances, therefore complicating symptom control (Torshin et al., 2024). Metabolism of vitamins is hence important not just for health but also for enhancing the quality of patients with chronic diseases. A personalized strategy addressing both metabolic pathways and individual health needs can lead to more effective intervention and patient outcome improvement, stressing the inseparable link between micronutrient metabolism and overall well-being (Figure 3.11).

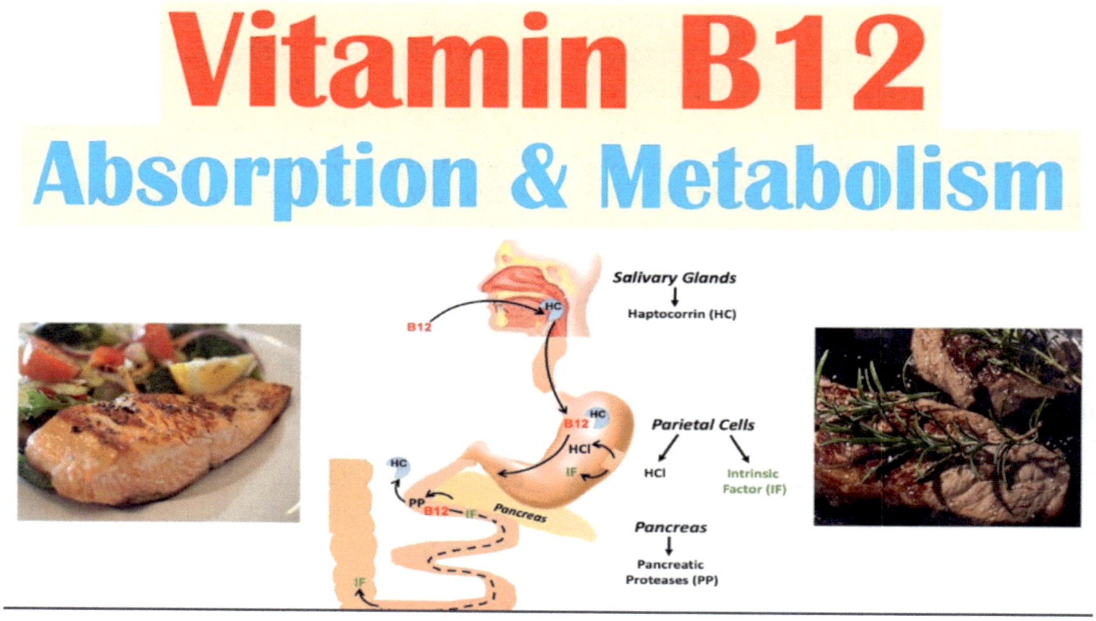

Figure 3.11. Pathway of vitamin B12 absorption and metabolism from dietary sources to intestinal uptake.

Source: https://external-content.duckduckgo.com/iu/?u=https%3A%2F%2Fi.ytimg.com%2Fvi%2FXbVX-s1t9_8%2Fmaxresdefault.jpg&f=1&nofb=1&ipt=9e70cff6b3d060d373ca23d808e27f59a61af996bdd114a69890c9c6b9c385ee.

3.4.1. Conversion of Vitamins to Active Forms

The metabolic conversion of vitamins to their biologically active forms is a critical aspect of micronutrient metabolism and contributes greatly to human health. The majority of vitamins are not biologically active in their food state; they must go through some biochemical conversions before they can be utilized within the body. Vitamin A, for instance, is synthesized from provitamin A carotenoids, which are common in plant foods, and must be converted to retinol to exert its physiological functions. Also, the B-vitamins, of major importance to energy metabolism, protein synthesis, and neural function, require enzymic conversions to be able to be transformed into their active coenzyme forms, e.g., thiamine pyrophosphate (B1) and pyridoxal phosphate (B6). Elucidation of these mechanisms of conversion becomes essential in the planning of interventions to treat vitamin deficiency, particularly as populations worldwide struggle with elusive hunger, where vitamin deficiencies persist even with caloric abundance (Strobbe et al., 2018). Biofortification represents a significant step in solving micronutrient deficiencies, particularly through enhancing the bioavailability of vitamins in terms of genetic and agricultural interventions. Biofortification involves the intentional alteration of the plants' natural metabolic processes to increase vitamin production. For example, through the application of biotechnology techniques, scientists aim at enhancing the yield of major B-vitamins in food staples, thus making the plant a more concentrated form of these micronutrients. With scientific research illuminating the complex biosynthetic pathways of these vitamins, , such as that of folate (B9), this paves the way for an integrated approach to the management of effective biofortification programs. Apart from attempting to reverse the tide of micronutrient deficiency diseases prevalent in developing countries, such success also highlights the need to embrace sustainable agricultural farming practices that are compatible with local food habits and health requirements (Blancquaert et al., 2016). The relationship between biofortification and vitamin conversion says more about the global nutrition strategies. While the final vitamin concentration in food can be optimized by biofortification, it is equally important to recognize the physiological pathways of converting such vitamins into action. As varied populations would include varied metabolic efficiencies based on genes and environments, the effectiveness of biofortified crops could vary widely among individuals. Accordingly, well-designed nutritional interventions based on these metabolic variations are required for optimal health benefits. At the same time, nutrition education regarding the importance of dietary diversity instead of sole reliance on biofortified foods will remain essential for achieving long-term micronutrient sufficiency. Lastly, an integrated approach of scientific intelligence, agricultural technology, and public health interventions is the only means to counter existing micronutrient metabolism problems among various populations (Blancquaert et al., 2016; Strobbe et al., 2018).

3.4.2. Role of Coenzymes in Metabolic Pathways

The role of coenzymes in metabolic pathways is key to the optimal functioning of many enzymatic reactions, particularly those involving micronutrients. Coenzymes are organic non-protein molecules that serve as integral cofactors needed for biochemical transformations. In metabolic pathways, they participate in redox reactions, and it becomes imperative for the conversion of substrates to products. For example, riboflavin, or vitamin B2, is converted to flavin mononucleotide (FMN) and flavin adenine dinucleotide (FAD), the coenzymes of most of the important enzymatic reactions, primarily in energy metabolism. As agents of electron transfer, they are vital in cellular respiration and in fatty acid oxidation. Thus, the availability of these coenzymes directly influences metabolic efficiency and energy production, and their importance is palpable in the overall context of micronutrient metabolism. An appreciation of coenzyme function in its totality is of great importance in the analysis of metabolic disorders resulting from micronutrient deficiency. Disorders , such as ariboflavinosis, which are caused by insufficient consumption of riboflavin, disrupt metabolic pathways that are greatly reliant on its coenzyme derivatives. This deficiency may impair metabolic activities by inhibiting the activity of central enzymes that are involved in energy formation and nutrient processing, ultimately triggering a series of wellness issues, including impaired growth, weakened immunity, and increased susceptibility to long-term illness. Additionally, it is advancing knowledge of coenzyme interactions in metabolic pathways that unlock doors for potential therapeutic interventions aimed at the correction of micronutrient deficiencies. By supplementing diets with coenzymes or their precursor vitamins, to some extent, it may be possible to relieve some of the undesirable health effects that arise from metabolic dysfunction. In addition to what they do for energy metabolism, coenzymes are also critical in a wide variety of anabolic and catabolic pathways. Coenzymes feature prominently in the biosynthesis of essential biomolecules like nucleotides and amino acids, highlighting their multifaceted contributions to cellular metabolism. For instance, during pig husbandry, optimal amounts of riboflavin are needed for best growth and health, with specific nutritional recommendations prescribed to ensure optimal supply at different stages of growth (Shastak and Pelletier, 2024). The dynamism of the metabolic processes equally illustrates coenzymes' function as significant crossroads, at the same time orchestrating a multitude of biochemical transactions. Last but not least, it is of paramount importance to comprehend the nonenzymatic interaction and micronutrient availability to formulate sound nutritional interventions that may enhance metabolic health and induce well-being among human and animal populations. The evidence gathered through studies, for instance, on post-bariatric surgery alterations (Dadson et al., 2025), highlights the importance of coenzymes in adaptive metabolic alterations and improvement, issuing an evidence-based call to action for their pivotal role in micronutrient metabolism (Figure 3.12).

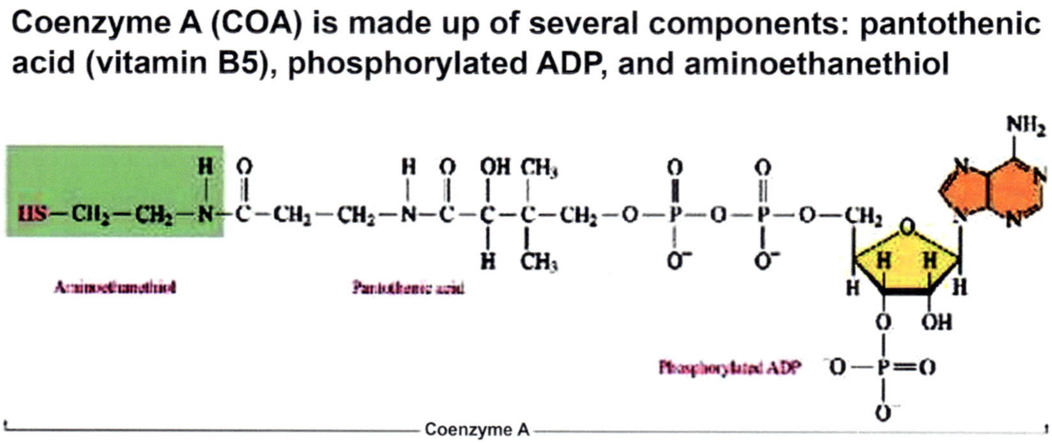

Figure 3.12. Structure of Coenzyme A showing its key components: Amino ethanethiol, pantothenic acid, and phosphorylated ADP.

Source: https://external-content.duckduckgo.com/iu/?u=https%3A%2F%2Fslidetodoc.com%2Fpresentation_image%2F57ad36dc938ea1935526e453361b1ac2%2Fimage-1.jpg&f=1&nofb=1&ipt=359ec2af872839ca9f7f2c38eea5e124a3b41b8dd3a0305d35fd94ddeea37965.

3.4.3. Effects of Deficiencies on Metabolic Processes

The role of micronutrients in the process of metabolism is thus crucial, as lack can lead to severe disruption of various biochemical reactions. For example, vitamins C and B-complex are pivotal to energy production because they serve as coenzymes in essential reactions that yield ATP. Deficiency in these micronutrients can disrupt cellular respiration, leading to a state of energy deficit typical of fatigue and impaired mental functioning. Apart from that, a few minerals like zinc and magnesium are needed for the activation of enzymes in metabolic activities. Their deficiency might lower the metabolic level, which may result in decreased thermogenesis and increased fat storage. Therefore, it is essential to comprehend the complex influence of micronutrient deficiencies on metabolic activity in designing effective dietary measures for overall wellness and metabolic function. Micronutrient deficiency not only impacts metabolism but also has far-reaching health consequences that can further exacerbate already existing conditions. The example of vitamin D deficiency and metabolic syndrome is a good example of such an impact. Vitamin D is an active agent in calcium metabolism, immune function, and insulin sensitivity. A deficiency in this nutrient has been associated with increased risk of type 2 diabetes, obesity, and cardiovascular disease. Concurrently, research indicates that micronutrient deficiencies may also reduce the body's ability to combat oxidative stress, leading to increased levels of reactive oxygen species and further causing impairment of metabolic functions. With these deficiencies becoming increasingly prevalent, especially in developing nations, they become an immediate public health concern that requires immediate action in the form of replenishing satisfactory levels of micronutrients among the populations. Strategies against micronutrient deficiency have spurred new methods, , such as food fortification and biofortification. The focus of such efforts is to enhance the nutrient value of staple foods, in the long run, a measure to counteract the risks of dietary deficiency. Biofortification employs many of the advances in plant biotechnology and applies them to increase the nutrient density of foods, which in turn provides a sustainable solution to improving nutritional status in low dietary diversity populations (Blancquaert et al., 2016). Similarly, fortification of common foods has been found useful in reducing deficiencies in developed countries; however, unequal access remains a problem, most significantly in rural and impoverished populations. Despite such advancements, prudence is necessary because evidence exists of adverse health impacts of excessive levels of vitamin supplementation among certain populations (Combet & Buckton, 2014). Solutions to micronutrient deficiencies require not only innovative farming but also sweeping public education initiatives regarding the importance of consuming a nutritionally well-balanced diet (Figure 3.13).

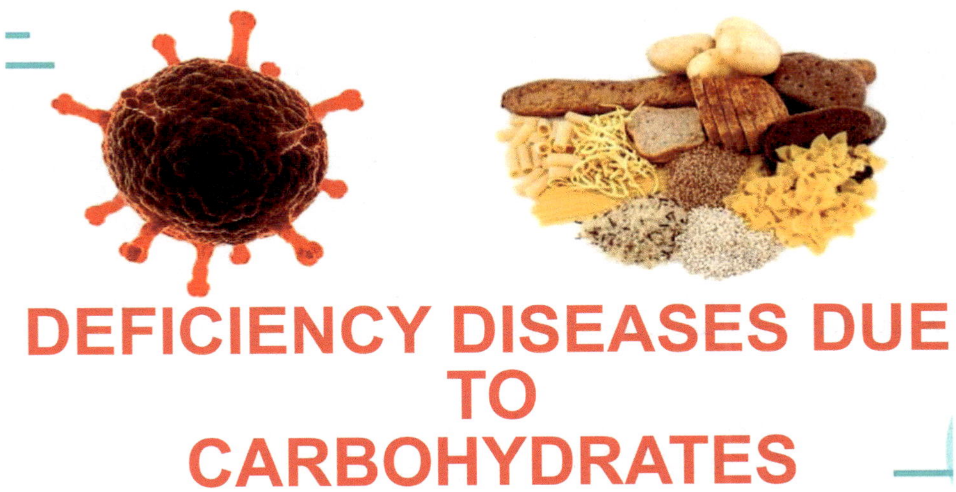

Figure 3.13. Carbohydrate deficiency and its link to related diseases.

Source:

3.5. Metabolism of Minerals

Mineral metabolism is a complex and critical part of human health, with very important influences on a number of physiological processes. Minerals , such as calcium, phosphorus, magnesium, and trace minerals are essential for attaining homeostasis, bone integrity, and cellular processes. Calcium and phosphorus, in particular, are of extreme importance for bone tissue mineralization, with vitamin D occupying a central regulatory position in this regard. The interaction of these minerals and vitamin D is quite significant, especially in the case of diseases , such as osteoporosis and osteoarthritis. Evidence shows that vitamin D affects the physiological activity of bone cells immediately, achieving good calcium-phosphorus homeostasis, necessary for overall metabolic activity and bone health (Sokolova et al., 2024). Consequently, an understanding of the precise mechanisms of mineral metabolism is crucial for developing useful therapeutic interventions to act against the consequences of mineral deficiency and associated diseases. In addition to calcium and phosphorus, fibroblast growth factor 23 (FGF23) has also been recognized as a significant regulator of mineral metabolism, particularly phosphorus homeostasis. As a key moderator of phosphatonin metabolism, FGF23 regulates phosphate levels within the body, demonstrating the enmeshed relationship of mineral and hormonal control. Its significance appears in children and adults alike, because the mechanisms for preserving mineral balance are greatly disparate by age. For example, in children, accurate mineral metabolism is vital for growth and development, particularly since they undergo endochondral ossification, a process of mineralizing long bones (Pons-Belda et al., 2023). The influence of FGF23 on vitamin D metabolism in children remains to be investigated extensively, but it is a relevant area that requires more studies, especially of conditions like rickets or chronic kidney disease, which interfere with normal mineral homeostasis.

The effects of disturbances in mineral metabolism are far-reaching and demand an integrative approach to micronutrient health. A lack of vital minerals like calcium and phosphorus can lead to osteoporosis, and trace element imbalance can disrupt enzymatic functions and metabolic activities in the body. For instance, a deficiency of vitamin D has been linked to defective calcium absorption, causing adverse effects on bone mineral density and skeletal status. As the mechanisms in mineral metabolism become better understood, it is important to integrate this knowledge into nutritional advice and clinical practice. Moreover, information from the genetic polymorphisms, including those affecting vitamin D receptor (VDR) activity, will be able to account for susceptibility of individuals to mineral disorders, thereby informing individualized dietary and therapeutic interventions on the basis of optimal micronutrient metabolism (Sokolova et al., 2024) (Figure 3.14).

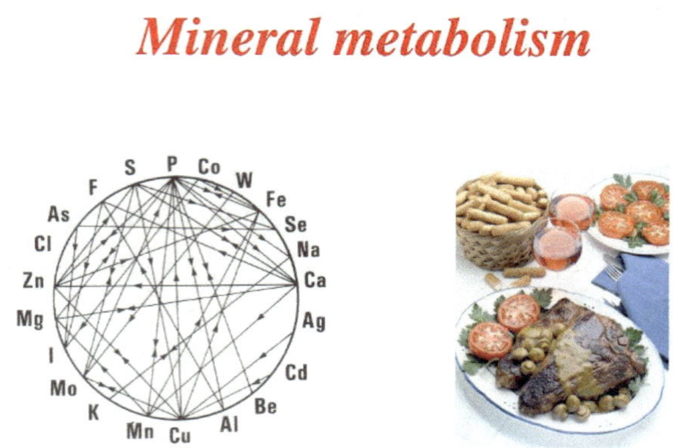

Figure 3.14. Diagram of mineral metabolism and dietary sources of essential minerals.

Source: https://external-content.duckduckgo.com/iu/?u=https%3A%2F%2Fimage2.slideserve.com%2F4493349%2Fmineral-metabolism-l.jpg&f=1&nofb=1&ipt=eebb6ae3c855ecbbbd3e33f727ee6a8a3a1596c23c6a049ff1ee3e9a22b3b8e2.

3.5.1. Bioavailability and Utilization of Minerals

Bioavailability is an important term used in mineral metabolism because it informs us of the extent to which minerals as a nutrient class are available for absorption and use by the body. Various factors influence mineral bioavailability, including food composition, the presence of inhibitors or enhancers, and certain physiological states. For instance, certain food fibers and plant phytates might be able to bind minerals like iron and zinc and reduce their absorption. Conversely, vitamin C is able to enhance iron absorption, illustrating the multifaceted relationship between dietary constituents in micronutrient metabolism. Given that contemporary diets emphasize convenience over nutrition, the role of bioavailability is more critical than ever, particularly in terms of creating deficiencies and their resulting health implications, which are increasingly being overlooked in the controversy surrounding modern dietary patterns (Combet & Buckton, 2014). The gut microbiota and its role in mineral bioavailability are a new area of research that underscores the complexity of micronutrient metabolism. Previous research has revealed that gut commensal microbes can significantly influence the absorption of key minerals , such as calcium, iron, and magnesium.

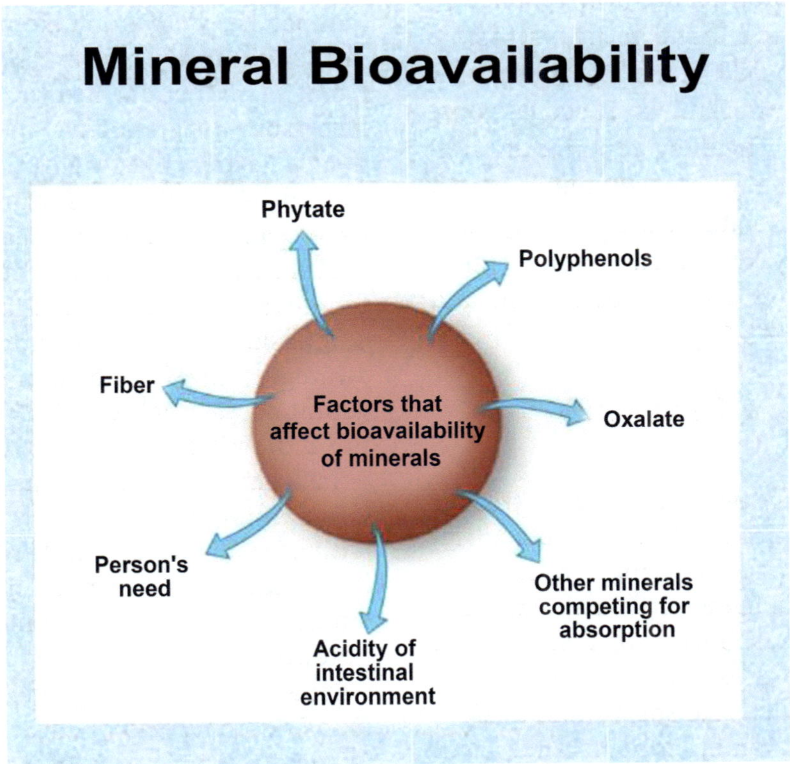

Figure 3.15. Key factors affecting mineral bioavailability in the body.

Source: https://external-content.duckduckgo.com/iu/?u=https%3A%2F%2Fimage3.slideserve.com%2F6173860%2Fmineral-bioavailability2-l.jpg&f=1&nofb=1&ipt=35ef9d3d053353b225b761c8cea38aa611794741df4d97c301ab083849b6cbf8.

The microbes are implicated in the biosynthetic pathways of certain vitamins and play a role in modulating the environment of the gastrointestinal tract, which affects the overall mineral absorption efficiency (Barone et al., 2022). This correlation implies that a healthy gut microbiome is not only vital for the absorption of nutrients but potentially for maximum utilization of minerals as well, thereby for general well-being and overall health. Such a finding invites more exploration into the possibility of how intervention through diet, like probiotics and prebiotics, could be a feasible option of maximizing mineral bioavailability. Maintenance of bioavailability and mineral utilization depends upon an integrated process involving diet, intestinal function, and lifestyle. In deficiency states, individually tailored interventions that combine nutrition education with microbiome-targeted regimens may become effective means of optimizing mineral absorption and preventing chronic disease. Further, understanding the interaction between mineral consumption balanced against bioavailability allows improved decision making in supplement versus whole food intake. Since over-reliance on supplements has been found to have possible ill effects like increased mortality and cancer risk among some groups, the most secure route to micronutrient sufficiency remains a well-diversified, nutritionally sufficient diet (Combet & Buckton, 2014). Healthy ways of integrating these findings may transform public health practice into micronutrient metabolism and optimization (Figure 3.15).

3.5.2. Interactions Between Different Minerals

These interactions between the different minerals play a significant role in the metabolism of micronutrients, and they affect absorption and bioavailability in living organisms. Calcium, magnesium, and phosphorus, for instance, are not only crucial to most body processes but also control each other's absorption. Excessive consumption of calcium, for instance, will inhibit magnesium and zinc absorption, which will lead to deficiencies of these nutrients. Such competition between minerals elucidates the importance of equal dietary intake. These interactions have to be considered, especially when talking about the nutritional adequacy of diets, as they can directly affect physiological well-being. A harmonious strategy of diet, taking such interactions into account, is indispensable in preventing micronutrient deficiency owing to inappropriate dietary practices or uncontrolled supplementation, as evidenced in the phenomenon of hidden hunger among hundreds of millions of individuals globally (Combet & Buckton, 2014). Moreover, the comprehension of synergistic and antagonistic interactions among minerals also accounts for the process of micronutrient metabolism in terms of its multifaceted nature. Certain minerals can interact to enable others to be absorbed, for example, vitamin C increases iron absorption by a tremendous amount. Conversely, high levels of one mineral can inhibit the absorption of another, , such as too much iron which can hamper the body's uptake of copper. Not only are such interactions clinically important from an individual health point of view, but also from a perspective of addressing public health issues like malnutrition and dietary illness. Mineral interaction complicates the development of dietary guidelines for optimal health because raising the intake of one nutrient tends to accumulate and affect others, thus emphasizing the role of integrated nutritional strategies to evaluate mineral intake in sum (Combet & Buckton, 2014). The potential for biofortification, which is applied for the enhancement of nutrient quality in staple foods, is an innovative approach to address issues with mineral interaction. Through this approach, optimization of the micronutrient content in staple crops , such as zinc and iron, could potentially offset deficiencies in consumers whose diets consist predominantly of these foods. Effective biofortification does require a nuanced understanding of the dynamics between minerals within the plant and its biochemical processes, particularly how one mineral affects another's uptake and function. Studies suggest that enhancing a single micronutrient, for example, by increasing zinc concentrations, may actually have some unforeseen effects on other minerals' bioavailability, making extensive studies of plant metabolism necessary. Having knowledge of such concepts, we can engineer crops not only to combat mineral deficiencies but also to maintain overall health through ensuring an even mix of minerals in the body, thus alleviating the problem of hidden hunger that plagues billions of people globally (Strobbe et al., 2018).

3.5.3. Consequences of Mineral Imbalances

The impacts of mineral imbalance are extensive and cumulative, with consequences on human health as well as crop and food production. In human nutrition, shortages of essential minerals , such as calcium, magnesium, and iron may lead to debilitating health issues , such as osteoporosis, anemia, and neuromuscular disorders. Research has also established that sub chronic manganese excess exposure worsens such imbalances to reduce the body's levels of required microelements, , such as potassium and copper, as confirmed by experiments conducted on Wistar rats fed with manganese-rich diets. This accumulation of manganese not only replaces these minerals but also damages the normal physiological functions, indicating the urgent need for a perfect balance of mineral intake to ensure overall well-being and metabolic functions (Kazakova et al., 2024).

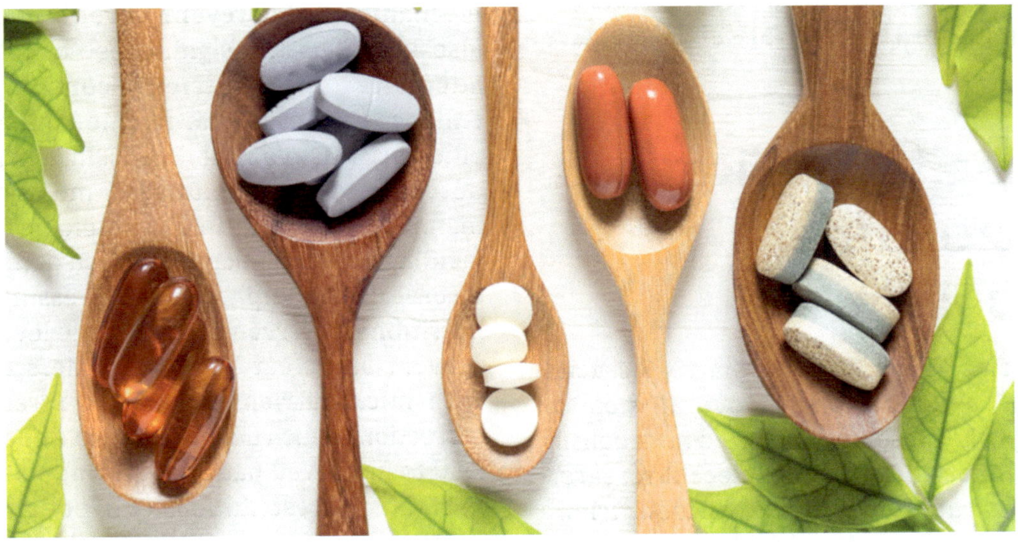

Figure 3.16. Common forms of mineral and vitamin supplements.

Source: https://external-content.duckduckgo.com/iu/?u=https%3A%2F%2Fdrvictorchan.com%2Fwp-content%2Fuploads%2F2023%2F08%2FMineral-Imbalances-A.png&f=1&nofb=1&ipt=9011bf4ff721e8d8875df6eb9b2c66f8ce49fdfe1475ac8948437a9aa2533920.

In agricultural systems, mineral imbalances pose serious disadvantages to growth of crops and nutrition status. Over-reliance on fertilizers, particularly in developing regions, usually prioritizes macronutrient application to the neglect of vital micronutrients. This deficiency, which has been documented in African soil conditions across various regions, , such as Ethiopia, results in extreme deficiencies of vital elements , such as zinc, boron, and copper. Not only are these dangerous to plant development and sustainability, but they also have an impact on human nutrition through the quality of staple foods. The inability of agriculture to regulate micronutrient levels effectively reveals a greater issue of food security because low nutrient content in crops can ultimately aggravate malnutrition among those who base their diet on such crops (Lowe et al., 2024).

Furthermore, the implications of the environmental effects of mineral imbalances cannot be overlooked. Soil erosion and over-farming, driven by the need for higher agricultural productivity, lead to the loss of micronutrients from the soil. The loss is not only an agricultural problem but has ecological implications too, as nutrient-rich soils play a crucial role in the conservation of biodiversity and ecosystem processes. Nutrient imbalance cascades can destabilize food webs and reduce the climate change resilience of agriculture. Accordingly, resolving such imbalances involves an integrated approach that interweaves human dietary requirements and environmentally sustainable agricultural practice, reconstructing the balance of minerals in soil and human health in order to secure a healthier future (Lowe et al., 2024) (Figure 3.16).

3.6. Health Implications of Micronutrient Metabolism

Micronutrient metabolism plays a very crucial role in the enhancement of overall health, particularly when it comes to thyroid metabolism and other endocrine disorders. Recent research has demonstrated that some micronutrient deficiencies , such as vitamin B12 and ferritin, have profound health implications, particularly in people with hypothyroidism. For instance, a case-control study identified that TSH was found to be elevated together with low levels of T4 in patients afflicted with hypothyroidism, with correlations between deficiencies in these micronutrients. The finding demonstrates the importance of assessing micronutrient status in patients with thyroid dysfunction to optimize their management and treatment protocols. Thus, the inclusion of routine micronutrient testing in practice can lead to more targeted interventions that address the underlying metabolic imbalance affecting thyroid function and overall health (Adam et al., 2025). The interplay between micronutrient metabolism and cardiometabolic health is becoming more widely regarded as key to understanding systemic health effects. Water T2 measurement as a metabolic balance biosensor, along with other predictive factors , such as age, body mass index (BMI), and pulse rate, has also been found to be promising in the evaluation of cardiometabolic health outcomes. Studies have established a close relationship between plasma water T2 and metabolic status, revealing that alterations in micronutrient metabolism directly influence cardiovascular and metabolic systems. This synergy between cardiometabolic markers and micronutrient status does not only illuminate mechanisms to prevent chronic disease but also identifies the significance of maintaining adequate micronutrient consumption to enhance cardiovascular function and metabolic efficiency (Cistola et al., 2025). In general, health outcomes of micronutrient metabolism are manifested via multiple physiological systems, yielding a direct linkage between deficiency and disease. They emphasize the pressing need for nutritional interventions at clinic levels to help prevent and treat health disorders associated with micronutrient deficiency. Screening and correction of such deficiencies have been found to lead to improved patient outcomes, particularly in complex presentations of hypothyroidism or cardiovascular disease. Ultimately, the interplay of micronutrients within metabolic processes reiterates the value of an orderly approach to health, with attention to prevention via extensive dietary analysis and individualized supplementation protocols to ensure maximum health and well-being among populations (Adam et al., 2025; Cistola et al., 2025).

3.6.1. Contribution to Health Promotion and Disease Prevention

Micronutrients play a crucial role in the prevention of disease and enhancement of health, influencing overall health and life expectancy. The shift in paradigms in nutritional science from merely preventing deficiency to maximizing health suggests this rising awareness. Specifically, vitamins and minerals influence physiological functions to minimize the risk of age-related chronic diseases. For instance, the lack of essential micronutrients has been linked with increased susceptibility to diseases , such as osteoporosis, intellectual impairment, and cardiovascular illnesses. With rising life expectancy, the need for adequate micronutrient intake acquires even greater significance, justifying the close link between diet, health condition, and healthy aging. This dynamic tale highlights how essential nutrients can protect against the body's changes that occur with age, focusing on their protective functions as dietary and lifestyle factors have more powerful roles in determining health alterations through time (Harris, 2012). Further, a few of the micronutrients are pivotal in specific metabolic pathways that control the body and maintain health.

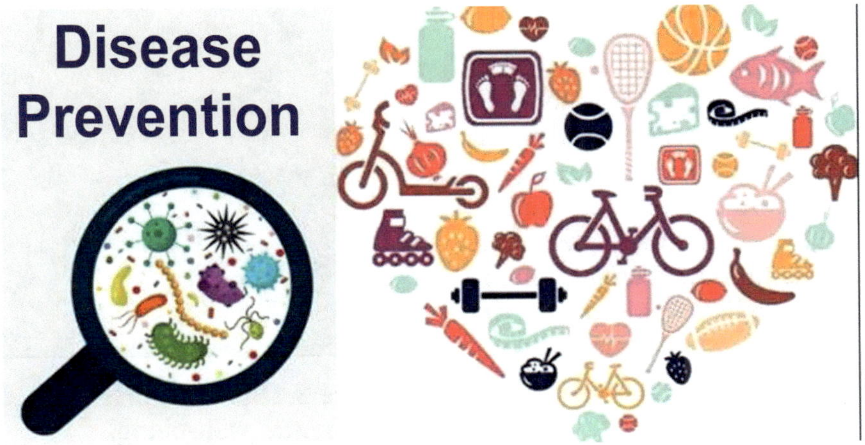

Figure 3.17. Promoting disease prevention through healthy lifestyle habits.

Source: https://external-content.duckduckgo.com/iu/?u=https%3A%2F%2Frn-journal.com%2Fimages%2Fcontent%2FHealthPromotionandDiseasePrevention-content_header_image-671.webp&f=1&nofb=1&ipt=eb2b9cf7296a091ce4ca731937dee34b54b7e8272e5fa1f75c5e8da0c8343073.

For example, B-vitamins play important roles in homocysteine metabolism, and folate and B12 deficiency have been found to be associated with homocysteine increase, a well-documented risk factor for cardiovascular disease. Antioxidant vitamins E and C, and dietary fats, have been suggested for cognitive function and the avoidance of neurodegenerative diseases, notably in vulnerable groups like the elderly. Evidence for such relationships highlights the essential role of micronutrients not only in facilitating physiological homeostasis but also in the modulation of chronic disease risk by mechanisms , such as oxidative stress reduction and inflammation. Later, understanding the preventive function of single micronutrients forms the basis of nutrition-driven strategies to enhance health and longevity (Anderson et al., 2011). This day's discussion of micronutrients further emphasizes their role in health promotion activities extending beyond individual dietary choice-making to the broader public health concerns. Initiatives dedicated to increasing micronutrient intake through food fortification and nutrition education reflect greater appreciation of the importance of adequate nutrient intake to population health. For instance, interventions targeting the supplementation of vitamins D and C and minerals like calcium and iron have been of interest due to their potential in improving the overall wellbeing of vulnerable populations. These interventions are imperative in addressing the conditions of public health issues like malnutrition, which compound the rates of chronic diseases. By integrating micronutrient considerations into health promotion programs, stakeholders can facilitate healthier communities and demonstrate that the strategic use of micronutrients in dietary habits is essential to disease prevention and successful health promotion (Harris, 2012) (Figure 3.17).

3.6.2. Impact of Deficiencies on Public Health

The impact of micronutrient deficiency on public health encompasses a wide range of physiological and societal consequences that can significantly hinder population wellbeing. An example is vitamin D deficiency, which affects skeletal health by compromising calcium and phosphate metabolism as well as immune regulation and susceptibility to chronic diseases. A number of studies have indicated correlations of low vitamin D levels with increased risk of autoimmune diseases, cardiovascular diseases, and metabolic disease , such as type 2 diabetes. Vitamin D deficiency remains a global problem, particularly within urban populations with restricted sun exposure and poor dietary vitamin D status, again emphasizing the need for public health interventions that encourage safe sun exposure as well as targeted supplementation measures that can effectively counteract such deficiencies (Ański et al., 2025). Likewise, the effects of zinc deficiency present a significant public health issue, particularly in developing nations where intake through diet is inadequate. Zinc is needed for numerous metabolic and physiological processes including immune function, growth, and cell maintenance. Five-year-old and younger children are particularly vulnerable since zinc deficiency is responsible for increased morbidity and mortality through greater vulnerability to disease and growth failure. The extensive impacts of zinc deficiency demand immediate action, and supplementary interventions, food fortification, and biofortification emerge as integral components of broader public health initiatives. These interventions can prevent the disabling health effects of zinc deficiency, resulting in healthier populations and reduced disease burden (Ciampo et al., 2024). Correcting micronutrient deficiencies is not only good for the health of individuals but also for societal health and economic well-being.

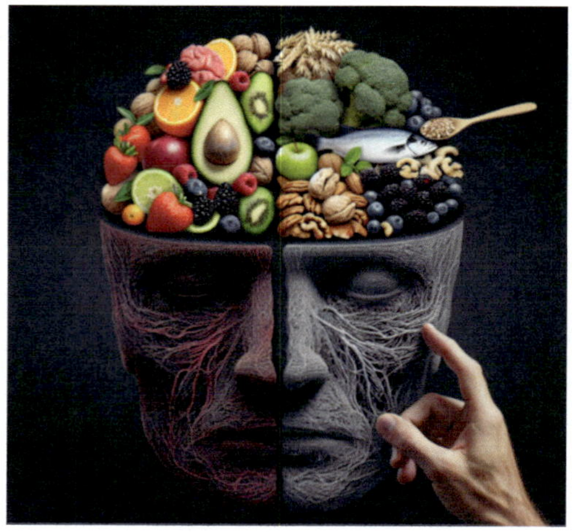

Figure 3.18. Nutrition's impact on brain health and mental well-being.

Source: https://external-content.duckduckgo.com/iu/?u=https%3A%2F%2Fmindfulharmonyoasis.com%2Fwp-content%2Fuploads%2F2024%2F05%2Fthe-impact-of-nutritional-deficiencies-on-mental-health-_pic-1-1024x585.png&f=1&nofb=1&ipt=93f3a957dc51654b93383d880604feeb32c122c3bb8a775b5fb8d79dfbed64a0.

The interplay between public health and micronutrient deficiencies is characterized by a complex matrix of causal determinants, including socio-economic status, diet, and healthcare access. For instance, deficit populations end up with higher healthcare costs and impaired workforce productivity due to illness and disability, representing significant economic burdens. Public health interventions must assume a multi-faceted approach to tackling such issues, , such as concerted action toward improved dietary diversity, food security, and awareness about micronutrients. Through the use of specific interventions, it is guaranteed that the widespread prevalence of micronutrient deficiencies is addressed, ultimately resulting in healthier societies and more sustainable economies (Ciampo et al., 2024; Sobi Ański et al., 2025) (Figure 3.18).

3.6.3. Importance of Micronutrient Supplementation

In global nutrition, micronutrient supplementation has emerged as an essential intervention for the control of disease-inducing deficiency and for general well-being. Vitamins and minerals are important micronutrients for many biochemical functions, but they are often consumed in insufficient quantities in most populations. The importance of micronutrient supplementation is especially real when one examines the effects of deficiency, including compromised immune function, growth stunting in children, and enhanced vulnerability to chronic illness. Zinc, for example, one of the most fundamental micronutrients, has a many-faceted role in physiological processes, from immune function to the regulation of glucose metabolism. These points emphasize the need to combat micronutrient deficiencies with effective supplementation efforts to improve health outcomes on a worldwide scale, not only personal health but also public health concerns regarding nutrition. Supplementation with zinc, especially, has been identified as universally relevant for overall health, given that zinc affects a myriad of life processes more than other micronutrients. Besides supporting child growth and immune resistance, the evidence indicates that a deficiency in zinc is correlated at a high level with diabetes and cardiometabolic disease risks. This correlation implies the potential for specific supplementation of zinc as a preventive strategy against such non-communicable diseases (NCDs). There is a broad consensus regarding zinc deficiency as a universal condition of health, yet procedures to assess zinc status at the population and individual levels are not established appropriately. Interventions to increase zinc intake, , such as supplementation, food fortification, and crop biofortification, are thus key. These interventions not only raise dietary zinc levels but also help to mitigate health disparities associated with zinc deficiency, ultimately resulting in healthier populations. The market for nutritional supplements is also affected by rising prices and declining availability of traditional nutrient ingredients, necessitating alternative ingredients being sought out. A suitable alternative is coconut, which is renowned for its better nutritional content and usability across industries, , such as animal husbandry and aquaculture. Coconut offers suitable macro and micronutrients for supplementation and the enhancement of growth and metabolic efficacy in livestock. The oil from coconuts has also been utilized to reduce greenhouse gas emissions in ruminants, in accordance with existing sustainability in agriculture. Although it holds promise, the use of coconut in bird diets is not yet common due to concerns with anti-nutritional factors. Nevertheless, the use of coconuts as inexpensive and nutrient-rich feeding material could enhance dietary diversity and resilience, a significant milestone in micronutrient supplementation programs (Mat et al., 2022; Lowe et al., 2024).

CLOSER LOOK

IMMUNE FUNCTION

Immune function refers to the body's ability to defend itself against harmful pathogens such as bacteria, viruses, fungi, and parasites. The immune system is a complex network of cells, tissues, and organs that work together to identify and eliminate threats while maintaining balance to avoid attacking the body's own cells. It is divided into two main components: innate immunity and adaptive immunity. The innate immune system is the first line of defense and includes physical barriers like the skin, as well as immune cells like neutrophils and macrophages that respond quickly to invaders. The adaptive immune system is more specialized and includes B cells, which produce antibodies, and T cells, which destroy infected or abnormal cells. This system also has "memory," allowing it to respond more effectively to pathogens it has encountered before, which is the basis for how vaccines work. Proper immune function is especially crucial during childhood, as children's immune systems are still developing. Nutrition, sleep, hygiene, physical activity, and stress levels all significantly influence immune health. Nutrients such as vitamin C, vitamin D, zinc, and protein are essential for supporting immune responses. When the immune system is weakened—due to malnutrition, illness, or medical treatments like chemotherapy—the body becomes more vulnerable to infections. Conversely, an overactive or misdirected immune system can result in autoimmune diseases, where the body attacks its own tissues. A closer look at immune function reveals that it is not only about fighting disease but also about maintaining balance and overall health. Supporting the immune system through healthy lifestyle choices, timely vaccinations, and regular medical check-ups is key to preventing illness and ensuring long-term well-being, particularly in children and other vulnerable populations.

SUMMARY

The complex role of micronutrients in metabolism suggests not only their need for maximal physiological functions but also the ruinous consequences of deficiencies. A comprehensive understanding of how micronutrients, , such as boron, affect plant physiology may create possibilities for improving crop yield and solving food insecurity issues. The findings from the transcriptome and proteome analysis of tobacco seedlings indicate that boron deficiency triggers extreme morphological and physiological changes, emphasizing the necessity for adequate micronutrient supply for growth and development (Lin et al., 2024). These findings are not only significant for enhancing agricultural cultivation but also for developing targeted interventions to counter micronutrient deficiencies in varied ecosystems. Further, the effect extends to human health, where micronutrient status has a major impact on performance and recovery, particularly in high-demand environments , such as military training. The reported decline in vitamin D and iron status among Marine Officer Candidates underscores the importance of monitoring micronutrient availability to optimize skeletal health and minimize injury risk during periods of high physical stress (Sekel et al., 2024). Such linking of micronutrient intake and effectiveness of operations emphasizes the importance of adequate nutrition in sustaining physical ability and overall health, particularly in populations undergoing rigorous training regimens. Ultimately, the study of micronutrient metabolism constitutes a focal nexus among agriculture, human well-being, and prevention. Intervention to address these dietary shortages offers potential for agricultural practice reform as well as public health. Knowledge gained from research on micronutrient responses, , such as those of boron in tobacco and the impact of vitamin D and iron in the military setting, can be leveraged to make decisions about strategies for improving micronutrient delivery systems. Encouraging interdisciplinary efforts between scientists, policymakers, and practitioners is therefore critical to contribute towards developing sustainable solutions that have the potential to advance crop productivity and human health and thereby provide a robust nutrition foundation for years to come.

To comprehend the intricacies of micronutrient metabolism, it is important to note the roles of some micronutrients, such as,, such as copper, vitamins A and D, to be mentioned among them, pertaining specifically to animal health and development. It was discovered that the transfer of the said micronutrients from the placenta and colostrum to piglets is very limited, hence the necessity for supplementation through diet. Supplementing sows with these essential nutrients in their diets or to lactating suckling piglets aims to enhance antioxidant metabolism, immunity, and microbiota development. However, research indicates that while such practices are capable of upwardly modulating micronutrient status in lactation, their impacts on oxidative stress responses and gut microbiota appear negligible on suckling and post-weaned piglets. This finding demonstrates a complex interaction between micronutrient supplementation and metabolic health during times of peak growth, with implications that additional research is needed (Galiot et al., 2025). Moreover, the timing of the micronutrient supplementation relative to the weaning stress phase is crucial for maximizing health outcomes in piglets. Weaning stress has been noted in the recent literature to have significant impacts on young farm animals' metabolic status of micronutrients, antioxidative ability, and gut microbiota composition. Remarkably, results vary with birth weight, and piglets of low birth weight are most benefited with certain micronutrient supplementation, particularly in gut microbiota growth. These results highlight the importance of understanding how nutrition interacts with stress and class of birth weight to affect metabolic and physiological neonatal pig health. Therefore, such interactions can be addressed by using well-timed interventions that may lead to improved health and growth performance based on farm practice management (Galiot et al., 2025). The metabolic function of micronutrients transcends the pig, as has been shown in trials with newborn calves from in vitro fertilization (IVP). Such calves, as large and heavy at birth as they are, have altered physiological parameters that can predispose them to clinical vulnerability. Trials spanning the first 24 hours of life have shown differences in critical parameters , such as blood gases, acid-based status, and functioning of vital organs. The heightened expression of enzymes within metabolic pathways likewise implies issues related to the energetic adaptability of IVP calves to their host environment. The significance of careful surveillance and potential nutritional intervention for these IVP calves is of utmost concern, particularly during the transition periods. Overall, these findings provide insight into the generalization of micronutrient metabolism in the context of neonatal vigor across various species, especially in circumstances in which there are technological advances in breeding.

References

1. Akubugwo, E. I., & Ugwuja, E. I. (2010). Impact of maternal *Helicobacter pylori* infection on trace elements (copper, iron and zinc) and pregnancy outcomes. https://core.ac.uk/download/pdf/87433.pdf (accessed on 13th June 2025).
2. Alengebawy, A., Abdelkhalek, S. T., Qureshi, S. R., & Wang, M. Q. (2021). Heavy metals and pesticides toxicity in agricultural soil and plants: Ecological risks and human health implications. *Toxics, 9*, 42–42. https://doi.org/10.3390/toxics9030042 (accessed on 13th June 2025).
3. Ali, H., Khan, E., & Ilahi, I. (2019). Environmental chemistry and ecotoxicology of hazardous heavy metals: Environmental persistence, toxicity, and bioaccumulation. *Journal of Chemistry, 2019*, 1–14. https://doi.org/10.1155/2019/6730305 (accessed on 13th June 2025).
4. Anderson, J. J. B., Garner, S. C., & Klemmer, P. (2011). Diet, nutrients, and bone health. https://www.semanticscholar.org/paper/4a9929f9c5946a1a1c45bd4577fbdb51d1f507a7 (accessed on 13th June 2025).
5. Ashwell, B. L., Baer, R., Bates, C., Berger, J., Bland, J., Brown, K., et al. (2013). Effect of zinc intake on serum/plasma zinc status in infants: A meta-analysis. https://core.ac.uk/download/9632973.pdf (accessed on 13th June 2025).
6. Dwyer, J. T., Wiemer, K. L., Dary, O., Keen, C. L., King, J. C., Miller, K. B., Philbert, M. A., Tarasuk, V., Taylor, C. L., Gaine, P. C. Jarvis, A. B., & Bailey, R. L. (2015). Fortification and health: challenges and opportunities. *Advances in nutrition (Bethesda, Md.)*, *6*(1), 124–131. https://doi.org/10.3945/an.114.007443 (accessed on 13th June 2025).
7. Ballou, E. R., Brown, A. J. P., Childers, D. S., Feldmann, J., et al. (2016). Host-imposed copper poisoning impacts fungal micronutrient acquisition during systemic *Candida albicans* infections. https://core.ac.uk/download/42130765.pdf (accessed on 13th June 2025).
8. Ballou, E. R., Brown, A. J. P., Childers, D. S., Potrykus, J., et al. (2014). Conflicting interests in the pathogen-host tug of war: Fungal micronutrient scavenging versus mammalian nutritional immunity. https://core.ac.uk/download/25497401.pdf (accessed on 13th June 2025).
9. Barone, M., Brigidi, P., D'Amico, F., & Turroni, S. (2022). Gut microbiome–micronutrient interaction: The key to controlling the bioavailability of minerals and vitamins? https://core.ac.uk/download/591963739.pdf (accessed on 13th June 2025).
10. Beane, K. E., Cicalo, C., Jeon, S., Kim, J., et al. (2021). Effects of dietary fibers, micronutrients, and phytonutrients on gut microbiome: A review. https://core.ac.uk/download/636391264.pdf (accessed on 13th June 2025).
11. Blancquaert, D., De Steur, H., Gellynck, X., Van Der Straeten, D., et al. (2016). Metabolic engineering of micronutrients in crop plants. https://core.ac.uk/download/84044241.pdf (accessed on 13th June 2025).
12. Dodd, F., Haskell-Ramsay, C., Jackson, P., Kennedy, D., et al. (2020). Acute and chronic effects of multivitamin/mineral supplementation on objective and subjective energy measures. https://core.ac.uk/download/305121296.pdf (accessed on 13th June 2025).

13. Donangelo, C., & King, J. (2012). Maternal zinc intakes and homeostatic adjustments during pregnancy and lactation. https://core.ac.uk/download/323080594.pdf (accessed on 13th June 2025).
14. ILO, J., & Famakinwa, A. (2022). Promoting millet, an underutilized crop. A review of food-based approach in combating micronutrient deficiency. *Revista Colombiana De Investigaciones Agroindustriales*, *9*(1), 66–78. https://doi.org/10.23850/24220582.4775/542924261.pdf (accessed on 13th June 2025).
15. Lin, J., Zheng, X., Xia, J., Xie, R., Gao, J., Ye, R., Liang, T., et al. (2024). Integrative analysis of the transcriptome and proteome reveals the molecular responses of tobacco to boron deficiency. *BMC Plant Biology, 24.* https://www.semanticscholar.org/paper/de15bf746ef0e7c69b8137ddc7634faa6adf60bf (accessed on 13th June 2025).
16. Liu, Q., Luo, D., Haase, J. E., Guo, Q., Wang, X. Q., Liu, S., Xia, L., et al. (2020). The experiences of health-care providers during the COVID-19 crisis in China: A qualitative study. *The Lancet Global Health, 8,* e790–e798. https://doi.org/10.1016/s2214-109x(20)30204-7
17. Lowe, N. M., Hall, A. G., Broadley, M. R., Foley, J., Boy, E., & Bhutta, Z. A. (2024). Preventing and controlling zinc deficiency across the life course: A call to action. *Advances in Nutrition, 15,* 100181–100181. https://doi.org/10.1016/j.advnut.2024.100181 (accessed on 13th June 2025).
18. Mat, K., Abdul Kari, Z., Rusli, N. D., Che Harun, H., Wei, L. S., Rahman, M. M., Khalid, H. N. M., et al. (2022). Coconut palm: Food, feed, and nutraceutical properties. *Animals, 12,* 2107–2107. https://doi.org/10.3390/ani12162107 (accessed on 13th June 2025).
19. Mochulska, O., Boyarchuk, O., Kinash, M., Vorontsova, T., & Volianska, L. (2021). The effects of vitamins A, E, D, disorders of their metabolism and the assessment of level of vitamin security in children (literature review). https://www.semanticscholar.org/paper/0f629341c23e0dd2ef8849a90bfadbf801dbcd44 (accessed on 13th June 2025).
20. Pons-Belda, O. D., Alonso-Álvarez, M. A., González-Rodríguez, J. D., Mantecón-Fernández, L., & Santos-Rodríguez, F. (2023). Mineral metabolism in children: Interrelation between vitamin D and FGF23. *International Journal of Molecular Sciences, 24.* https://www.semanticscholar.org/paper/26a455103ee29c91ef67f779390e0681075aee33 (accessed on 13th June 2025).
21. Shastak, Y., & Pelletier, W. (2024). Exploring the role of riboflavin in swine well-being: A literature review. *Porcine Health Management, 10.* https://www.semanticscholar.org/paper/f91fc160a68ee15bbd8521a866aca36b5679101b (accessed on 13th June 2025).
22. Sokolova, A., Berbets, O., Fediv, B., & Sokolov, B. (2024). Correction of vitamin D deficiency and the role of BsmI (rs1544410) VDR gene polymorphism in mineral metabolism related to cartilage regeneration in osteoarthritis. *Cell and Organ Transplantology.* https://www.semanticscholar.org/paper/bd0f176116e484575ac00af44fbdf530b8eee158 (accessed on 13th June 2025).
23. Wilson, R. B., Liang, Y., Kaushal, D., & Carr, A. (2024). Molecular pharmacology of vitamin C and relevance to health and obesity—A narrative review. *International Journal of Molecular Sciences, 25.* https://www.semanticscholar.org/paper/2d6b7804b3b55fcdfefb851e0c4cfc110c09f517 (accessed on 13th June 2025).

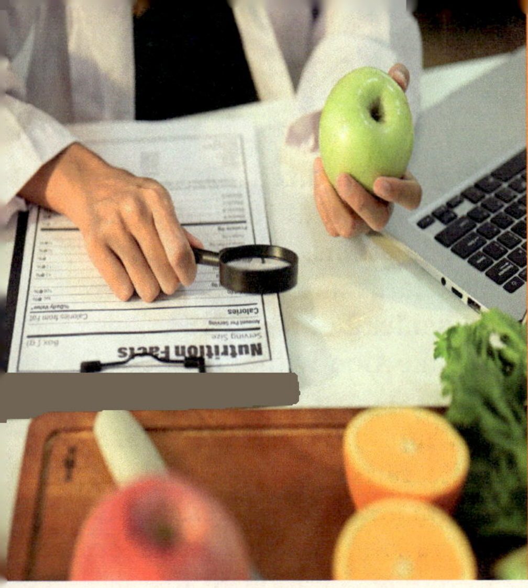

Chapter 4
NUTRITIONAL ASSESSMENT

Contents

Introduction....107
4.1. Types of Nutritional Assessment....111
4.2. Dietary Assessment Methods....115
4.3. Anthropometric Measurements....119
4.4. Biochemical Analysis....123
4.5. Factors Influencing Nutritional Status....128
4.6. Applications for Nutritional Assessment....131
Summary....137
References....139

Introduction

The contribution of nutritional assessment in health care cannot be overemphasized because it plays a critical role in the evaluation of the health status of a patient. Nutritional assessment involves a methodical process of calculating intake from diet, nutritional need, and patient health as a whole. This involves a process encompassing various techniques, including clinical evaluation, dietary questioning, biochemical assessment, and anthropometric measurements. Through the implementation of these methods, health professionals are able to identify malnutrition, deficiencies, and other nutritional problems that have an impact on overall health and enable effective interventions to be formulated. For instance, studies have shown that compliance with specific dietary regimes, , such as the Mediterranean diet, can play a significant role in altering health outcomes among various populations, including individuals with chronic illnesses like cancer (Giaginis et al., 2022), which underscores the importance of thorough nutritional assessment. An integral part of the assessment of nutrition is the measurement of nutritional status and intake using standardized tools. Mini Nutritional Assessment (MNA) is one tool that can be employed in identifying individuals at risk for malnutrition. Proof has revealed that a great majority of certain populations, , such as blind and visually impaired individuals, exhibit a linkage between nutritional status and oral health, as indicated by the number of teeth intact and total teeth functioning (Samnieng et al., 2015). This link emphasizes intervention by way of nutrition at an early stage in connection with individuals' specific states of health. Thus, utilization of quality diet assessment can come a great distance toward early detection of potential nutritional concerns, facilitating on-time and appropriate interventions that enhance patient wellness. Finally, integration of nutritional data into care plans is crucial for optimizing patient outcomes. Practitioners must interpret data obtained from nutritional assessments to create individualized nutrition care plans that address identified nutritional imbalances or deficiencies. For instance, in chronic disease-at-risk populations, the implementation of dietary modifications based on nutritional assessment can lead to improved health-related quality of life. In patients with breast cancer, adherence to diet by consuming a healthy diet is not only linked to better nutritional status but also promotes recurrence-free survival (Giaginis et al., 2022). Thus, holistic nutritional evaluation becomes essential in guiding healthcare decisions, ultimately reestablishing the role of nutrition as a vital component of disease management and prevention treatment (Figure 4.1).

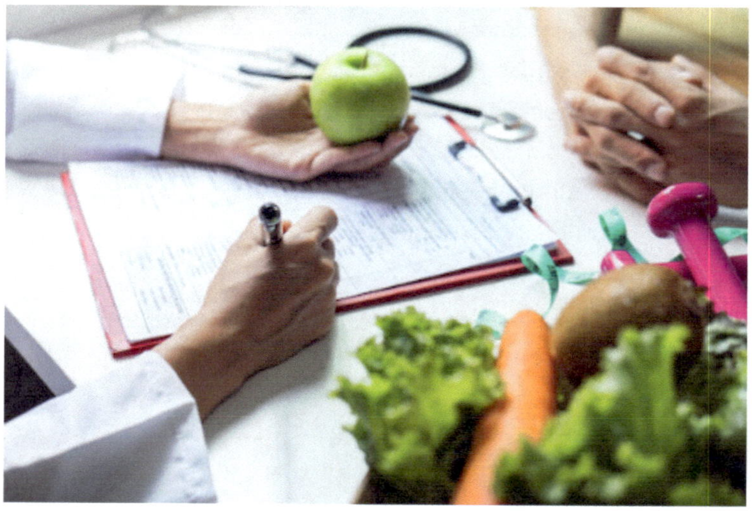

Figure 4.1. Clinical nutrition assessment and dietary counseling.

Source: https://external-content.duckduckgo.com/iu/?u=https%3A%2F%2Fwww.nursingcenter.com%2Fgetattachment%2Fcd2a74d3-6d34-45c6-8e7e-01011d98a387%2FABCDs-of-the-Nutritional-Assessment.aspx&f=1&nofb=1&ipt=d9ab927d79f98d6557281ba4a27677be3c4301840b3a9d57d12dd1d4b3fc7992.

Definition of Nutritional Assessment

Nutritional evaluation is a significant procedure employed in evaluating individuals' dietary intake, nutritional status, as well as overall health. It is a comprehensive evaluation that aims to identify deficiencies or excess of nutrients responsible for health disorders. It often employs several methods, including dietary history interviews, anthropometric measurements, biochemical tests, and clinical examinations. From the application of these methods, health professionals can gain critical information about an individual's eating habits, overall body health, and any diseases that may affect nutritional status. This information is valuable in the development of customized nutrition programs that address individual needs, enabling individuals to achieve and maintain optimal well-being. The core mandate of nutritional assessment is not only to diagnose nutritional deficits but also to provide meaningful recommendations that ensure improved health outcomes for different populations and, in the process, establish its relevance in clinical nutrition and public health practice. By way of addition, the definition of nutritional assessment extends beyond the simple appraisal and entails ongoing monitoring of nutritional status with a view to altering dietary plans accordingly.

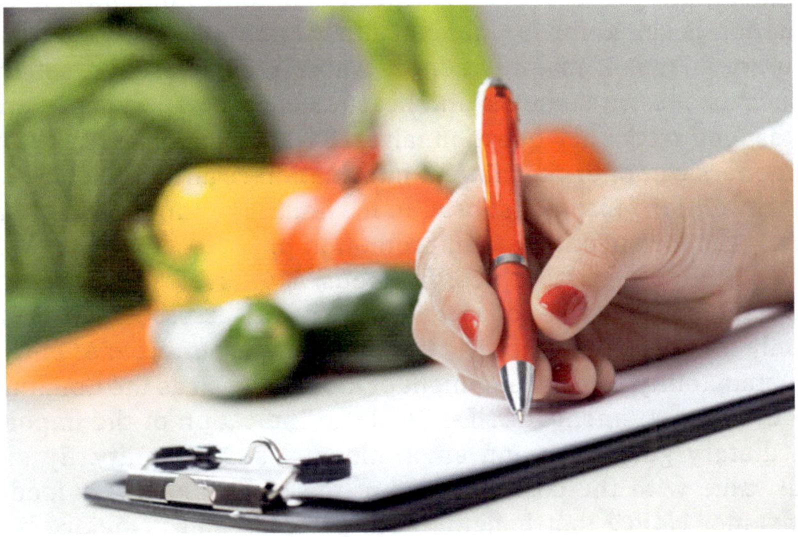

Figure 4.2. Nutritional planning with fresh vegetables.

Source: https://external-content.duckduckgo.com/iu/?u=https%3A%2F%2Fmilehighspine.com%2Fwp-content%2Fuploads%2Fnutritional_assessment.jpg&f=1&nofb=1&ipt=4443480b23c757494bdb5167e6aa995342cfe2be91f8258e8a45d5104269f927.

This dynamic relationship realizes that nutritional needs can change for varying reasons, , such as aging, disease progression, and lifestyle changes. For instance, to treat diseases , such as gastroparesis, a detailed nutritional assessment can be employed to choose appropriate dietary intervention for alleviating symptoms as well as nutrition adequacy. Experts realize that dietary management, coupled with appropriately selected pharmacologic therapies, is crucial to effectively treating such complexities (Schol et al., 2021). Continual monitoring enables timely nutritional regimen adjustment, maximizing quality of life and therapeutic effectiveness in individuals. Comprehensively, the adaptive nature of nutritional assessment resonates with the idea of personalized medicine by closely connecting dietary intervention to individual health patterns. Beyond its benefits in the clinic, nutritional assessment is a valuable asset in public health and preventive programs. By combining population-level nutritional information, health organizations are able to view widespread deficits and act accordingly. Large-scale nutritional surveys, for example, are able to determine trends of malnutrition among specific populations so targeted community-based interventions can be created to address those deficits. Furthermore, research consistently determines that nutritional status influences overall health, mental and cognitive health included (Livingston et al., 2020). Thus, achieving nutritional needs through the use of efficient assessment methods can lead to enhanced health outcomes as well as reduced healthcare expenses. As healthcare systems around the globe strive to adopt more integrated approaches, integrating holistic nutritional assessment becomes increasingly important in advancing individual and public health agendas (Figure 4.2).

Importance of Nutritional Assessment in Health

Nutritional assessment is one of the most important areas for understanding diet and health status interaction. As nutrition emerges as a dominant factor in non-communicable disease prevalence, dietary intake evaluation is called for in public health planning. It allows medical practitioners to identify people who are at risk of malnutrition or whose dietary practices place them at risk for chronic diseases , such as obesity, diabetes, and heart disease. By applying a variety of assessment instruments, , such as food frequency questionnaires, 24-hour dietary recalls, and anthropometric assessments, practitioners can offer meaningful information regarding dietary habits. Armed with such information, interventions may be tailored to maximize health benefits, rendering nutritional assessment a critical basis for effective health promotion practice, particularly among groups with dietary concerns and limited access to healthy foods. Moreover, the integration of nutritional evaluation and environmental concerns adds its worth to health assessment. Research illustrates that dietary habits not only influence one's health but also form part of broader environmental matters like pollution and sustainability. The development of models , such as the Combined Nutritional and Environmental Life Cycle Assessment (CONE-LCA) is an indication of the importance of achieving a balance between dietary guidelines and environmental sustainability. By aligning the cost in terms of nutritional value with the cost in terms of the environment for food, stakeholders can foster informed consumer choice that benefits both personal and planetary health. For instance, emerging indices like the Health Nutritional Index (HENI) capture the cost of health of food selection so that one can make informed nutritional diet choices that benefit nutritional health as well as sustainability at once, highlighting the core place of integrative nutritional analysis in contemporary paradigms of health. Moreover, socio-economic effects of nutritional assessment cannot be dismissed since they are the basis of the efficacy of public health interventions and policies. Detection of nutritional deficiency in diverse groups has the tendency to respond to health inequalities and inform resource allocation for specific interventions. The development of the relationships between nutrition, economic status, and availability of wholesome food sources gives policymakers leverage to design programs that can enhance the food environment, especially among at-risk populations. Breaking down barriers to healthy eating through targeted public health initiatives has the ability to reduce rates of diet-related disease and improve the well-being of a community overall. Thus, as a component of sustainable development, nutritional assessment is recognized as one of the most influential factors in defining fair health outcomes and hence it is required that policymakers and health practitioners prioritize and implement effective nutritional assessment methods in policies and practice, taking into consideration the inter-linkage between environmental sustainability, health, and nutrition as defined by recent research (Stylianou, 2018) and programs (Harris et al., 2013).

Overview of Methods Used in Nutritional Assessment

Nutritional evaluation employs various means to ascertain the diet pattern and nutritional status of groups of people. Anthropometry is one of the important methods where there is systematic measurement of body size, weight, and body composition. It is a simple tool employed to ascertain malnutrition, and it exists in various forms , such as body mass index (BMI), waist circumference, and skinfold thickness. Anthropometric measurements are of very high significance, especially in vulnerable populations , such as children, where growth and development should be the prime priority. The literature has established the utility of these measurements in the prediction of health outcomes, as evidenced in studies conducted for Bangalore that found 68% malnutrition among school children, indicating that proper measuring techniques need to be used in nutritional assessment (Hasan, 2010). The other large method of nutritional assessment is dietary assessment, which measures food and nutrient intake through various mechanisms, including 24-hour recall, food frequency questionnaires, and diet diaries. These attempts to derive a total picture of individuals' or populations' food practices. Each instrument has its weaknesses and strengths, e.g., the 24-hour recall yields precise dietary information but is prone to dependence on memory and will not necessarily capture regular consumption. Despite these limitations, dietary evaluation tools are essential to the detection of nutrient inadequacy and to guiding public health intervention. The use of technological innovation, , such as mobile health apps, has further refined these tests so that they can now be more easily and accurately provided in real time. Biochemical tests, otherwise considered the gold standard for the assessment of nutrition, provide quantitative measures of nutrient content within biological tissues like blood, urine, or tissue. These readings are particularly useful in the diagnosis of specific nutrient toxicities or deficiencies not discernible through diet intake data alone. One's serum concentration of vitamins and minerals, for example, is a direct measure of nutritional status. In conjunction with anthropometric and food intake data, biochemical measurements can be extremely useful in a total assessment of nutritional status. Such a multi-faceted approach is required to address complex conditions like malnutrition, which, as evidenced in children researched in Bangalore, has long-term implications for both intellectual development and future work capacity (Hasan, 2010). The intersection of different approaches to appraisal renders nutritional intervention for different populations more precise and effective (Figure 4.3).

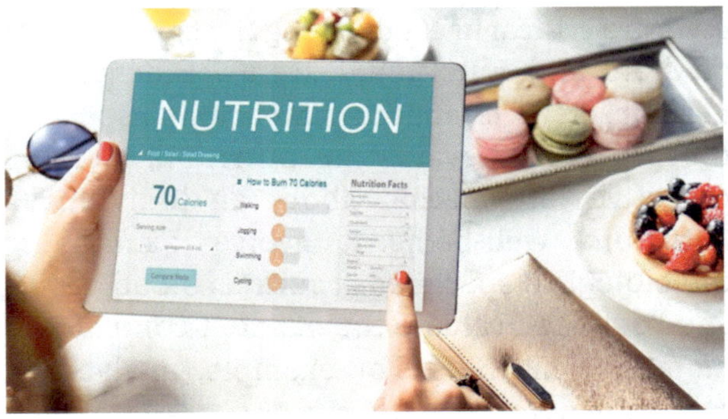

Figure 4.3. Digital nutrition tracking and calorie assessment.

Source: https://external-content.duckduckgo.com/iu/?u=https%3A%2F%2Fwww.nutritionfact.in%2Fwp-content%2Fuploads%2F2023%2F03%2FNutritional-Assessment.jpg&f=1&nofb=1&ipt=086108a6b57d0c5cc6a3902dc8d7a0441d9b60e2a5de06441d7cad1f04456726.

4.1. Types of Nutritional Assessment

A comprehensive examination of nutritional assessment requires a well-explicated tour of its various approaches, each of which is meant to solve particular clinical or investigative requirements. The most employed approach is the dietary assessment, which is typically used in three primary forms: 24-hour dietary recall, food frequency questionnaires, and weighed food records. The 24-hour dietary recall entails asking the participants to report everything they have eaten and drunk over the last 24 hours, giving a point-in-time picture of what and how much is being eaten. Food frequency questionnaires, in contrast, quantify usual consumption over long periods and are therefore particularly useful for wide-scale research. Weighed food records take more effort but are precise in supplying food intake data and can identify inadequacies in nutrients among people. All these methods, although possessing strengths and limitations of their own, are critical in establishing the consumption of diets and nutritional status. Biochemical measurement is another important aspect in the process of evaluating nutrition, yielding objective information about an individual's nutritional well-being. It involves quantifying the biological specimens , such as blood, urine, and tissue to evaluate the nutrient content and metabolic markers. For example, analysis of blood can determine deficits or excesses of vital vitamins and minerals, and analysis of urine generally indicates the degree of hydration as well as electrolyte equilibrium. The addition of biochemical tests has the effect of greatly enhancing dietary assessment precision by providing a physiological aspect to reported dietary intake. These tests are particularly useful to identify covert deficiencies that are not evident from diet recall. Thus, they are employed to construct the pillars of personalized nutrition programs and thereby improve public and private health outcomes. Lastly, anthropometric measurements supply vital information in supporting nutritional diagnosis by measuring physical parameters of body composition. These standard procedures under this class include height and weight measurement, body mass index determination, skinfold thickness, and bioelectrical impedance analysis. These methods are of utmost importance in assessing growth, obesity, and nutritional status for a broad spectrum of populations. As an example, BMI is often applied as a simple screening tool to categorize individuals into being underweight, normal weight, overweight, or obese. More sophisticated techniques like dual-energy X-ray absorptiometry (DEXA) provide accurate details regarding fat distribution and lean body mass, which add to the information on health risks based on various body compositions. With the inclusion of dietary and biochemical assessment, anthropometric measurements give a more comprehensive view of nutritional status, hence enabling more successful interventions to be planned and executed (Figure 4.4).

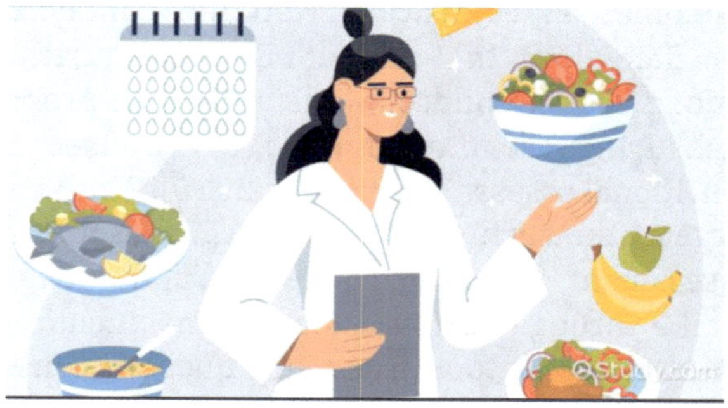

Figure 4.4. A nutritionist guiding healthy eating and meal planning.

Source: https://external-content.duckduckgo.com/iu/?u=https%3A%2F%2Fstudy.com%2Fcimages%2Fvideopreview%2Fvideopreview-full%2Fm6lp6e7cou.jpg&f=1&nofb=1&ipt=0d684537ca8963b6d08cd24190ba84d3c53b658c686d1feadd657fc11ae5123c.

4.1.1. Dietary Assessment Methods

In nutritional assessment, dietary intake and nutritional status are vastly dependent on dietary assessment methods. Through the years, traditional methods , such as food diaries and 24-hour recalls were used to yield information about people's diet. These two methods are usually respondent-based on memory and effort, resulting at times in inaccuracies. As an alternative to a digital method of increasing the reliability of dietary intake, researchers have increasingly turned to digital technology, including smartphone apps that allow consumers to photograph meals. Investigations have established that photo-based dietary surveys, e.g., the NutriNote Gama app, are very good compared to conventional methods, including weighing food. In assessing these new methods, it is crucial to consider their precision and satisfaction of users, as evidenced in the satisfactory comments from the participants of the Nutrinote Gama application (Budiningsari et al., 2024). In addition to computer-based tools, specific assessment tools , such as the Mini Nutritional Assessment (MNA) and Seniors in the Community: Risk Evaluation for Eating and Nutrition (SCREEN-14) contribute to an overall assessment of food habits and nutritional risk. They provide insightful information regarding the nutritional well-being of the elderly and patients with specific dental diseases. A comparative study of patients with implant-supported prostheses and patients with natural dentition reported that both sets of patients had a normal nutritional status as indicated by the MNA scores. Therefore, discrepancies were noted, , such as higher Body Mass Index (BMI) in the implant group, which indicates their unique vulnerability to nutritional insufficiency, particularly in the variety of foods consumed and fruit consumption as measured by SCREEN-14 (Homsi et al., 2024). These differences identify the necessity of using multiple dietary assessment methods to reflect the multifactorial nature of nutrition. Furthermore, the utilization of both standard and new dietary assessment methods could further enhance the process of nutritional consumption evaluation across different populations. The use of multiple methods to determine nutritional intake allows scientists to compare findings, thereby being more confident in the data collected. For instance, combining computer-based photo evaluation with a three-day food diary could depict a broader image of what an individual eats and their eating habits. This multi-modal approach enables researchers to identify individualized dietary needs and tailor interventions, accordingly, resulting in improved nutrition outcomes. As technologies continue to progress, the horizon for better dietary assessment methods is broad and full of promise, with better evaluations of nutrition and health in different populations. All these advances will play a significant role in guaranteeing effective public health interventions aimed at correcting nutritional inadequacies and better overall eating habits.

4.1.2. Anthropometric Measurements

Anthropometric measures are a fundamental part of nutritional status assessment and provide crucial information about body structure and growth patterns. Height, weight, and body mass index (BMI) are some of the measures that offer useful information about the nutritional status of the body in a person. Specifically, in child populations, these measures can ascertain whether or not a child is well-nourished, at risk of malnutrition, or stunted or wasted. As kids develop, their MUAC also has changed needs, and continuous surveillance by means of anthropometric measurements is critical in ensuring healthy growth. Continuous observation through measurement of MUAC helps caregivers and healthcare providers implement adequate interventions where necessary, hence being a key determinant of long-term health status. Mid-upper arm circumference (MUAC) measurement has been a widely applied methodology employed under anthropometric assessment, particularly among facilities that cover children with disabilities. This is a fast and simple measurement that can be applied to diverse clinical settings. A meta-analysis of studies from 24 nations concluded that MUAC has increasingly been utilized as part of nutritional assessment. The heterogeneity in measurement method and cut-offs, however, suggests an aspect of non-standardization that can compromise the comparability of findings between studies. The review indicated that although MUAC also has the potential to identify malnourished children, particularly those with disabilities, there is a need to standardize the measures to facilitate effective nutritional surveillance and planning for intervention (Hayes et al., 2023). In addition to MUAC, the implementation of other nutritional screening tools together with anthropometric measurement provides a more effective way of identifying malnutrition among children.

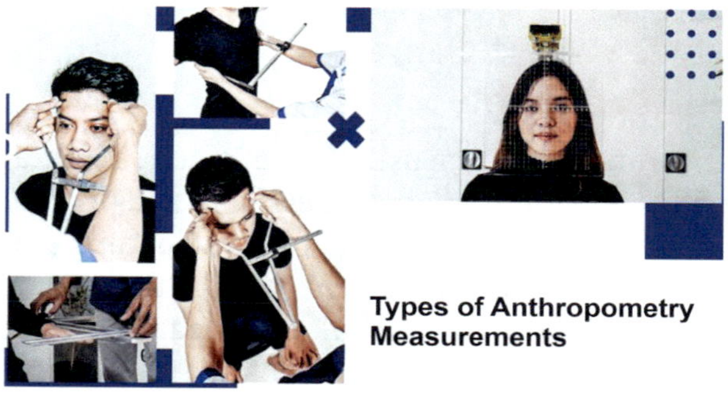

Figure 4.5. Different methods of anthropometric measurement.

Source: https://external-content.duckduckgo.com/iu/?u=https%3A%2F%2Fsoloabadi.com%2Fwp-content%2Fuploads%2F2018%2F12%2Ftypes-of-anthropometry-measurements.jpeg&f=1&nofb=1&ipt=7da98615a4c8ca309760d01bbd5658ab473547b191dbfa0beba0cd0dd0bb803a.

For instance, one comparison study contrasted the efficiency of four screening instruments with standard anthropometric measurements. It revealed that even though anthropometry remained a cornerstone of nutritional evaluation, tools like STRONG Kids were highly sensitive and specific to identify malnutrition risk. However, each tool demonstrated varying strengths in detection ability, and therefore, appropriate selection according to specific situational needs and population characteristics is essential. Because the burden of childhood malnourishment continues to increase globally, it is important to make use of a combination of anthropometric evaluations and screening tools when it comes to early and effective preventive interventions in nutritional assessment (Sayed et al., 2023) (Figure 4.5).

4.1.3. Biochemical Analysis

In the realm of nutritional assessment, biochemical analysis plays a crucial role in defining individual diet requirements and overall health status. Biochemical analysis is able to measure the required nutrients and metabolites, and the entire profile of one's nutritional status can be viewed. Because biochemical markers can reflect food intake or physiological response, they prove very effective in identifying deficiencies and excesses of individual micronutrients. Evidence indicates that qualitative and quantitative methods of determining adequacy of nutrient intake are obviously essential to successful personal and population assessment. For micronutrients that yield sufficient information to calculate an average nutrient requirement (ANR), determining the probability and confidence of adequacy is possible. By systematic analysis of methods, these biochemical tools enhance our ability to make inferences about nutrient adequacy in both environments, ultimately informing dietary recommendations and interventions that are tailored to specific health goals. Furthermore, biochemical analysis is central to the overall understanding of food quality and consumer behavior. The place of traditional foods cannot be discounted in nutrition assessment because such food groups often stand for cultural preference intertwined with nutrient patterns. Consumer beliefs in this respect are complex and driven by both sensory perceptions and experience. Studies on traditional food certification, in this case, that of the protected denomination status, illustrate the importance of the measurement of sensory quality to explain consumer food selection. Sensory properties of such foods are reliant on their production process and therefore biochemical examination gains importance to relate such production methods to nutritional quality. By recognizing the relationship between typical food properties and biochemical composition, nutritionists are better placed to recommend that consumers make healthier options that honor cultural heritage as well as enhance food variety. Finally, the use of biochemical analysis in nutritional evaluation emphasizes the role of societal determinants influencing food habits. Socio-economic status and cultural tradition, among others, can have implications for nutrient intake and food selection. Biochemical tests can reveal underlying inadequacies that normal dietary practices may not be correct. To this extent, a focus on maximizing micronutrient supplementation through diet is at the heart of things, as highlighted in more recent studies. The mechanism of assessing adequacy of diet has to accommodate to respond to local trends and to fit into the socio-political determinants of food intake. As the significance of traditional food cultures grows, it is essential to identify their nutritional implications through biochemical examination to plan effective public health actions and interventions to provide improved nutritional status among various populations, hence a nutrition-aware society.

4.2. Dietary Assessment Methods

Nutritional assessment methods are significant instruments of nutritional assessment, providing information on group and individual diet intake. The traditional methods, , such as food diaries, 24-hour recalls, and food frequency questionnaires, have widely been used due to their capacity to provide dietary data. These methods often contain inherent biases, , such as recall bias and social desirability bias, which lead to reported errors in dietary intake. As scientists strive to maximize the validity of these measurements, new tools have entered the stage. The use of Artificial Intelligence (AI) in dietary assessment methods is of major promise since it offers innovative solutions for overcoming traditional limitations and optimizing the accuracy of dietary data collection. Using advanced statistical models and algorithms, AI-based methods provide an effective way to assess nutritional intake in relation to health endpoints (Cofre et al., 2025). AI-assisted dietary analysis software has been developed to compensate for the limitations present in conventional methods. Technologies, including image-based and motion sensor-based technology, can easily acquire real-time dietary data without overburdening the user. Image-based instruments use advanced food recognition technologies that classify and measure the volume of food, which is less susceptible to errors than human recording. Concurrently, motion sensor-based instruments track eating behavior by evaluating movement, hence providing accurate data on actual consumption patterns. These technologies not only enhance user experience by their simple-to-use interfaces but also yield data that is generally recall bias-free, making it easier for valid conclusions about dietary intake and impact on health (Phalle and Gokhale, 2025). Besides the potential advantages of AI-based approaches to dietary assessment, further evidence is needed to fully endorse their use in diverse populations. Currently, literature illustrates the effectiveness of these tools in certain groups; yet evidence with larger sample sizes and other populations is required to determine generalizability. In addition, there is still a moderate risk of bias in most current studies, primarily related to confounders (Cofre et al., 2025). While AI technologies improve, their integration into nutrition care practice holds a promising future for increasing dietary assessment accuracy and ultimately better health outcomes. For these methods to achieve standard application in clinical settings, ongoing validation studies and explorations of their implementation among diverse populations will be crucial in determining their role as an essential component of nutritional assessment (Figure 4.6).

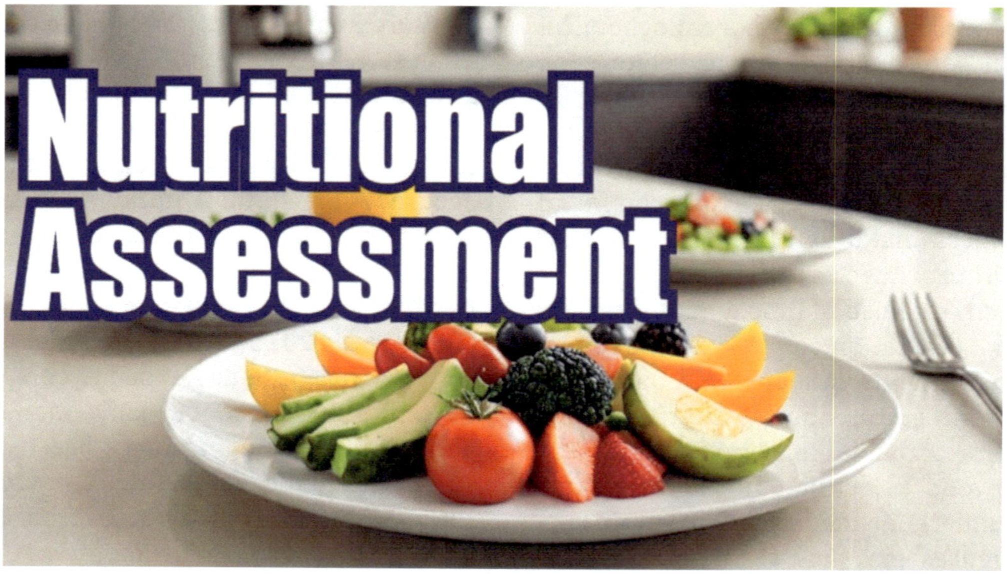

Figure 4.6. Nutritional assessment through balanced dietary choices.

Source: https://external-content.duckduckgo.com/iu/?u=https%3A%2F%2Fi.ytimg.com%2Fvi%2FJpG1fYSQ3UA%2Fmaxresdefault.jpg&f=1&nofb=1&ipt=644e796cb53d2d8d3f7e04b0c243bef3343e69cd53bcf87ceba997008bda7284.

4.2.1. 24-Hour Dietary Recall

The 24-hour recall diet method is one of the most important nutrition assessment tools that function by obtaining complete information about an individual's dietary history for the previous day. The approach provides the researchers with a snapshot of what people consume, and based on it, to can determine gaps in food and overall diet quality. In particular, studies highlight the value of remembering not just numbers but diversity in foods, which can have robust implications for health. For instance, the comparative evaluation of acute childhood malnutrition utilized the 24-hour dietary recall to separate tribal and non-tribal food patterns, demonstrating significant information on nutritional status and variety of intake (Shahadat et al., 2025). Thus, the recall method is a cornerstone of nutritional evaluation that can be applied to population-level and personalized dietary advice. In regard to the evaluation of the validity of the 24-hour dietary recall, it is pertinent to mention the effect of context and demographics on feeding habits. For example, a focused study on lactating women in rural settings established that socio-demographic traits played a major role in feeding patterns and nutrition knowledge, presenting direct correlations with breastfeeding and the nutritional status of infants (Hulamani et al., 2025). By using this recall procedure, researchers could compare the influence of maternal knowledge and food intake on child development and growth, thereby showing the variety of approaches. Furthermore, the ability of the 24-hour recalls adapting to various populations and environments makes them available in public health nutrition studies to allow for tailored intervention conducive to meeting the demands of certain communities. Reliability and validity of 24-hour dietary recall are vital in ensuring credible information in nutritional research. Nevertheless, participant recall bias and accuracy in reporting must be surmounted. Research conducts multiple recalls or confirms data with food frequency questionnaires in order to become more precise. Furthermore, cultural differences in food behavior can lead to variation in the interpretation of portion sizes and food types, rendering interviewer training precise and prompts standardized. In mothers' and children's research, as in malnutrition and diet research, this extremely specialized research methodology is required in order to determine specific eating deficiencies that can induce intervention steps (Hulamani et al., 2025; Shahadat et al., 2025). In summary, while the 24-hour dietary recall is a potent tool in nutritional assessment, its dependability hinges on strict application and surroundings awareness to ensure the quality and consistency of the data obtained (Figure 4.7).

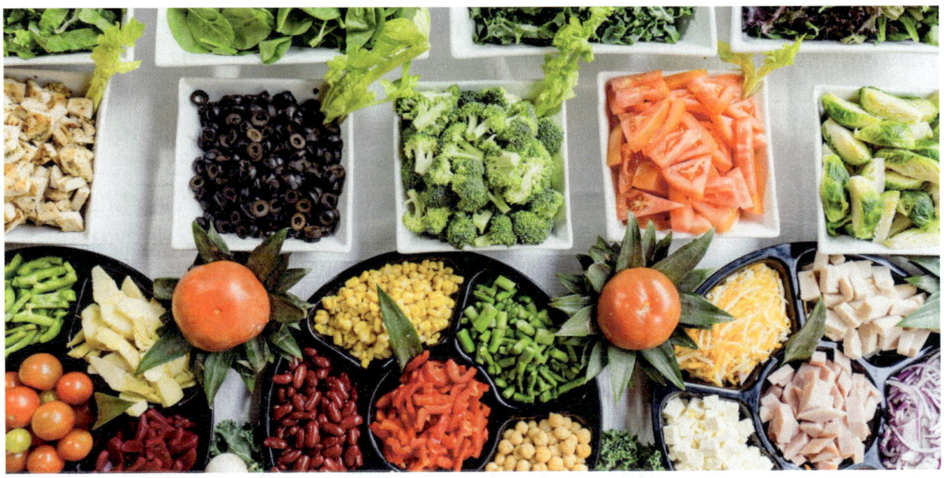

Figure 4.7. A variety of fresh, nutritious ingredients for a balanced diet.

Source: https://external-content.duckduckgo.com/iu/?u=https%3A%2F%2Fopenlab.ncl.ac.uk%2Fassets%2Fproject-cover-intake24-large.jpg&f=1&nofb=1&ipt=0c20b952804731cfe0d9e6359a0693c38a123e37ef2e4b60d2cce4cd5395ef1b.

4.2.2. Food Frequency Questionnaires

Food frequency questionnaires (FFQs) are a valuable tool in nutritional measurement by offering data on the frequency of consumption of foods over a period of time. They are typically designed in a way where the respondent can tick the frequency with which they consume various food items, ranging from daily to less than once a month. FFQs have gained popularity as they are fairly easy to administer and are able to capture patterns of consumption that can influence health outcomes. In contrast to detailed diet recalls, which require precise weight measurements and instantaneous recall, FFQs can be answered on a rushed basis, making them a suitable instrument in large-scale epidemiologic research. They also enable an inquiry into long-term dietetics in populations, with the result being enhanced public health data. Though they are handy, they should be aware of their limitations, particularly for precision and potential misreporting, which can affect the validity of results in studies of nutritional intake and health associations. Scalability is one of the most important advantages of FFQs, as they allow researchers to ascertain eating habits across various populations with ease. For example, FFQs have been used in studies with adolescents in an effort to establish dietary habits and their associations with health, which can be particularly beneficial when implementing focused interventions. Through the Polish teens' study, the short food frequency questionnaire form (SF-FFQ4PolishChildren) was instrumental in obtaining diet information, hence it enabled one to evaluate the nutrition knowledge and lifestyle behaviors (Hamu et al., 2018). These were not only necessary for the understanding of existing dietary patterns but also instrumental in creating focused education programs to support better nutritional behavior among vulnerable populations. FFQs are, therefore, capable of being used as an essential part of public health programs aiming to address diet-related issues at a population level. Nevertheless, FFQ validity has been determined to vary in different studies, with evidence indicating underreporting upon comparing self-reported data with objective biomarkers. An investigation of how self-reported food diets gathered with FFQs, 24-hour recalls, and food diaries compare has shown significant differences, particularly regarding energy intake, where FFQs have a higher tendency to underreport nutritional consumption compared to other methods (Park et al., 2018). Underreporting is of concern in accurately determining the nutritional status of populations, thus impacting clinical practice and public health intervention. In an effort to enhance the validity of inferences made from FFQs, scientists may complement such measurements with other methods of estimating diet or employ innovative statistical strategies to adjust for measurement error. Lastly, as a foundation of the world of nutritional assessment, acknowledging FFQ limitations and formulating methods of minimizing such inbuilt flaws are imperative in the endeavor for nutritional science and public health intervention.

4.2.3. Diet Diaries

Among the nutritional assessment tools, diet diaries are an effective way of quantifying dietary habits longitudinally. As opposed to single-meal dietary recall or food frequency questionnaires that rely on participants' self-report and memory, diet diaries provide a systematic approach to tracking food intake on a day-to-day basis. This method allows one to record one's food, beverages, and snacks for a period, hence allowing for greater accuracy of diet self-reporting. Moreover, diet diaries can counteract recall errors related to biases, particularly in populations where chronic energy underreporting and overreporting can skew results. With the addition of temporal nuances of food consumption and meal habits, diet diaries contain information regarding eating habits that are essential to nutritional quality and their impact on health outcomes, thus forming an integrative model for dietary behavior assessment. The use of diet diaries is also evident while assessing their use in the determination of chrono nutrition habits. Recent research highlights that the approach utilized for collecting dietary data has a significant impact on the results of diet and health consequences. A careful investigation with questionnaires and diet diaries, for example, reported varying results with respect to diet quality and obesity markers, underlining consistency in methodology as being crucial in nutrition science. Specifically, the use of complete food diaries was unrelated to diet quality or obesity to any appreciable extent, whereas questionnaire results had indicated potential risks associated with the frequency and timing of eating. Therefore, through the utilization of diet diaries, not only is the dataset enriched but also allows researchers to factor in the time dimension of consumption, capturing a more comprehensive view of the complex dynamics involving dietary patterns and health status, as was exemplified by the analysis of EI misreporting. Diet diaries are also pivotal in enhancing nutritional outcomes, particularly among vulnerable populations , such as the elderly. Empirical evidence from food diaries has shown significant improvements in nutritional status when eating therapy is supplemented by structured recording methods, , such as the Protein-enriched MED Diet or PROMED-EX trials. The trials used food diaries for months to look at differences in dietary quality and nutrient intake between the groups, leading to improved understanding of nutritional sufficiency and eating compliance. The positive results mentioned in such studies, including increased consumption of essential nutrients, testify to the strength of diet diaries in guiding effective dietary interventions. Diet diaries not only facilitate accurate nutritional assessment but also are integral to the preparation and evaluation of individualized dietary interventions for the promotion of lifelong health and well-being, particularly in risk groups for undernutrition and associated comorbidities (Figure 4.8).

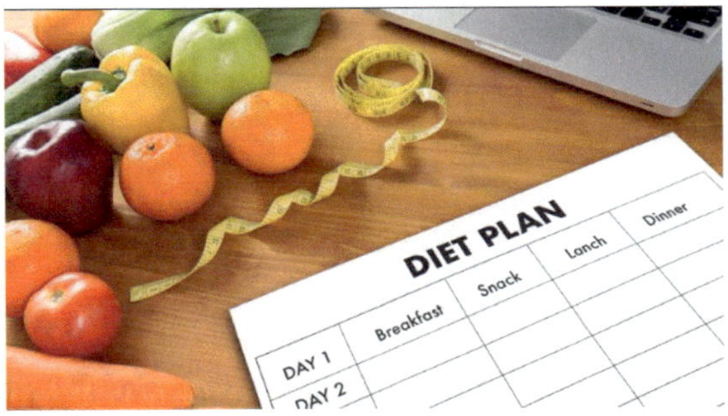

Figure 4.9. Meal planning with fruits and a structured diet chart.

Source: https://external-content.duckduckgo.com/iu/?u=https%3A%2F%2Fimages.indianexpress.com%2F2017%2F11%2Fdiet-plan.jpg&f=1&nofb=1&ipt=acf1576a30361a3f88bf89d59e1b8b359510e67dfd9168210d5e02779da14fa7.

4.3. Anthropometric Measurements

Anthropometric measurements play a significant role in the field of nutritional assessment as they provide quantifiable data about the body composition and growth pattern of an individual. The commonly used parameters for these measurements are height, weight, body mass index (BMI), skinfold thickness, and waist circumference. Based on these indicators, health workers can ascertain the nutritional status of individuals and identify potential deficiencies or excesses that may influence their well-being. Particularly, the nutritional status of mothers and children can be charted using these measurements because they indicate not just the physical development of children but also their dietary patterns and how maternal health contributes to patterns of growth (Gümüş et al., 2024). Ultimately, anthropometric measurements are fundamental tools for assessing the success of nutritional and public health interventions. Comparison of anthropometric data not only quantifies personal health but also makes it possible to detect overall trends in groups of people. For instance, the use of z-score indicators in the examination of nutritional status among children within particular population groups shows extensive disparities in health outcomes. Studies , such as those on Kamar children in Chhattisgarh depict how certain anthropometric measurements show instant public health problems, particularly among disadvantaged sections (Kanwar et al., 2024). By systematic quantification of growth and health indicators, researchers can develop targeted interventions to combat malnutrition and its dangers. This not only creates a better image of regional health challenges but also underscores the demand for evidence-based policies that aim to improve nutritional levels across different communities. Moreover, anthropometric measurements are essential indicators of observing growth over time, allowing for early detection of possible health issues. Periodic monitoring allows detection of trends, divergence, or plateaus of growth, possibly necessitating medical attention or lifestyle modifications. In maternal and child health, understanding the interconnectedness of growth patterns is required, as evidenced by studies that confirm the link between the nutritional status of mothers and the health status of their offspring (Gümüş et al., 2024). Because they are done with standard methods, these measures generate uniform information that can be used to guide healthcare professionals and policymakers to act appropriately on the nutritional needs of at-risk populations. In summary, anthropometric measurements form the foundation in nutritional assessment, informing clinical practice and guiding public health interventions towards enhanced health outcomes for the individual and the population (Figure 4.10).

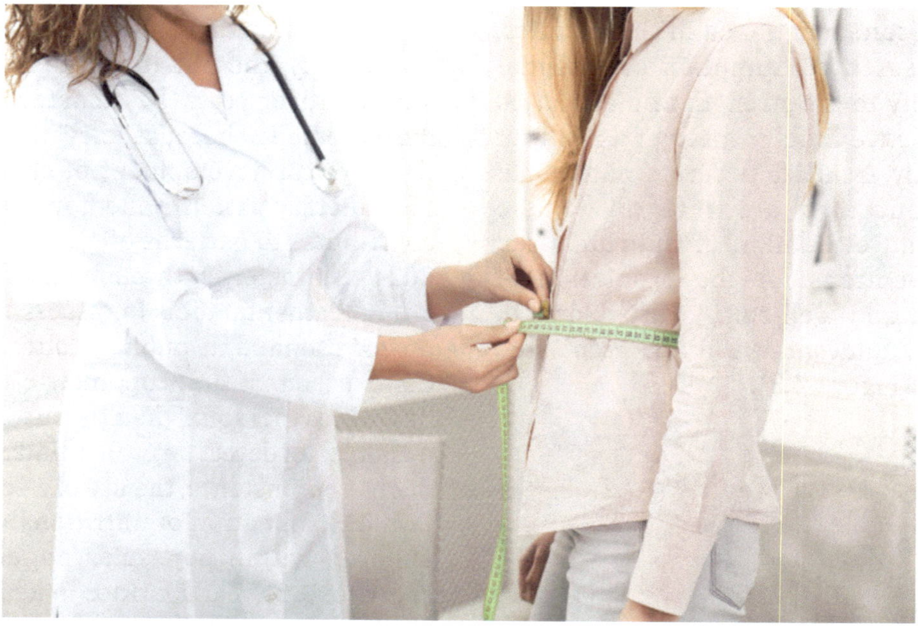

Figure 4.10. Measuring waist circumference for nutritional assessment.

Source: https://external-content.duckduckgo.com/iu/?u=https%3A%2F%2Fwww.verywellhealth.com%2Fthmb%2FXVHR1MCE8iZyvohYNBKNKPW6sTY%3D%2F5760x3840%2Ffilters%3Ano_upscale()%3Amax_bytes(150000)%3Astrip_icc()%2Fnutritionist-measuring-bmi-of-patient-in-office-1092685108-5c83551a8c00442da4561f2f5a5de7b5.jpg&f=1&nofb=1&ipt=b0ee98135d634b76e5a601c4a9c06d09d31e2147d9ff3d5148724fe3640a40b0.

4.3.1. Body Mass Index (BMI)

Body Mass Index (BMI) is one of the widely applied measures in nutritional assessment and provides a simple numerical value characterizing the body fat content of an individual based on height and weight. BMI may be utilized by health workers to classify weight as underweight, normal weight, overweight, and obese, which can easily permit population screening and determination of health risk associated with body composition. In pediatric populations, for instance, BMI is an important marker utilized in monitoring development and growth. It has been noted that a change in a child's BMI can reflect global health status as well as nutritional status and thus inform dietary intervention and public health policy choice for preventing childhood obesity and its ensuing health consequences (Hegde et al., 2025). However, the shortcomings of BMI must be considered, as it does not differentiate between lean mass and fat mass, leading to misperceptions regarding one's health. Once again, while BMI is such a vital screening measure, it is imperfect. Recent research gives evidence that BMI might not focus on important details regarding body composition, , such as variations in muscle weight and fat distribution, which could give a more accurate picture of an individual's health status. For example, athletes could have high BMI levels that place them in the overweight or obese category, yet they possess low body fat percentages. Accordingly, BMI cut-off values must be reevaluated, particularly for groups that show variations in body build, age, and ethnicity (Wu et al., 2024). This implies that health practitioners need to come up with a more holistic approach to interpreting BMI scores in relation to other measurements in terms of anthropology and performance indicators. This kind of overall assessment can lead to more individualized nutritional advice and intervention methods. The incorporation of additional measures in addition to BMI gives an improved analysis of a person's health profile. The use of combined anthropometric indicators, including waist circumference and body fat percentage, in conjunction with BMI, can also reveal the divergence between healthy individuals and individuals at risk of chronic disease development. This is particularly important in the context of the obesity epidemic, as the identification of at-risk populations is better performed through this multi-dimensional approach. With health guidelines always evolving, the need for enforcing comprehensive strategies for assessing nutritional status will always be in the limelight. With the enhancement of the use of BMI by additional assessments, health practitioners are better equipped to improve their productivity in producing effective nutritional intervention as well as general health and wellness, with the knowledge that BMI should not be the sole parameter for qualification of specific medical interventions and treatments (Wu et al., 2024) (Figure 4.11).

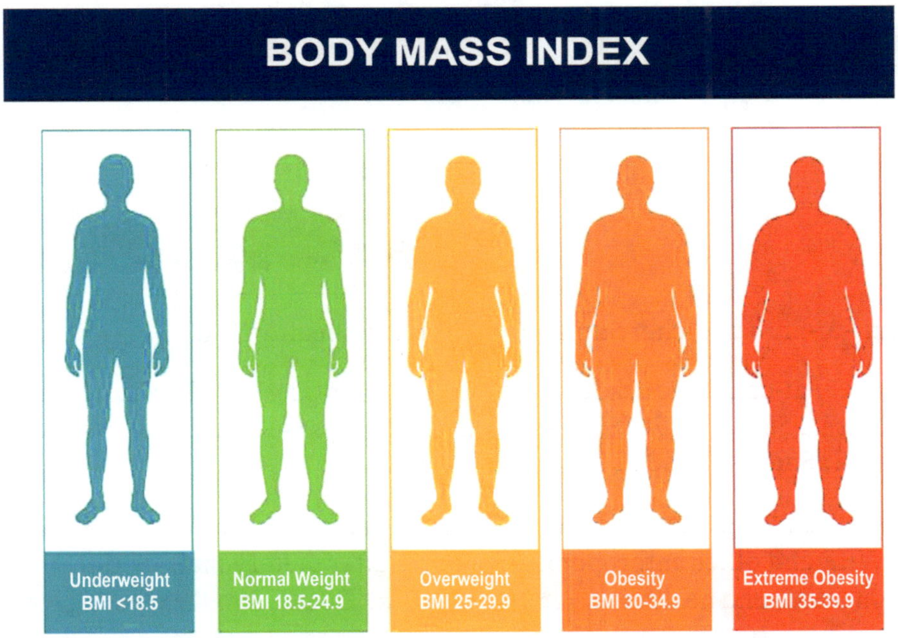

Figure 4.11. BMI chart categorizing weight status by body mass index ranges.

Source: https://external-content.duckduckgo.com/iu/?u=https%3A%2F%2Ffindhealthtips.com%2Fwp-content%2Fuploads%2F2022%2F11%2Fbody-mass-index-bmi-chart-1.jpg&f=1&nofb=1&ipt=57386ee76a5353b0283261bdd7b79520624c0d2909cb81e5af14d364df7b88b1.

4.3.2. Waist-to-Hip Ratio

Waist-to-hip ratio (WHR) is a key anthropometric measurement under nutritional assessments, particularly in determining body fat distribution and associated health threats. Unlike body mass index (BMI), which provides a rough estimate of body weight relative to height, WHR offers a more distinguishing notion of fat distribution. This measurement is derived by dividing waist circumference by hip circumference, enabling one to directly measure central adiposity. Higher WHR implies a higher ratio of visceral fat and is associated with increased risk of metabolic syndrome, cardiovascular diseases, and some cancers. Therefore, incorporating WHR into nutritional assessment has the potential to enhance the ability to identify those at high health risk and allow more targeted dietary intervention to decrease fat, particularly around the abdominal region, to effectively counteract the risk. There is evidence that the health consequences associated with the waist-to-hip ratio are of particular concern in at-risk groups, , such as children with cerebral palsy and young women with breast cancer.

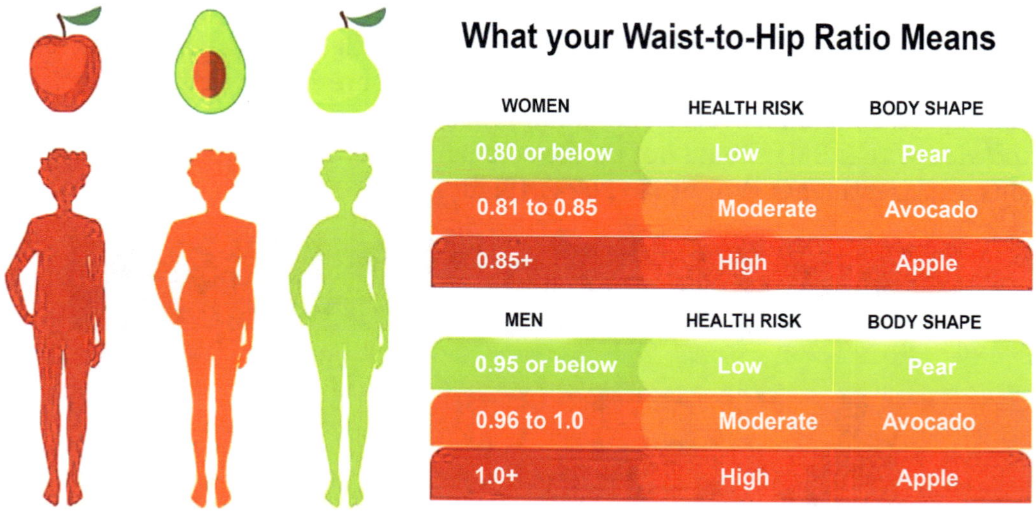

Figure 4.12. Waist-to-hip ratio chart links body shape to health risk.

Source: https://external-content.duckduckgo.com/iu/?u=https%3A%2F%2Fhealthjade.net%2Fwp-content%2Fuploads%2F2017%2F01%2Fwaist-hip-ratio.jpg&f=1&nofb=1&ipt=3bcfc4484f9ae7faed412c96262d3ba174b5ad4e4fb6d301127dc70f35f23492.

For instance, a study comparing malnourished children with cerebral palsy showed substantial improvement in WHR and other anthropometric indices after dietary intervention, thereby suggesting improved nutrition status and health markers (Fatima et al., 2024). Similarly, young women with breast cancer showed alarming trends for WHR, indicating the need to implement specialized nutritional interventions in combating obesity and corresponding cardiovascular risk (Aés et al., 2024). These findings demonstrate the utility and use of WHR as a primary metric in diverse populations, outside of its conventional applications, underscoring the importance of preventive care in maximizing health and survival across different stages of life and disease statuses. Practically speaking, applying the waist-to-hip ratio to include in comprehensive nutritional evaluation protocols allows health professionals to create individualized health plans. Effective nutritional interventions can be designed not only to maximize overall global dietary intake but also to specifically address the lowering of central obesity, based on WHR values. Knowing the correlation of WHR with various health outcomes, nutritionists and dietitians are now capable of prescribing lifestyle modifications like food alteration and exercise routine that are determined by individual requirements. Furthermore, baseline WHR measurements can be repeated regularly to be employed as a principal component of ongoing nutritional assessment, directing indicated intervention based upon trends in body composition. Therefore, the waist-to-hip ratio emerges as an important asset in allowing for a more delineated strategy to enhance nutritional health and decrease the risk of disease (Figure 4.12).

4.3.3. Skinfold Thickness Measurements

Skinfold thickness test is a component of nutritional evaluation and gives valuable information regarding the composition of fat in the body. The method involves the periodic measurement of skinfolds at various body locations and utilizing the measurements to make an approximation of the total body percentage of the person. While the method is inexpensive and straightforward, a degree of expertise is required so that standardization and consistency of reading can be ensured. Skinfold measurement is of great value in sport and clinical settings, where measurements of body composition taken over time can be used to inform training and dietary schemes. The convenience of skinfold measurement has ensured its popularity despite the availability of newer techniques like bioelectrical impedance analysis and dual-energy X-ray absorptiometry. Skinfold thickness measurements were found to be reliable by many studies, citing their correlation with other body composition measurement methods. For instance, research showed that skinfold and underwater weighing (UWW) give similar measures of body percentage fat, further validating the hypothesis that skinfold measurement is an adequate surrogate for the estimation of body adiposity (Kaplan et al., 2009). Besides, the accuracy of skinfold measurements allows clinicians to assess regional variations in fat deposition, potentially of crucial significance to the health risk for an individual. Note should, however, be taken of the limitation of techniques , such as the influence of variables , such as hydration state, exercise, and the technical competence of the technician, which may introduce variability to results. Finally, nutritional evaluation of pediatric populations via skinfold measurements is both challenging and rewarding. Due to the spurts of growth and hormonal changes that occur during childhood and adolescence, regular and precise skinfold assessment can be critical to the observation of patterns of growth and body composition. A study of children with pediatric Crohn's disease reveals the influence of drugs on certain skinfold thickness measurements, indicating that some drug has an effect on body fat distribution in children (Andrews et al., 2018). The results underscore the use of skinfold thickness measurements in children's nutritional evaluation to enable specific interventions ensuring healthy development and body composition. As the field evolves, increasingly accurate measurement methods and translational use of research will further enhance the utility of skinfold measurements in both clinical and sport nutrition practice.

4.4. Biochemical Analysis

Biochemical testing constitutes one of the pillars of the field of nutritional assessment, providing important information regarding an individual's nutritional status and metabolic health. Through the quantitative measurement of specific biochemical markers in body fluids , such as blood and urine, healthcare providers can identify nutritional deficiencies, excesses, and imbalances that may have significant health consequences. For instance, some of the major markers, like hemoglobin and serum albumin levels, have been compared to long hospital stays and recovery times in children. It has been observed that malnourished children have significantly lower levels of these markers, thus becoming extremely vulnerable to infection and complications during the healing process (Ali et al., 2025).

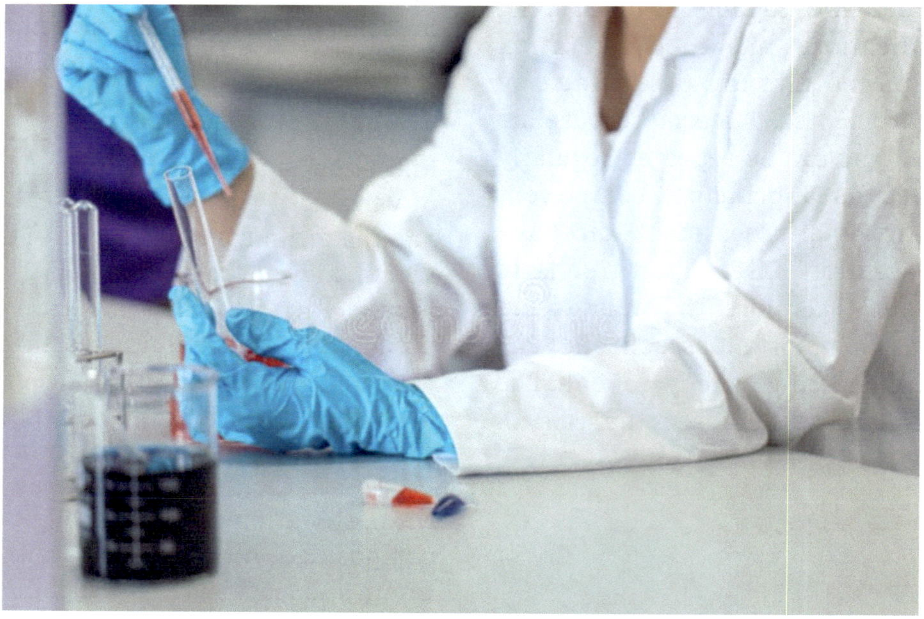

Figure 4.13. Biochemical analysis conducted in a laboratory setting.

Source: https://external-content.duckduckgo.com/iu/?u=https%3A%2F%2Fthumbs.dreamstime.com%2Fb%2Fbiochemical-analysis-chemical-analysis-lab-background-biochemical-analysis-chemical-analysis-lab-n-134290011.jpg&f=1&nofb=1&ipt=f73cf18ff2c253c65d205d26c57ba432deb74055ab19964b6409275894da853b.

Therefore, applying regular biochemical testing in hospitals can contribute to the early detection of nutritional problems to enable specific interventions that enhance patient outcomes. In addition, the effectiveness of nutritional treatments can be greatly improved using precision nutrition strategies that involve biochemical testing. While conventional approaches tend to apply high standards to everyone regardless of their variations, precision nutrition uses an individual's own characteristics and biochemical information to make personalized diet recommendations. Through consideration of factors like genetics, composition of gut microbiota, and current eating habits, health professionals can develop better management plans for health disorders like obesity and malnourishment in populations with different levels of heterogeneity. Recent systematic reviews have critically assessed the impact of such tailored interventions and emphasized the relevance of biochemical markers in evaluating outcomes like body mass index (BMI) and weight change (Huey et al., 2025). This increases the likelihood of success through providing a dynamic image of how one's biochemistry will react to dietary intervention. In summary, the use of biochemical analysis in nutrition evaluations not only informs us more precisely regarding individual diets but also helps in creating customized nutritional methods. As more evidence is emerging on the link between some biochemical markers and health outcomes, clinicians can utilize this evidence in order to implement improved assessment approaches. The realization that some deficiencies, , such as serum albumin and vitamin D deficiencies, cause prolonged recovery and increased morbidity proves the critical significance of their identification through biochemical testing at an early stage (Ali et al., 2025). Embracing a more individualized approach, founded on rigorous biochemical testing, will serve to optimize nutritional interventions, ultimately resulting in improved health outcomes in diverse populations (Figure 4.13).

4.4.1. Blood Tests for Nutrient Levels

Tests of blood levels of nutrients form a significant component of nutritional assessment, as they provide highly valuable information regarding the health status of an individual. The tests examine numerous biomarkers in the blood, , such as the concentration of vitamins, minerals, and macronutrients, which can indicate any deficiency or excess. For instance, a deficiency in vitamin D may result in bone health issues, while high levels of cholesterol can be a sign of cardiovascular issues. Ongoing monitoring of these levels enables health practitioners to personalize dietary guidance and intervention more effectively. Moreover, blood analysis can reveal underlying medical issues that are not revealed by dietary analysis alone, and therefore, are an integral part of a comprehensive nutritional assessment. Consequently, understanding the interpretation of blood test results is essential for effective management of health as well as personalized nutrition. The accuracy and validity of blood tests for nutritional composition can play a significant role in clinical decisions. The time taken for the sample, fasting, and laboratory practices is all essential to achieve accurate results. Blood samples following overnight fasting usually give more reliable data regarding nutrient composition since the consumption of food affects the levels of certain biomarkers. In addition, variations in the procedures used in the laboratory can lead to differing results, which highlights the importance of standardization of testing protocols. Interpretation for the patient must, however, consider individual circumstances, including age, gender, and overall health status. Monitoring overtime may provide data on the effectiveness of dietary change or supplementation. Therefore, a subtle comprehension of these tests is necessary for both healthcare professionals and patients to make wise choices regarding nutritional well-being. The implications of blood tests for nutrient status reach beyond personal health; it can also advise public health programs and dietary recommendations. From the analysis of population-wide excesses or deficiencies of nutrients, health agencies can formulate interventions specifically designed to enhance general nutritional status. For instance, if most of the population shows low iron levels, public health can include education on dietary sources of iron or promotion of fortified foods. Furthermore, awareness of correlations between blood nutrient levels and disease can drive research into preventive practices, perhaps reducing the cost of healthcare for diet-related diseases. Here, not only is the testing of blood diagnostic, but also a means to promote communal health. In that sense, they are at the heart of both individual dietary practice and public health policy.

4.4.2. Metabolic Marker Urine Tests

Metabolic marker urine testing has become a valuable tool in nutrition evaluation for various populations. The test provides a non-invasive means of obtaining vital metabolic information by collecting data without invading the inside of the body. Quantifiable markers found in urine, , such as electrolytes, glucose, and ketones, provide valuable information regarding metabolic states and deficiencies and excesses. For instance, the presence of elevated blood glucose may indicate uncontrolled diabetes or carbohydrate metabolism disorder, while abnormal ketone levels may uncover inappropriate dietary carbohydrate or energy metabolism derangements. Based on these metabolic results, healthcare practitioners can design individualized dietary interventions to correct diagnosed inadequacies and increase general well-being.

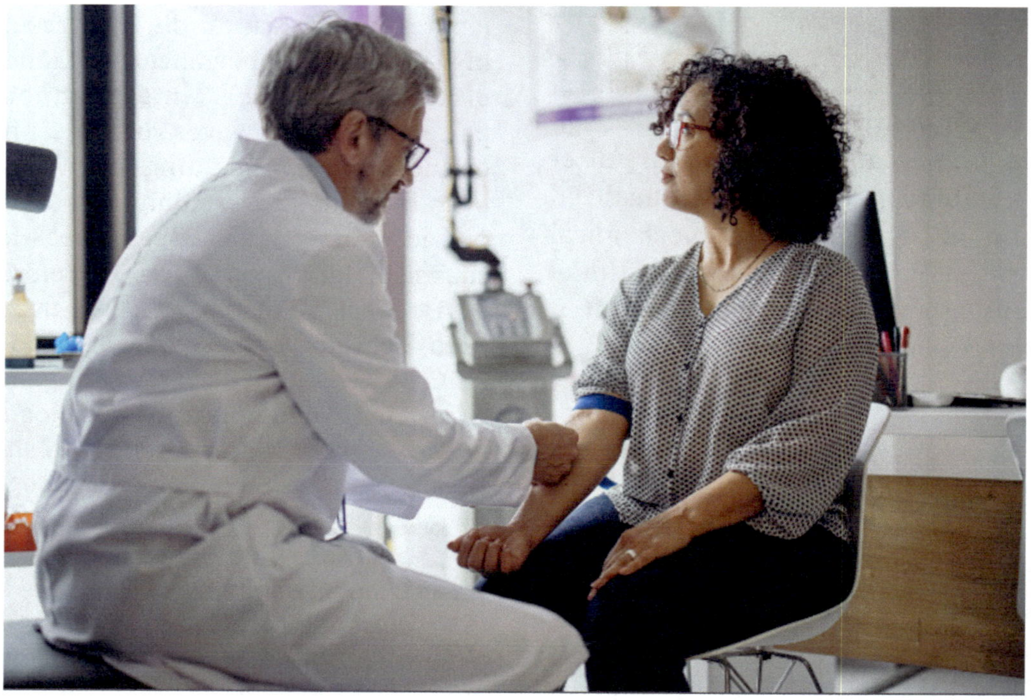

Figure 4.14. Doctor preparing patient for blood sample collection.

Source: https://external-content.duckduckgo.com/iu/?u=https%3A%2F%2Fimages.ctfassets.net%2Fyixw23k2v6vo%2F3ElbAEspFt2CTAGQ1gdnWJ%2Fd36d415c0c1d6ec281d74a148b75acef%2FGettyImages-1394005030-3000x2000.jpg&f=1&nofb=1&ipt=85fd24ad070d15e97176df382acfd378c8d95fa5b8a13ff2ac3b5e4b178376b6.

When in the clinical setting, urine analysis is generally more desirable than blood analysis due to the convenience and practicality of the method. The dipstick method, as applied in studies with cattle, demonstrates this point. One study conducted on buffaloes discovered that urinary tests could be utilized to identify metabolic disorders due to inadequate living conditions and poor nutrition. Proteinuria and ketonuria levels indicated dietary insufficiencies, pointing out the relationship between nutrition and health status for the group. These analyses not only inform the health profession concerning the acute status of health in the subjects but also form a foundation for general interventions for community health. Therefore, urine analysis for metabolic markers is a significant part of nutritional assessment, with actionable data that can lead to improved diet. Secondly, the incorporation of urine analysis within routine health checks can encourage an early intervention strategy for health and nutrition management. Through continuous monitoring of metabolic indicators, practitioners can identify trends and changes in nutritional status over time, facilitating early intervention. For instance, the early detection of abnormal metabolic indicators in human populations can induce lifestyle interventions prior to the establishment of serious diseases. In the research carried out with buffaloes, between urine abnormalities and feeding habits, the importance of enhancing nutritional management strategies was highlighted. In this respect, urine tests not only yield instantaneous information to the dietitian concerning the food intake relevant to the immediate state of health but also to long-term nutritional enhancement. With more evidence coming in on the accuracy of such tests in different populations, their application in the field of nutritional assessment keeps expanding in importance in both human and veterinary medicine in the formulation of future dietary recommendations and health policy (Figure 4.14).

4.4.3. Tissue Biopsies for Nutrient Status

The use of tissue biopsies as a method of assessing nutrient status has been identified for its ability to provide direct information about the biochemical body environment. Compared to traditional serum or plasma biomarker quantifications, tissue biopsies provide the ability to analyze particular nutrient concentrations in multiple tissues, i.e., muscle and fat. This approach allows for more accurate evaluation of nutrient metabolism and utilization, reflective of the cellular nutritional status of the body rather than relying on systemic markers themselves. This is particularly critical in defining the status of malnutrition or insufficiency in nutrients, which is not always apparent through standard blood work. The significance of this method is in creating tailored nutritional interventions that are personalized to the needs of an individual and therefore enhance the effectiveness of treatment and better health outcomes, a theme being explored in established literature regarding biomarkers of nutrients and their impact on patient health (Denno et al., 2016). For metabolic conditions , such as type 2 diabetes, the tissue biopsy is pivotal in unraveling the complex interrelation between exercise, diet, and metabolic health. A study on the role of nutritional status during training involving exercise uncovered the fact that changes in skeletal muscle function are deeply linked with nutrient availability and utilization during exercise. For instance, the analysis of muscle biopsies revealed differences in gene expression for lipid metabolism and oxidative capacity, illustrating how exercise performance and metabolic regulation in diabetic patients can be impacted by nutrient status. This illustrates that tissue biopsies may be able to guide not only the acute nutrient status to clinicians but also how nutritional maneuvers would optimally individualize exercise programs to maximize clinical outcome (Calders et al., 2020). In addition, the integration of tissue biopsy testing into nutritional assessment is a milestone in the practice of personalized medicine. As the need for individualized dietary counsel continues to evolve, tissue biopsies allow healthcare professionals to create interventions that are more precisely aligned to an individual's individualized metabolic profile. Through the evaluation of certain nutrients at the cellular level, clinicians can identify targeted mechanisms for overcoming deficiencies and elevating overall well-being. The personalized insight gained from this method aids in comprehending the varying body tissues' response to levels of nutrients, thereby improving the development of effective nutritional plans. Thus, the application of tissue biopsies in nutritional diagnostics not only explains the intricacy of interaction in nutrient metabolism and absorption but also emphasizes the importance of individualized diet intervention in optimizing patient outcomes under varied health conditions (Denno et al., 2016).

4.5. Factors Influencing Nutritional Status

Nutrition status in man is complicated and influenced by several physiological, psychological, and environmental variables. Physiologically, sex and age are grossly influential on nutritional needs and absorptive capacity. For instance, elderly individuals require less energy and have disrupted metabolism, which can lead to malnutrition if their food intake is not correctly altered. Psychological factors are also a key determinant, as conditions , such as depression or anxiety can drastically impair appetite and food intake. The home setting, socio-economic status, and access to healthy foods can also have a marked effect on diet quality being consumed and therefore on nutritional status. All of these explain the complexities of nutritional evaluation and highlight the necessity of a holistic approach in diet and health outcome evaluation. Existing medical conditions and chronic illnesses are pivotal in influencing nutritional status, especially among the surgical and critically ill populations. Malnutrition aggravates the seriousness of these conditions, which translates into poor outcomes for surgery, extended hospitalization, increased morbidity and mortality rates. For example, conditions , such as liver disease or cancer, immediately impair nutrient absorption, altering metabolism and increasing nutritional requirements. Furthermore, comorbidities often necessitate drug therapies that will either exacerbate nutritional deficiencies or negatively interact with portions of the diet. It has been shown that thorough nutrition assessment and tailored intervention are necessary in combating these effects and ensuring optimal health. The inclusion of preoperative nutritional care can greatly enhance the outcomes of surgery, positioning tailored nutrition in the clinical environment as a necessity (Herc et al., 2024). Education level, economic stability, and healthcare access are all important social determinants of population nutritional status. Individuals from lower socioeconomic groups typically lack easy access to nutritious foods, contributing to food insecurity and malnutrition. Education is also a large part of it, with people not knowing anything about nutrition making unhealthy food choices because of misinformation or not having resources. Geographical location also determines access to fresh fruits and vegetables and whole foods as opposed to processed foods, directly influencing the quality of diet. Nutritional assessment must intervene on these social determinants to create impactful interventions. Population-based interventions focused on educating communities regarding nutrition, as well as increasing access to healthy foods, are important in decreasing disparities and improving the nutritional status at the population level (Ravaioli et al., 2023) (Figure 4.15).

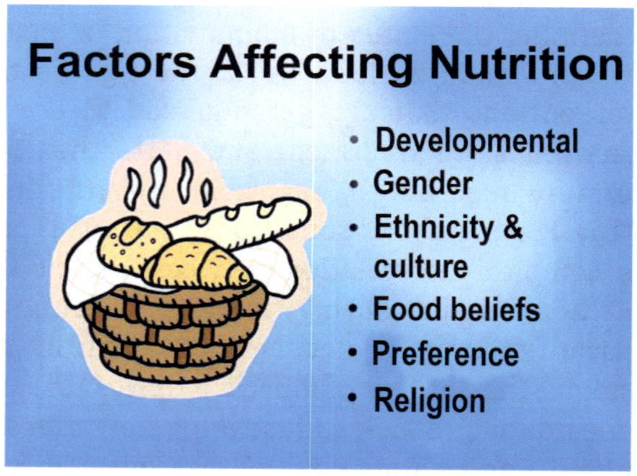

Figure 4.15. Various personal and cultural factors affect nutrition.

Source: https://external-content.duckduckgo.com/iu/?u=https%3A%2F%2Fimage.slideserve.com%2F1138883%2Ffactors-affecting-nutrition-l.jpg&f=1&nofb=1&ipt=909755625192178f3aead477dfaeab37a32d28aac8fee2fec3e14e071952c25d.

4.5.1. Socioeconomic Status

The socioeconomic status (SES) construct has significant impacts on diets and nutritional status through income, education level, and employment status. Individuals with lower SES most often experience many factors that limit their ability to use nutrient-dense food. On limited budgets, families may have to accept cheaper foods high in calories and sugars and fats but low in nutrients. This has profound health implications, particularly in children, who are especially susceptible to the effects of poor nutrition. There is a suggestion to be made that SES has an unpleasant correlation with nutrition, indicating that impoverished children are more likely to suffer from food insecurity and ultimately develop higher rates of dental cures and obesity (Cheever et al., 2025). Therefore, SES is the most important area that must be tackled in nutritional assessment and intervention to improve global public health. The SES effect also extends beyond food availability; it impacts what one knows and does about diet. Education level dictates how much of a person's understanding of nutrition and health. People who are more educated tend to have greater knowledge of nutritional standards as well as proper food intake practices, which eventually leads to good health outcomes. On the contrary, poor education tends to produce poor nutrition as the person may not recognize the long-term effects of his/her diet (Huey et al., 2025). The interventions that aim at enhancing nutritional awareness among low SES groups need to account for these educational disparities. Interventions to provide available, informative resources can bridge knowledge disparities and make it possible for people to make better choices and, therefore, avoid the adverse effects of low SES on health. Finally, incorporating precision nutrition methods into addressing nutritional disparities by SES might enhance intervention effectiveness. Precision nutrition is concerned with individualized eating recommendations developed with a multitude of personal aspects in consideration, , such as genetics, medical conditions, and lifestyle. Through the identification that food reactions vary among individuals, and more importantly among different SES groups, being targeted, interventions can more effectively induce healthier eating habits (Huey et al., 2025). Personalized nutrition approaches have been shown to induce more diet change in underserved populations because they address specific problems these populations face. Thus, infusing nutritional screenings with increased focus on SES and applying precision nutrition approaches can potentially enhance the effectiveness of public health initiatives to improve nutrition and health outcomes in diverse socioeconomic populations.

4.5.2. Cultural Food Habits

Cultural food habits are part of nutritional assessment and consider the social, historical, and environmental contexts under which food is chosen. These habits determine what populations and families consume, and their nutrient composition and health. For example, meals in these cultures focus on locally grown produce that vary significantly from culture to culture. Food systems in different societies can shape not only available foods but also preparation methods and eating manners. Nutritionists and health practitioners benefit from this cultural view by needing to address these differences while developing effective nutrition plans. By not grasping the cultural significance of food, nutritional assessments can overlook significant dietary factors influencing health status and assist in perpetuating health inequities and countering the effectiveness of interventions planned to assist low-income families (Dowler, 2008). When it comes to addressing cultural eating patterns, attention needs to be taken to existing disparities in food access and how this influences nutritional status. Low-income family members are frequently denied access to good-quality foods that accommodate their cultural preferences. This situation contributes to health inequalities, as documented through obesity and malnutrition among the populations. Moves , such as the Acheson Inquiry recognize the need for targeted policies beyond personal efforts, which require comprehensive approaches embracing the diversity of cultural practices within low-income environments. Placing strong emphasis on culturally responsive nutritional planning can help end poverty and unhealthy living cycles, resulting in healthier societies in the long term. These considerations call for cultural sensitivity in public health initiatives, complementing arguments advocating for differentiated dietary assessment that is respectful and sensitive to cultural foodways (Dowler, 2008).

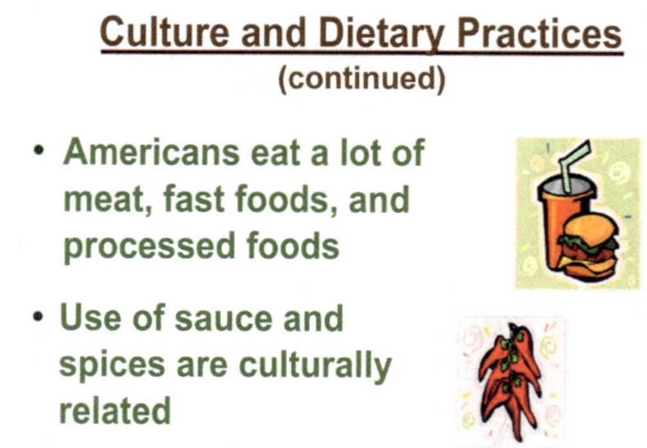
Culture and Dietary Practices
(continued)
• Americans eat a lot of meat, fast foods, and processed foods
• Use of sauce and spices are culturally related

Figure 4.16. Cultural influences on food choices and seasoning preferences.

Source: https://external-content.duckduckgo.com/iu/?u=https%3A%2F%2Fimage2.slideserve.com%2F4399733%2Fculture-and-dietary-practices-continued1-l.jpg&f=1&nofb=1&ipt=6ee5e11191b2a63a9419f4d6848c0e1f8d8a76901f051cbfdc645e81f01c5371.

Furthermore, the relationship between global health policies and cultural dietary practices emphasizes the complexity of achieving sustainable food security and nutrition goals. The Sustainable Development Goals (SDGs), particularly SDG 2 (Zero Hunger) and SDG 6 (Clean Water and Sanitation), reflect growing recognition of interdependent food and water security in various cultural contexts. However, a lack of adequate advancement in such realms warrants coordination amongst global initiatives towards confronting imbalances appropriately. Climatic issues and increasing requirements for food and water resources compound intricacies in these goals. Therefore, integral strategies that accommodate cultural dietary patterns become a necessity. Through familiarity with food culture and local food systems, stakeholders can create evidence-informed interventions that appreciate cultural diversity while enhancing nutritional security and sustainability in ways that align with global health objectives (Figure 4.16).

4.5.3. Age and Gender Differences

The interplay among age and gender distinctions significantly influences nutritional status and dietary needs, the requirements for effective nutritional assessment. As life ages, metabolic rates, physiological needs, and disease susceptibility are modified. For instance, children require a higher percentage of the required nutrients to boost development and growth, while older adults may require adjustments for decreased metabolism as well as the potential for chronic health ailments. Gender further complicates nutrition needs because females and males eat differently and have different tastes, which affect their nutrient intake. Moreover, women's hormonal fluctuations during menstruation, pregnancy, and menopause could result in differences in the demands for nutrients, necessitating gendered dietary guidelines, which must be evaluated rigorously during nutritional assessment to produce optimal health benefits. The impact of mental health on food intake also varies with age and gender, affecting the nutritional assessment of patients who have illnesses , such as SMI. Studies indicate that people with SMIs, including schizophrenia and major depressive disorder, eat poorly, favoring high intakes of unhealthy macronutrients and excess calories. These are especially prevalent in young adults, who may be at a crossroads to set up eating habits they will have for the rest of their lives, and older adults, who may already have established nutritional habits. More specifically, schizophrenic patients have much higher intakes of energy and unhealthy fats compared to healthy controls. This underscores the importance of age- and gender-specific nutritional evaluations since both are major determinants of dietary habits and health status and can cause inequalities in nutritional status across groups (Firth et al., 2018). Nutritional assessment methods must also consider the evolving epidemiologic patterns of disease , such as non-alcoholic fatty liver disease (NAFLD) with strong age- and gender-predominant patterns. Studies ascertain that while the prevalence of NAFLD increases with increasing age, the disease is significantly higher in men than in women, indicating the role of gender in the pathogenesis and manifestation of this disease. Additionally, available information stipulates that adults and, more especially, youth with pre-existing metabolic abnormalities can develop NAFLD irrespective of being overweight or obese, complicating the nutritional picture further. With age, alterations in body composition and insulin resistance may also affect the progression of NAFLD. By incorporating age- and gender-stratified measures into nutrition assessment, clinicians are better placed to identify vulnerable populations and implement targeted interventions to reduce associated complications from poor nutritional status (Wong et al., 2017) (Figure 4.18).

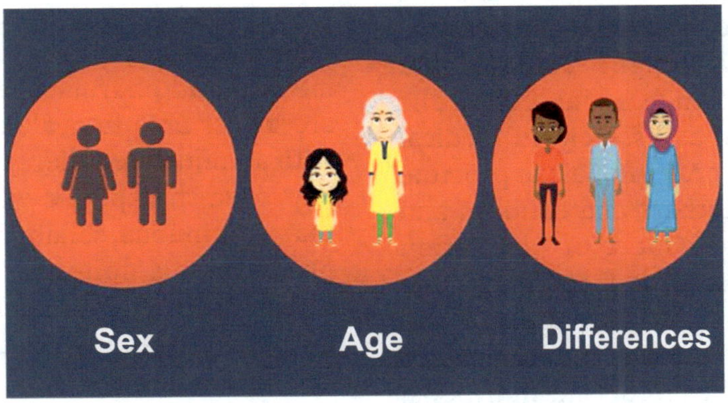

Figure 4.18. Demographic factors like sex, age, and cultural differences.

Source: https://external-content.duckduckgo.com/iu/?u=http%3A%2F%2Faea365.org%2Fblog%2Fwp-content%2Fuploads%2F2018%2F03%2FSex-Age-Differences-graphic.png&f=1&nofb=1&ipt=60234b503b9ae17ce52351693852263331 05f0e4c6944f465eb11bb64d80e47a.

4.6. Applications for Nutritional Assessment

In the evaluation of the broad uses of nutritional assessment, one of the most important functions is the role it has in public health program planning and dietary research. Nutritional assessments provide essential information on patterns of intake and nutritional status that serve as the foundation for designing successful interventions for a given population. For instance, the identification of usual intake distributions with improved diet assessment , such as the SIMPLE macro enhances research through precise data on micronutrient deficiency and eating patterns. The technique employs a strong statistical model that is capable of assisting researchers in estimating the typical nutrient intake distributions, revealing vital information that can be employed to guide public health policy as well as neighborhood health interventions for diet enhancement and intervention (Luo et al., 2020). Consequently, effective nutritional assessment not only illuminates the current status of dietary intake but also guides the ways of enhancing aggregate population health. Another significant application of nutritional assessment is the clinical management of obesity, particularly in women of reproductive age. Since the prevalence of obesity is on the rise and has the potential to have a remarkable impact on maternal and child health outcomes, nutritional assessment protocols are now gaining traction among healthcare providers to inform preventive and intervention strategies. Obstetricians and gynecologists, for instance, employ these assessments to monitor food intake and weight patterns in pregnancy to minimize risk factors associated with obesity in the mother, including gestational diabetes and delivery complications. FIGO guidelines emphasize tracking BMI and diet habits before pregnancy and during pregnancy to maintain healthy weight control and nutritional adequacy (McAuliffe et al., 2020). The inclusion of nutritional assessment in medical practice enables health professionals to promote healthier results for mothers and children and thus assume a central aspect of population health. Lastly, nutritional assessment finds a role at the intersection of policy development and health education. Complete assessment enables policymakers to ascertain appropriate nutritional deficiencies in populations, which may be used to inform specific educational intervention that plugs those gaps. Dietary intake analysis can identify population-specific deficiencies, such as,, such as underconsumption of iron in certain populations, leading to the creation of fortification programs, , such as those illustrated using the SIMPLE-Iron macro. These new schemes can be effectively capable of addressing micronutrient deficiencies ascertained from nutritional assessments, thereby improving the health status at large levels (Luo et al., 2020). The resultant health education schemes resulting from these assessments empower individuals with knowledge about healthy eating habits, effectively illuminating various communities. The nutritional assessments are, thus, not only symptomatic but also catalysts for broader systemic enhancements in improving public health and nutrition.

4.6.1. Patient Care and Clinical Settings

Patient care success in a clinical setting needs extensive nutrition evaluations, particularly among patients with chronic diseases like inflammatory bowel disease (IBD). These patients are likely to be managing complex drug regimens that raise the likelihood of drug interactions due to other self-medication practices, , such as the use of nutritional supplements to correct malabsorption issues. A critical issue in this context lies in the lack of pharmaceutical monitoring, which can potentially help alleviate adverse events and enhance patient compliance with clinical therapy guidelines. By employing an interdisciplinary strategy that encompasses both medical and pharmaceutical specialists, clinics are better able to evaluate patient compliance with administered therapy, leading ultimately to improved therapeutic outcomes. It is essential that continuous collaboration between health professionals follows, as this maintains a safety culture that aims at the efficacy of nutritional therapy in follow-up consultation for the management of IBD (Fleischmann et al., 2025). Anthropometric assessments are still a fundamental part of nutritional assessment in clinical practice, yet the reliability of such measurements has not been properly resolved. Medical anthropometric measurement errors can very much affect the accuracy of nutritional data and thus render effective patient care and the identification of health risks difficult. An examination of technical errors of measurement (TEM) indicates that despite the majority of measurements showing fair reliability between professionals, considerable variation exists between those with more experience and less experienced practitioners. For example, hand length and adductor pollicis thickness measurements revealed unacceptable error ranges, demonstrating the critical need for repetitive training and adherence to standardized protocol. It is only through ongoing educational campaigns that the accuracy and clinical utility of anthropometric data can be maintained so that medical professionals are able to access accurate information for the effective diagnosis and management of patients (Rodrigues et al., 2025). Incorporating systematic nutritional assessment in daily clinical practice, in addition to enhancing patient care, also benefits overall health results. The interconnection between medication management and nutritional assessment provides a broader perspective on the health status of a patient. Hence, installing systematic assessment protocols, , such as frequent anthropometric measurements and regular medication reviews, becomes necessary. These steps enable health professionals to identify potential nutritional deficiencies or imbalances that are particularly critical in chronically ill individuals. Furthermore, through patient sensitization and education on their nutritional needs, healthcare teams can ensure greater participation rates among their care plans. Lastly, a keen focus on patient-centered nutrition assessment within clinical settings is accountable for the development of individualized interventions, which are key to offering acceptable and sustainable health outcomes (Fleischmann et al., 2025; Rodrigues et al., 2025) (Figure 4.19).

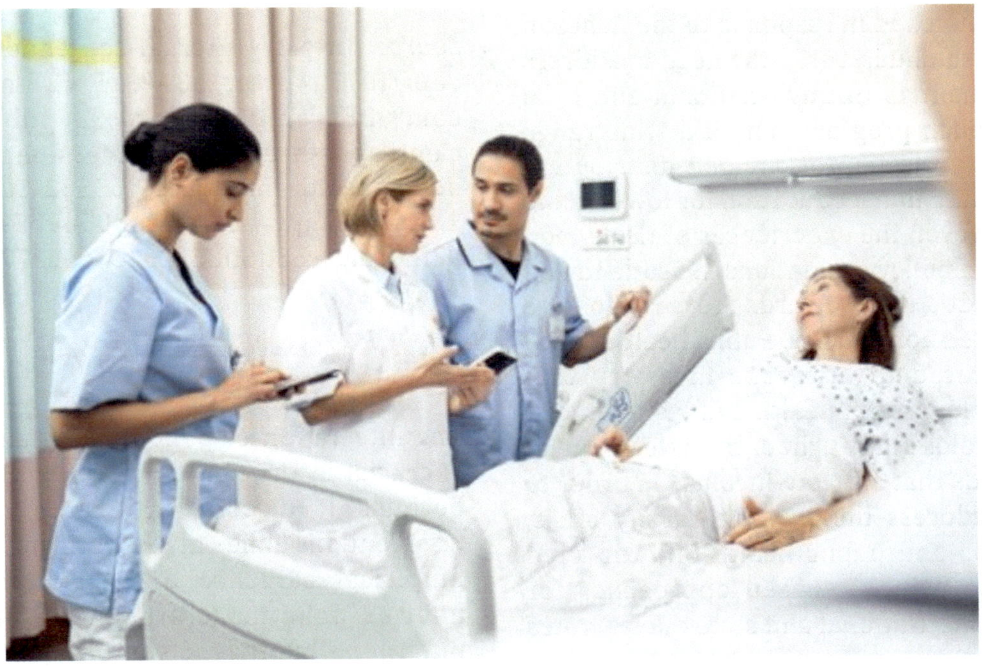

Figure 4.19. The medical team performing bedside patient evaluation.

Source: https://external-content.duckduckgo.com/iu/?u=https%3A%2F%2Ftse1.mm.bing.net%2Fth%3Fid%3DOIP.l9wfMRxm7mBwQaZa9PJG-AHaE8%26cb%3Diwc2%26pid%3DApi&f=1&ipt=15c2769e73a974e5295c88d728a968e4dcb8f7a8ea671cc1403ea753de24dce1.

4.6.2. Public Health Initiatives

Public health initiatives play an important role in the solution of nutritional disparities in society, particularly among the marginalized. Governments and organizations have realized that diseases , such as obesity and food poverty, are not only personal issues but are embedded in the injustices of the system. Experiments in the UK demonstrate that poorer families experience more of poor nutritional status, which can lead to child and adult obesity. Given focused efforts over the past decade to minimize such health disparities, comprehensive policy frameworks that effectively address such needs strategically have been lacking. This deficiency calls for an integrated approach that not only addresses immediate nutritional requirements but also fosters long-term change in the accessibility and education of food and thereby build healthier communities. Interventions against nutritional disparities have led to the development of personalized public health interventions. Programs that aim to improve access to healthy food are necessary where economic limitations limit healthy options. For instance, several programs have been launched in response to the Acheson Inquiry, which underscored the need to address health inequalities through national and local initiatives. Such programs entail a wide range of activities, from improving food distribution systems to nutritional education for low-income people. However, the experiences of these food and nutrition policy evaluations in Scotland and Wales suggest a shift towards more responsive and integrated approaches. Public health policy is better placed to intervene in a way that benefits the long-term health and well-being of such households in the light of the heterogeneity of households that are 'low-income.' In order to effectively address the existing obesity crisis, policymakers and public health officials need to prioritize evidence-based approaches for their programs. National and state obesity rates analyzed indicate that existing policies might not be doing a sufficient job of fighting the crisis as it is. The research community needs to pose fundamental questions that may guide subsequent policy action through the prism of emerging solutions that seek to address the root determinants of unhealthy diet. To this end, it becomes more evident that a complex strategy that involves intervention at the upstream level is needed. By focusing on broad public health interventions, there is the potential to create effective long-term change that not only improves individual well-being but also sets the foundation for a healthier community food and lifestyle environment (Juliano et al., 2005; Dowler, 2008) (Figure 4.20).

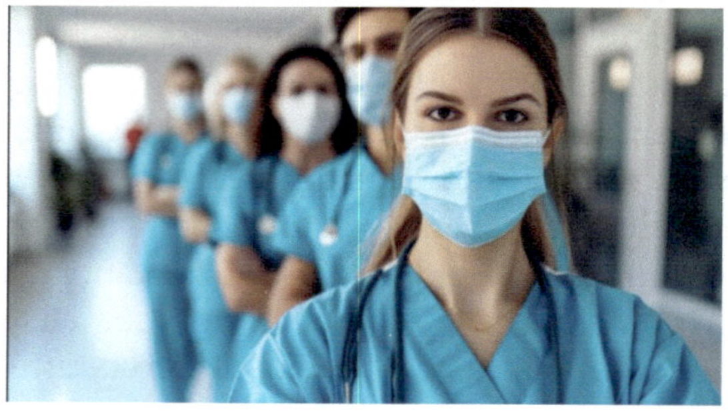

Figure 4.20. Healthcare workers supporting public health initiatives.

Source: https://external-content.duckduckgo.com/iu/?u=https%3A%2F%2Fimg.freepik.com%2Fpremium-photo%2Fpublic-health-campaigns-healthcare-professionals-leading-public-health-initiatives_765582-10555.jpg&f=1&nofb=1&ipt=b11b92cd30549b59e32afa09942f21eafaec55d6ff86de61e469c877b4f9aa50.

4.6.3. Research and Policy Development

The integration of policymaking and research is crucial in the field of nutritional evaluation because it directly influences meaningful interventions aimed at promoting public health. Empirical evidence derived from research informs policymakers of dietary needs and nutritional deficiencies that are prevalent among populations. This is, particularly, critical in devising programs aimed at alleviating food insecurity, thereby contributing to sustainable food systems. Evidence-based policy recommendations can guide resource allocation choices so that the measures applied to enhance nutritional analysis are both effective and cost-effective. By a scientific analysis of the outcomes of implemented policies, research can help rebalance approaches so that they are more in tune with population needs, emphasizing the interactive nature of ongoing inquiry and policy adjustment in the context of nutrition.

The incorporation of ontology-based innovative approaches in nutrition research reinforces the policy's evidence base. From contemporary studies, the construction of ontologies , such as the ontology for nutritional epidemiology (ONE), is pivotal in alleviating the complexity in data integration and enhancing research output accuracy in this area. The systematic organization of nutritional data allows for a more natural understanding of the interactions between disparate dietary determinants and their health implications, which can prove crucial for guiding effective policy interventions. These frameworks allow for extensive reviews of existing standards and recommendations, allowing researchers to gain insights that reveal nutritional immunization deficits as well as conditions necessitating targeted interventions. Through the use of such resources, policymakers can develop more educated policies that address the multidimensionality of nutritional challenges in multi-faceted populations. A key aspect of successful policymaking is the capacity to consolidate fragmented research into effective plans of action. On the basis of various case studies, addressing multifaceted nutrition issues requires the coordination of various stakeholders, including government agencies, non-profit organizations, and business executives. Moreover, international programs to optimize fisheries management, shown through working papers of the International Sustainability Unity, demonstrate how research programs adopting a collaborative approach have been capable of overcoming obstacles in terms of nutritional shortages and food supply security (Harris et al., 2013). By being proactive in participating in multi-disciplinary research and adopting findings within policy programmers, actors are capable of optimizing resilience in food systems as well as promoting sustainable modes. This kind of strategy not only enables comprehensive nutritional assessment but also supports foresight policies that boost population health gains in a more multi-faceted world.

CLOSER LOOK

NUTRITION

Nutrition is the science of how food affects the body's growth, development, and overall health. It involves the intake of nutrients—such as carbohydrates, proteins, fats, vitamins, and minerals—that are essential for energy production, cellular repair, immune function, and disease prevention. Proper nutrition is crucial throughout all stages of life, from infancy to old age. A balanced diet supports optimal body function, maintains a healthy weight, and reduces the risk of chronic illnesses like heart disease, diabetes, and cancer.

Macronutrients (carbohydrates, proteins, and fats) provide the energy necessary for daily activities and physiological functions. Carbohydrates are the body's primary energy source, while proteins are vital for tissue growth and repair. Fats support brain function, hormone production, and nutrient absorption. Micronutrients—vitamins and minerals—are equally important, though required in smaller amounts. For instance, iron is essential for oxygen transport in the blood, while vitamin D helps maintain healthy bones and immunity. Hydration is another key aspect of nutrition. Water aids in digestion, nutrient transport, temperature regulation, and toxin elimination. Malnutrition—both undernutrition and overnutrition—can lead to serious health problems. Undernutrition may result in stunted growth, weakened immunity, and developmental delays, especially in children. Overnutrition, often due to poor dietary habits and sedentary lifestyles, contributes to obesity and related diseases.

Cultural, economic, and psychological factors also influence nutritional choices. Education about healthy eating habits, food accessibility, and mindful consumption plays a critical role in improving nutritional outcomes. In clinical settings, nutrition therapy is often used to manage conditions like diabetes, kidney disease, and eating disorders. The nutrition is foundational to health and well-being. A well-balanced, varied, and nutrient-dense diet, paired with an active lifestyle, is key to disease prevention, longevity, and quality of life.

SUMMARY

The increasing incidence of frying food consumption in China has been recognized as a major risk factor for the increasing CVD burden, with studies showing an estimated relationship between increased frequency and the occurrence of CVD events, , such as coronary heart disease and stroke. The research estimates that the phenomenal 127.6 grams of per-week fried food consumption in 2031 will further exacerbate the public health crisis in this region, warranting dietary guidelines with emphasis on reducing such unwholesome sources of food (Wang et al., 2025). This brings into focus the exceedingly crucial function of effective nutrition education and policy change to impart healthier eating habits among people. Furthermore, understanding how dietary antioxidants and body mass index (BMI) interact contributes vital information for the evaluation of stroke risk and prevention. Research on the Composite Dietary Antioxidant Index (CDAI) in U.S. adults affirmed a strong interaction between antioxidant intake and BMI status, with results showing that higher levels of dietary antioxidants can provide stronger protective effects against stroke, particularly in those of greater BMI. This nuanced interrelation between nutritional variables and demographic factors can be used to better shape public health policy and dietary advice, tailoring it to specific groups who may be at increased risk (Li et al., 2024). Such incorporation of such evidence into public health policy, therefore, may potentially improve stroke prevention, which will translate into improved health outcomes across a range of different populations. In integrating evidence from different nutritional evaluations, it is evident that intervention towards dietary practices is critical to counter the risks of chronic diseases. The evidence of the harmful impacts of fried foods on heart health and the protective capacity of dietary antioxidants shows the complexity of nutrition's role in disease prevention. Therefore, public health players should advocate for comprehensive strategies that not only promote a healthy diet but also empower communities against the risk of consuming unhealthy diets. Collaborations among healthcare workers, policymakers, and educational institutions are necessary to translate effective nutrition interventions that lead to long-term changes in behavior, hence reducing the disease burden of diet-related noncommunicable diseases (Li et al., 2024; Wang et al., 2025). By such concerted effort, it is possible to pave the way for healthier future generations, placing priority on the importance of continued nutritional surveillance and adaptive interventions.

A clear understanding of nutrition assessment is important to evaluate the nutritional status of individuals in various populations. Central to this evaluation lies the definition of sarcopenia, which has been revolutionized over the past few years. Specifically, the European Working Group on Sarcopenia in Older People 2 (EWGSOP2) laid out a complex approach, emphasizing the crucial role of both low muscle strength and low muscle mass as vital markers of health state. This definition, in two parts, aims to render the determination of those at risk for sarcopenia more specific, especially among the elderly, where muscle loss is strongly linked to adverse health outcomes. The overlapping of sarcopenia and broader nutritional conditions , such as malnutrition and cachexia, underscores the need for sensitive assessments that can capture functional and structural features of muscle health, as indicated in more current research (Sánchez-Rodríguez et al., 2019). Additionally, the role of nutrition assessment extends beyond individual health to involve public health considerations and regulatory settings. The European Food Safety Authority (EFSA) also participates in establishing databases providing ready access to information on food safety and chemical risks. One of these databases is OpenFoodTox, which consolidates risk assessments for various substances present in foods and provides an organized approach to investigating human health risks. By facilitating the sharing of the relevant toxicological information and reference points, the OpenFoodTox supports researchers as well as healthcare professionals making sound nutritional choices. The EFSA needs to be aware of both the health risks suggested by the ingestion of food as well as the diet counseling required for the future direction for enhanced risk communication as well as decision-making (Dorne et al., 2017). Finally, the integration of nutrition assessment with broader health and safety control is obviously apparent in dialogue between scientific research and policymaking. Challenges posed by various definitions of health-related conditions like sarcopenia and malnutrition emphasize the necessity for a harmonized approach that would increase clarity and ensure consistency in assessments. Global organizations' joint ventures aim to generate international definitions, therefore making clinical research and practical use in clinics easier. The invocation of expert panels in answering such issues is proof of constructive action towards the encouragement of the quality of public health results. As nutritional assessment continues to change, these regulatory views will eventually contribute to a more holistic approach to nutrition's role in health maintenance and disease prevention (Sánchez-Rodríguez et al., 2019).

References

1. https://core.ac.uk/download/47325.pdf Dowler E. Symposium on 'Intervention policies for deprived households' Policy initiatives to address low-income households' nutritional needs in the UK. *Proceedings of the Nutrition Society.* 2008;67(3):289-300. doi:10.1017/S0029665108008586 (accessed on 13th June 2025).
2. Ambayo, H., Bouwman, J., Bronselaer, A., De Baets, B., et al. (2019). An ontology to standardize research output of nutritional epidemiology: From paper-based standards to linked content. https://core.ac.uk/download/222452585.pdf (accessed on 13th June 2025).
3. Andrews, H., Chao, C., Gupta, N., Leu, H., et al. (2018). Thiopurines are negatively associated with anthropometric parameters in pediatric Crohn's disease. https://core.ac.uk/download/323074673.pdf (accessed on 13th June 2025).
4. Branca, F., Garcia-Alvarez, A., & de Groot, C. P. G. M., et al. (2009). Overview of methods used to evaluate the adequacy of nutrient intakes for individuals and populations. https://core.ac.uk/download/pdf/29248327.pdf (accessed on 13th June 2025).
5. Cappuccio, F., Hilton, S., McKay, C., Perkins-Porras, L., et al. (2003). Behavioral counselling to increase consumption of fruit and vegetables in low-income adults: Randomized trial. https://core.ac.uk/download/44324.pdf (accessed on 13th June 2025).
6. Ravaioli, F., De Maria, N., Di Marco, L., Pivetti, A., Casciola, R., Ceraso, C., Frassanito, G., Pambianco, M., Pecchini, M., Sicuro, C., Leoni, L., Di Sandro, S., Magistri, P., Menozzi, R., Di Benedetto, F., & Colecchia, A. (2023). From Listing to Recovery: A Review of Nutritional Status Assessment and Management in Liver Transplant Patients. *Nutrients, 15*(12), 2778. https://doi.org/10.3390/nu15122778 (accessed on 13th June 2025).
7. Cheever, V. J., Mohajeri, A., Patel, K., Burris, R. C., & Hung, M. (2025). Impact of free sugar consumption on dental caries: A cross-sectional analysis of children in the United States. *Dentistry Journal, 13.* https://www.semanticscholar.org/paper/c7346ab66492611b60f07d8bd7ff073c5aed0e7c (accessed on 13th June 2025).
8. Cofre, S., Sanchez, C., Quezada-Figueroa, G., & López-Cortés, X. A. (2025). Validity and accuracy of artificial intelligence-based dietary intake assessment methods: A systematic review. *The British Journal of Nutrition.* https://www.semanticscholar.org/paper/309473b7a8811c9deab1916b5e9ba2607d4340a1 (accessed on 13th June 2025).
9. Denno, D. M., Musser, C. A., Nelson, Z. C., Tarr, P. I., et al. (2016). Chapter Five. Systematic review results by biomarker classifications. https://core.ac.uk/download/70385873.pdf (accessed on 13th June 2025).
10. Fatima, R., Fatima, I., Yousaf, F., Kaynat, W., Ikram, N., Ansar, S., & Khan, M. A. (2024). Dietary modifications for the malnourished children with cerebral palsy. *Journal of Health and Rehabilitation Research.* https://www.semanticscholar.org/paper/0af11dcea4c4d86160d15cb11a848575425f9e75 (accessed on 13th June 2025).
11. Firth, J., Stubbs, B., Teasdale, S., Ward, P. B., Veronese, N., Shivappa, N., Hébert, J. R., et al. (2018). Diet as a hot topic in psychiatry: A population-scale study of nutritional intake and inflammatory potential in severe mental illness. *World Psychiatry, 17,* 365–367. https://doi.org/10.1002/wps.20571 (accessed on 13th June 2025).

12. Fleischmann, D., Binder, B., Huss, M., Elger, T., Wolf, C., Loibl, J., Tews, H., et al. (2025). Interprofessional approach to personalized medication management and therapy optimization in IBD care. *Frontiers in Medicine, 12.* https://www.semanticscholar.org/paper/563e57325 7af38b9cc868252bc4e2fe81fe9e737 (accessed on 13th June 2025).

13. Gedil, M., & Menkir, A. (2020). An integrated molecular and conventional breeding scheme for enhancing genetic gain in maize in Africa. https://core.ac.uk/download/286455309.pdf (accessed on 13th June 2025).

14. Giaginis, C., Kavantzas, N., Mantzorou, M., Papandreou, D., et al. (2022). Adherence to Mediterranean diet and nutritional status in women with breast cancer: What is their impact on disease progression and recurrence-free patients' survival? https://core.ac.uk/download/543115426.pdf (accessed on 13th June 2025).

15. Gümüş, A. B., Köktürk, S. N., Yardımcı, H., Uzun, A. K., & Koç, N. (2024). The association between maternal and child nutritional status: Evidence from a social pediatrics outpatient clinic. *Turkish Journal of Pediatric Disease.* https://www.semanticscholar.org/paper/38cd0a 7add72af9f0c6f95a1a96b055da2ec9327 (accessed on 13th June 2025).

16. Harris, C., Agnew, D., Leotte, F., Arthur, R., Walmsley, S., Davies, T., & Peatman, T. (2013). Fisheries and aquaculture and their potential roles in development: An assessment of the current evidence. https://core.ac.uk/download/75777502.pdf (accessed on 13th June 2025).

17. Hasan, I. (2010). A study of prevalence of malnutrition in government school children in the field area of Azad Nagar, Bangalore, India. https://core.ac.uk/download/pdf/289449.pdf (accessed on 13th June 2025).

18. Herc, A., Koczkodon, K., Krompiewski, M., Marcinkowska, D., et al. (2024). Nutritional treatment of patients in the perioperative period–Literature review. https://core.ac.uk/download/620863354.pdf (accessed on 13th June 2025).

19. Juliano, C., Segal, L. M., Earls, M. J., Glendening, P. N., & Hearne, S. A. (2005). *F as in Fat: How Obesity Policies Are Failing in America, 2005.* https://core.ac.uk/download/71351405.pdf (accessed on 13th June 2025).

20. Li, X., Hu, X., & You, C. (2024). Interactive effects of composite dietary antioxidant index with body mass index for the risk of stroke among U.S. adults: Insight from NHANES 2001–2018. *Frontiers in Nutrition, 11.* https://www.semanticscholar.org/paper/7768b7a2ccaca51a7636 529edecfc3387fef66dc (accessed on 13th June 2025).

21. Livingston, G., Huntley, J., Sommerlad, A., Ames, D., Ballard, C., Banerjee, S., Brayne, C., et al. (2020). Dementia prevention, intervention, and care: 2020 report of the Lancet Commission. *The Lancet, 396*, 413–446. https://doi.org/10.1016/s0140-6736(20)30367-6 (accessed on 13th June 2025).

22. Luo, H., Dodd, K. W., Arnold, C. D., & Engle-Stone, R. (2020). Introduction to the SIMPLE Macro, a tool to increase the accessibility of 24-hour dietary recall analysis and modeling. *Journal of Nutrition, 151*, 1329–1340. https://doi.org/10.1093/jn/nxaa440 (accessed on 13th June 2025).

23. Machado, G., Pinheiro, C., & Rodrigues, L. (2018). Cheese: Food perception and food choice. https://core.ac.uk/download/187759553.pdf (accessed on 13th June 2025).

24. Phalle, A., & Gokhale, D. (2025). Navigating next-gen nutrition care using artificial intelligence-assisted dietary assessment tools—A scoping review of potential applications. *Frontiers in Nutrition, 12.* https://www.semanticscholar.org/paper/cdcc2c41b6d7b1a8f8d42dd6411b3f89f306a293 (accessed on 13th June 2025).

25. Sánchez-Rodríguez, D., Marco, E., & Cruz-Jentoft, A. J. (2019). Defining sarcopenia: Some caveats and challenges. *Current Opinion in Clinical Nutrition & Metabolic Care, 23*, 127–132. https://doi.org/10.1097/mco.0000000000000621 (accessed on 13th June 2025).

26. Schol, J., Wauters, L., Dickman, R., Drug, V., Mulak, A., Serra, J., Enck, P., et al. (2021). United European Gastroenterology (UEG) and European Society for Neurogastroenterology and Motility (ESNM) consensus on gastroparesis. *United European Gastroenterology Journal, 9*, 287–306. https://doi.org/10.1002/ueg2.12060 (accessed on 13th June 2025).

27. Stylianou, K. (2018). Nutritional and environmental impacts of foods on human health. http://deepblue.lib.umich.edu/bitstream/2027.42/147641/1/kstylian_1.pdf (accessed on 13th June 2025).

28. Wang, A., Ao, Y., Liu, X., Wan, X., Pan, Z., Jiao, J., & Zhang, Y. (2025). Potential impact of the time trend of fried food consumption on the cardiovascular disease burden in China. *Food & Function.* https://www.semanticscholar.org/paper/eb27b67a57b18dd369ce659c8f0c1a0848058c1c (accessed on 13th June 2025).

29. Wu, Y., Li, D., & Vermund, S. H. (2024). Advantages and limitations of the Body Mass Index (BMI) to assess adult obesity. *International Journal of Environmental Research and Public Health, 21.* https://www.semanticscholar.org/paper/1f20eaebe4c1c273e27a3589ad269b70bf1fa8dd (accessed on 13th June 2025).

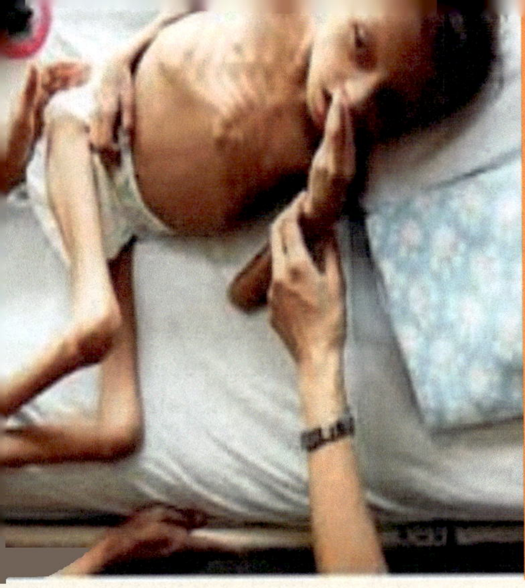

Chapter 5

PROTEIN-ENERGY MALNUTRITION (PEM)

Contents

Introduction....143
5.1. Causes of Protein-Energy Malnutrition....146
5.2. Types of Protein-Energy Malnutrition....150
5.3. Symptoms and Health Effects....154
5.4. Populations at Risk....157
5.5. Diagnosis of Protein-Energy Malnutrition....161
5.6. Treatment and Management....165
Summary....171
References....173

Introduction

The integrative method of addressing the complex issue of protein-energy malnutrition (PEM) begins with an understanding of its many-sided nature, because it is a significant global health concern, particularly in the Third World. PEM is caused by a discrepancy between the body's nutritional needs and nutrient intake from dietary sources, leading to inadequate protein and energy consumption. The impact of PEM extends far beyond physical health to cognitive and psychological development. Vulnerable populations, including young children and infants, are at high risk, as their childhood years require adequate nutritional advantages for optimal growth and improved health status. Examination of PEM is hence of extreme significance to public health, as it is linked with other determinants in health and socioeconomics that assist in producing malnutrition-poverty cycles. One area of inquiry that is applicable here is the study of the impact of PEM on recovery from acute health events, , such as strokes. Research studies, , such as those involving adult rats, provide pertinent data on how dietary deficiencies after such incidents stall recuperative processes. The studies on PEM illustrate essential parallels between human conditions and animal models, as evidenced by results demonstrating spectacular variations in health outcomes in relation to different protein content in diets. For instance, one study highlighted that a 0.5% protein diet led to spectacular cognitive impairment, in comparison to situations among human stroke patients with malnutrition (Ramos et al.). This association underscores the paramount significance of proper nutrition in facilitating recovery, thereby emphasizing the necessity of targeted intervention to avert and treat PEM. Understanding the broader consequences of PEM also necessitates examination of where it overlaps with other health conditions, , such as anemia, among vulnerable populations. Studies show that severe anemia, which is usually a result of associated malnutrition, heavily imposes on health service utilization and increases mortality rates among children, particularly in malaria-endemic areas (PL et al., 2002). The establishment of risk factors, including educational levels of parents and nutritional levels, offers an extensive framework for developing effective anemia control programs that also target PEM. As the connections between malnutrition, anemia, and overall health effects fall into place, public health measures must take into consideration the systemic and interconnected nature of such conditions. Ultimately, the management of PEM not only impacts an individual's health but also greatly impacts community health facilities and resources (Figure 5.1).

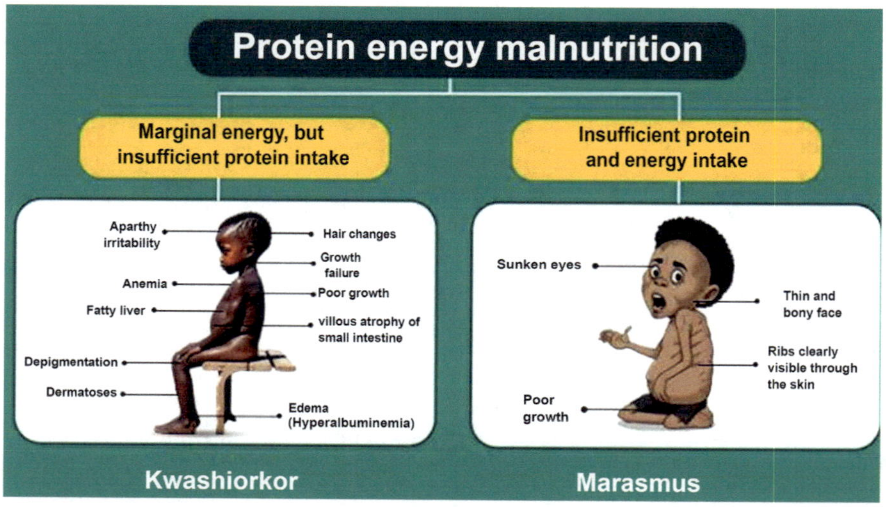

Figure 5.1. Comparison of Kwashiorkor and Marasmus in protein-energy malnutrition.

Source: https://media.geeksforgeeks.org/wp-content/uploads/20240603182016/Protein-Energy-Malnutrition-.webp.

Definition of Protein-Energy Malnutrition

Protein-Energy Malnutrition (PEM) is a serious public health problem that comprises the inappropriate consumption of protein and energy, leading to adverse health outcomes. PEM encompasses a series of disorders, which are most commonly encountered in vulnerable populations , such as children, the aging population, and people with chronic illnesses. Its presentation can range from mild to severe, based on the extent and duration of the nutritional impairment. The clinical presentation of PEM is weight loss, growth retardation, wasting of muscles, and immune impairment, leading to increased risk of infections and longer recovery times. PEM has been identified by the World Health

Organization as a key concern with a focus on dealing with it comprehensively through nutrition interventions in order to reduce its consequences on health and development, especially where there is resource limitations. Through comprehension of the nature and extent of PEM, medical professionals are able to better treat the nutritional requirements of infected groups with a view to enhancing overall health outcomes. Central to the comprehension of PEM is its categorization into various types, that is, marasmus and kwashiorkor. Marasmus is typically brought about by severe energy deficiency, resulting in muscle wasting and weight loss, while kwashiorkor is largely brought about by protein deficiency with sufficient calorie intake, which presents edema, fatty liver, and discoloration of skin and hair. The two diseases reflect distinct metabolic responses to malnutrition and demonstrate the complexity of PEM. It is important to be able to differentiate between the two for proper diagnosis and treatment. Clinical assessments usually include measurement of dietary intake, anthropometric assessment, and biochemical markers of nutritional status. Through the interaction between clinical assessment and public education about proper nutrition, health workers are able to implement efficient interventions against PEM so that individuals can be provided with the needed nutrients to maintain a healthy balance of physiology, thus averting long-term ailments associated with chronic undernutrition. The effects of PEM are not only short-term health consequences but also have a significant bearing on social, economic, and development results. In kids, the effects can be long-term, affecting cognitive growth, education, and overall adult economic productivity. In populations with a high prevalence of PEM, there is also the risk of having inter-generation cycles of malnutrition that perpetuate poor socio-economic status and health. In addition, PEM contributes to the healthcare burden, overloading those already stretched health system resources, particularly in low- and middle-income nations where it is more common. Resolution of PEM, thus, requires application of a multi-faceted approach with improved food security, better access to quality diet food, and nutrition education on balanced diets, as well as addressing the socio-economic determinants causing malnutrition. As the world continues to address malnutrition, comprehension of the complexities of PEM is still vital in developing efficient interventions and fostering universal improvements in health in these affected areas (Figure 5.2).

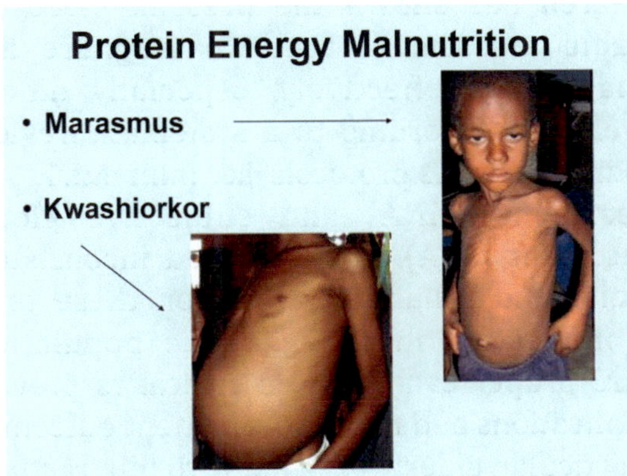

Figure 5.2. Clinical presentation of Kwashiorkor and Marasmus.

Source: https://external-content.duckduckgo.com/iu/?u=https%3A%2F%2Fimage3.slideserve.com%2F6859191%2Fprotein-energy-malnutrition-l.jpg&f=1&nofb=1&ipt=2dc289a6f3ea4522c6a6113dc714a28fe6d5b8e36da5ae8ce5e36c6b8454ce06.

Importance of the Topic in Global Health

The global health implications of PEM are extensive, particularly given its universality among vulnerable populations, , such as children and the elderly. In addition to sabotaging short-term health outcomes, causing an increase in morbidity and mortality, PEM also has lasting impacts on mental development and physical ability. Its impact is of greatest concern in developing countries, as it worsens the poverty-disease nexus, sabotaging socioeconomic progress. Effective interventions that target PEM thus have key roles to play in broadening public health programs internationally. The World Health Organization is eager to emphasize the need for targeted nutritional programs to combat these deficiencies because adequate nutrition lies at the heart of health, irrespective of life stages. Combating PEM is not only vital to an individual's well-being but also to the stability and development of society at large. Research has shown the pressing need for reliable assessment tools to diagnose and manage PEM effectively, especially among the elderly. According to a systematic review, existing diagnosis protocols, i.e., mini nutritional assessment (MNA) and subjective global assessment (SGA), demonstrated inconsistent validity and reliability. However, these tools are ineffectual in the geriatric population, where proper evaluation is critical to prevent complications and to improve patient outcomes. In particular, elderly patients with hip fractures show high levels of malnutrition that make their recovery process challenging and raise mortality risks. The incidence of malnutrition among this population reflects an immediate void in effective nutritional screening. Consequently, there is a need to promote diagnostic precision and availability so that global health programs can decrease the PEM burden in high-risk groups (Craven et al., 2017). Moreover, the economic effects of PEM extend beyond direct health care expenditure to influence productivity and quality of life. Nutritional deficiencies in older adults, for example, have been linked with poorer functional recovery and higher complication rates in the course of hospital stay. The link reinforces the importance of nutritional intervention, particularly following acute health occurrences like hip fractures. The literature indicates that the treatment of malnutrition not only improves health outcomes but also turns out to be cost-effective, leading to better resource utilization within healthcare organizations. One study reported that focused nutritional therapy resulted in noteworthy improvement in nutritional status and functional recovery of elderly patients after hip fracture (Malafarina et al., 2017). This underscores the necessity of international health policy that places a focus on nutrition because preventing and curing PEM can yield healthier and more resilient populations, eventually boosting economic security and public health.

5.1. Causes of Protein-Energy Malnutrition

The complex mesh of etiology of Protein-Energy Malnutrition (PEM) essentially rests in the socio-economic and cultural determinants influencing the diet of individuals with their eating habits. Socio-economic status of the family, in the majority of communities, influences the quality of eating a diverse range of food items. For instance, lower-income families may compromise with cheaper, calorically dense foods instead of more expensive, nutrient-dense foods, resulting in an imbalance favorable to malnutrition. Moreover, socio-cultural perceptions of food will also have an impact on feeding habits and intake, particularly in lactating mothers. It has been proven that the education level of the mother plays an important role; mothers who possess higher levels of nutrition knowledge will be able to provide children with proper nutrition, hence reducing the risk of PEM. As such, these socio-cultural forces must be tackled so that the risk factors of Protein-Energy Malnutrition for vulnerable populations can be mitigated (Akinpelu, 2015). The second most important aspect for the development of PEM is the eating habits adopted in the early childhood years. Children require specific feeding patterns that promote good development and growth; any inconsistency with what is recommended can lead to harmful nutritional deficiencies. The period of complementary food introduction, for example, is critical; it has been established that children who delay complementary feeding, particularly after the age of six months, are at higher risk of malnutrition. Inadequate breastfeeding also matters; children who are not breastfed do not receive the necessary nutrients that are vital to their growth. The interplay between such feeding patterns, coupled with the incidence of illness or dietary limitation within households, underscores the need for interventions aimed at shaping healthy infant feeding behavior (Mohammed, 2019). Last but not least, the contribution of health-related complications cannot be overstated in PEM causative theory. The children with underlying health problems and those with repeated infections are particularly vulnerable to malnutrition, as these conditions also increase their nutritional requirements. Such illnesses may impair nutrient intake, and infections may add to the loss of nutrients, entering a vicious cycle of disease and malnutrition. For instance, institutional children have been found to be at higher risk of PEM due to the compounding nature of such health problems. Also, fluctuations in economic status or environmental issues, such as food shortages or natural disasters, may disrupt food availability, causing it to become even more challenging for families to provide adequate nutrition for children. Therefore, it is important to address health issues with nutritional education and socio-economic assistance to reduce the incidence of Protein-Energy Malnutrition (Mohammed, 2019) (Figure 5.3).

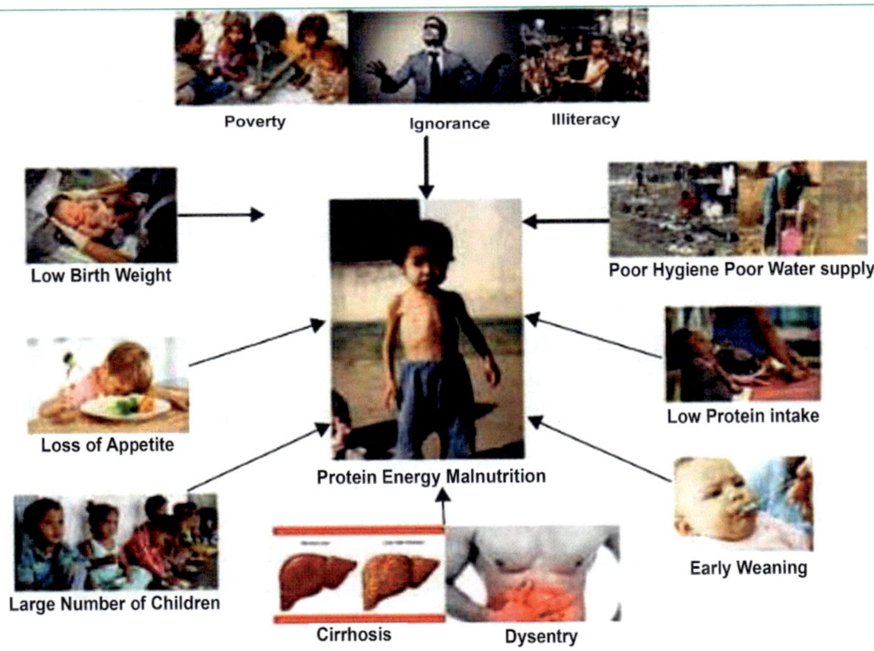

Figure 5.3. Factors leading to and resulting from protein energy malnutrition.

Source: https://external-content.duckduckgo.com/iu/?u=https%3A%2F%2Fimg.brainkart.com%2Fimagebk34%2FqY5yKAd.jpg&f=1&nofb=1&ipt=5b8149e700dc1a7d1a5bfe8a3d55cce4968577a77ff2eaf89cda0b469d9b624d.

5.1.1. Insufficient Dietary Intake

Inadequate intake is the major precipitant of PEM in susceptible populations , such as the elderly and patients with chronic disease. Nutrition adequacy is essential for the maintenance of optimal body composition as well as for metabolic function. Several factors are responsible for low intake, including age-related physiological change, or the disease-imposed metabolic demand , such as cancer. As age advances, alterations in gastrointestinal function impair food digestion and nutrient absorption, and this perpetuates a cycle exacerbating the nutritional deficiency and incidence of malnutrition in the elderly (Rémond et al., 2015). Furthermore, individuals with chronic diseases also have lower appetites and higher caloric needs caused by the metabolic distress of their illnesses, and this makes their nutrition more complicated and renders them more susceptible to PEM. At a broader level, poor dieting can worsen illnesses where they exist, producing a chain reaction of deteriorating health. For example, cancer patients usually end up being malnourished due to the interaction of several factors that consist of the adverse effects of cancer treatment, mental issues, and social resistance to food intake (Beretta et al., 2016). These issues not only compromise their potential to meet nutritional needs but also have negative consequences , such as increased hospital stays and poorer treatment results. The severity of the condition may necessitate an intense probe into nutritional needs, employing established assessment strategies to identify and address individual dietary deficiencies. Therefore, a focused strategy on nutritional intervention is essential, with such patients being provided with individualized dietary advice and intervention in order to counteract the risks posed by inadequate intake and PEM. Ultimately, dealing with inadequate dietary intake must go beyond identification and involve the effective application of dietary measures appropriate to the individual. For the elderly and patients with chronic diseases, nutritional interventions must consider the unique challenges of decreased appetite, changes in digestive ability, and increased nutritional demands. Practitioners must collaborate to craft adequate nutritional policies that not only consider aging and disease-related issues but also patients' psychosocial circumstances. The integration of good nutritional support interventions, through the utilization of fortified food or artificial nutritional approaches, can be instrumental in rebuilding adequate levels of nutrients, enhancing quality of life, and reducing the overall burden of Protein-Energy Malnutrition (Rémond et al., 2015; Beretta et al., 2016). Developing a solid framework of understanding and response for inadequate dietary intake is thus necessary in mitigating the impact of PEM on vulnerable populations.

5.1.2. Socioeconomic Factors

Understanding socioeconomic determinants influencing PEM will help in developing effective interventions. At the core lies poverty, where income limitations within the household make families lack the resources to provide adequate nutrition. Educational disparities compound this issue by impairing parents' knowledge of children's nutritional requirements. Poorer families often face barriers like limited access to healthcare, poor knowledge of child health, and lack of support systems, all of which significantly contribute to the incidence of malnutrition. Environmental conditions and hygiene are also negatively impacted in poor environments, further increasing children's vulnerability to malnutrition. Through taking these socioeconomic factors into account, interventions can be targeted at improving dietary consumption and health for vulnerable populations, as underscored by many studies that attest to the interrelatedness of economic factors and nutritional well-being (Stephen, 2015). In addition to material poverty, population factors entwine with socioeconomic status to form a complex setting for malnutrition. Young maternal age and below-average maternal education, for instance, have been directly linked with increased rates of PEM among children. Young and uneducated mothers are most likely to lack proper knowledge of children's diet and good infant-feeding practices, leading to poor dietary intakes. It is also observed through evidence that their offspring are more likely to be in poor nutritional status if mothers possess a body mass index below desired values, demonstrating the inter-generational aspect of malnutrition. Moreover, large family households have very little to share with all dependents, and therefore, the nutrition available to each child is not sufficient. Such population characteristics, particularly those related to the socioeconomic gradient, generate widening disparities in PEM incidence and demand public health interventions that consider individual and community-level indices (Ahmed, 2015). Seasonal variation in food availability also renders the socioeconomic background of PEM more complex. In the majority of regions, particularly in those characterized by cyclical agricultural cycles, chances to access energy-dense foods can vary significantly from season to season, thus exposing low-income populations to risks. For example, during rainy periods, food production problems are compounded by vulnerability to disease spreading in low-lying territories can cause poor dietary intake, resulting in higher malnutrition levels. Alternatively, dry-season food scarcity could compel households to consume poorer and less diverse diets, also contributing further to PEM risk. Evidence has established the high association of these seasonal characteristics with sociodemographic traits and has suggested that interventions must include agricultural assistance in addition to nutritional education. Managing the above seasonal socio-economic determinants can increase resilience to malnutrition by a considerable amount and overall health outcomes for children (Stephen, 2015) (Figure 5.4).

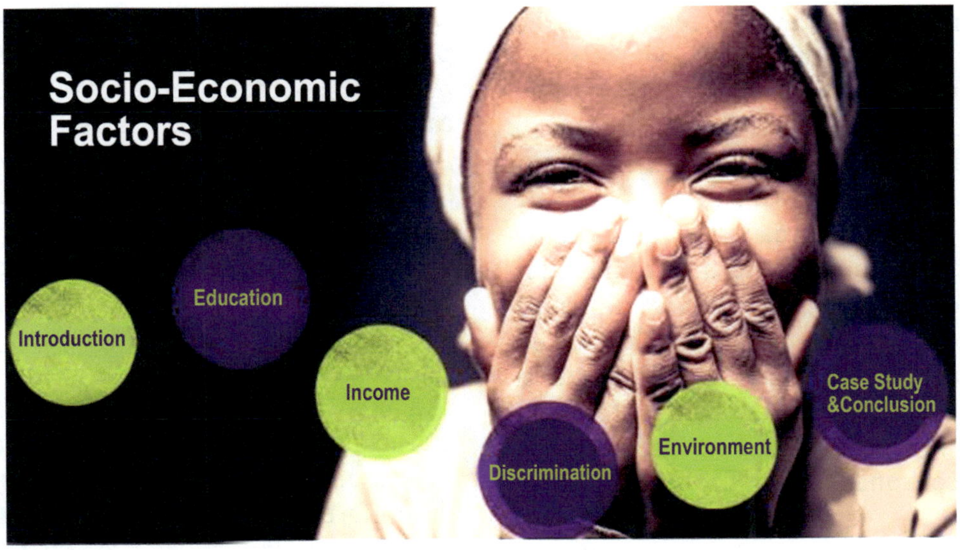

Figure 5.4. Key socio-economic factors influencing well-being.

Source: https://external-content.duckduckgo.com/iu/?u=https%3A%2F%2F0901.static.prezi.com%2Fpreview%2Fv2%2Frksze5ef755w32azqxx6owxao36jc3sachvcdoaizecfr3dnitcq_3_0.png&f=1&nofb=1&ipt=4cb3e1b46ff41be7307e01524218e36fb0354121b19f6bd3d8db56c8337b5bb3.

5.1.3. Health Conditions Affecting Nutrient Absorption

Nutrient absorption is a significant process whose efficiency can be greatly impaired by various diseases to cause PEM. GIT plays a key role in nutrient breakdown and absorption, and any decline in its efficiency will result in significantly compromised nutritional status, particularly among the elderly. Aging affects GIT through mechanical breakdown of food, changes in gastrointestinal motility, and interference with the linings of the intestines' ability to absorb basic nutrients. With compromised GIT, older people are more susceptible to malnutrition, which in turn exacerbates related health conditions, demonstrating a vicious circle of deteriorating health. Management of these age-related changes is a solution to designing efficient eating recommendations for the elderly group with a focus on maximizing nutrient availability and utilization through balanced food intake and meal planning (Rémond et al., 2015). In addition to age-related impairment, other chronic diseases might hinder nutrient absorption and enhance the risk for protein-energy malnutrition. Conditions like celiac disease, inflammatory bowel disease (IBD), and diabetes impair the body's ability to digest and absorb nutrients. For example, damage to the small intestine occurs with the ingestion of gluten in celiac disease, resulting in reduced mineral and vitamin absorption. Consuming specialized diets is often required with long-term malabsorption and resultant severe nutrient deficiencies. Similarly, diabetic patients can get gastroparesis, characterized by delayed gastric emptying and affects nutrient absorption. With these complexities, clinicians are duty-bound to understand the multi-faceted nature of nutrient absorption impairments in placing high priority on adequate nutritional assessment and individualized management programs in consonance with the unique health concerns of the patient (Agarwal et al., 2025). In addition, the psychosocial factors entailed in diseases that affect nutrient absorption cannot be overlooked. Mental health status, social isolation, and socioeconomic status are factors that can heavily influence eating habits and food choices. Depression and anxiety, for instance, may suppress appetite, result in poor intake of nutrients, and contribute to malnutrition. Moreover, residents of residential aged care facilities usually experience several morbidities that exacerbate their risk of nutritional issues. As has been documented, almost half of all individuals in such settings are malnourished due to factors in appetite and food consumption, which suggest that there is an urgent need for both physical and mental well-being to go together. The implementation of robust nutrition strategies in such settings, with a multidisciplinary model highlighted, can suppress the impact of psychosocial issues on nutrient absorption and promote overall health outcomes among vulnerable individuals (Agarwal et al., 2025).

5.2. Types of Protein-Energy Malnutrition

The classification of PEM comprises several types, primarily kwashiorkor and marasmus, which are quite distinct in their clinical presentation and etiology. Kwashiorkor is primarily protein-deficiency with adequate calorie supply, which results in presentation , such as edema, hepatomegaly, and skin lesions. This type is largely prevalent in developing nations where protein in the diet is missing, and this reflects the significance of well-nourished nutrition during early life. Conversely, marasmus is a severe protein and calorie deficiency, leading to severe weight loss and muscle wasting. Children suffering from marasmus are growth-retarded and weak and appear emaciated. It is important to learn about the differences between these PEM conditions in order to give them proper diagnosis and treatment because their treatment approaches significantly differ and need individualized nutritional care to recover and prevent long-term morbidity. Moreover, PEM globally is typically compounded by socio-economic factors like poverty, food insecurity, and political instability. Famine-stricken areas or areas of conflict can have extremely high levels of PEM, particularly among the vulnerable , such as children and the elderly. Economic factors play important roles in the absence of nutrition and having access to sufficient and nutritious food becomes an issue for the majority. It is the interaction between market forces, food policy, and local farming that directly affects the community food security and nutrition level. For instance, countries with compromised agricultural systems may be unable to provide adequate dietary diversity, leading to poor intake. Meeting these socio-economic determinants is important in an effort to effectively counteract PEM through concerted interventions through policy reforms in food, community-based programs of support, and educational interventions aimed at instilling better eating habits in the target populations. Managing PEM also includes taking a broader approach by integrating medical and nutritional interventions, particularly where concomitant disease exacerbates malnutrition. For example, among populations with chronic illness, disease effects , such as cancer further complicate nutritional uptake and dietary absorption, as evidenced by chemotherapy-induced nausea and vomiting (CINV) that can seriously impair food consumption (Isenring et al., 2016). Similarly, focused care and intervention among vulnerable individuals , such as the elderly or the poor, are paramount in improving overall health outcomes.

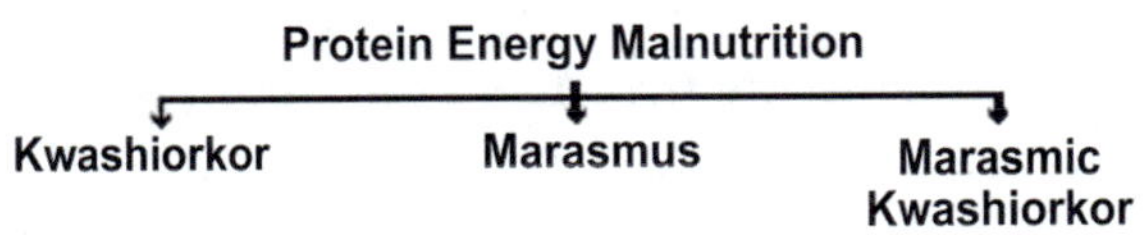

Figure 5.5. Types of protein energy malnutrition: Kwashiorkor, Marasmus, and Marasmic Kwashiorkor.

Source: https://external-content.duckduckgo.com/iu/?u=https%3A%2F%2Fimg.brainkart.com%2Fimagebk35%2FHO4LlXi.jpg&f=1&nofb=1&ipt=339d16773a817ed356f659a35efa78663e6b9c715cc24489a9800219e2551707.

Education in relation to nutrition, accessible dietary supplements, and improving food security programs are among the primary factors in controlling PEM. From a health context, an understanding of the nuances of forms of PEM, such as, , such as the complex balance of nutrition needs, and their broader socio-economic contexts can significantly contribute to maximum outcomes for the subject populations and individuals (Boland and Brautigam, 2010) (Figure 5.5).

5.2.1. Kwashiorkor

Kwashiorkor is a severe protein-energy malnutrition (PEM) whose key feature is the deficiency of protein, often in infants weaned from breast milk to a low-protein but relatively high-carbohydrate diet. It most commonly occurs after a sudden dietary change, whereby poor protein intake leads to typical clinical manifestations of edema, irritability, and failure to thrive. Besides the physical condition, kwashiorkor also causes permanent developmental and cognitive damage in children, making their future life as well as health more complex. Socio-economic status, agriculture work, and lack of proper knowledge about proper nourishment increase their prevalence in areas with lower socio-economic status, rendering it difficult to escape the cycle of malnourishment and disease. The pathophysiology of kwashiorkor illustrates the complex interaction between protein nutrition and overall health. While the main etiology is protein malnutrition, it can be pointed out that kwashiorkor often includes low energy consumption, providing an indicator of the multicausal etiology of malnutrition. It is a classic example where the condition of undernourishment creates metabolic changes affecting not only growth but also immune processes and overall metabolic activity. Disturbed metabolism can result in hypoalbuminemia and hypoproteinemia, conditions which are commonly found in patients with the syndrome. Thus, while rehabilitation of protein deficiency is of prime concern, kwashiorkor is treated by a comprehensive approach incorporating consideration of the broader nutritional well-being, energy, and micronutrient requirement to effectively reestablish well-being and prevent relapse. Kwashiorkor also invites us to examine prevailing nutritional paradigms and policies in a critical manner. The historical background of a protein crisis illustrates a naive idea that identifies a lone dietary offender in protein without considering variables interacting to cause malnutrition. In achieving a solution to kwashiorkor, as Cicely Williams's writing intimated, one must have an expansive understanding of variables causing food deficiencies and malnourishment and not merely supplement dietary protein. Such a perception urges researchers and policymakers to look into the fundamental causes driving malnutrition, with an eye to the fact that primary as well as secondary causes must be addressed in order for intervention to succeed. Indeed, sole focus on protein intake may deflect scrutiny from larger-scale, systemic issues , such as food availability, poverty, and education that play an important role in explaining the prevalence of kwashiorkor. Multidimensional consciousness of such kind is necessary to create long-term global strategies in the battle against protein-energy malnutrition effectively (Eddy, 1977; Johansson et al., 2015).

5.2.2. Marasmus

Marasmus, the most severe of the PEM diseases, affects primarily infants and young children due to poor caloric intake. Marasmus is characterized by a critically significant loss of body fat and muscle tissue. Marasmus patients typically have a wasted appearance, protruding ribs, and tight, adherent skin over the bones, demonstrating the extremely severe catabolism of the body in the process of dismantling stored energy depots. Malnutrition has several causes, with socio-economic insecurity, limited diet variety, and disease being among the most prominent factors. These root causes must be addressed in the case of Marasmus since multi-dimensional interventions have the strong influence of improving nutritional status, particularly among vulnerable populations (Dukhi, 2020). In addition to the Marasmus individual, wider public health dynamics are involved. Marasmus children have delayed development and impaired immunity, making them increasingly susceptible to infection. This self-perpetuating cycle—such that malnutrition leads to illness, and illness exacerbates malnutrition—presents gigantic challenges for the health infrastructures in low-resource settings. With increasing malnutrition burden, nutrition education and investments in health facilities are critical. Early intervention, especially during the first 1000 days of life, when growth is most rapid, can prove highly effective in preventing such detrimental effects and promoting healthier outcomes (Dukhi, 2020). Intensive methods which target not only the consumption of food but also health care and community education are necessary so as to effectively intervene. Recent advancements in the understanding of alternative sources of nutrition indicate new directions for reducing the prevalence of Marasmus. For instance, breakthroughs in the production technology of mycoprotein, which is a high-protein food product produced from fungi, can provide cheap and viable sources of food in malnutrition-endemic regions. Current studies indicate that the substitution of conventional meat with mycoprotein can yield similar health benefits, , such as improved cholesterol profiles and lower glycemic responses, along with being environmentally sustainable. Such a protein substitute could decrease reliance on animal proteins, which might be less accessible in poor communities. The inclusion of mycoprotein in nutrition plans for combating Marasmus may thus not only alleviate acute deficiency but also provide long-term nutritional security and health among vulnerable populations (Figure 5.6).

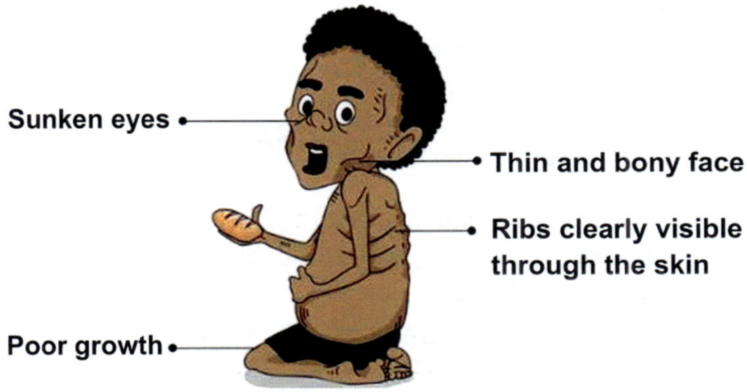

Figure 5.6. Key signs and symptoms of marasmus in children.

Source: https://external-content.duckduckgo.com/iu/?u=https%3A%2F%2Fimages.medindia.net%2Fpatientinfo%2F950_400%2Fsymptoms-and-signs-of-marasmus.jpg&f=1&nofb=1&ipt=9b2cc1f9e192d1e20ad4d62be179f5c920e1a53397d13f0dc3c709f804288c72.

5.2.3. Mixed Forms of PEM

PEM is a range of clinical syndromes resulting from the inadequate intake of nutrients, particularly protein and calories. Of the various forms of PEM, mixed forms are particularly important since they typically reflect a combination of marasmus and kwashiorkor. Marasmus involves a serious deficiency of energy and leads to significant weight loss and wasting of muscles, while kwashiorkor is primarily caused by protein deficiency despite adequate calories and comes with edema and liver fat. The combination of these types makes treatment more challenging since the nutritional needs can be vastly different. Therefore, detection of overlap in signs is critical for accurate diagnosis and effective intervention, particularly among vulnerable populations , such as children and the elderly who are likely to present signs of both forms at the same time. Outcomes of combined types of PEM have ramifications on the broader society because these micronutrient deficiencies often happen in contexts of socioeconomic constraints and food insecurity. The likelihood of obtaining mixed PEM is heightened in regions of chronic poverty, political instability, or natural disasters, where the right diet becomes significantly limited. In addition, financial limitations could deter the availability of high-quality sources of protein, compelling people to adopt cheap, calorie-dense, but nutritionally deficient foods. This condition not only exacerbates malnutrition rates but also sustains a cycle of poverty and health problems, , such as increased susceptibility to infection and delayed recovery from illness. Because of this, it is important to treat the underlying cause of food insecurity to avoid the burden of mixed PEM. Also, the COVID-19 pandemic has revealed the weakness of global food systems and their impact on nutritional status in various mixed forms of PEM. During lockdown and self-quarantine, people are most likely to have food availability and delivery in terms of disruptions, hence higher malnutrition levels. The literature indicates that sufficient protein intake is essential for efficient immune function, therefore making people with PEM at risk of infection (Iddir et al., 2020). As highlighted in earlier research, micronutrient status compounds these weaknesses by augmenting infection risks and inflammation, further embedding malnutrition (Agarwal et al., 2025). The hidden complexity of compound PEM, combined with ripple impacts of a crisis like the pandemic, justifies the need for holistic health responses championing nutrition security, forward-looking community health responses, and policies that reduce inequalities underlying food access.

5.3. Symptoms and Health Effects

The symptoms of PEM are varied and can have significant effects on the overall health of an individual. In the majority of circumstances, PEM subjects typically exhibit immense weight loss with decrease in muscle mass and body fat and possibly decrease in physical strength and resistance to disease. Clinically, it is marked by a range of signs including fatigue, weakness, and general lack of vigor, particularly in older individuals. Malnutrition in elderly care settings is associated with increased levels of infections, falls, and other clinical disturbances that compromise quality of life. Such severity of symptoms typically requires a multi-dimensional diagnostic and treatment approach, and thus there is considerable priority placed on comprehensive nutritional assessment as part of routine health screening in the elderly (Agarwal et al., 2025). The health consequences of PEM extend beyond mere weight loss, as they encompass a series of physiological dysfunctions. Older patients undergo changes in the gastrointestinal tract which compromise nutrient absorption, exacerbating the deleterious impacts of malnutrition (Rémond et al., 2015).

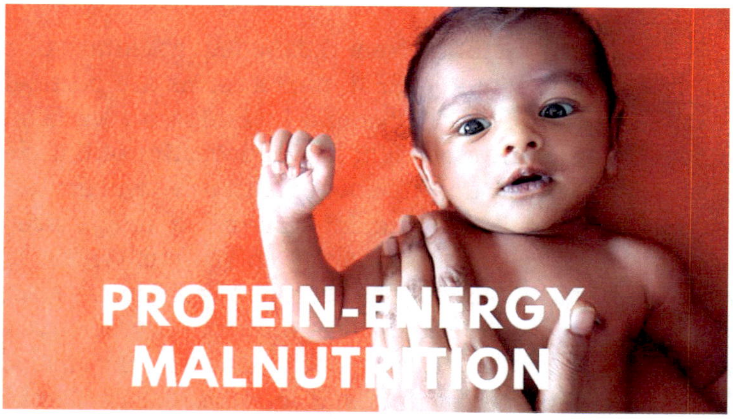

Figure 5.7. Infants show signs of protein-energy malnutrition.

Source: https://external-content.duckduckgo.com/iu/?u=https%3A%2F%2Fallhealthbenefitsof.com%2Fwp-content%2Fuploads%2F2022%2F02%2FProtein-Energy-Malnutrition.png&f=1&nofb=1&ipt=7b2e81870d42377ab2d65fee9d53b196b93e714fbb9126bae21f7b64c2bc9cac.

The decline in gastrointestinal function not only compromises digestive proficiency but also leads to the absence of vital vitamins and minerals, which play crucial roles in maintaining systemic health. As such, malnutrition is more prone to developing a number of diseases, including cardiovascular disease, skeletal disorders, and compromised immune response. The interaction between malnutrition and these conditions can render it a vicious cycle in which ill health further inhibits optimal nourishment, highlighting the need to correct PEM in vulnerable populations with all due haste. The social and economic consequences of PEM also cannot be overlooked. The added healthcare cost of managing malnutrition complications weighs it down on the healthcare system, particularly in long-term care centers where malnutrition is prevalent (Agarwal et al., 2025). With increasing hospital admissions and longer recovery times from illness, the demand for medical resources goes up, making sustainability in health provision an issue. Therefore, efficient nutrition guidelines must be implemented. These protocols have to be multidisciplinary in nature in order to address not only nutritional intake but also what influences appetite and food absorption, thereby decreasing the comprehensive health effect of PEM among populations (Rémond et al., 2015). Effective management strategies can enhance the quality of life and lower the total healthcare demand for malnutrition (Figure 5.7).

5.3.1. Physical Symptoms

The physical presentation of PEM is multifaceted, a reflection of the extreme impact of subnormal intake of nutrients on body functions. PEM patients may have remarkable loss of weight, where there is depletion of subcutaneous fat and muscles. This is more evident in children, who experience growth retardation and a compromised immune system, thereby making them susceptible to infections. The presence of edema, or swelling due to fluid accumulation, is a diagnostic symptom that occurs in another form of PEM, particularly in kwashiorkor, which is an advanced form of PEM. It is often accompanied by an enlarged belly, indicating pathology of the liver and depletion of protein reserves necessary for fluid balance. These signs point toward the necessity of nutritional rehabilitation for reversing health and preventing long-term malnutrition effects. In addition to weight loss and edema, the physical presentation of PEM can contribute to additional complications that affect the overall health and quality of life. Dermatologic presentations, such as alopecia and cutaneous lesions, are evident, which is also aggravated by the impaired immune response. The skin may become dry, scaly, or pigmented, impairing its protective role against microorganisms. Besides, one can feel fatigue and weakness and, most importantly, have their psychosocial status impacted negatively, thus being unable to participate in activities of daily living and social functioning. These symptoms also show failure of the system as the body must reallocate available resources towards prioritizing essential over non-essential functions.

The combination of these physical symptoms highlights the immediate necessity of treating PEM, as they are detrimental individually and collectively represent a vicious cycle of deteriorating well-being, as explained in the Global Burden of Diseases, Injuries, and Risk Factors Study 2015 (Kassebaum et al., 2016; Vos et al., 2016). The effects of these physical symptoms extend far beyond the individual, to influence public health dynamics within communities and nations. Excessive levels of PEM can strain healthcare systems and economic development as a labor force can become increasingly disabled by malnutrition sickness. Moreover, since children composed such a large proportion of those affected, future generations are left with a diminished capacity to thrive. The connection between physical PEM symptoms and overall health effects is demonstrated by studies that link malnutrition with increased disability-adjusted life years (DALYs), which reveal the need for sustainable interventions. Effective nutrition programs and policies that aim at prevention and rehabilitation must be accorded a high level of priority to avoid the adverse effects of PEM, ultimately improving health markers and contributing towards economic stability (Kassebaum et al., 2016; Vos et al., 2016).

5.3.2. Psychological Effects

The psychological effects of PEM are really profound and extensive, with serious consequences for an individual's general health and quality of life. Malnutrition is not just physiological; it also damages a person's emotional and mental functioning. For one, victims of PEM are more prone to anxiety and depression, not only due to their physical state but also because malnutrition comes with the social implication of being "weak" or "sickly." Such social isolation leads to low self-esteem and feelings of loneliness. Moreover, cognitive impairment due to malnutrition, such as difficulty concentrating and memory loss, exacerbates these emotional problems, creating a vicious cycle that does not allow for recovery and overall well-being. Moreover, the contribution of PEM in hindering mental health is quite significant in special vulnerable groups , such as the elderly. As suggested in the literature, malnutrition in older individuals is exceedingly prevalent, and studies have established that virtually half of all residents in aged care facilities have this condition (Agarwal et al., 2025). Malnutrition and mental health are highly interdependent, and aging will typically lead to the loss of appetite and altered taste, leading to inadequate nutritional status. x

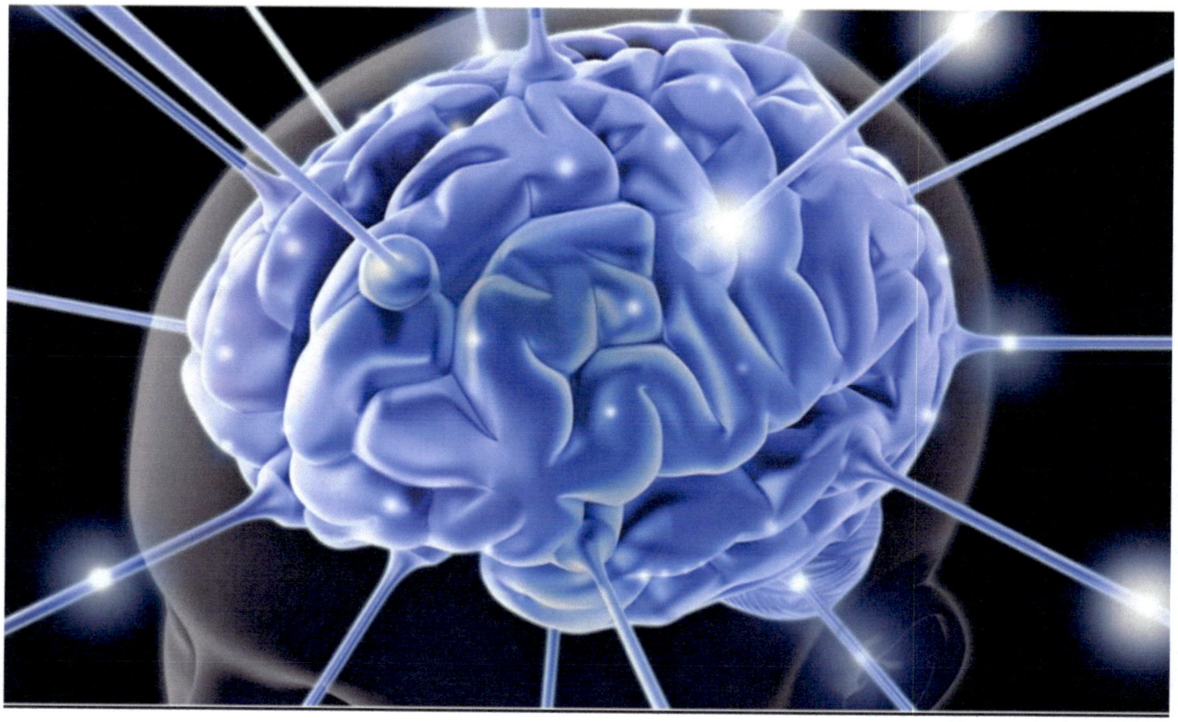

Figure 5.8. Illustration of brain activity and neural connections.

Source: https://external-content.duckduckgo.com/iu/?u=http%3A%2F%2Ftherapyjoker.com%2Fwp-content%2Fuploads%2F2019%2F01%2FPsychologycover-1000x600.jpg&f=1&nofb=1&ipt=2942915c85e42f0702dd712e94c2a1ba282ee27f96f96fd13e1e80ad2c3f19aa.

The decline in gastrointestinal function not only compromises digestive proficiency but also leads to the absence of vital vitamins and minerals, which play crucial roles in maintaining systemic health. As such, malnutrition is more prone to developing a number of diseases, including cardiovascular disease, skeletal disorders, and compromised immune response. The interaction between malnutrition and these conditions can render it a vicious cycle in which ill health further inhibits optimal nourishment, highlighting the need to correct PEM in vulnerable populations with all due haste. The social and economic consequences of PEM also cannot be overlooked. The added healthcare cost of managing malnutrition complications weighs it down on the healthcare system, particularly in long-term care centers where malnutrition is prevalent (Agarwal et al., 2025). With increasing hospital admissions and longer recovery times from illness, the demand for medical resources goes up, making sustainability in health provision an issue. Therefore, efficient nutrition guidelines must be implemented. These protocols have to be multidisciplinary in nature in order to address not only nutritional intake but also what influences appetite and food absorption, thereby decreasing the comprehensive health effect of PEM among populations (Rémond et al., 2015). Effective management strategies can enhance the quality of life and lower the total healthcare demand for malnutrition (Figure 5.7).

5.3.3. Long-Term Health Implications

PEM has significant long-term health impacts going beyond simple acute nutritional deficiencies. PEM generally leads to a decrease in the overall health status of individuals, particularly the elderly and the multi-morbid. Residential aged care (RAC) facilities are a case in point, with studies indicating that up to half of their residents are malnourished. Factors , such as decreased appetite, poor diet, and impaired nutrient absorption are the reasons behind this shocking statistic. Therefore, malnutrition is linked with a host of adverse health outcomes, including increased susceptibility to infection, increased risk of falls, and increased incidence of pressure ulcers. These complications not only increase healthcare costs but also lead to severely compromised quality of life among affected individuals, making proper intervention methods a necessity within this group (Agarwal et al., 2025). Physical effects of PEM are only the tip of the iceberg; long-term consequences also affect cognitive functions, particularly among vulnerable groups , such as children and the elderly. It has been found through research that there is a link between nutritional status and cognitive functioning, with the importance of highlighting that poor nutrition can negatively influence brain functioning. In children, for example, poor food intake can hinder academic growth, since their brain development depends on acquiring necessary nutrients. The consequences of the relationship can cause lasting impacts on education and even future economic prospects. For the elderly who are malnourished, cognitive impairment may manifest as increased loss of memory and increased susceptibility to dementia. Nutritional treatment can therefore be important in avoiding these long-term cognitive issues, emphasizing the importance of comprehensive nutrition interventions (Woodhouse & Lamport, 2012). In light of the important health outcomes of PEM, active nutrition management is imperative. Implementing systematic screening and assessment processes in healthcare settings, including RAC settings, will have a significant effect on patient outcomes. Multi-disciplinary intervention techniques have shown merit in the improvement of not only the residents' nutritional status but also prevention against deterioration due to malnutrition. Individually planned meals, modification of food service, and ongoing nutritional support based on the specific needs of the individual are included. Integration of holistic nutrition principles can enable the early identification of at-risk patients and early intervention, hence avoiding related health complications. Through coordinated efforts to treat nutrition prior to other factors, healthcare providers can substantially restore people's physical and mental health, plagued with PEM, resulting in healthier communities ultimately (Agarwal et al., 2025).

5.4. Populations at Risk

Risk groups for PEM also include the elderly, who have special problems that contribute to their risk. There are changes in gastrointestinal physiology with age, in a way that decreases the intake and absorption of nutrients. With a decrease in mechanical functions, gastrointestinal motility, and chemical digestion, the ability of the elderly to consume and utilize adequate nutrition is impaired, thereby increasing the risk for malnutrition. These conditions create a vicious cycle in which malnutrition exacerbates existing health problems and leads to organ dysfunction, particularly that of the nervous, musculoskeletal, cardiovascular, immune, and skin systems (Rémond et al., 2015). Therefore, consideration of older adults' special nutritional needs is significant in order to mitigate the negative health effects of malnutrition and support a better quality of life for this population. Further, the elderly are at risk of such events as hip fractures, which compromise their nutritional status further. Research indicates that malnutrition among patients who have hip fractures is prevalent in the elderly, with some research claiming that nearly 19% of the patients according to some definitions are malnourished, while this reaches up to 45% according to extended definitions. Poor nutrition not only hinders recovery but also puts postoperative complications and death at greater risk, with a study showing a 30% mortality rate one year after hip fracture (Malafarina et al., 2017). This further highlights the need for nutritional assessment and intervention among this patient population. By putting nutritional rehabilitation at the center of recovery, health care providers can significantly improve the recovery outcome and quality of life among older individuals. Aside from the elderly, children and individuals with chronic illness are also special populations. In children, PEM causes growth impairment and developmental delays, significantly impeding physical and mental growth. In patients suffering from chronic diseases , such as diabetes or cancer, the metabolic burden of these diseases can enhance the risk of nutritional deficiency, making them more vulnerable to PEM. These patients require specialized nutrition management to treat and avert malnutrition. There is a need for education and dietary counseling to ensure proper nutrition among these patients so that they receive optimal protein and energy levels for staying healthy. Therefore, holistic nutritional interventions that consider the special needs of vulnerable population groups are essential to reducing the incidence of PEM and overall health outcomes (Figure 5.9).

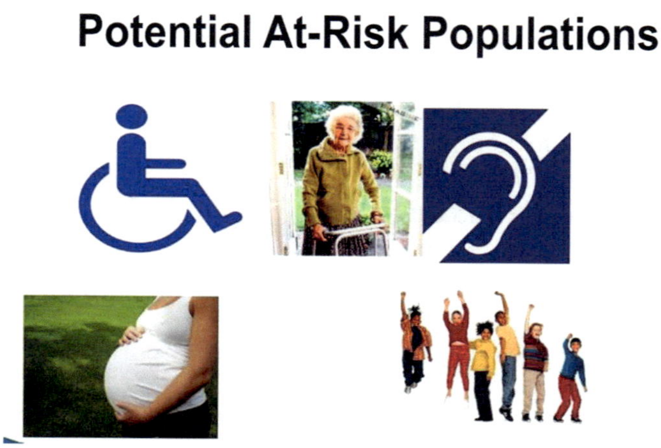

Figure 5.9. Populations are at higher risk for health and nutritional challenges.

Source: https://external-content.duckduckgo.com/iu/?u=https%3A%2F%2Fimage3.slideserve.com%2F7030143%2Fpotential-at-risk-populations-l.jpg&f=1&nofb=1&ipt=3659172438f028d1381b3ced5aeb8531de96d642a729c1c842e258810bd1d5ff.

5.4.1. Children and Infants

In regard to the impact of PEM on children and infants, one must also consider the heterogeneity of nutrition. The nutritional state of children is also contingent upon whether mothers have sufficient knowledge about dietary requirements and whether diet consumed is sufficient. A study in the Puskesmas Banyudono I area concluded that over half of the mothers exhibited a medium level of knowledge with respect to proper foods. Despite this consciousness, there were still a remarkable majority of infants lacking adequate nutrition, with a high percentage being malnourished. This shows the utmost necessity for not just nutrition education among the mothers but also access to quality foods for their infants. Implications of findings suggest that enhancing mother education will not suffice to combat PEM, meaning broader modifications within the food supply system and socioeconomic benefits to families must occur (et al., 2016). Beyond immediate health concerns, PEM is also a marker of growth, cognitive development, and overall health being hindered in children. The World Health Organization identifies protein-energy malnutrition as a priority in developing nations, where it is still prevalent among children and infants. The seriousness of the disease necessitates strategic intervention to improve dietary practices. For instance, the formulation of complementary foods based on locally available raw materials at the community level presents a potential solution to raise protein and energy status among malnourished infants. Evidence indicates that home-prepared preparations are capable of significantly improving the nutritional content of diets having higher protein and energy density compared to traditional diets (Abiodun et al., 2020). Not only do such practices meet current nutritional gaps, but also induce long-term food practices in communities, hence guaranteeing long-term gains in health. Prevention of PEM among children and infants must similarly be addressed through an integrated approach involving education, resource allocation, and community intervention. As nutritional deficiencies can adversely affect developmental milestones and overall health, early action is crucial. Complementary food formulation programs with a focus on using local ingredients have the potential to offer both economic and nutritional gains to families. With active involvement from the local community in production and consumption, it is possible to establish resilience to malnutrition. As demonstrated by the recent study, the production of these nutritionally informative commodities not only meets children's dietary needs but also increases focus on the importance of balanced diet. This holistic approach would thus be a highly important step towards reducing PEM's impact on vulnerable groups (Abiodun et al., 2020).

5.4.2. Elderly Individuals

With progressive age, the likelihood of developing PEM is significantly higher, particularly in older patients with one or more concomitant illnesses , such as chronic kidney disease (CKD). With aging and CKD together, typically metabolic alterations and body composition changes occur, culminating in malnutrition. For the elderly patient, already potentially compromised in terms of nutrient intake and utilization, the development of CKD merely aggravates these issues, putting them at higher risk of malnutrition pathology. Nutritional guidance for CKD typically involves decreased protein content, which might be at odds with geriatric guidance recommending greater ingestion of protein to counteract malnutrition pathology. Therefore, establishing balance among these nutritional orders is crucial in maintaining the nutritional status and overall health of elderly CKD patients to control both PEM and CKD progression optimally (Cacciapuoti et al., 2024). Furthermore, the implications of protein-energy malnutrition extend beyond physical health to affect the quality of life in the elderly. Malnourishment in older people can lead to lower muscle mass, loss of strength, and increased frailty, all of which perpetuate the deficiencies of aging. These physical deficiencies can add to the susceptibility of falls and resulting injury, making further recovery and rehabilitation even more difficult. Malnourishment has also been known to impair cognitive function because essential nutrients are key to maintaining proper brain function. The malnutrition-cum-compromised-vulnerability-to-infections association also holds increased threats of mortality within this patient group. Thus, PEM remediation is of extreme importance not only for physical wellness but also for retaining mental as well as emotional stability (Osatogbe, 2024).

To efficiently fight protein-energy malnutrition, individualized nutrition intervention is of extreme importance in the elderly. These interventions should involve careful assessments of nutritional status, functional capacity, and individual health status to establish personalized nutrition plans. For instance, the use of high-quality protein foods , such as lean meats, milk, and legumes can be used to promote nutritional improvement and malnutrition prevention. Furthermore, regular monitoring of nutritional status with the use of Geriatric Nutritional Risk Index can enable timely adjustment of dietary regimens based on changing health status. In summary, PEM management in the elderly requires an interdisciplinary practice that is more than mere dietary management but also interprofessional practice to provide the best possible aging (Cacciapuoti et al., 2024) (Figure 5.10).

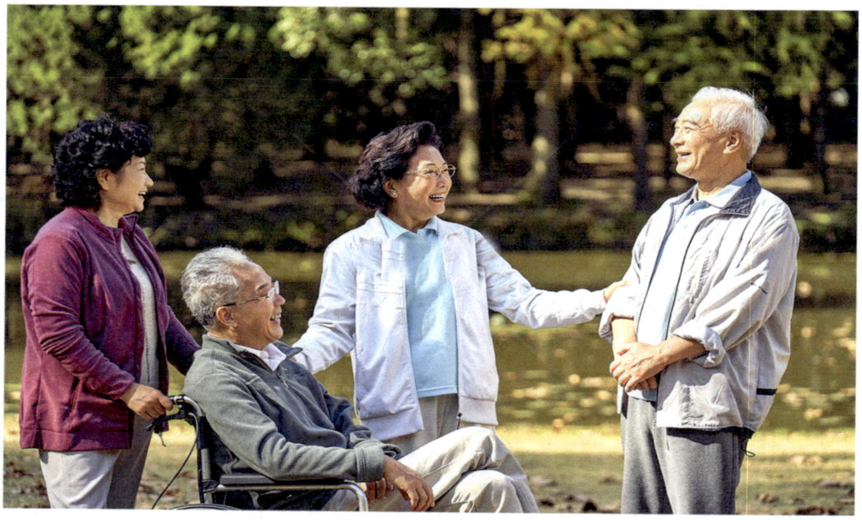

Figure 5.10. Elderly people enjoy social interaction in the park.

Source: https://external-content.duckduckgo.com/iu/?u=https%3A%2F%2Fwatermark.lovepik.com%2Fphoto%2F20211209%2Flarge%2Flovepik-elderly-people-walking-and-chatting-in-the-park-picture_501700423.jpg&f=1&nofb=1&ipt=fc1a1761c453d668bb90081345551243a90b1c489362dea2a4fcf53ce3e15daf.

5.4.3. Individuals in Low-Income Countries

Low-income populations suffer from tremendous PEM adversity, more or less impacting their development, growth, and well-being. Malnutrition is either in the form of undernutrition or overnutrition, while undernutrition predominates in poor areas where low caloric and protein intake is a common phenomenon. According to the World Health Organization, this form of malnutrition is among the most critical global health threats, with insufficient diet intake or ill health that prevents proper utilization of nutrients. The majority of low-income regions have citizens involved in a situation of food lack underpinned by economic instability, climatic change, and inadequate healthcare access. The combination of these factors leads to a condition where hunger and malnutrition are endemic, and global health interventions need to focus on preventing these persistent conditions among vulnerable populations (Arega et al., 2014). In ascertaining diet sufficiency, the socio-economic setting has the authority of deciding on individuals' nutritional status in poor countries. Egyptian studies illustrate the direct influence changes in economic conditions, including incomes and distribution, play on diet and nutritional status (Eid et al.). Low-income families, for instance, consume cheaper foods with more calories and less or no essential nutrients, which exacerbates PEM. To this end, the relationship between income increases and diet quality signifies that even modest improvements in economic means may not immediately translate into improved nutrition due to current constraints , such as food costs and availability. Hence, policy directives must consider both the micro and macroeconomic factors, and it becomes all the more crucial for comprehensive strategies for enhanced food security and ensuring that vulnerable groups attain requisite energy and protein to sustainably combat malnutrition (Eid et al.). Protein-energy malnutrition among low-income nations can only be reversed by a multi-faceted assault that considers not merely short-term nutrition needs but also long-term socio-economic development. Interventions must include improving access to quality, affordable food, promoting sustainable agriculture, and education investment in nutrition. Furthermore, public health programs must educate people on the importance of breastfeeding and nutrition needs of children and pregnant women because they are at greater risk of malnutrition. Engaging communities in the development of culturally appropriate nutrition education programs also has the capacity to empower individuals to make healthier food choices, enhancing resilience against PEM. Lastly, collaboration among governments, nongovernmental organizations, and communities plays a pivotal role in designing sustainable approaches dealing with malnutrition issues by focusing on the underlying issues while promoting overall health and well-being for individuals in low-income countries (Arega et al., 2014).

5.5. Diagnosis of Protein-Energy Malnutrition

Diagnosis by the clinician of PEM is quite crucial, especially with its association with negative health consequences. Diagnosis of PEM is made using various means, with emphasis on exact assessment of nutritional status. The Malnutrition Inflammation Score (MIS) and Global Leadership Initiative on Malnutrition (GLIM) criteria are some tools used in this regard. The MIS provides a comprehensive examination that is sensitive to the levels of inflammation as well as nutrition status among patients, particularly those undergoing renal therapy. Conversely, GLIM criteria strive to provide a standardized platform for identifying malnutrition across diverse populations. With these measurements, healthcare providers are able to distinguish effectively the occurrence of malnutrition, thereby implementing corresponding interventions to advance patient outcomes and overall health status among susceptible groups (Leal-Escobar et al., 2025). Interestingly, sensitivity and specificity of the different methods determine the actual-day applicability of the methods in clinical practice. The author has recently conducted a study on the efficacy of the GLIM criteria in patients on peritoneal dialysis and reported that the criteria were 65.8% sensitive and 61.6% specific in comparison to the MIS. While these results indicate some level of concordance between the two techniques, the GLIM criteria did not outperform the MIS in diagnosing PEM. The challenge of making precise diagnoses for malnutrition emphasizes the necessity of further research to optimize existing criteria and possibly generate new diagnostic tools dedicated to specific clinical groups. Having agreed and appropriate diagnostic protocols in place is essential to facilitate timely and effective intervention, particularly in the context of acute care where malnutrition is present (Leal-Escobar et al., 2025). Adding further complexity to the clinical PEM diagnosis scenario is how the interaction between malnutrition and comorbidities affects each other and obscures true measurement. For instance, studies indicate that patients suffering from conditions , such as cervix cancer carry a high prevalence of protein-energy malnutrition, with coexistent conditions complicating their management. Studies indicate that among hospitalized cervical cancer patients, nearly 20% have protein-energy malnutrition, which elevated their risk of death considerably. This interaction calls for the importance of comprehensive diagnostic approaches with both malnutrition and other coexistent diseases in mind. With these complexities, advances in diagnostic methods and criteria are essential in order to ensure accurate identification and treatment of PEM, especially in high-risk populations where treatment may alter clinical course (Figure 5.11).

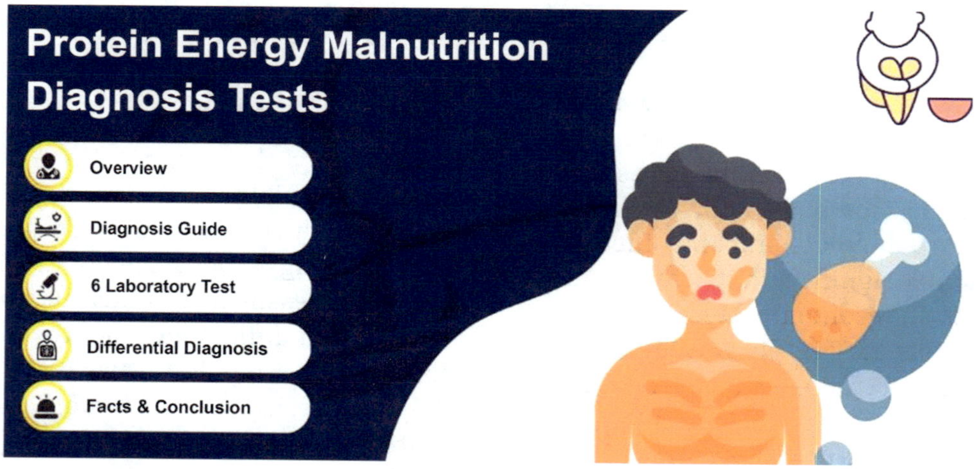

Figure 5.11. Diagnostic steps for identifying protein-energy malnutrition.

Source: https://external-content.duckduckgo.com/iu/?u=https%3A%2F%2Fimages.drlogy.com%2Fassets%2Fuploads%2Fimg%2Fadmin%2Fhealth_blog%2Fprotein-energy-malnutrition-diagnosis.webp&f=1&nofb=1&ipt=e482d844ec0cc5e494587b44e4103dcdd5a52d0d2c15c4a152a5b9f8606c331c.

5.5.1. Clinical Assessment Methods

Clinical assessment measures employed in diagnosing PEM play an essential role in determining the appropriate nutritional interventions that individuals require. Full assessment typically begins with nutritional risk screening for classifying patients at risk of malnutrition upon hospital admission. This is a significant first step because it enables health care professionals to identify individuals who may require further assessment. With this, a thorough assessment should then be conducted, including subjective and objective criteria. These may include medical history, food intake patterns, and physical exams that altogether give a general view of the patient's nutrition. Such systematic screening tools have been found to play a vital role in creating an effective treatment plan based on patient-specific needs, eventually promoting better patient outcomes through the early identification of malnutrition (Rudd et al., 2020). While assessing Protein-Energy Malnutrition, standardized clinical assessment tools need to be used, which can yield valid information. Anthropometric measures, including body mass index (BMI), mid-upper arm circumference, and skinfold thickness, are significant predictors of body composition and cellular mass. Additionally, extensive laboratory studies may detect biochemical markers of malnutrition, e.g., serum albumin levels, which identify the patient's protein status. Evaluations of mental and functional status are also pertinent, as these influence a patient's compliance with nutritional management.

Through access to these diverse measurement methods, healthcare providers can produce a multi-dimensional picture of a patient's nutritional status, thereby enhancing the formulation of personalized dietary interventions for combating PEM (Rudd et al., 2020). A multidisciplinary treatment approach to PEM enhances clinical outcomes significantly. Multidisciplinary teamwork among dietitians, doctors, nurses, and allied health professionals is imperative in the development and execution of effective nutritional care plans derived from the comprehensive assessments carried out. Through the use of multiple specialists, the process offers an assurance that all the determinants of a patient's health, physical to psychological, are considered in the nutritional care plan. Besides, the establishment of reasonable lines of communication among the healthcare team offers an improvement in the quality and continuity of care. Such a multimodal strategy not only reduces the risk of malnutrition complications but is also linked with shorter hospital stays and improved patient quality of life, thereby validating the importance of strict clinical assessment methods for efficient management of protein-energy malnutrition (Reber et al., 2019).

5.5.2. Laboratory Tests

Diagnosis of PEM is often made by interpreting a sequence of laboratory investigations that determine the nutritional and metabolic status in subjects with PEM. Laboratory investigations provide useful information about the physiological derangement from protein and energy deficiency. The levels of hormones , such as T3, T4, and TSH in serum, are significant laboratory parameters that are of prime importance for analyzing metabolic function and control of energy. A study revealed that PEM-affected children had dramatic falls in the concentration of serum T3 and T4, but not that of TSH, reflecting an adaptive response to malnutrition, potentially obscuring pre-existing pathophysiological abnormalities (Ahmed et al., 2018). Thus, laboratory tests are useful not only in the diagnosis of PEM but also in monitoring the effectiveness of therapeutic management, demonstrating dynamic interaction between endocrine function and nutrition. Also, tests conducted in a laboratory are not only endocrine evaluation, as biochemical protein and other nutritional status metabolic parameters measurements are also included. Particularly, serum albumin and prealbumin levels are of particular concern because they reflect visceral protein status and the body's ability to make proteins. In PEM patients, abnormally low serum albumin is also a frequent finding, indicating a compromised nutritional status that can be of clinical significance, , such as in the development of impaired wound healing and infection susceptibility. Furthermore, drawing complete metabolic panels can provide insight into electrolyte imbalance, liver function, and kidney function, all of which are very important in PEM patient management. Thus, identification of certain laboratory abnormalities is significant as these markers enable clinicians to tailor interventions according to the biochemical status and clinical presentation of the patient. Development of experimental models to simulate PEM also underscores laboratory evaluation with an understanding of mechanisms of malnutrition and how it influences the ability to recover. For instance, one study established nutritional models in rats to replicate situations equivalent to mild to moderate PEM. Within this study, these researchers evaluated how different protein levels impacted metabolic condition and nutritional insufficiency through measurement of change in liver fat reserve, body weight, and serum proteins (Ramos et al.). Through their connection of laboratory findings to behavioral recovery outcomes, these models enlightened the significant relationship between nutrition and functional recovery, highlighting the significance of rigorous testing protocols. Together, these experimental approaches and lab techniques advance the understanding of PEM, offering opportunities for increased diagnostic and therapeutic interventions in the fight against this widespread health affliction.

5.5.3. Nutritional Screening Tools

Nutritional screening tools are important tools in identifying at-risk persons for PEM, particularly among vulnerable groups , such as the aged, high-risk patients, or hospitalized patients. These tools enable early identification and treatment, which is essential for optimizing health outcomes.

Among the numerous screening techniques, the Mini Nutritional Assessment (MNA) and the Subjective Global Assessment (SGA) are premier tools. It is revealed through research that while the MNA has moderate predictive validity to assess mortality risk and poor physical functioning, it is marked as very low in concurrent validity, indicating inconsistencies in diagnosing PEM accurately (Craven et al., 2017). Detailed screening approaches that are reliable and applicable to all continue to be the need of the hour in a bid to address the negative effects of malnutrition, especially due to the rising aging population globally. The consequences of undiagnosed or inappropriately managed PEM are severe, with ensuing increased morbidity and health costs. Observational studies in RAC facilities have found it estimated that about half of all RAC residents are malnourished, predominantly secondary to multifactorial factors on appetite and nutrient absorption (Agarwal et al., 2025). Thus, utilization of reliable nutritional screening tools becomes a top priority not only for diagnosis but also for the utilization of early nutritional interventions.

A holistic screening method can enhance care quality overall among the elderly, without compromising on ensuring that malnutrition is identified early and addressed. Systematic screening practices implemented in these settings can serve as a basis for preventive care, and deficiency of nutrients can be addressed prior to manifesting as full-fledged health complications. The ability of nutrition screening tools to counteract PEM is reliant on the validation and development of effective measures that are able to cross populations, particularly in independently living or community-residing older adults. While the present measures like the MNA and SGA have widespread application, their capacity is constrained by a pressing requirement for additional research aimed at enhancing their effectiveness and specificity in determining the risk of malnutrition (Craven et al., 2017). In addition, multidisciplinary care teams will need to be involved in planning well-thought-out nutritional intervention that involves routine screening, individualized intervention, and ongoing monitoring. Such an interface between medical practitioners will enable improved health promotion and quality of life in high-risk populations. Only by a commitment to comprehensive evaluation and validation of screening tools can we hope to decrease the appalling incidence of PEM and resultant complications (Figure 5.12).

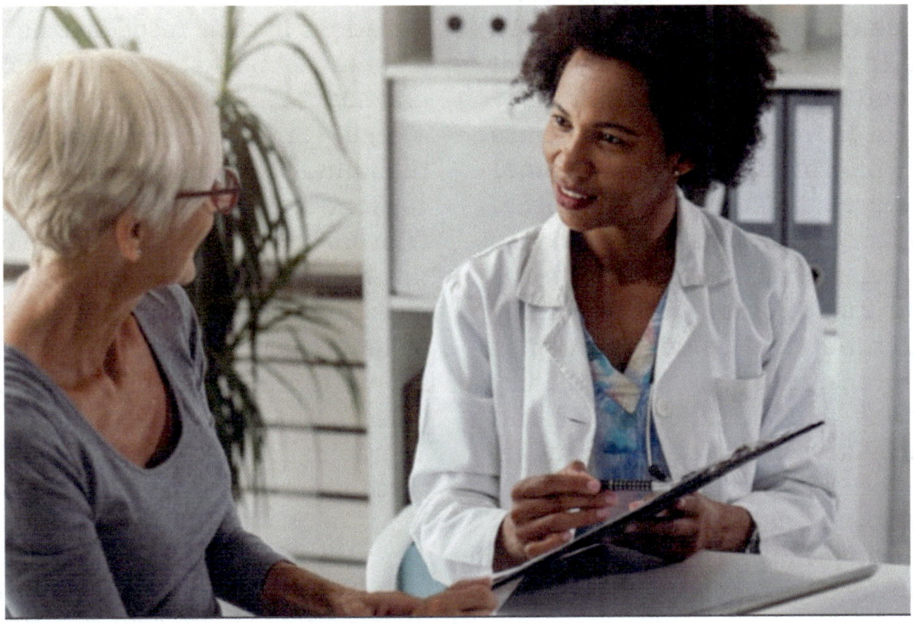

Figure 5.12. Nutritional consultation between the patient and healthcare provider.

Source: https://external-content.duckduckgo.com/iu/?u=https%3A%2F%2Fwww.beckydorner.com%2Fwp-content%2Fuploads%2F2021%2F01%2FiStock-1211390807.jpg&f=1&nofb=1&ipt=0e96c38d488676731a1ac1c0285e7ffddef77c024ca8f0725aa9ba1c4bb808a2.

5.6. Treatment and Management

Management and treatment of PEM depend on a multifactorial strategy emphasizing nutritional repletion and therapy of pathologies. The evidence suggests that nutritional treatment must be tailored to the individual patient's health condition, food desire, and degree of malnutrition. Early diagnosis and detection of PEM are crucial, particularly among patients at high risk, e.g., cancer patients. For instance, treatment of PEM in patients with multiple myeloma not only improves nutrition but has the ability to substantially influence clinical outcome, as reflected in outcomes indicating such patients have higher chances of all-cause mortality if diagnosed with accompanying PEM (Gebremedhen et al., 2025). Thus, screening for nutrition in clinical practice regularly is paramount to intervention planning for the purposes of optimizing health and functional recovery. The treatment of PEM most often involves enteral and parenteral nutrition, respectively, depending on whether the individual can accept oral food. Enteral nutrition is typically preferred with the presence of a functional gastrointestinal tract to deliver nutrients directly for optimal recovery of energy as well as protein synthesis. Parenteral nutrition would then be necessary when there is compromised gastrointestinal function, like in the majority of cancer disease conditions that may hinder proper nutrient absorption.

Evidence is in favor of patients, for example, of cholangiocarcinoma with PEM having increased complications and the therapeutic effectiveness being subsequently optimized through early nutritional rehabilitation (Gebremedhen et al., 2025). In such a situation, vigilant attention to food consumption and therapy modification based on individual response can result in improved clinical outcomes as well as lowered healthcare expenditure through fewer hospitalizations. Moreover, the psychological factors that influence PEM and its management cannot be overlooked. Family and patient education and emotional support are essential to ensure adherence to dietary recommendations and treatment regimens. Health care providers must engage patients in discussions focusing on the significance of nutrition to their general treatment, especially for those enduring chronic illnesses , such as multiple myeloma or cholangiocarcinoma. Creating a supportive atmosphere for discussing dietary requirements and restrictions supports a common view of management, hence enhancing patients' self-efficacy in handling their PEM. Lastly, a holistic approach to combining medical, nutritional, and psychological management is inevitable for effective treatment of PEM and optimization of long-term patient outcomes.

5.6.1. Nutritional Rehabilitation

The process of nutritional rehabilitation is crucial in treating PEM, particularly among vulnerable groups , such as children and the elderly. Nutritional rehabilitation is a structured process of restoring the normal nutritional status by means of certain diet-based treatments with emphasis on increased protein and energy intake. Successful rehabilitation is typically started with an appropriate assessment of the patient's nutritional needs, followed by the creation of an individualized meal plan incorporating high-quality protein foods and energy-dense foods. This approach aims at the specific needs of the individual, facilitating recovery and promoting overall well-being. This individualized strategy is necessary, as standardized therapy may not be equally effective for all patients with PEM because of variations in their respective health conditions and nutritional status. New developments with oral nutritional supplements (ONS) have played a significant role in optimizing nutritional rehabilitation effectiveness. Notably, a new concentrated high-protein energy-dense ONS with 60% whey protein content has entered the market, offering significant potential to meet the energy and protein requirements of malnourished patients. The product has been shown to enhance compliance and optimize muscle protein synthesis, both being key to improving nutritional, functional, and clinical outcomes.

Clinical experience confirms the effectiveness of such an innovative dietary intervention, as attested to through improved anthropometric measures and functional capacity in rehabilitation patients. Such findings demonstrate that healthcare professionals can better address problems commonly faced in treating patients suffering from protein-energy malnutrition, particularly those with diminished appetite and increased nutritional needs consistent with the presence of certain underlying conditions (López-Gómez et al., 2024). Further, the global prevalence of protein-energy malnutrition points to the necessity of effective nutritional rehabilitation programs among the population. Low socioeconomic areas have a very high prevalence of PEM, and they demand specific health interventions with respect to specific local issues. For instance, South Asia has been identified as a region where the highest prevalence of PEM is found, and it particularly targets young children. It is necessary to implement age-relevant nutritional strategies in order to effectively tackle this widespread condition. Moreover, being aware of regional differences in nutritional deficiencies, as presented by the Global Burden of Disease Study, can guide public health policies that work towards reducing the effects of malnutrition. Therefore, nutritional rehabilitation must be responsive to individual and context factors to create effective interventions in achieving significant health gains in populations with protein-energy malnutrition (Ji et al., 2024) (Figure 5.13).

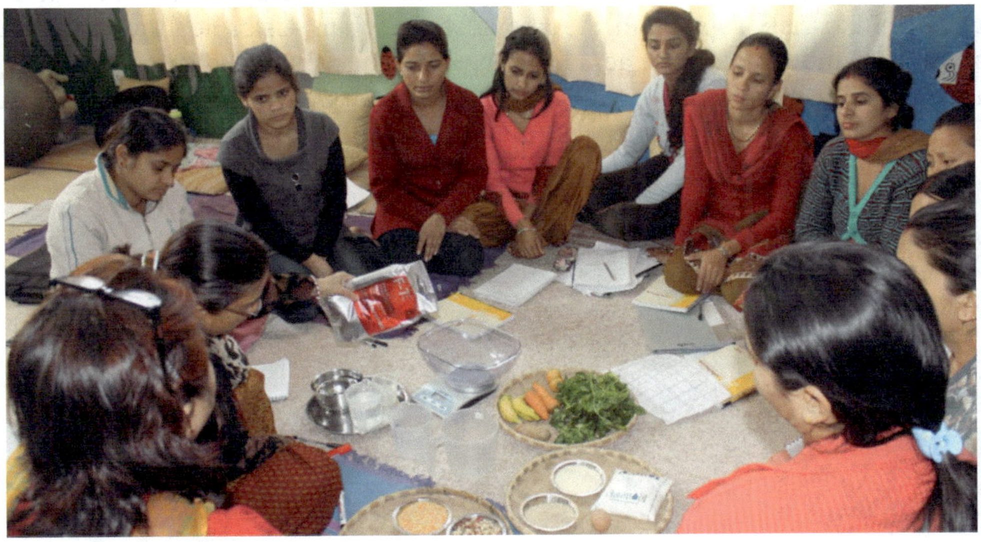

Figure 5.13. Women participating in a community nutrition education session.

Source: https://external-content.duckduckgo.com/iu/?u=https%3A%2F%2Fnepalyouthfoundation.org%2Fwp-content%2Fuploads%2F2021%2F10%2FRmoSvufA-e1647644266304.jpeg&f=1&nofb=1&ipt=1624559dd0dfb541a9686e058e5374a1c0f9493a94ac03e46cd7ceeebd2f9d38.

5.6.2. Medical Interventions

Effective medical management of PEM is critical in the reversal of the deleterious effects of inadequate protein and caloric supply. PEM management entails a multifaceted strategy that includes nutritional restoration, pharmacotherapy, and supportive care. Tailored feeding protocols based on individual requirements are crucial since they consider the patient's age, co-morbidities, and severity of malnourishment. In addition, collaboration among health professionals of varying specialties is also an important factor in developing an intervention plan that considers the entire health of the patient. Multidisciplinary collaboration leads to a holistic approach to all facets of medicine, from comorbidities like diabetes, with improved patient outcomes and quality of life as seen in patients with severe PEM (Elendu et al., 2024). Pharmacologic management can also be integrated with nutritional rehabilitation in PEM patients. Mineral and vitamin supplementation will restore individual deficiencies that are so common following malnutrition, including iron, vitamin D, and zinc, which are necessary for immune response and health. Also, correcting the underlying systemic cause , such as inflammatory disease or infection is necessary to maximize nutritional status. Among children, a recent historical study cites the identification of significant independent risk factors for PEM, , such as physical activity and household income, as indicative of the reality that medical interventions must include social and environmental determinants of health (Deng et al., 2024). Clinicians are able to better treat both the acute and chronic effects of PEM among their patients by using particular pharmacological supports coupled with nutritional therapy. Moreover, continuous monitoring and evaluation of those treated for PEM are imperative to ensure the success of interventions implemented. Regular checks allow timely changes in dietary and pharmacological interventions based on progress and response to intervention by individuals. In the case of long-term cases or those that are complex with other health issues, continuous screening will help in assessing the likelihood of relapsing to malnutrition. The creation of a nomogram model to estimate PEM risk, as seen in the above studies, can assist healthcare workers in early identification of such individuals and adjust interventions accordingly. Later, through proper and preventive medical management, adversity with PEM can be minimized, improving patient health outcomes and reducing healthcare expenses (Elendu et al., 2024; Deng et al., 2024) (Figure 5.14).

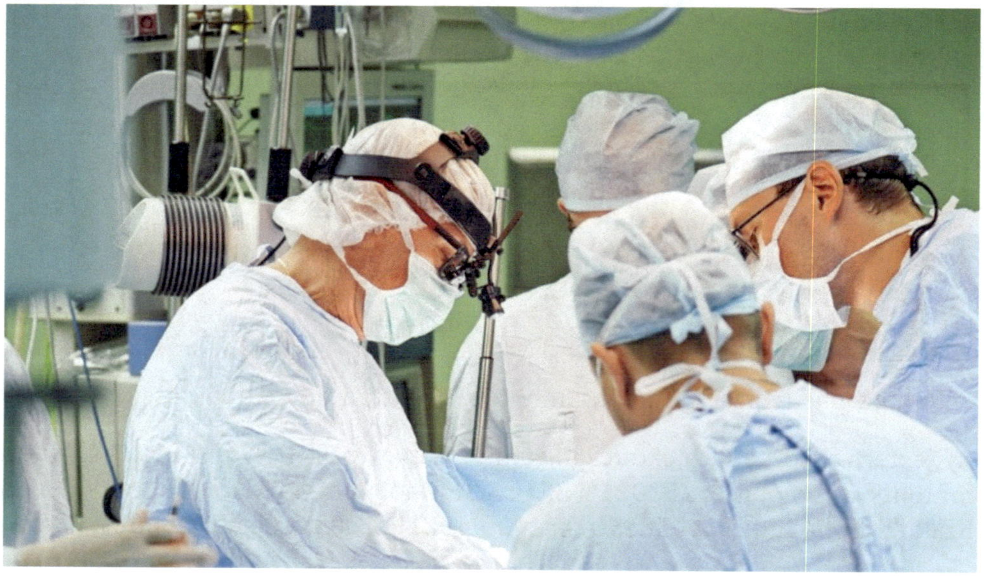

Figure 5.14. Surgeons performing a medical procedure in an operating room.

Source: https://external-content.duckduckgo.com/iu/?u=https%3A%2F%2Fcomhealthpro.org%2Fwp-content%2Fuploads%2F2023%2F02%2Fmedical-intervention-1080x628.jpg&f=1&nofb=1&ipt=1667ef9170730b24b6df474ab537739526aa4e6e0c730cc986b842040bbb69fe.

5.6.3. Community-Based Programs

Programs working at the grassroots level play a vital role in addressing PEM, particularly in impoverished regions where malnutrition is extremely high. Such programs aim to work at the grassroots level and mobilize communities to bring into focus as well as address the malnutrition-related problems. A fine example is the intervention being carried out by Child Family Health International (CFHI) in La Paz, Bolivia, where the organization has launched sustainable healthcare initiatives for malnourished children. Using exhaustive needs assessment processes, CFHI has made the crucial linkages between health, nutrition, and poverty and launched tailored interventions designed to address better eating habits and health education among communities. This community-based strategy not only targets short-term nutritional requirements but also enables families to build long-term strategies that can break the cycle of malnutrition in their communities. The effect of community-based programs spills over beyond direct health benefits; they also make significant contributions to wider socio-economic advancements. By enabling local communities through knowledge and resources, these programs assist in building resilience against the cycle of poverty commonly linked with malnutrition. For instance, when individuals and households acquire knowledge of nutrition and appropriate consumption habits, they can develop healthy eating habits that enhance well-being. This is critical for the first 1,000 days of a child's life, which is the most crucial period for growth and development. Combating malnutrition during this period can yield tremendous long-term benefits in terms of reducing healthcare costs and improving productivity at the community level. Thus, community-based programs address both the symptoms and causes of PEM effectively, producing healthier people and better economic stability for susceptible groups. Secondly, the collective effort aspect of community-based programs makes them more efficient in fighting malnutrition. Community-based programs are usually collaborative ventures between local governments, NGOs, and community actors. Using multiple resources and abilities, collaborations facilitate comprehensive solutions to malnutrition that can be adapted to local situations. For instance, community health workers may integrate nutrition education into broader health promotion activities so that households are getting end-to-end support for both their nutritional and health requirements. Such complementarity is not only optimizing intervention impacts, but it is also evoking collective action and social solidarity among populations. As emphasized by international health organizations, , such as the World Health Organization, inter-organization partnerships are instrumental in spearheading systemic change in the war against malnutrition, particularly in nations with high levels of severe acute malnutrition and poverty (Sandoval et al., 2014; Dukhi, 2020).

CLOSER LOOK

DIETARY INTAKE

Dietary intake refers to the amount and types of food and nutrients consumed by an individual over a specific period. It is a key factor in maintaining health, supporting growth and development, and preventing nutritional deficiencies or chronic diseases. An optimal dietary intake provides the body with essential macronutrients (carbohydrates, proteins, and fats) for energy and body function, as well as micronutrients (vitamins and minerals) needed for metabolic processes, immunity, and cellular health.

The quality and quantity of dietary intake are influenced by various factors such as age, gender, activity level, health status, culture, and socioeconomic conditions. For example, children, pregnant women, and athletes have higher nutritional needs, while elderly individuals may require fewer calories but more nutrient-dense foods. A balanced dietary intake typically includes a variety of fruits, vegetables, whole grains, lean proteins, and healthy fats, while limiting added sugars, sodium, and processed foods.

Monitoring dietary intake is important in both clinical and public health settings. It helps identify nutritional gaps, assess risks of malnutrition or obesity, and guide dietary planning and interventions. Common methodazs include food frequency questionnaires, 24-hour dietary recalls, and food diaries. In medical nutrition therapy, accurate assessment of dietary intake is crucial for managing conditions like diabetes, hypertension, obesity, and gastrointestinal disorders.

Poor dietary intake—whether due to overconsumption or underconsumption—can lead to serious health consequences. Overeating energy-dense, nutrient-poor foods contributes to obesity, heart disease, and type 2 diabetes, while inadequate intake may result in deficiencies such as anemia, scurvy, or rickets. The dietary intake is a fundamental aspect of nutrition and health. Ensuring a well-balanced, adequate, and culturally appropriate diet is essential for promoting wellness, preventing disease, and supporting a high quality of life.

SUMMARY

PEM is a chronic international public health problem that impacts vulnerable populations, including children and pregnant women in low- and middle-income countries. The severity of PEM necessitates a multi-variable approach since its prevalence is influenced by nutritional impairments, socioeconomics, and healthcare. Adjustment of these variables is necessary in developing impactful interventions that can alleviate the malnutrition burden. A significant focus on enhancing food intake, through micronutrients , such as zinc, is capable of reinforcing nutritional status and health results. Systematic reviews commend the efficacy of zinc supplementation in increasing serum/ plasma concentration, as well as put demands on further research to confirm these findings in mixed populations (Ashwell et al., 2013). Evidence from various programs aimed at responding to PEM, , such as the PEM Scheme in South Africa, indicates both the potential success and failure of current interventions. Despite being subscribed to by large numbers of health facilities, evidence indicates that there remains inadequate coverage and targeted support for malnourished subjects. Challenges, through inappropriate training of healthcare workers and lack of consistent monitoring, are barriers to the effectiveness of such efforts. In spite of this, some encouraging findings have been found, with weight-for-age Z-scores being improved in enrolled children, suggesting that formal approaches may lead to beneficial outcomes when strictly implemented (Dhansay et al., 2003). Lastly, PEM resolution is not only the concerted effort of healthcare systems but also community-based action to facilitate awareness and education regarding nutritional health. By putting greater weight on the need for collaboration between various stakeholders, government, medical practitioners, and non-governmental organizations, the fight against PEM can be further strengthened. Collective effort must be directed toward stronger nutrition education, overcoming socio-economic disparity, and increased provision of essential food supplements and health care. Hence, it will become important to formulate specific policies that incorporate comprehensive nutrition strategies in a bid to shatter the cycle of malnutrition and offer healthier avenues for future generations.

PEM impacts various physiological processes in a very significant manner, particularly when it is associated with stress caused by conditions , such as global ischemia. Research has established that PEM can potentially enhance systemic inflammatory responses, which can facilitate impaired recovery following neurological insults. Specifically, the findings indicate that PEM causes an abnormal acute-phase response characterized by increased levels of positive acute-phase proteins , such as alpha-2-macroglobulin, in addition to a decrease in negative acute-phase proteins , such as albumin. These changes in protein synthesis and core temperature fluctuations are significant, as they can have ramifications on the healing process as a whole and the body's ability to respond to ischemic events, rendering recovery strategies challenging and calling for unique nutritional interventions (Smith et al., 2025). The connection between PEM and neuroplasticity is an area that warrants exploration. Experiments demonstrate that malnutrition can alter the hippocampal expression of plasticity-related proteins, those being critical for cognitive rehabilitation following a stroke. For instance, lower concentrations of such critical markers as brain-derived neurotrophic factor (BDNF) and growth-associated protein-43 (GAP-43) suggest a compromised capacity for neuroplastic adaptations following ischemic injury. Although there was some indication of enhanced expression in individual cases under stress conditions after PEM, the overall maintenance of neuronal integrity remained unchanged by previous malnutrition states (Prosser-Loose et al., 2025). The complex interplay between nutritional status and cognitive recovery after stroke comes through in these results. Although there is new information coming through, there remain significant hurdles to the investigation of the role of PEM in established animal models for ischemia. Experiments in rat and gerbil models revealed that while PEM did not exacerbate ischemic neuronal injury, it did induce variability in metabolic parameters , such as blood glucose and acid-base status, important variables to be kept constant in experimental protocols. Such fluctuation can obscure the observation of how nutritional deprivation influences ischemic damage, hence complicating interpretation. Thus, the study emphasizes the use of nutritional therapy in treatment protocols for brain ischemia with the realization that PEM can be treated to enhance recovery pathways and enhance neurological rehabilitation strategies beyond clinical interventions (Prosser-Loose et al., 2025).

References

1. Ahmed, Z. (2015). Prevalence and seasonal variation of severe childhood protein calorie malnutrition in Khartoum: Implication for brain function. https://core.ac.uk/download/76979779.pdf (accessed on 13th June 2025).
2. Akinpelu, A. O. (2015). Socio-cultural predictors of protein energy malnutrition among breast-feeding mothers in Osogbo Metropolis, Nigeria. https://core.ac.uk/download/234687215.pdf (accessed on 13th June 2025).
3. Ashwell, B. L., Baer, R., Bates, C., Berger, J., Bland, J., Brown, K., et al. (2013). Effect of zinc intake on serum/plasma zinc status in infants: A meta-analysis. https://core.ac.uk/download/9632973.pdf (accessed on 13th June 2025).
4. Beretta, G. D., Caccialanza, R., Cereda, E., Gavazzi, C., et al. (2016). Nutritional support in cancer patients: A position paper from the Italian Society of Medical Oncology (AIOM) and the Italian Society of Artificial Nutrition and Metabolism (SINPE). https://core.ac.uk/download/74324933.pdf (accessed on 13th June 2025).
5. Boland, M., & Brautigam, A. (2010). Economic analysis of options for food aid policy in Honduras. *International Food and Agribusiness Management Review, 13*(2), 51-68.(accessed on 13th June 2025).
6. Craven, D. L., Isenring, E., Kelly, J. T., Marshall, S., et al. (2017). A systematic review and meta-analysis of the criterion validity of nutrition assessment tools for diagnosing protein-energy malnutrition in the older community setting (the Macro Study). https://core.ac.uk/download/196605412.pdf (accessed on 13th June 2025).
7. Dukhi N. Global Prevalence of Malnutrition: Evidence from Literature [Internet]. Malnutrition. IntechOpen; 2020. Available from: http://dx.doi.org/10.5772/intechopen.92006(accessed on 13th June 2025).
8. Eddy, T. P. (1977). An error of medicine? Kwashiorkor and the "protein gap." *Tropical Doctor, 7*, 28–32. https://www.semanticscholar.org/paper/a62988883e476186631fb34c9c5b7956a90f811e (accessed on 13th June 2025).
9. Iddir, M., Brito, A., Dingeo, G., Sosa, S., Samouda, H., La Frano, M. R., & Bohn, T. (2020). Strengthening the immune system and reducing inflammation and oxidative stress through diet and nutrition: Considerations during the COVID-19 crisis. *Nutrients, 12*, 1562–1562. https://doi.org/10.3390/nu12061562 (accessed on 13th June 2025).
10. Isenring, L., Kiss, N., Marx, W., McCarthy, A., et al. (2016). Chemotherapy-induced nausea and vomiting: A narrative review to inform dietetics practice. https://core.ac.uk/download/196601603.pdf (accessed on 13th June 2025).
11. Ji, S., Zhou, Y., Zhao, Q., Chen, R., & Su, Z. (2024). Trends in three malnutrition factors in the global burden of disease: iodine deficiency, vitamin A deficiency, and protein-energy malnutrition (1990-2019). *Frontiers in nutrition, 11*, 1426790. https://doi.org/10.3389/fnut.2024.1426790(accessed on 13th June 2025).
12. Johansson, J., Sahin, C., Pestoff, R., Ignatova, S., Forsberg, P., Edsjö, A., Ekstedt, M., et al. (2015). A novel SMAD4 mutation causing severe juvenile polyposis syndrome with protein losing

enteropathy, immunodeficiency, and hereditary hemorrhagic telangiectasia. *Case Reports in Gastrointestinal Medicine, 2015.* https://www.semanticscholar.org/paper/2d836c18a393661 46ff9767ea55dcb9bbabb0e92 (accessed on 13th June 2025).

13. Kassebaum, N. J., Arora, M., Barber, R. M., Bhutta, Z. A., Brown, J. C., Carter, A., Casey, D., et al. (2016). Global, regional, and national disability-adjusted life-years (DALYs) for 315 diseases and injuries and healthy life expectancy (HALE), 1990–2015: A systematic analysis for the Global Burden of Disease Study 2015. *The Lancet, 388*, 1603–1658. https://doi.org/10.1016/s0140-6736(16)31460-x (accessed on 13th June 2025).

14. Lai, J. C., Tandon, P., Bernal, W., Tapper, E. B., Ekong, U. D., Dasarathy, S., & Carey, E. J. (2021). Malnutrition, frailty, and sarcopenia in patients with cirrhosis: 2021 practice guidance by the American Association for the Study of Liver Diseases. *Hepatology, 74*, 1611–1644. https://doi.org/10.1002/hep.32049 (accessed on 13th June 2025).

15. Woodhouse, Allison and Lamport, Ph.D., Mark A. (2012) "The Relationship of Food and Academic Performance: A Preliminary Examination of the Factors of Nutritional Neuroscience, Malnutrition, and Diet Adequacy," *Christian Perspectives in Education*, 5(1). Available at: https://digitalcommons.liberty.edu/cpe/vol5/iss1/1 (accessed on 13th June 2025).

16. Malafarina, V., Reginster, J. Y., Cabrerizo, S., Bruyère, O., et al. (2017). Nutritional status and nutritional treatment are related to outcomes and mortality in older adults with hip fractures. https://core.ac.uk/download/pdf/212756692.pdf (accessed on 13th June 2025).

17. Mohammed, Z. M. E. (2019). The risk factors contributing to protein-energy malnutrition among children under five years old at Bashair Teaching Hospital Khartoum Sudan 2018. https://core.ac.uk/download/287126278.pdf (accessed on 13th June 2025).

18. Murray, C. J. L., Ikuta, K. S., Sharara, F., Swetschinski, L. R., Robles Aguilar, G., Gray, A. P., Han, C., et al. (2022). Global burden of bacterial antimicrobial resistance in 2019: A systematic analysis. *The Lancet, 399*, 629–655. https://doi.org/10.1016/s0140-6736(21)02724-0 (accessed on 13th June 2025).

19. Prosser-Loose, E. J. (2025). Effects of protein-energy malnutrition on outcome of global cerebral ischemia. https://core.ac.uk/download/226140493.pdf (accessed on 13th June 2025).

20. Reber, E., Gomes, F., Vasiloglou, M. F., Schüetz, P., & Stanga, Z. (2019). Nutritional risk screening and assessment. *Journal of Clinical Medicine, 8*, 1065–1065. https://doi.org/10.3390/jcm8071065 (accessed on 13th June 2025).

21. Rudd, K. E., Johnson, S. C., Agesa, K. M., Shackelford, K. A., Tsoi, D., Kievlan, D., Colombara, D. V., et al. (2020). Global, regional, and national sepsis incidence and mortality, 1990–2017: Analysis for the Global Burden of Disease Study. *The Lancet, 395*, 200–211. https://doi.org/10.1016/s0140-6736(19)32989-7 (accessed on 13th June 2025).

22. Smith, S. (2025). Effects of protein-energy malnutrition on the inflammatory response to global brain ischemia. https://core.ac.uk/download/226129722.pdf (accessed on 13th June 2025).

23. Souza Filho, P. F., Andersson, D., Ferreira, J. A., & Taherzadeh, M. J. (2019). Mycoprotein: Environmental impact and health aspects. *World Journal of Microbiology and Biotechnology, 35.* https://doi.org/10.1007/s11274-019-2723-9 (accessed on 13th June 2025).

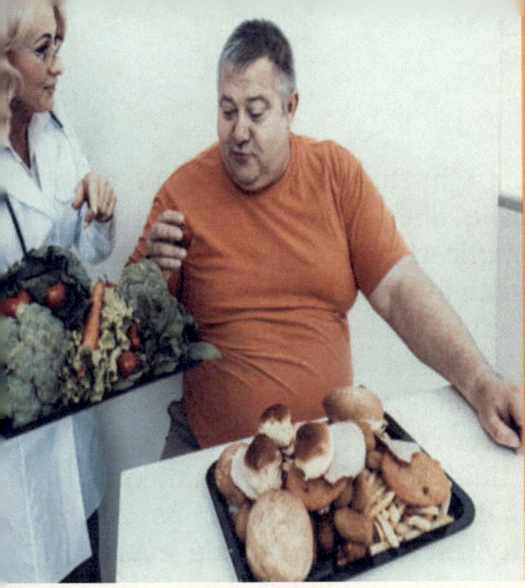

Chapter 6

OBESITY AND OVERNUTRITION

Contents

Introduction....175
6.1. Causes of Obesity....178
6.2. Health Consequences of Obesity....182
6.3. Nutritional Aspects of Overnutrition....186
6.4. Societal Impact of Obesity....190
6.5. Prevention Strategies....194
6.6. Treatment Options....198
Summary....204
References....206

Introduction

The overview of the intertwined problem of obesity and overnutrition opens doors for critical thinking regarding their influence on public policy and health at the individual level. Obesity, defined as pathological excess body fat, has become an epidemic at a global level, transforming the health landscape into fundamental ways. Obesity is not merely an outcome of individual decisions but influences complex networks of socioeconomic determinants, cultural transformation, and environmental exposure. The rising rate of obesity has driven an attendant increase in associated health problems, such as type 2 diabetes, cardiovascular disease, and cancer of various kinds. Hence, the solution to obesity requires a holistic approach that connects health, economic, and social contexts, emphasizing the necessity to study the causes and consequences of the public health problem of obesity. Compounding the obesity problem is overnutrition, an activity of overspending on nutrients in amounts greater than the body requires. This is especially concerning in a time when food insecurity is contrasted withcontrasted with increased numbers of obesity. The irony that underprivileged groups have poor access to good food while others eat too much explains a broader system imbalance. Research has confirmed that the negative impacts of overnutrition not only affect individual welfare but also have implications for social organization. For instance, Fróna et al., (2019) highlights the interdependence of food security and diet modes, shedding light on how imbalanced patterns of consumption have broad implications for public health and the environment. It is crucial to understand these dynamics to develop effective intervention schemes to fight obesity and encourage better lifestyle choices in communities. In obesity and overnutrition, their converging pathways and what this foretells for future generations must be considered. As a case point, gestational diabetes mellitus (GDM) is a classic example of how these conditions unfold in high-risk groups, for instance, in pregnant women. Obesity and advanced maternal age increase the risk of GDM, which further affects both child and maternal health outcomes. Consequently, the long-term effect is experienced over generations since children born to GDM mothers are themselves at high risk of obesity and metabolic disease. Plows et al. (2018) identify the need to understand and treat GDM in the context of the obesity epidemic and demand more effective prevention and treatment measures. In the process, the introduction sets the stage for a critical examination of the intertwined narratives of obesity and overnutrition, stressing the imperative to have an intersectoral and multidisciplinary approach to address these basic public health concerns.

Definition of Obesity and Overnutrition

In public health, obesity is best simply described as a surplus of body fat that is unhealthy. The World Health Organization uses body mass index (BMI) measures to describe obesity, with individuals who have a BMI of 30 or higher considered obese. This classification offers a less complicated method of estimating weight against height, but it doesn't consider fluctuations in muscle mass and disparities in fat distribution. Excessive obesity rates are not only a health issue in one individual, but also a public health concern for the entire world, with socioeconomic influences and environmental factors exacerbating its prevalence. As the course of obesity advances, associated health dangers, cardiovascular disease, diabetes, and certain cancers, rise to justify efforts at joined-up public health intervention with early intervention and prevention of obesity and its complications to address an increasingly severe threat to contemporary health systems (Li et al., 2020). Overnutrition, which may co-exist with obesity, is an excessive consumption and intake of nutrients, in particular calories, producing overweight and obesity. This situation may be caused by an imbalance in dietary patterns, where dietary trends consist of high-calorie, low-nutrient foods compared to nutrient-rich, healthier foods. The impacts of modern food systems, defined by the prevalence of processed and fast food, combine with socioeconomic determinants, reinforcing the overnutrition cycle. Interestingly, overnutrition is not simply the consequence of hyper-caloric intake but also hyper-consumption of specific macronutrients, i.e., sugars and fats, leading to metabolic disturbances. Thus, the remedy for overnutrition entails a change in behavior towards healthy dietary practices and food policies favoring intake of varied, nutrient-dense foods (Béné et al., 2018). Effective obesity and overnutrition control also lie in their socio-environmental determinants. Socioeconomic status, food access, marketing practice, and culture all have a significant influence on dietary patterns and on the health consequences. In the particular context, low-income communities are confronted with the impossibility of being able to get healthy food and instead end up consuming highly processed foods that contribute to obesity. Besides that, marketing practices for unhealthy food disproportionately affect vulnerable groups, further widening the gaps in health consequences. In order to address these problems, policymakers must devise strategies that create equitable access to nutritious food sources, improve nutrition education, and promote public awareness regarding the dangers of obesity and overnutrition. Such an intersectoral approach has the ability to drive the creation of healthier environments and improved population health gains among at-risk communities (Li et al., 2020) (Figure 6.1).

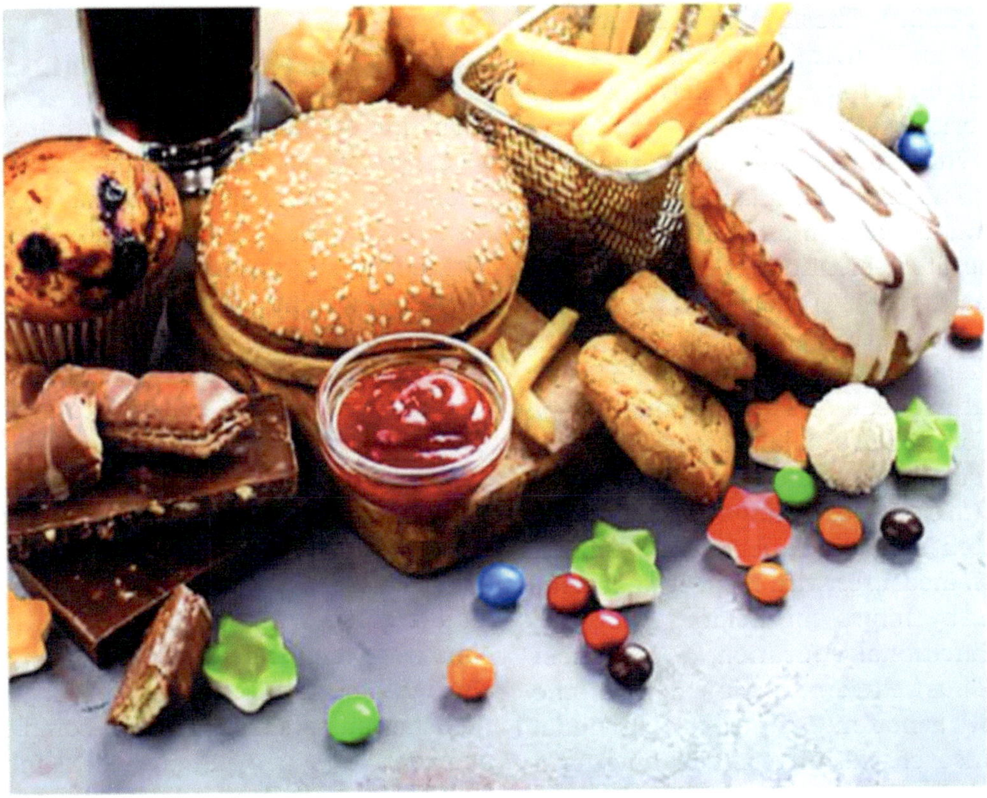

Figure 6.1. Foods high in sugar and fat contribute to overnutrition.

Source: https://external-content.duckduckgo.com/iu/?u=https%3A%2F%2Fwww.dailypioneer.com%2Fuploads%2F2021%2Fstory%2Fimages%2Fbig%2Fovernutrition-is-not-health-giving-2021-11-01.jpg&f=1&nofb=1&ipt=424e82264728d470c46a08fecfc12b2c6e7f92b5de1d924e90444af2237af936.

Importance of Addressing the Issue

The rising incidence of obesity and overnutrition comes into the limelight due to its severe ramifications for public health as a whole, but particularly for women of childbearing age. As research gives more significance to the preconception phase, it becomes crucial to address weight management and nutrition prior to pregnancy. Inadequate attention to these matters not only sacrifices maternal health but also jeopardizes harsh repercussions to newborn outcomes. The shocking evidence of a link between obesity and gestational diabetes, pre-eclampsia, and neonatal complications serves as a clarion call to healthcare professionals to play an active role. They undertake these steps in the form of initiating discussions about health, nutrition, and effective weight reduction management methods, as illustrated by the FIGO Pregnancy Obesity and Nutrition Initiative. In doing so, practitioners can make a notable contribution toward decreasing the threats posed by obesity, thereby ensuring healthier pregnancies along with future well-being for generations to come (Jacob et al., 2020). Obesity and overnutrition are not only an individual health issue but also a social one that becomes worse over time. This crisis in public health is tightly connected with noncommunicable diseases (NCDs) , such as cardiovascular disease, which are a tremendous burden on global healthcare systems. The afore-mentioned evidence given in global health policy reports shows a clear intent towards reducing premature NCD death through focusing on the risk factors of obesity. The task that is ahead of us is intimidating, as the number of cardiovascular deaths continues to rise, particularly in middle- and lower-income countries. With countries aiming at a 25% decline in NCD-related mortality, effective application of prevention measures with respect to obesity, for example, by improving health policy and supplying nutritional education, is of utmost relevance. Thus, extreme action against the rise in obesity is not only critical for individual health but also crucial in terms of long-term public health (Joseph et al., 2017). Further, the importance of fighting obesity and overnutrition is again balanced by broader implications for socioeconomic health. The expenses and weights of obesity, including increased healthcare expenditures, lost productivity, and decreased quality of life, underscore the importance of tackling this epidemic. Implementing more extensive strategies that focus on public education, community intervention, and food security can drastically alter the trend of obesity rates. Such population-level health determinants have considerable influence in shaping people's choices and behaviors regarding diet and physical activity. By promoting a culture that supports healthier lifestyles, organizations and governments can mitigate the dire threats posed by obesity, ultimately leading to healthier populations and reduced healthcare burdens in the future. Thus, recognizing and responding to the complex status of obesity is critical in formulating a long-term, sustainable public health policy (Joseph et al., 2017).

6.1. Causes of Obesity

The increase in obesity is a result of the rising occurrence of overnutrition, characterized by too much caloric intake with inadequate physical exercise. Urban life, driven by the advancement of technology, has led to sedentary culture that leads to weight gain. Fast food culture, coupled with intense marketing of high-calorie foods, has a profound impact on what and how much individuals consume. These categories of diet fads not only contribute to calorie consumption but also predispose the body to foods high in sugar and fat, which are well established to promote weight increase. Moreover, processed foods' ease often gets ahead of more traditional diets filled with whole, high-nutrient foods, making it difficult to maintain a healthy weight and thus leading to obesity. It requires a balanced perspective on this complex interplay to craft effective public health interventions directed at arresting the obesity crisis. Besides eating habits and lifestyle, genetic and metabolic conditions also determine the tendency of a person to become overweight. Genetic factors can predispose a person to obesity because some individuals have a diminished metabolic rate or a certain pattern of appetite control that predisposes them to overeating. Metabolic variations will usually affect how well the body is able to metabolize food into energy and how much energy is wasted by physical movements. The effect of hormonal imbalances, including insulin resistance and leptin imbalance, are important factors that could induce obesity. In addition, research shows that there is a connection between overnutrition and other metabolic diseases , such as non-alcoholic fatty liver disease (NAFLD), which would complicate weight regulation and result in obesity (Wong et al., 2017). Therefore, the management of obesity requires a multi-faceted approach that considers genetic factors as well as environmental factors. Psychological factors and socio-economic status also play an important role in the complexities of obesity. Emotional eating, which is commonly used as a stress or anxiety relief measure, will result in calorie overconsumption, keeping the cycle of weight gain going. Social conditions like poverty or limited access to health care can limit one's ability to become healthier, making things worse. Providing individuals with knowledge about nutrition and providing them with healthy food and physical activity can retard such consequences. In the urban context, where access to fresh produce can be limited in food deserts, broad-based community health measures must be implemented to increase access to healthy choices. Finally, understanding the interplay among psychological, social, and economic determinants is essential in building effective interventions to arrest the epidemic of obesity and confront the urgent issue of overnutrition (Longo et al., 2019) (Figure 6.2).

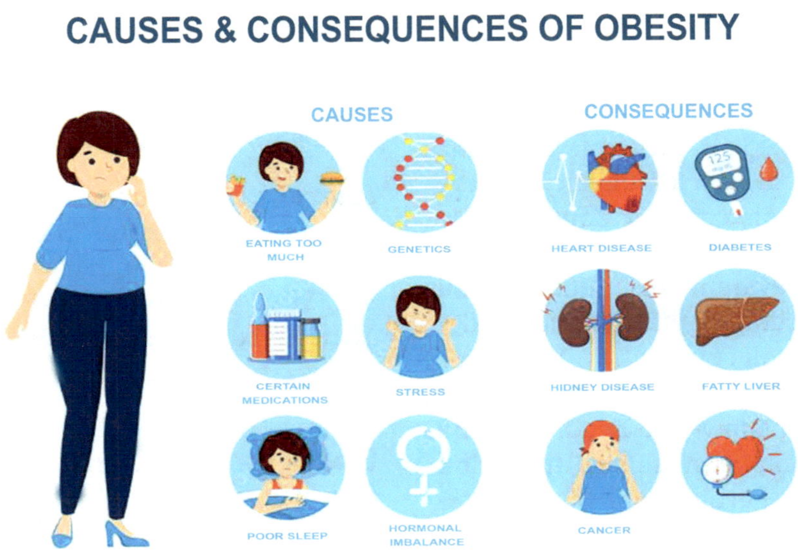

Figure 6.2. Causes and health consequences associated with obesity.

Source: https://external-content.duckduckgo.com/iu/?u=https%3A%2F%2Fas2.ftcdn.net%2Fv2%2Fjpg%2F02%2F45%2F93%2F81%2F1000_F_245938135_7fTlT46F6zs2Kp58Da9owApFuvqThPcf.jpg&f=1&nofb=1&ipt=2b20c87506565cc963ca8c6b4b30b523dcafed1b6bf38575402f7be18f0cda7f.

6.1.1. Genetic Factors

The role of genes in obesity and overnutrition has been an area of considerable research in recent history, primarily because researchers are attempting to uncover the complex relationship between genes and the environment. Variation in certain genes has been found to be major determinants of susceptibility to obesity. For instance, polymorphism in genes , such as FTO and MC4R, is associated with increased body mass index (BMI) and fat deposition. These genetic predispositions have an effect on energy balance, appetite, and metabolism, indicating how genetic characteristics cross with lifestyle factors in the causality of obesity. Nonetheless, it is worth noting that genetic predisposition does not work alone; rather, it works in collaboration with environmental factors , such as eating habits and exercise levels, rendering the causality of obesity complicated. This complex relationship is used to put emphasis on tackling obesity within a framework that considers both genetic and lifestyle factors (Wong et al., 2017). Moreover, studies show that genetic factors have the capability of shaping how individuals respond to dietary intake and physical activity. The International Agency for Research on Cancer finds that there are probable epigenetic and microbiota factors that impact an individual's nutritional interactions in relation to genetic profile. For instance, some people with certain genetic markers can metabolize fats or carbohydrates in a different way, which influences their weight status despite equal dietary consumption. This variation highlights the multifactorial nature of obesity, where certain genetic profiles render some people more prone to weight gain from high-calorie diets that are prevalent in modern food environments. Accordingly, genetic susceptibility may be the principal culminating factor for the rising prevalence of obesity, particularly among developing and low- and middle-income countries experiencing fast dietary transition (Romieu et al., 2017). Furthermore, the evidence noted from observing the global rising obesity epidemic can support that the concept of obesity having its genetic susceptibility enhanced by environmental factors is correct. Even though genetic factors are significant, they are not enough to account for the rising incidence of obesity, particularly in populations undergoing nutrition transition. Diet environmental alterations, such as increased availability of highly processed foods and sweetened beverages, interact with genetic risk factors to enhance the danger of obesity. Hence, whereas genetics confer susceptibility to obesity, they are strongly influenced by lifestyle habits, , such as dietary habits and physical activity. Significantly, the complexity of these interactions underpins the search for personalized strategies that acknowledge genetic susceptibility alongside lifestyle modification as an element of the solution to obesity and overnutrition (Wong et al., 2017) (Figure 6.3).

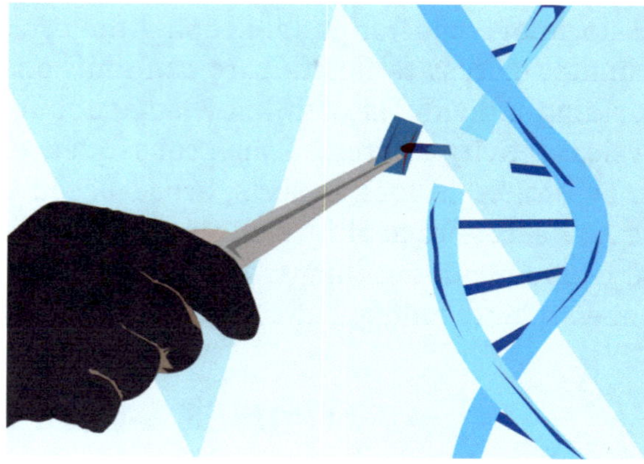

Figure 6.3. Illustration of genetic modification through DNA editing techniques.

Source: https://external-content.duckduckgo.com/iu/?u=https%3A%2F%2Fimages.elearncollege.com%2Fwp-content%2Fuploads%2F2022%2F08%2FGENE345TICS-02.jpg&f=1&nofb=1&ipt=68b107ff6f2ffd766ff681b5441806ba28ea56cc1b0631aa87a71d4e8a2c67ea.

6.1.2. Environmental Influences

The risk factors for overnutrition and obesity are multifactorial and cannot be neglected. Urbanization has brought about tremendous dietary changes with fast food and processed food ruling the market due to affordability and accessibility. Urban availability of high-calorie, low-nutrient foods has been challenged with increased calorie intake and obesity. Secondly, advertising plays a central role in food selection, mostly for poor food options. The social trend is reinforced by the working families' time constraint that renders fast food attractive by virtue of convenience. Studies have shown that low-income families are especially vulnerable to these impacts, as they might prioritize cost and convenience over the quality of nutrients and thus adopt poor dietary habits and an ensuing rise in obesity (Jacob et al., 2020). Besides nutritional impacts, physical inactivity is also augmented by environmental determinants typical of urbanization. Neighborhood planning has an impact on the ability of the residents to engage in regular physical activity; the lack of park spaces, pathways, or recreational facilities deters exercise and outdoor activity. It is indicated by a study that individuals who live in neighborhoods with inadequate access to fresh fruits and vegetables or safe spaces for physical activity are susceptible to obesity and other disorders of health (Wong et al., 2017). Thus, city planning and promoting access to recreational spaces are important. Advances in constructing community infrastructure could encourage a healthy lifestyle, consistent with public health recommendations for increased physical activity and thereby reducing obesity prevalence. The interplay between genes and the environment must be considered when addressing obesity and over nutrition. While genetic susceptibility to weight gain can make significant contributions to risk, the modern environment can impose added risks. Overnutrition and hence excessive levels of obesity are notably prevalent in populations with a trend towards sedentary lifestyle and negative metabolic responses to caloric intake. But environmental modifications, such as improved access to nutritious food and more physical activity have the ability to offset such genetic risks (Jacob et al., 2020). Population-based public health intervention aimed at both environmental and behavioral changes is essential in combating obesity, with interventions that may individually be tailored to account for community-specific challenges and strengths. These combined efforts will eventually result in healthier lifestyles, reducing obesity rates as well as the associated health effects (Figure 6.4).

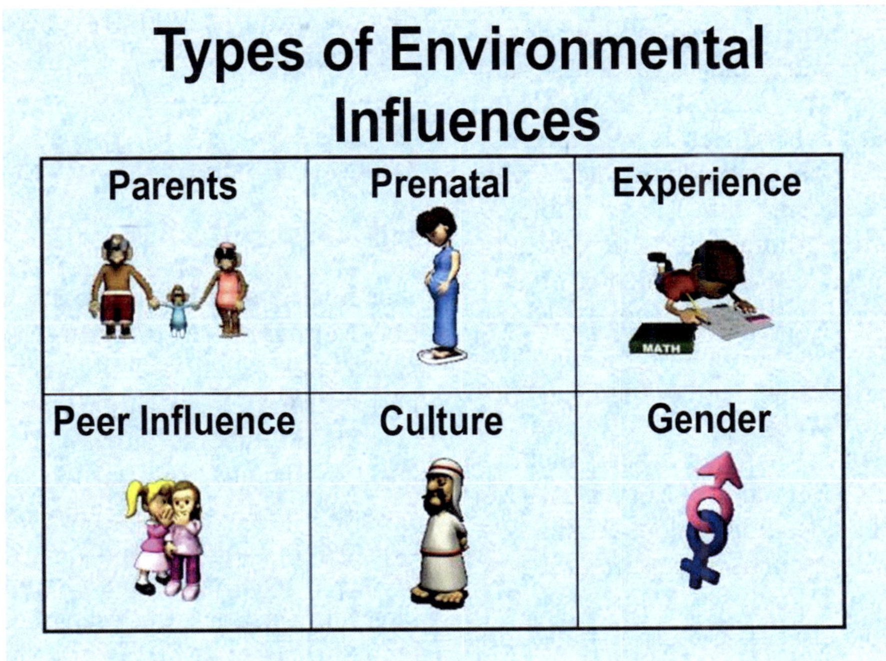

Figure 6.4. Environmental factors influencing human development.

Source: https://external-content.duckduckgo.com/iu/?u=https%3A%2F%2Fimage.slideserve.com%2F388768%2Ftypes-of-environmental-influences-l.jpg&f=1&nofb=1&ipt=995601398fc7c249028151419db9b2e3e981b81b67fbd7df7a8eb87235a9bcac.

6.1.3. Behavioral Patterns

It is essential to understand patterns of behavior related to obesity and overnutrition in order to develop successful interventions. Lack of physical activity, where children spend long amounts of time sitting, is a major reason for weight increase and poor eating habits. Children in general have a concerning movement away from physical activity, with more screen time than playing outdoors. This trend can contribute to excessive deposition of body fat as well as unfavorable cardiometabolic-related consequences. As mentioned, physical inactivity and poor dietary habits are the primary causal risk factors of obesity, with implications that interventions aiming at increased activity levels and improved diet in vulnerable populations are essential (Karava et al., 2023). With the early recognition of these cycles, targeted interventions can be designed to disrupt such patterns, thus reducing obesity and associated health issues. Early nutritional exposures should not be placed too prominently in terms of establishing future behavior patterns. Maternal prenatal and lactational overnutrition have been found to make offspring more susceptible to obesity, leading to pathological behaviors akin to addiction. So profound is the influence of fetal programming on modified gene expressions ensuing through the mechanism of enhanced caloric intake during development to shape neural circuits mediating reward and behavior that the downstream consequences include susceptibility to obesity and obesity disorders throughout life. Furthermore, the inflammatory responses that develop as a consequence of hypercaloric intake further complicate the interrelationship between maternal nutrition and offspring behavior, thus rendering understanding of such relationships essential to well-adjusted health strategies (Línez et al., 2018). Understanding such patterns allows for early interventions that are potential reducers of subsequent risk associated with obesity. Socioeconomic and cultural influences also play a critical function in influencing behavior patterns linked to overnutrition and obesity. Poorer households may suffer from food insufficiency and limited access to quality food sources, leading to reliance on low-cost, high-energy food. Such dependence not only causes nutritional imbalances but also instills a pattern of overnutrition among family members. In addition, social norms about food intake and body image both facilitate and prevent pathological behavior. Societies that make it "normal" to have sedentary living and eat non-nutritious foods can do so without even realizing it by perpetuating harmful patterns. Being aware of these background influences is crucial to developing universal health policies that are sensitive to environmental and cultural-influenced behavioral patterns. This plan highlights the significance of community-based initiatives in supporting healthier living among diverse groups and preventing the obesity epidemic better.

6.2. Health Consequences of Obesity

The health effects of obesity extend beyond body appearance, affecting physical health, mental health, and overall quality of life. Obesity has a strong link with chronic diseases , such as type 2 diabetes and heart disease, and it imposes an enormous burden on the healthcare system worldwide. Obesity also predisposes one to many complications , such as high blood pressure, dyslipidemia, and some cancers. The interconnectedness between obesity and chronic kidney disease (CKD) is the most prominent. As Li et al. (2020) posits, as obesity increases, the risk of developing kidney impairments also rises, highlighting the urgent need for prevention and intervention. These connections serve as reminders that obesity's effects are not merely at the individual level but have implications on public health as well, necessitating ambitious measures in stemming this rapidly expanding epidemic. Another critical factor in the health consequences of obesity is its influence on gestational diabetes mellitus (GDM). Obese individuals, especially women, have a higher risk of developing GDM, which poses serious threats to maternal and neonatal health. Overweight and obesity are risk factors that lead to insulin resistance in pregnancy, causing abnormal glucose tolerance and chronic hyperglycemia. As outlined in Plows et al., (2018), the outcomes of GDM include heightened risk of type 2 diabetes in the mother and the child, as well as danger of macrosomia and complication at birth.

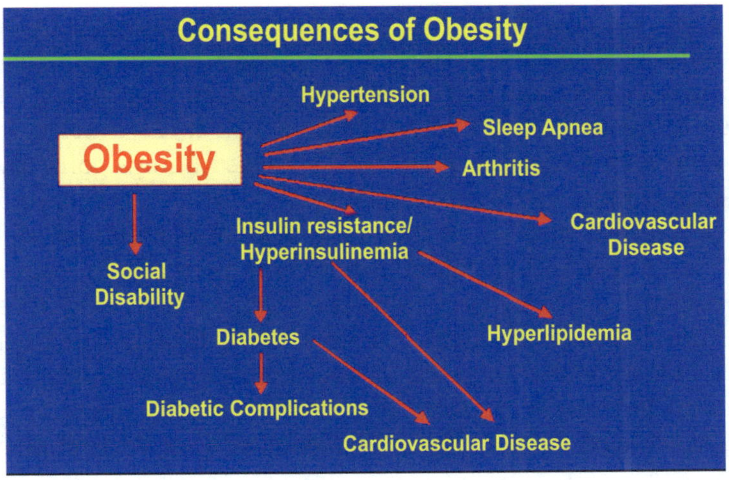

Figure 6.5. Health complications arising from obesity.

Source: https://external-content.duckduckgo.com/iu/?u=https%3A%2F%2Fimg.medscapestatic.com%2Ffullsize%2Fmigrated%2Feditorial%2Fconferences%2F2002%2F1440%2Fcu01.fig02.gif&f=1&nofb=1&ipt=92e39eb372491e099901ee6808b4194496404b7ee59f8e33c2ebf6ceeb5a25fd.

All these interconnected conditions highlight prevention of obesity before and during pregnancy as a major preventive strategy. Understanding the multi-dimensional consequences of obesity, and more specifically on maternal health, can guide public health policy and tailored treatment plans. Finally, the psychological and social factors of obesity contribute significantly to its impact on health. Individuals with obesity carry with them stigma and discrimination that lead to mental diseases , such as depression and anxiety. The social connotation of obesity is expressed in so many different forms, from affecting job opportunities, relationships, to the individual's self-esteem. Further, the relationship between obesity and mental disorders can create a cycle of viciousness wherein psychological distress aggravates eating behavior and results in further weight gain. These psychological aspects need to be targeted to provide satisfactory obesity treatment and must be addressed through an integrated approach involving physical and psychological care. In order to address the obesity epidemic comprehensively, stakeholders need to prioritize mental health services and community support systems that support healthier living and overall well-being (Figure 6.5).

6.2.1. Physical Health Risks

Its increasing rate among children is a serious physical health issue that carries extensive consequences for adulthood. In that context, the World Health Organization has corroborated the fact that obese children are likely to become obese adults, thereby accelerating the risk of developing non-communicable diseases (NCDs) , such as type 2 diabetes, cardiovascular disease, and certain cancer forms in adulthood (Di Cesare et al., 2019). These chronic conditions not only reduce the well-being of individuals suffering from them but also impose tremendous burdens on health systems around the world. Furthermore, the long-term consequences of obesity in childhood can generate sustained disease complications of health, leading to a vicious cycle of poor health that is hard to break. Effective interventions and policies directed at the environmental causes of obesity are critical in mitigating these risks and ensuring healthier futures for the next generation. Physical inactivity is a critical risk determinant of obesity, multiplying the risks associated with overnutrition significantly. Evidence has it that a lack of participation in physical activity is directly associated with increased overweight and obesity in children. Specifically, a Ghana-based study identified that children engaged in sport activities less than three times a week were 44% more likely to be obese or overweight (Aryeetey et al., 2017). These findings point towards the importance of building environments conducive to physical activity as an integral part of obesity prevention policy. Society and schools must make sure that programs supporting active living are developed, adopting physical education in the curriculum and making recreational space available. The more physically active opportunities are added, the more the negative health impact of sedentary lifestyles can be reduced, resulting in lower childhood obesity rates. In addition to the immediate health risks of the individual, obesity and overnutrition also lead to psychological and social issues that enhance physical issues. Overweight children and youth typically experience discrimination and harassment and thus are isolated, develop low self-esteem, and suffer from mental illnesses , such as depression and anxiety. These mental issues can create a feedback loop, making it more challenging to create good habits and reestablish an unhealthy pattern of sedentary lifestyle behaviors. The interdependence of physical and mental health makes it essential that interventions are holistic, addressing both aspects of health. Promoting a holistic strategy to the control of obesity, including mental as well as physical interventions for health, can lead to more effective solutions and improve overall well-being among young individuals affected by overnutrition and the attendant hazards (Di Cesare et al., 2019).

6.2.2. Psychological Effects

The psychological effect of overnutrition and obesity extends far beyond mere physical health concerns and drastically affects mental health. Obese individuals experience higher levels of anxiety and depression, which in turn lead to an ongoing cycle of emotional consumption and weight gain. Stigmatization of obesity results in isolation, low self-esteem, and uselessness, all adding to mental health issues. Studies have shown that individuals with obesity are likely to undergo discrimination in most settings, , such as the workplace and healthcare facilities, which will enhance the psychological burden. This complex pattern of social judgment and individual experience enhances the need for an interdisciplinary approach towards solving the psychological impacts of obesity, giving a lot of weight to mental health care as well as physical health care (Li et al., 2020). Also, the biological factor is exacerbated by the interaction between obesity and psychological effects. Appetite and satiety centers in the hypothalamus are controlled by emotional state, and hence psychological distress has a correlation with overeating. Emotional eating is a gateway method of access for most that subsequently leads to caloric consumption due to unpleasant emotions rather than real hunger. This behavioral response can create a feedback loop where increased weight heightens mental illness issues, which presents a daunting challenge to the impacted individuals. Efforts to break this circle should recognize the role of mental health professionals and nutritionists in the development of individualized programs that address not only food intake but also interventions for efficient depression and anxiety management (Petticrew et al., 2019). In understanding the interrelatedness of obesity, overnutrition, and mental illness, effective interventions must be systems-based. It enables a holistic conceptualization of how economic, psychological, and social determinants affect overall health in individuals with obesity. Establishing an enabling environment that minimizes stigma and facilitates healthy lifestyle change can enable resilience against obesity's psychological impacts. Engagement in community support networks, psychotherapy, and tailored nutritional advice can help individuals take charge of both their weight and their mental health simultaneously. Thus, the psychological impact of obesity is not only an ethical responsibility but also a factor to consider in the development of successful prevention and treatment programs (Li et al., 2020) (Figure 6.6).

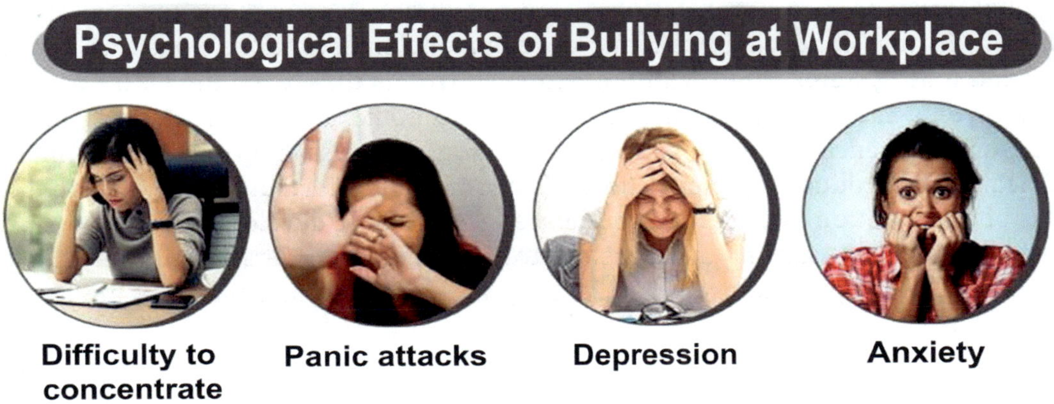

Figure 6.6. Psychological effects of workplace bullying include anxiety, depression, panic attacks, and difficulty concentrating.

Source: https://external-content.duckduckgo.com/iu/?u=https%3A%2F%2Fimages.medindia.net%2Fpatientinfo%2F950_400%2Fpsychological-effects-of-bullying-at-workplace.jpg&f=1&nofb=1&ipt=40c352fcb77712493c1acf35fc7bf1438ce1c0a78328abb44a5c9ae08dc28071e.

6.2.3. Economic Implications

The economic impacts of obesity and overnutrition are widespread and diverse, ranging beyond individual health results to impact more general organizational features of society. Greater levels of obesity are linked with increased costs for health care, since obese individuals tend to require more medical attention for chronic illnesses , such as diabetes, cardiovascular disease, and certain cancers. The financial cost is felt both at the individual and state levels, accounting for significant levels of public health spending. Effective management of obesity requires forward planning, in the form of public campaigns and preventative treatment, which costs significantly. Furthermore, the economic productivity of the individuals concerned can be decreased through absence and compromised performance at work, accounting collectively for national economies. This creates a negative cycle where negative health consequences reduce the effectiveness of the workforce, contributing to economic problems in the society (Haddad et al.). In developing societies, the shift towards overnutrition accelerates economic hazards, particularly in the backdrop of ongoing urbanization and rising incomes. The food transition, whereby increased consumption of processed food is noted, usually leads to lifestyle changes that are convenience-oriented and not based on nutritional value. This shift affects economic development through its role in accelerating the rate of chronic diseases, which in turn stretch healthcare resources. The relationship between food consumption, economic well-being, and health indicates the complex dynamics of determinants influencing society. Policy intervention encourages healthier food chains and diet education holds significant roles to steer populations towards improved diets. Evidence is required to disentangle such complexities and to create beneficial strategies, requiring joint effort on the part of policymakers, healthcare workers, and researchers to inform interventions aimed at altering harmful trends in foods and encouraging more desirable economic prospects (Haddad et al.). The broader challenges of achieving food and nutrition security are most evident in nations like Ghana, where undernutrition and overnutrition coexist, suggesting more pervasive economic implications. Challenges , such as poverty, global warming, and urbanization of the population render the landscape of nutritional health difficult, in turn hindering economic development. Interventions , such as investment in agriculture and food systems, and social protection programs that reach the entire population are required to reverse the impacts of malnutrition on economic development. Such interventions not only ensure resilience for marginalized populations but also help local economies through enhanced health and productivity. Nourishment-sensitive policy formulation will be able to reduce the impacts of malnutrition and create a good base for upcoming development programs. Ensuring that one is committed to learning and reacting to the complex drivers of food insecurity will be of great importance to optimize economic stability and growth, particularly in low- and middle-income countries.

6.3. Nutritional Aspects of Overnutrition

Overnutrition, characterized by excessive caloric intake and dietary imbalance, is a major cause of rising obesity globally. The fact should be noted that overnutrition is not merely overconsumption but consists of a complex interplay between eating patterns, lifestyle, and determinants of socioeconomic factors. The majority of individuals end up consuming high-calorie, low-nutrient foods through increased availability and aggressive marketing of processed foods. Moreover, a sedentary lifestyle further aggravates the condition, as a lack of physical activity reduces energy expenditure, contributing to more weight gain. The effects of overnutrition go beyond mere weight gain; they bring in an array of health conditions , such as type 2 diabetes, cardiovascular disease, and other metabolic disorders that compromise public health and overwhelm healthcare systems globally. While the importance of macronutrient balance, carbohydrate, protein, and fat, persists in the nutrition controversy, the rising prevalence of micronutrient deficiencies among overnourished individuals cannot be ignored. In an ironic twist, calories consumed in excess by individuals can put them in danger of a deficiency of essential vitamins and minerals, placing a dual burden of obesity and malnutrition. For instance, a high-refined-sugar and fat diet will displace the intake of fruits, vegetables, and whole grains that are crucial to overall well-being. Depletions may cause exacerbation of chronic disease threats through effects on immune response, bone health, and metabolic function. For example, cardiovascular diseases remain a pertinent threat associated with food choice, paving the way for comprehensive policies targeted towards a balanced diet and preventive care interventions aimed at addressing obesity as well as undernutrition simultaneously

(Joseph et al., 2017). Enhancing the nutritional aspect of overnutrition must be achieved through a multisectoral approach encompassing public health interventions, community-based interventions, and educational interventions in an attempt to support enhanced dietary behavior. Highlights of effective strategies include increasing access to healthy food in low-income areas, initiating nutrition education in schools, and supporting policies to limit marketing of unhealthy foods to children. These measures not only enhance a healthy food environment but also empower individuals to make healthful food choices, with attendant improved health status across groups. Additionally, harmonizing health policies and socioeconomic determinants reveals the promise to diminish the burden of disease of conditions entailing overnutrition. In our quest to battle the acute issue of obesity, fixing the nutritional determinants of overnutrition must remain on the agenda of public health (Luyckx et al., 2018) (Figure 6.7).

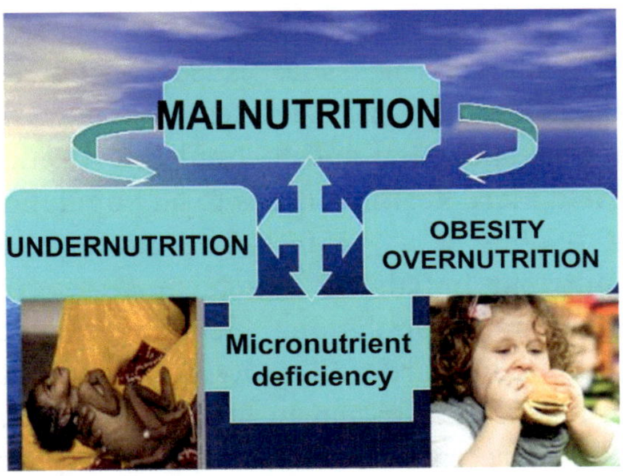

Figure 6.7. Types of malnutrition: Undernutrition, overnutrition, and micronutrient deficiency.

Source: https://external-content.duckduckgo.com/iu/?u=https%3A%2F%2Fi.pinimg.com%2Foriginals%2Fef%2Fc2%2F13%2Fefc213a241ec5aa001d21e2044a174ab.jpg&f=1&nofb=1&ipt=68c20f9346ec9ea315a47a0d5d7442dbc108d9df42f02273fea0f742c84bf5a1.

6.3.1. Excess Caloric Intake

Caloric overconsumption has been identified as a primary cause of the worldwide epidemic of obesity, which has garnered serious interest from scientists and public health professionals. When individuals consume more calories than they expend through physical activity and metabolic processes, excess energy is retained in the body in the form of fat, leading to an increase in BMI. Research has proven that the consumption of food at a fast rate can lead to caloric overconsumption. For example, one longitudinal study uncovered that people who consumed their meals at a faster rate consumed more calories than those who ate at a slower pace by significant margins and that this correlation with eating speed and excess caloric consumption was related to BMI gain over time (Kabata et al., 2025). This finding highlights the complex interaction between caloric consumption and energy balance, which indicates that cautious eating habits need to be adhered to in order to reduce the likelihood of obesity. Also, environmental factors contribute maximally towards excessive caloric intake in modern society. The commonality of calorically dense but nutritionally poor foodstuffs and extensive marketing campaigns suggest an environment to facilitate overnutrition. Subsidization of healthy food has been put forward as a potential solution to this trend; evidence indicates that the steps can exert significant impact on food consumption and purchasing habits by encouraging individuals to make healthier choices (Comini et al., 2024). The impact of subsidies is, nonetheless, temporary, as evidenced by decreased consumption of healthier foods upon elimination of economic incentives. Thus, while promoting healthier food consumption and sustainable eating habits is important, understanding the drivers behind caloric overconsumption is imperative to the construction of appropriate public health interventions that will be able to reduce obesity. Finally, minimizing excess caloric consumption involves a multi-dimensional approach that involves not only personal behavior change but also food environment changes. Health promotions encouraging balanced meals and healthy ways of living can empower people to make better choices. Further, nutritional literacy campaigns that educate consumers on caloric content and the hazards of overconsumption can heighten the awareness of consumers of caloric content and its consequences. By fostering a culture of health and moderation, communities are in a better place to restrict the risks associated with excessive caloric intake. Lastly, combining individual responsibility with social support systems can be the type of environment where individuals will be less likely to fall victim to overnutrition and therefore really address the growing epidemic of obesity.

6.3.2. Nutrient Imbalance

In the current public health setting, nutrient imbalance is a major contributory factor to the overnutrition and obesity epidemic. Imbalance in nutrients is a condition where the consumption of macronutrients and micronutrients is not proportional to each other and thus creates varying conditions, including obesity. Nutrition imbalance is normally associated with excessive food intake of energy-dense foods that are low in nutrient and insufficient food intake of nutrients , such as vitamins and minerals. This is an alarming trend because it results not only in weight gain but also in malnutrition, thereby exacerbating cognitive dysfunction and compromised health outcomes. The effects of diet on general health are of the utmost significance, and especially so in at-risk populations, where poor dietary choices can literally make or break academic and health achievement. The primary link between nutrition and intellect reveals that unless children get the necessary nutrients to facilitate maximum brain performance, their performance at school can be severely compromised, once more perpetuating the disadvantageous cycle typically associated with overnutrition and obesity (Woodhouse & Lamport, 2012). Moreover, the consequences of unbalanced nutrients extend far beyond matters of personal health; they represent grave social and economic problems as well. The concomitance of conditions , such as obesity and malnourishment, has emerged as an evolving process in various socioeconomic settings. Evolving countries are developing the double burden of undernutrition and obesity, thus complicating their health situation. This combination of disease could worsen existing inequalities, with wealthier groups enjoying easier access to nutrient-rich food and consequently further excluding poor groups. Hence, policymakers are under pressure to fill these gaps with innovative nutritional interventions that target both overweight adults and malnourished children.

Conditional cash transfer (CCT) schemes, for instance, have been suggested as potential solutions but must be properly administered to avoid adverse effects in advanced transition environments. The issues caused by nutrient imbalance emphasize the necessity of equitable resource allocation and focused interventions to yield more health benefits to all populations (Aitsi-Selmi et al., 2009). The consequence of nutrient imbalance affects most severely among some populations, including children, whose bodies are still growing and require well-balanced nutrition in order to grow and think correctly. Nutritional lack at critical developmental stages has long-lasting effects, leading to poor academic performance and vulnerability to a variety of disease conditions. When combined with overconsumption of high-calorie, low-nutrient foods, children are caught in a vicious malnutrition-obesity cycle. These habits not only undermine their immediate health but also their eventual productivity and well-being. It is important that education and public health programs emphasize the importance of well-balanced diets as well as dispelling myths about nutrition. By creating awareness of the right mode of eating and access to healthy food, one can mitigate the adverse effects of nutrient imbalance and promote better health outcomes for and educational gains of future generations (Woodhouse & Lamport, 2012) (Figure 6.8).

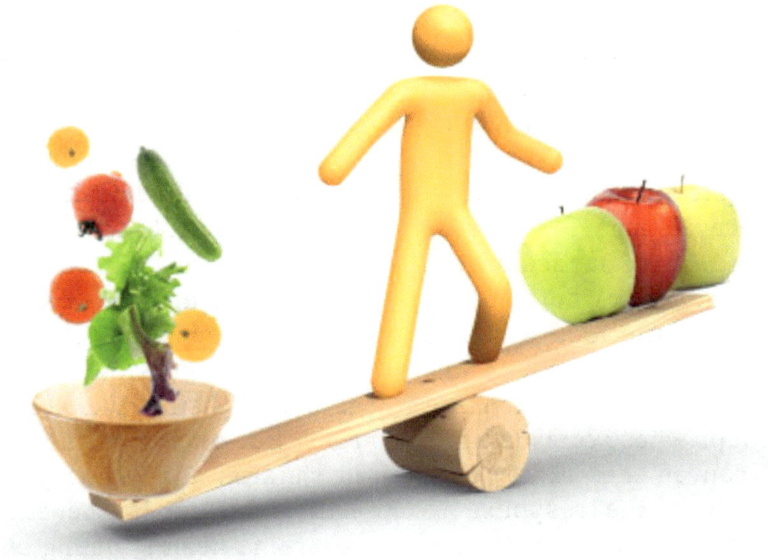

Figure 6.8. Nursing diagnosis chart for imbalanced nutrition less than body requirements.

Source: https://external-content.duckduckgo.com/iu/?u=http%3A%2F%2F4.bp.blogspot.com%2F-TAr_b4G12ig%2FUCFHASmzUAI%2FAAAAAAAAAJw%2FRAKZIl3Bvqs%2Fs1600%2Fnursing_diagnosis_imbalanced_nutrition_less_than_body_requirements.jpg&f=1&nofb=1&ipt=a356a07bd918c426d2d08e8a5e8a2979477a9e2a8a00ba5982383cf6e0f56178.

6.3.3. Role of Processed Foods

Processed foods form a pivotal part to the contemporary universe of obesity and overnutrition, having a broad effect on diet and nutritional well-being. They are usually rich in fat, sugar, and salt, resulting in excessive caloric intake combined with an absence of essential nutrients that produce an imbalance favorable for weight gain. For instance, processed food snack foods, soft beverages, and fast foods, which are now more accessible and advertised, have revolutionized traditional eating patterns to lead to reliance on convenient but nutritionally poor foods. This, thus, exposes those who consume processed food to increased risks of obesity, chronic diseases, and poor overall health outcomes. Current public health interventions lay much emphasis on policymaking against the avoidance of excessive intake of processed foods to combat the rising prevalence of obesity and promote healthier dietary habits among at-risk populations (Joseph et al., 2017). The contribution of processed foods towards obesity cannot be exaggerated in view of their connection with metabolic disturbance and inflammation. The research has proved that processed food diets distort regular appetite cues and metabolism, causing individuals to become stuck in overeating. Due to the fact that most of these foods use additives and preservatives, they can alter gut microbiota, an essential modifier of metabolic health, inducing inflammation and conditions of obesity. Further, increasing evidence has emerged that confirms that overconsumption of high-fructose corn syrup and trans fats found in the majority of processed foods can expand insulin resistance, which is a leading cause of Type 2 diabetes. This disturbance of metabolism highlights the importance of creating greater public awareness of the consequences of consuming processed foods and its broader health impact (Bourke et al., 2016). While tackling the obesity crisis, it becomes a necessity to investigate the socio-economic factors behind the prevalence of processed foods. Poor communities, in particular, are likely to suffer from food deserts where healthy foods are unavailable and the food available is processed food. The advertisement by the food industries further fuels this condition as it targets vulnerable groups whose consideration may lie in cost and convenience rather than nutrient value. Therefore, the response to the role of processed foods in obesity and overnutrition requires an integrated system with education, policy reformulation, and empowerment of the community. Facilitating greater access to healthier food and generating awareness on nutrition can empower people to make informed decisions to support overall health in spite of the dominance of a market for processed foods (Joseph et al., 2017).

6.4. Societal Impact of Obesity

The social impact of obesity extends way beyond personal health, penetrating numerous spheres of life nowadays, like economics, education, and public policy regarding public health. As obesity prevalence increases, healthcare spending skyrockets, placing an enormous load on the public purse. Up to $190 billion in the United States alone, both direct healthcare expenditure and indirect costs , such as lost productivity, is the estimated economic cost of obesity. Such economic implications compel policymakers and healthcare executives to put interventions targeting the reduction of obesity on high priority, but the success of such programs is subject to large dependence on public awareness and community participation. Accordingly, the necessity to address obesity supersedes personal preference; it necessitates a public commitment by society to promote environments in support of healthier lifestyles and dietary habits as a response to resisting an expanding public health problem endangering generations yet to come. Schools are key combat zones for resisting obesity and determining social health and diet-related behaviors. Schools by their very nature play a unique role in that they are responsible for children's education as well as their intake of nutrition during early ages. But an increasing incidence of obesity in children and young people has unveiled a critical lacuna in the education curriculum regarding healthy eating and physical activity. Adoption of integrating comprehensive nutrition education and physical activity programs in school curriculum can significantly impact long-term lifestyle choices, reducing obesity rates in the process. Nevertheless, these programs are constrained by insufficient funding, limited resources, and coercion to observe standardized tests. Ensuring that the schools consider students' health equal to their performance is crucial in developing a generation that considers nutrition and physical activity to be central aspects of a healthy life (Erenstein et al., 2022). Moreover, cultural discourses surrounding food consumption and the body play a significant role in dramatically influencing society's perception concerning obesity. The expansion of ultra-processed food has multiplied unhealthy diet patterns, as societal demands continue to reinforce unrealistic body ideals that ironically increase both overnutrition and undernutrition. The contrast routinely serves to heighten stigma against obese individuals, further isolating them and perpetuating cycles of discrimination. The discourse of health and wellness increasingly must deconstruct those culture norms and address the systemic issues that reinforce unhealthy lifestyle habits. Academics posit that sustainability is critical in reshaping food systems with the perspective that the notion of healthy diets needs to go beyond the focus on calories to encompass broader aspects of environmental and social well-being (Béné et al., 2018). Obesity's multiple causes necessitate a response in coming up with effective strategies in improving health equity and developing environments for fostering healthier behaviors (Figure 6.9).

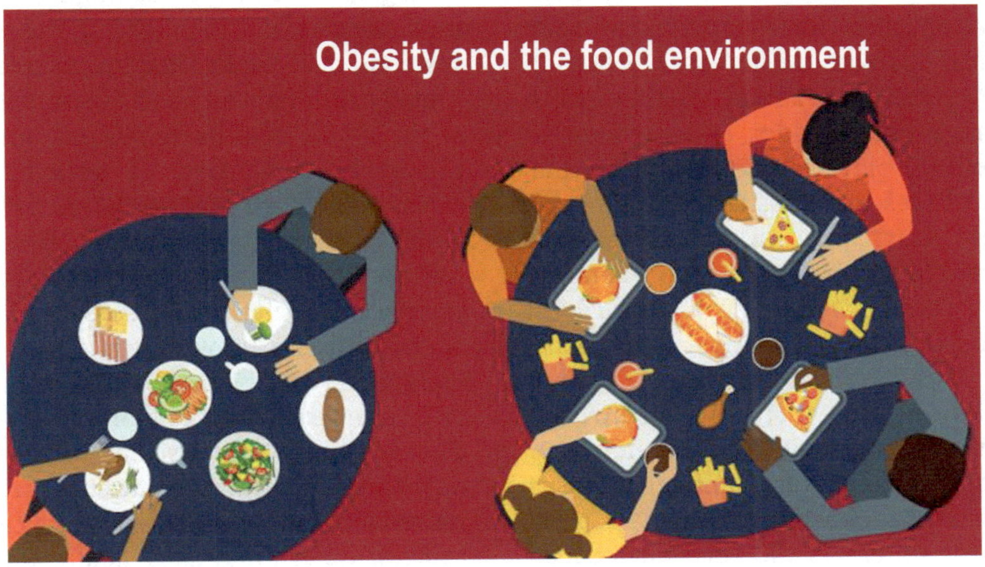

Figure 6.9. Impact of food environment on dietary choices and obesity.

Source: https://external-content.duckduckgo.com/iu/?u=https%3A%2F%2Fukhsa.blog.gov.uk%2Fwp-content%2Fuploads%2Fsites%2F33%2F2017%2F03%2F6.3206_PHE_TH_Health-Matters_Obesity_Online.png&f=1&nofb=1&ipt=dbfdb810d1dafc67335c41793fd025b8be42f0c29d5a8d26278e5a6703ace193.

6.4.1. Stigmatization and Discrimination

Discrimination and stigmatization of the overweight and obese are central culprits, exacerbating their ailments and hindering access to the medical care they need. Individuals regard larger sizes as indicators of laziness, low willpower, and poor decisions, a context where individuals are devalued and discriminated against. This stigmatization is not just expressed in social interactions but also in healthcare, where the obese individual can be provided with inferior or biased care. Evidence shows that a number of regression analyses demonstrate how the variables like self-objectification and negative affect predict lower medical care satisfaction among bigger women, pointing to the need for a healthcare system that considers the unique needs of the group and strives for the creation of a more inclusive setting (Koutsouros, 2003). The impacts of discrimination are not confined to the experience at an individual level; they influence public health interventions overall intended for obesity and overnutrition management. In the majority of the world, particularly sub-Saharan Africa, there exists a paradox where individuals can end up stigmatizing obesity yet idealizing large body sizes. In Nigeria, for instance, nearly 45% of the population believe that obesity is an esteemed attribute, demonstrating the complex dynamics between cultural perceptions and health effects (Chigbu, 2018). This dualism makes the evolution of effective counter-obesity interventions difficult since stigmatization might discourage individuals from accessing help or complying with preventive treatment practices. Therefore, it is essential to tackle these social dynamics in order to establish an environment in which people can seek healthier lifestyles without necessarily fearing judgment or ostracism. In addition, public health interventions must consider and respond to the complex interplay between social norms, individual attitudes, and obesity-induced health inequalities. Internalization of stigmatizing attitudes can lead to negative self-concept and reduced mental well-being in those with a background of obesity. For most individuals, such negative self-concept prevents healthy behavior and sustains further overnutrition in a self-perpetuating cycle. The distinction of female gender, urban dwelling, and older age as variables with higher obesity rates and perceptual distortion only reiterates the need for focused educational campaigns in order to change body size perceptions and foster an environment of inclusiveness in health communication (Chigbu, 2018). Successful multipronged interventions are required in order to overcome stigmatization and discrimination and finally improve the discourse surrounding health in obesity.

6.4.2. Impact on Healthcare Systems

The rising level of obesity and overnutrition imposes enormous burden on the healthcare system worldwide. The two conditions lead to increased chronic conditions , such as type 2 diabetes, cardiovascular diseases, and their attendant complications, hence rising medical care demands. For instance, gestational diabetes mellitus (GDM), potentially caused by maternal obesity, is harmful not just to mothers but also to their children, entering a cycle of complications that can potentially last long after the mother has given birth. Approximately 16.5% of pregnancies are complicated by GDM, and the higher the rate of obesity, the higher this rate is likely to become, leading to greater difficulties for healthcare professionals to address the problem. Rising such preventable conditions impose enormous pressure on healthcare resources, necessitating more holistic management strategies leading to overall system inefficiencies and highlighting the necessity of systemic changes directed towards resolving the root causes of obesity and overnutrition (Plows et al., 2018). Healthcare systems must address the growing burden of noncommunicable diseases caused by obesity. Current global health policy goals aim to reduce such impacts, and the goal is to reduce premature mortality due to noncommunicable diseases by 25% by 2025. Such successes, however, hinge on successful integration of evidence-based health policies and interventions. Control of obesity-related diseases like cardiovascular diseases requires not only customized patient care but also integrated public health interventions across societal determinants of health and systemic impediments. Socioeconomic determinants, the ability of health policies, and the access to health care are determinants that have a strong impact on health outcomes. The development of healthcare systems to tackle these complex challenges will therefore be at the center of turning around the trend of rising cases of obesity and advancing population health (Joseph et al., 2017). The influence of obesity on healthcare systems is supported by the expenditure on chronic diseases. Excessive treatment costs of obesity diseases lead to greater economic loads on the patients and on the health-care services. Since patients require ongoing medical treatment, from preventive practices to surgery and drug therapy, medical costs are high. In the majority of regions, particularly among middle- and low-income countries, resources are already limited, and increased requirements for chronic disease control could immobilize available infrastructures. This cost pinch risks diverting both funds and attention away from other significant healthcare sectors, ultimately impairing overall quality of care. A prevention and early intervention intersectoral approach can relieve these pressures while building healthier populations, reducing expenditure in the long run, and making healthcare systems more resilient to the growing threat of obesity and overnutrition (Joseph et al., 2017) (Figure 6.10).

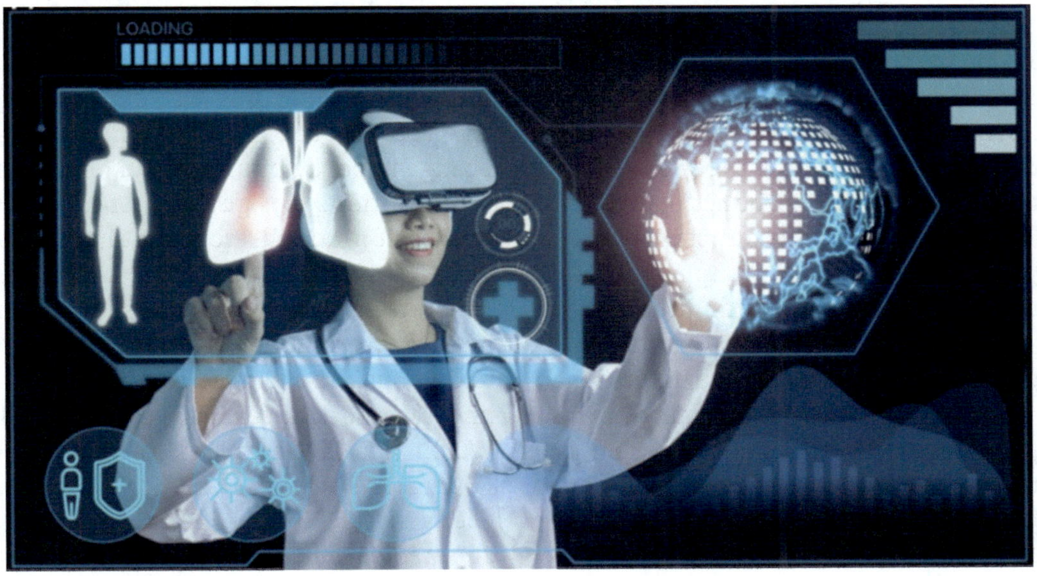

Figure 6.10. VR and AI integration in advanced medical diagnostics.

Source: https://external-content.duckduckgo.com/iu/?u=https%3A%2F%2Fares.decipherzone.com%2Fblog-manager%2Fuploads%2Fckeditor_ai-medical-staff.jpg&f=1&nofb=1&ipt=3db76c7a05933194e84b0af2989caf0af7af14236ab640a9067c5a5d29e0ecab.

6.4.3. Influence on Productivity and Workforce

The intersection of obesity, overnutrition, and organizational productivity is a critical area to address, particularly as world population trends shift and dietary intake improves. A surplus of highly processed foods leads to poor diets, which further leads to an explosion of diet-related chronic disorders , such as obesity and diabetes. Not only do these ailments have direct health implications for individuals but alfor on organizational productivity. Obese workers are susceptible to increased rates of absenteeism, reduced motivation, and decreased overall workplace performance. Because productivity in the work force directly correlates with worker well-being, it is apparent that it is essential to fight against obesity and promote healthier diets in order to help build a more productive and efficient work force today. It is important that organizations recognize the importance of nutrition in the workplace because a healthier workforce can lead to lower healthcare costs and improved employee morale. The obesity problem is also connected with the broader issues of food production and distribution networks. With a growing population and shifting wealth distributions, the required diets also shift. Existing food systems are under pressure to produce high-quality food with the minimum environmental impact while satisfying the increasing demand for healthy food. Systems that fail to deliver such demands may inadvertently promote conditions like obesity, which in turn affect workforce productivity. Actually, the complexity of the food chain, fueled by climatic factors and economic factors, underscores the necessity of simplifying food production along nutritional specifications. Sustainable strategies must be developed to provide affordable access to healthy foods since this not only impacts the health of individuals but also has ripple effects on workforce productivity (McClements et al., 2020; Binns et al., 2021). Technological innovation holds the key to stemming the epidemic of obesity as well as improving productivity in the workforce. Robotics, biotechnology, and artificial intelligence provide the possibility for creating a stronger food production system with emphasis on quality and nutrition. These technologies can simplify food supply chains, hence making it easier for individuals not to consume unhealthy food products that contribute to obesity. Further, the engagement of stakeholders across the food chain during technological development and utilization is critical in order to foster acceptance as well as adherence to healthier eating patterns. By focusing on technology solutions that promote healthy eating and sustainable access to food, organizations can create an employee workforce that is not only more engaging but productive as well, hence contributing to improved outcomes for both workers and businesses during rising rates of obesity (McClements et al., 2020; Binns et al., 2021).

6.5. Prevention Strategies

Effective prevention intervention is of great concern in solving the increasing pandemic of obesity and associated hazards of over nutrition. Prevention interventions have to be multidimensional and include education, community intervention, and policy actions. Education plays a critical role in sensitizing people toward healthy food choice and physical activity. Interventions may be specifically initiated in schools, the workplace, and in community spaces to disseminate population-specific information. Also, engaging people in the creation of supportive settings that promote eating well and regular physical activity is necessary. For instance, local governments can have easy access to municipal parks and recreation facilities, thereby encouraging residents towards outdoor and physical activities. From such a culture of health, such prevention measures can significantly reduce the rate of obesity and enable sustainable change in behavior among the population. Policy interventions by governments can increase prevention actions to counteract obesity and over nutrition. Governments can implement regulations on food labels, marketing, and pricing to promote healthier diets. For example, taxing sugar beverages can deter consumption and promote alternatives, as concluded in World Health Organization and World Dental Federation suggestions for sugar reduction (Zeng et al., 2025). These attempts can be supplemented with food labeling regulations demanding open and transparent information about food products. By placing the information in the public domain, consumers are in a position to make intelligent decisions, hence contributing towards healthier eating habits. Moreover, starting education campaigns that explain the long-term health effects of consumption of a balanced diet can generate awareness and stimulate significant public behavior towards food consumption. Further, cooperation between various sectors in the formulation of an all-encompassing framework for preventing obesity is necessary. This involves cooperation between healthcare providers, schools, not-for-profit organizations, and food manufacturers to coordinate efforts for healthier living. For example, healthcare providers can do routine screening and counseling of target populations to identify people who would benefit by personalized nutrition guides and changes in lifestyle. Secondly, food manufacturers' reformulation of products with reduced sugar and fat content can have population-level effects on dietary practices. Use of these approaches in combination can enhance prevention effectiveness as an overall measure. Also, as noted in research examining the risk factors of breast cancer, identification and management of both modifiable and non-modifiable factors within a community are necessary in order to design effective prevention measures tailored to individualized community needs (García-Sancha et al., 2025) (Figure 6.11).

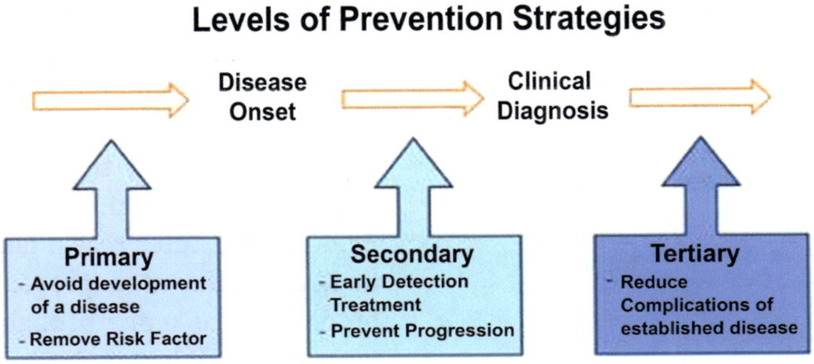

Figure 6.11. Three levels of disease prevention: Primary, secondary, and tertiary.

Source: https://external-content.duckduckgo.com/iu/?u=https%3A%2F%2Fedblogs.columbia.edu%2Fpcore%2Ffiles%2F2017%2F04%2Fprevention_strategy-1nr9qp0.jpg&f=1&nofb=1&ipt=47694e96f0c5db13c69d7085fbc8e0dea9d596d65bf1ce03bcb26bec184c01fa.

6.5.1. Public Health Initiatives

Public health interventions have a key function to fulfill in prevention against the rising epidemic of overnutrition and obesity, particularly among susceptible populations , such as children. Public health interventions aim to promote an environment supportive of healthier lifestyle patterns through education and community. Through promotion of dietary alteration and physical exercise, public health interventions strive to reduce the occurrence of obesity and lower its associated health risks. Evidence suggests that early intervention is critical because the formation of healthy habits during childhood can have a lasting effect on long-term health outcomes. There is therefore a pressing need for well-directed interventions that resonate with the distinct developmental and cultural contexts of each community in a bid to address the dual burden of malnutrition effectively. In Thailand, for instance, rising levels of overweight children under the age of five, as shown by national child development survey data, highlight the need for public health response that is integrative. Sanji Suresh's acknowledgment of the double burden of malnutrition highlights how socio-demographic factors can complicate health interventions. Public health initiatives must account for such factors in their response so as to adjust their approach accordingly and tackle both undernutrition and overnutrition. Strategies might include enhanced access to healthy diets, education in healthy eating habits, and encouragement of safe spaces for physical activity. These multi-component strategies are essential to reversing desperate trends since they also increase overall health equity for the groups at risk from obesity and undernutrition. Alignment of policy frameworks supporting public health action is essential to long-term success against obesity and overnutrition. Multiagency partnerships and collaborations among government agencies, NGOs, and community stakeholders can maximize resource utilization and enable experiential learning. Interventions like community-based nutrition programs, school health programs, and urban design to enable active living can be integrated into broader health agendas. Furthermore, public health messaging can effectively communicate the risk associated with obesity and promote positive behavioral changes among various populations. As Sanji explores potential solutions, it should be mentioned that obesity prevention needs to be addressed in terms of the multifaceted interaction between diet, physical activity, and the environment. By this holistic approach, societies can have a chance to establish robust health systems to effectively counter the epidemic of obesity (Hong et al., 2020; Tembo, 2024).

6.5.2. Educational Programs

Establishment of education programs in nutrition awareness is important to prevent the rising prevalence of obesity and overnutrition among adolescents. Schools provide a good forum for these interventions because they could reach a large proportion of youth, particularly in early stages. Through the inclusion of comprehensive nutrition education within the curriculum, students can be taught more about eating well, the importance of exercise, and the implications of poor eating. These courses must not only teach but also engage students in hands-on activities, , such as cooking classes or participative workshops, that will reinforce learning as well as retention. Research has indicated that well-conceived educational interventions can significantly influence food consumption habits and food attitudes among adolescents, hence influencing healthier lifestyle choices that decrease the risk of obesity and associated health consequences (Abeje et al., 2024). Additionally, encouraging inter-professional cooperation among teachers, health professionals, and families can augment the effectiveness of health education interventions for preventing overnutrition. Multidisciplinary teams can offer an integrated response to nutrition education, incorporating not just individual eating behavior but also deeper socio-economic determinants of food preference and availability. For instance, workshops could be offered to parents in developing skills in meal planning and food budgeting for healthy foods. The community itself also has the ability to offer a support network outside the school, in turn affecting habitual behavior within the home and the community. This overall strategy acknowledges the fact that overnutrition is a complex issue and therefore needs collective action to bring sustainable change among teens. Evidence indicates that if families are included in health education programs, better health outcomes are more probable, indicating the importance of community alliances in these programs (Potera, 2004). Finally, constant evaluation and updating of curricula of educational programs are necessary to ensure ongoing effects and relevance in preventing obesity and overnutrition. The programs need to be monitored periodically to assess their effectiveness and the students' retention of the knowledge. Through feedback from the students, parents, and teachers, developers of programs can gain areas where improvements are required and make changes to curricula in response to current health trends and community needs. Also, applying evidence from studies of dietary behavior, , such as the high degree of association between physical inactivity and overnutrition among adolescents, can be applied to program modifications according to specific risk factors that are present in different groups (Abeje et al., 2024). The objective is not just to bring about short-term behavioral change but also sustainable health outcomes, which ensures that constant improvement is an important component of such educational programs. Overall, such responsive and dynamic education programs are critical to the challenge of reversing the accelerating trend toward obesity and providing healthier options for young people (Figure 6.12).

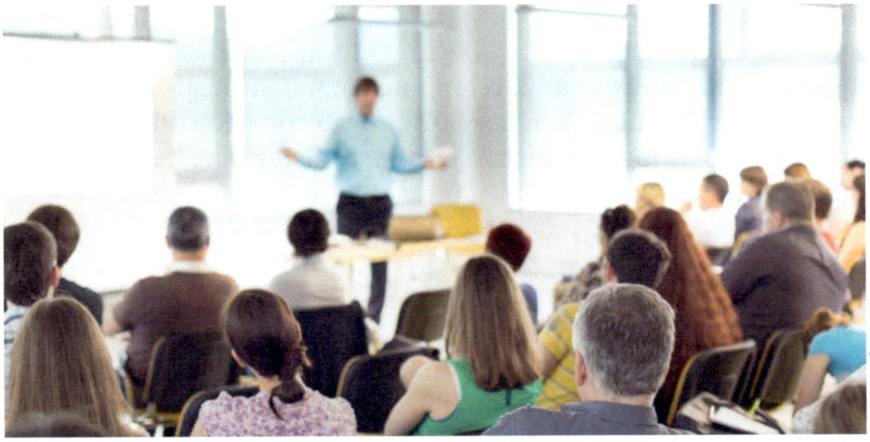

Figure 6.12. Participants attending an in-person training or educational seminar.

Source: https://external-content.duckduckgo.com/iu/?u=https%3A%2F%2Fwww.constructionbusinessowner.com%2Fsites%2Fdefault%2Ffiles%2Fmain_image%2Fmain-training.jpg&f=1&nofb=1&ipt=156bd28e40f0ef289b426f26cb9c86589bf2be183b4b682a331f005e44432002.

6.5.3. Community-Based Interventions

Community-based interventions have emerged as an essential strategy to prevent obesity and overnutrition, particularly in the era of mounting health issues. They aim at engaging local communities in addressing unhealthy diet and physical inactivity through unified efforts that consider the particular cultural and environmental context of the community. For instance, projects may add community gardens, culinary lessons, or exercise challenges, all of which support healthier lifestyles for participants. By engaging in individuals and making them feel a sense of investment in health interventions, communities are more able to sustain attitude and behavior changes related to nutrition and health. This hands-on engagement is critical not just for short-term outcomes but also for fostering long-term health improvement in the population. In addition, the success of community-based interventions could be attributed to their focus on inclusivity and personalized approaches based on specific requirements of individual communities. Research has shown that in the event that social determinants of health , such as income inequity and access to healthy foods are targeted, then interventions become more likely to reduce obesity rates. For example, adopting policies supporting increased access to fresh produce and fruits in food deserts has a significant impact on eating healthily among vulnerable populations. Building partnerships among local groups, health care providers, and policy makers optimizes this intervention reach and resources, which facilitate integrated support for members of the community. As the literature indicates, such collaborative efforts are uneven in effect but bring home the imperative of aligning strategies with meeting diverse community contexts and preferences (Haddad et al.). The shifting food landscape suggests the imperative for community health interventions that put education and awareness regarding nutrition first. Many populations are faced with problems emanating from the food pattern change characterized by increased consumption of processed foods, which in most instances is responsible for the rising incidence of obesity-related conditions. In light of this tendency, interventions must entail educational components that inform individuals about better dietary habits and the importance of physical activity. In addition, scholars have posited that the inclusion of different stakeholders, , such as local leaders and community members, in the policy-making process is essential to develop meaningful strategies that target the underlying drivers of obesity and overnutrition (Tembo, 2024). Prioritizing such collaborations can enable community-based programs to be game-changers in transforming food choices and ultimately enhancing population health outcomes.

6.6. Treatment Options

While managing the complex issue of overnutrition and obesity, consideration of the variety of treatments suitable for the individual patient needs and choice is essential. Regardless of the management strategy, its efficacy is not merely based on clinical success but also on the attitude of the patient toward his or her health. Evidence suggests that drivers of patient preferences play a significant role in healthcare professionals (HCPs) designing individualized management plans. Emotional well-being, support systems, and readily available resources are significant determinants of which treatment options patients will find acceptable and viable.

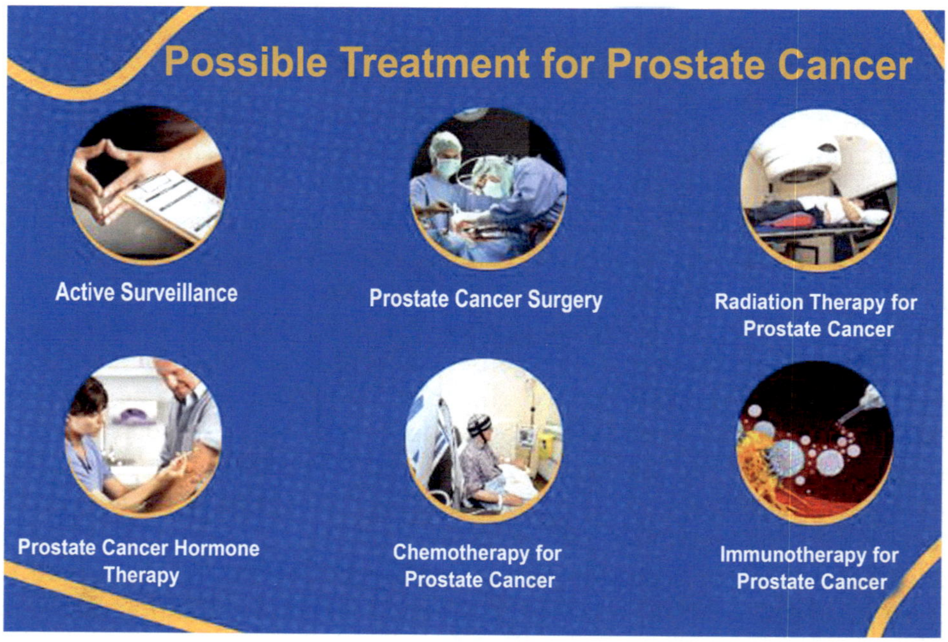

Figure 6.13. Treatment options for prostate cancer.

Source: https://external-content.duckduckgo.com/iu/?u=https%3A%2F%2Factchealth.com%2Fimages%2Fprostate-possible.png&f=1&nofb=1&ipt=436334f8a76f3c827b77ce52b36ac360497bffa276f2dbf27c26f2ca9beb970d.

The recognition of this information affirms the value of HCPs in building open communication with patients to provide a more personalized obesity treatment that can lead to improved adherence and obesity-related disorder outcomes (Craig et al., 2025). Pharmacotherapy and surgery provide two noteworthy paths to the management of obesity. Existing evidence points to concern regarding the long-term safety of medications for WL and surgery being at the top of the agenda of PLwO, as well as their healthcare providers. Specifically, the ACTION-China study points to a significant concern over the safety of these interventions, since a considerable percentage of PLwO have doubts about the effectiveness of medication compared to other interventions. Moreover, the majority of PLwO indicate that weight regain after surgery is a major risk, reflecting the subtle complication of patient attitudes toward these interventions. These conclusions necessitate careful consideration of the benefits and drawbacks of drug and surgical treatments to guarantee that treatment is not merely science-based but also aligned with patient worry and expectations regarding long-term outcomes (Luo et al., 2025). Incorporation of support systems into treatment planning remains crucial to facilitating effective weight management.

Research shows that patient decision-making for obesity treatment is significantly influenced by family, friends, and HCP emotional support. The importance of the necessity to address psychological concerns as well as interventions in physical terms by health practitioners to enhance the effectiveness of treatment is vital. By receiving extensive training on how obesity is a chronic condition needing ongoing management, HCPs can set patients' fears regarding treatment aside and bring about an understanding of the complexity involved. Encouraging a culture of patient engagement and empowerment of their care decisions leads to higher compliance and sustainable lifestyle changes, driving successful outcomes in the battle against obesity and overnutrition (Craig et al., 2025) (Figure 6.13).

6.6.1. Lifestyle Modifications

Lifestyle modifications are also an important part of fighting over nutrition and obesity because they assist an individual in making correct choices about their health. Daily exercise and a healthy diet are the basis for effective control of weight. Having a minimum of 150 minutes of moderate-intensity aerobic activity every week, together with muscle-strengthening exercises, aids in maintaining a healthy weight and keeping it there. In addition, incorporating healthy foods rich in fiber, vitamins, and minerals and reducing intake of processed food and added sugars can facilitate significant health improvements. Successful lifestyle interventions target not only weight loss but well-being overall, thereby reducing the prevalence of obesity-related diseases and fostering a long-term commitment to health. Lifestyle influences extend beyond individual behavior to wider household and community settings. Evidence highlights how maternal pregnancy health, in particular maternal overweight, can have long-term impacts on child health, , such as adiposity and metabolic disorders (Gaillard, 2015). Therefore, a large variety of interventions that address pregnant women in terms of nutrition and physical well-being can have significant intergenerational impact. Along with this, creating environments to support healthy eating habits and a physically active life is crucial. Societies can implement policies that offer access to quality food, safe spaces for physical exercise, and programs to educate families about the requirement of balanced living. Targeting the socio-environmental determinants of health is an important element in bringing the era of obesity to a close. Lastly, the integration of lifestyle change into public health policy is imperative to the elimination of obesity and overnutrition. Understanding the physiological and psychological foundations of food choices makes it possible to develop personalized interventions that account for patient preferences and challenges. Investigations into epigenetic factors have more recently highlighted the mechanisms by which nutritional programming and maternal regulation may affect susceptibility to obesity

(Campión-Zabalza et al., 2012). By the identification of potential epigenetic biomarkers and the setting up of patient-specific dietary recommendations based upon these, healthcare providers are better able to manage obesity's complex mechanisms. Thereafter, an integrated approach involving education, community reinforcement, and individualized interventions will be likely to be more effective in creating positive life change among diverse populations and eradicating the endemic prevalence of obesity and its attendant health implications (Figure 6.14).

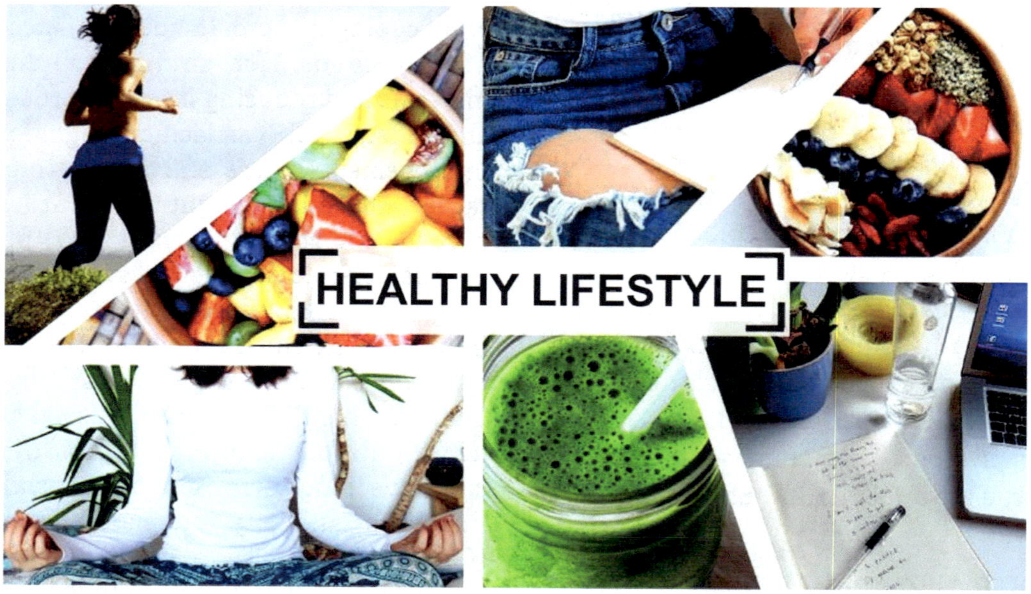

Figure 6.14. Core elements of a healthy lifestyle.

Source: https://external-content.duckduckgo.com/iu/?u=https%3A%2F%2Fwww.manomaya.in%2Fassets_web%2Fimages%2Fhealthy-lifstyle-modification.jpg&f=1&nofb=1&ipt=ace7b075c5e4438a7414d4d762e39258abedaa96810746238ced9e2e370436fa.

6.6.2. Medical Interventions

Medical interventions against obesity and overnutrition must be multifaceted, integrating pharmacologic therapies, behavioral modifications, and, when indicated, surgery. For individuals whose body mass index (BMI) exceeds levels that are prescribed, medical providers often prescribe weight reduction medications as a component of complete therapy. Such drugs, , such as orlistat and phentermine-topiramate, have been found to help to achieve significant weight loss with the aid of dietary adjustments and physical exercise. However, while being highly effective, extremely few people with obesity receive ongoing prescriptions for such medications, indicating poor utilization and accessibility of such interventions. This inconsistency is most often a result of neglect by medical professionals in managing weight and stigmatization of obesity, and therefore patients avoid seeking the necessary medical attention. In addition, behavioral management plays an important role in weight management strategies by placing importance on changing meal patterns and increased physical exercises. Cognitive-behavioral therapy (CBT), dietetics counseling, and structured exercise regimens play an important role in enabling individuals with methods to modify their lifestyle. The worth of such interventions is emphasized by studies indicating that long-term success in weight loss relies significantly on maintenance of behavior change. In addition to one-to-one counseling, group therapy and community-based support programs supplement the effectiveness of behavioral methods by enhancing responsibility and motivational encouragement among clients. It's important to place these interventions within the cultural environments and economic realities that people live in, in a manner that they are made available and interpretable (Zhang et al., 2025). Hence, a robust combination of medical and behavior interventions can possibly create a synergistic effect, making the total impact of obesity therapy stronger. In certain cases, bariatric surgery can be the optimal treatment for individuals with severe obesity, particularly when other treatment options have not worked. Surgery, , such as gastric bypass and sleeve gastrectomy, is aimed at decreasing stomach capacity for food consumption by a significant degree, leading to immense weight loss along with remission of obesity-associated comorbidities. Research shows that patients undergoing bariatric surgery generally experience dramatic decreases in conditions , such as type 2 diabetes, hypertension, and cardiovascular disease, highlighting the great health benefits associated with surgery (Zhang et al., 2025). Despite the potential benefits, candidates must undergo rigorous screening processes, including psychiatric testing and dietary planning, to maximize their chances of surgical success and health outcomes. Thus, incorporated in a consideration-based way in the overall framework of obesity therapies, medical treatments in the forms of surgical treatments can offer pioneering solutions to those who have been facing the problems of obesity and overnutrition (Figure 6.15).

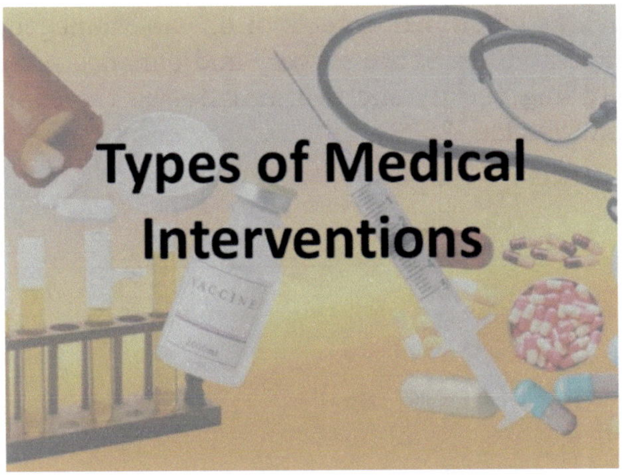

Figure 6.15. Types of medical interventions and tools.

Source: https://external-content.duckduckgo.com/iu/?u=https%3A%2F%2Fcdn.slidesharecdn.com%2Fss_thumbnails%2Ftypesofmedicalinterventions-140912105754-phpapp01-thumbnail-4.jpg%3Fcb%3D1410520086&f=1&nofb=1&ipt=d14f52b12e7dd89d945fd803027e6b5e33c093db01f4706d834afecfd8a91ab1.

6.6.3. Surgical Options

Surgical options are now a significant aspect of treating obesity and over nutrition, particularly in individuals who cannot shed significant weight by just altering their lifestyle. Bariatric surgery entails various procedures that seek to facilitate weight loss through the alteration of digestive processes. Gastric bypass, sleeve gastrectomy, and adjustable gastric banding are surgeries that can readily reduce caloric intake and improve metabolic health. The medical impact of these surgeries will be to induce extensive weight loss, which will decrease obesity-associated diseases , such as type 2 diabetes, high blood pressure, and sleep apnea. As obesity rates continue to grow, these surgeries are increasingly being accepted as medically required procedures rather than only being elective procedures, indicating a shift towards surgical treatment in healthcare systems. In addition, selection for undergoing surgical treatment is generally made on the basis of a comprehensive evaluation process. Bariatric surgery candidates typically undergo psychological testing, dietary counseling, and physical exams to ensure that they are prepared for the radical lifestyle changes that follow surgery. Long-term success from surgery also largely depends on patients eating properly and exercising regularly. Studies indicate that patients who are actively engaged with post-operative care have improved outcomes, including effective weight management and enhanced quality of life. This integrated type of care increases the success of surgery and indicates the value of an interdisciplinary approach to practice in addressing obesity and overnutrition and meeting the general public health demand to address this expanding epidemic. Along with the advantage of surgical interventions, there are certain inherent risks and pitfalls that must be tackled. Like any other surgical procedure, bariatric surgery carries the risk of infection, nutritional deficiencies, and complications related to anesthesia. Additionally, the psychological impact of rapid weight reduction may lead to the formation of new challenges, , such as changed social habits and the possibility of issues related to body image. Therefore, pre- and post-operative care systems like counseling and support groups play an important role in the success of the patient. Through the treatment of physical as well as emotional aspects of obesity management, healthcare providers are able to optimize the outcome of bariatric surgery and enhance patient well-being, setting out a holistic approach to controlling obesity and overnutrition in the contemporary world (Foering, 2018; Balalakshmi and Unnikrishnan, 2023).

CLOSER LOOK

OBESITY EPIDEMIC

The obesity epidemic is a global public health crisis characterized by a significant and rapid increase in the number of individuals who are overweight or obese. Obesity is defined as an excessive accumulation of body fat that presents health risks, typically measured using Body Mass Index (BMI). A BMI of 30 or higher is classified as obese. The rise in obesity rates over the past few decades has affected people of all ages, genders, and socioeconomic backgrounds, with especially alarming trends in children and adolescents. The causes of the obesity epidemic are multifactorial. Key contributors include poor dietary habits, such as high consumption of processed foods, sugary beverages, and fast food, which are often calorie-dense but nutrient-poor. Additionally, sedentary lifestyles, with increased screen time and decreased physical activity, play a major role. Environmental and societal changes—like urbanization, limited access to healthy foods, and aggressive marketing of unhealthy products—further promote weight gain.

Obesity is more than a cosmetic concern—it significantly increases the risk of chronic diseases such as type 2 diabetes, cardiovascular disease, hypertension, stroke, and certain cancers. It also impacts mental health, leading to conditions like depression, low self-esteem, and social stigma. The economic burden of obesity is substantial, including higher healthcare costs and loss of productivity. Combating the obesity epidemic requires a multi-level approach. Public health strategies must promote healthier food environments, encourage physical activity, implement nutrition education, and regulate food marketing. At the individual level, lifestyle modifications involving balanced diets and regular exercise are key. In some cases, medical or surgical interventions may be necessary. The obesity epidemic is a serious and growing threat to global health. Addressing it effectively demands coordinated efforts across governments, communities, healthcare systems, and individuals.

SUMMARY

The research on obesity and overnutrition reveals a complex interplay between higher caloric consumption and micronutrient insufficiency, particularly in vulnerable populations like children and adolescents. The meta-analysis of numerous studies reveals that overnutrition is not merely a condition of excess weight but is also associated with increased risk of iron deficiency. Evidence suggests that children who are obese have a much higher likelihood of developing iron deficiency than their counterparts who are overweight, and this suggests that issues of overnutrition are not exclusive to caloric excess. This association is important because it underlines the significance of achieving a higher understanding of nutritional status encompassing macronutrients and crucial micronutrients (Tan et al., 2024a). Additionally, the report points out that attention to the effects of overnutrition in public health policymaking is required. As the rate of obesity rises worldwide, the conventional view of nutrition that entails the quantity of food consumed must yield to a worldwide approach where both quantity and quality are taken into consideration. The reverse link between iron deficiency and obesity, and the absence of strong associations with zinc or vitamin A deficiency, requires further study into the dynamics of micronutrient consumption in relation to high-calorie intake. Understanding such dynamics is essential in the design of interventions that address not only obesity but overall health for affected populations (Tan et al., 2024b). Finally, the understanding that overnutrition and deficiencies of key micronutrients can be concurrent necessitates reconsideration of nutrition guidelines and education approaches. The double burden is a severe public health issue that must be solved through intersectoral interaction among healthcare, education, and food policy sectors. The fixing of the complexities of obesity and overnutrition requires a paradigm shift that brings together prevention of caloric excess with prevention of inadequate intake of micronutrients. Finally, measures toward promoting balanced diets, enriched with both macronutrients and micronutrients, are crucial toward building healthier populations and alleviating the long-term effects of overnutrition and its associated deficiencies (Tan et al., 2024a).

The rise of obesity and overnutrition has become an issue of utmost public health importance, particularly in youths and children. One of the major contributing factors to this rise is maternal obesity, which has been proven to impact on the metabolic health of the child through the medium of changing the FTO gene expression. In a study involving female Sprague Dawley rats, exposure to high-fat diet during pre-mating and lactation resulted in offspring with greater expression of hypothalamic FTO and more fat content. This suggests that early nutrition can program individuals for hyperphagia and adiposity that would subsequently result in obesity in later life (Bravard et al., 2011). These findings highlight the importance of addressing maternal health and nutrition as key factors in cutting down on obesity risk trajectories for the offspring. Childhood obesity is not merely the result of unhealthy diets and a sedentary lifestyle but is also shaped by social and environmental determinants to a decisive extent. Rural South African studies have found poor trends in the nutrition of children that are contributing to increased levels of overweight and obesity. The study highlighted the fact that shifts in socioeconomic statuses and food patterns, where increased amounts of processed foods emerged, were central to this epidemic. Some demographic trends were reported to report a higher prevalence of concurrent overweight and obesity in girls compared to boys, as well as rising metabolic disease risk factors like pre-hypertension and dysglycemia (Pedro, 2017). These findings underscore the urgent need for targeted public health interventions to address the demands of the complex condition of obesity in diverse settings, particularly for vulnerable populations. Lastly, the relationship between food habits and obesity offers important lessons for prevention approaches. Research shows that the types of food that a person consumes, , such as high sugar and saturated fat foodstuffs, have a strong association with the body mass index (BMI) and other assessments of obesity. Dietary variation among rural adolescents exhibits gender inequality, where adolescent girls tend to take more unhealthy fat, leading to excess overweight and other metabolic diseases. This calls for meticulous comprehension of nutrition knowledge and intervention schemes devoted to healthier food among risk groups , such as adolescents. Lastly, addressing the intertwined nature of obesity, lifestyle, and eating habits becomes critical in developing robust solutions to turn around the burgeoning obesity epidemic (Pedro, 2017).

References

1. Ah Hong, S., Benedict, L., Kasemsup, V., McKinley, M., et al. (2020). Case 2: The double burden of malnutrition: Challenges and opportunities in Thailand. https://core.ac.uk/download/428271144.pdf (accessed on 13th June 2025).
2. Aitsi-Selmi, A.; Benova, L.; Sholkamy, H.; Marmot, M.; (2009) Addressing the double burden of malnutrition in Egypt: do conditional cash transfers have a role? Presented at: IUSSP Scientific Panel on Health Equity and Policies in the Arab World: International Seminar on Social and Health Policies for Equity: Approaches and Strategies, London, UK.(accessed on 13th June 2025).
3. Ansong, R. S., Koryo-Dabrah, A., Setorglo, J., Steiner-Asiedu, M., et al. (2022). Food and nutrition security situation in Ghana: Nutrition implications for national development. https://core.ac.uk/download/544237341.pdf (accessed on 13th June 2025).
4. Aryeetey, R., Lartey, A., Marquis, G. S., Nti, H., Colecraft, E. K., & Brown, P. (2017). Prevalence and predictors of overweight and obesity among school-aged children in urban Ghana. *BMC Obesity, 4.* https://doi.org/10.1186/s40608-017-0174-0 (accessed on 13th June 2025).
5. Acharya TA. Recent Research Trends in Medical and Health Sciences [Internet]. 1st ed. Balalakshmi C, Unnikrishnan P, editors. Lucknow: MKSES Publisher; 2023 [cited 2023
6. Béné, C., Oosterveer, P., Lamotte, L., Brouwer, I. D., de Haan, S., Prager, S. D., Talsma, E. F., et al. (2018). When food systems meet sustainability–Current narratives and implications for actions. *World Development, 113*, 116–130. https://doi.org/10.1016/j.worlddev.2018.08.011 (accessed on 13th June 2025).
7. Binns, C., Lee, M. K., Maycock, B., Torheim, L. E., Nanishi, K., & Duong, D. T. T. (2021). Climate change, food supply, and dietary guidelines. *Annual Review of Public Health, 42*, 233–255. https://doi.org/10.1146/annurev-publhealth-012420-105044 (accessed on 13th June 2025).
8. Bourke, C. D., Berkley, J. A., & Prendergast, A. J. (2016). Immune dysfunction is a cause of malnutrition. *Trends in Immunology, 37*, 386–398. https://doi.org/10.1016/j.it.2016.04.003 (accessed on 13th June 2025).
9. Campión-Zabalza, J., Cordero, P., Martinez, J. A., Milagro-Yoldi, M., et al. (2012). Interplay of early-life nutritional programming on obesity, inflammation and epigenetic outcomes. https://core.ac.uk/download/83573772.pdf (accessed on 13th June 2025).
10. Chigbu, C. (2018). Epidemiology of adult obesity in Enugu Southeast Nigeria. https://core.ac.uk/download/161997128.pdf (accessed on 13th June 2025).
11. Craig, H., Alsaeed, D., Al Ozairi, E., Norris, S., Holian, J., Kennedy, C., Heneghan, H., et al. (2025). Factors influencing patients to choose one obesity treatment over another: A qualitative study. *International Journal of Obesity.* https://www.semanticscholar.org/paper/4ce5efb17e1ef5e3f27c4bc7a240c6ec7a626d8a (accessed on 13th June 2025).
12. Di Cesare, M., Sorić, M., Bovet, P., Miranda, J. J., Bhutta, Z. A., Stevens, G. A., Laxmaiah, A., et al. (2019). The epidemiological burden of obesity in childhood: A worldwide epidemic requiring urgent action. *BMC Medicine, 17.* https://doi.org/10.1186/s12916-019-1449-8 (accessed on 13th June 2025).

13. Erenstein, O., Jaleta, M., Sonder, K., Mottaleb, K. A., & Prasanna, B. M. (2022). Global maize production, consumption and trade: Trends and R&D implications. *Food Security, 14*, 1295–1319. https://doi.org/10.1007/s12571-022-01288-7 (accessed on 13th June 2025).

14. Foering, A. (2018). Pediatric type II diabetes mellitus: Examining the upward trend. https://core.ac.uk/download/158970346.pdf (accessed on 13th June 2025).

15. Fróna, D., Szenderák, J., & Harangi-Rákos, M. (2019). The challenge of feeding the world. *Sustainability, 11*, 5816–5816. https://doi.org/10.3390/su11205816 (accessed on 13th June 2025).

16. Gaillard, R. (2015). Maternal obesity during pregnancy and cardiovascular development and disease in the offspring. https://core.ac.uk/download/43291211.pdf (accessed on 13th June 2025).

17. García-Sancha, N., Corchado-Cobos, R., & Pérez-Losada, J. (2025). Understanding susceptibility to breast cancer: From risk factors to prevention strategies. *International Journal of Molecular Sciences, 26.* https://www.semanticscholar.org/paper/a3d3e3bcfdf6cf1612633b1b5975db58caa72384 (accessed on 13th June 2025).

18. Karava, V., Dotis, J., Kondou, A., & Printza, N. (2023). Malnutrition patterns in children with chronic kidney disease. *Life, 13*, 713–713. https://doi.org/10.3390/life13030713 (accessed on 13th June 2025).

19. Koutsouros, V. M. (2003). Predictors of large women's satisfaction with health care. https://core.ac.uk/download/234122099.pdf (accessed on 13th June 2025).

20. Woodhouse, Allison and Lamport, Ph.D., Mark A. (2012) "The Relationship of Food and Academic Performance: A Preliminary Examination of the Factors of Nutritional Neuroscience, Malnutrition, and Diet Adequacy," *Christian Perspectives in Education*, 5(1). Available at: https://digitalcommons.liberty.edu/cpe/vol5/iss1/1(accessed on 13th June 2025).

21. Longo, M., Zatterale, F., Naderi, J., Parrillo, L., Formisano, P., Raciti, G. A., Béguinot, F., et al. (2019). Adipose tissue dysfunction as determinant of obesity-associated metabolic complications. *International Journal of Molecular Sciences, 20*, 2358–2358. https://doi.org/10.3390/ijms20092358 (accessed on 13th June 2025).

22. Luyckx, V. A., Tonelli, M., & Stanifer, J. W. (2018). The global burden of kidney disease and the sustainable development goals. *Bulletin of the World Health Organization, 96*, 414–422D. https://doi.org/10.2471/blt.17.206441 (accessed on 13th June 2025).

23. Pedro, T. M. (2017). The association of nutrition on body composition and metabolic disease risk in rural South Africa children and adolescents. https://core.ac.uk/download/188769708.pdf (accessed on 13th June 2025).

24. Petticrew, M., Knai, C., Thomas, J., Rehfuess, E., Noyes, J., Gerhardus, A., Grimshaw, J., et al. (2019). Implications of a complex perspective for systematic reviews and guideline development in health decision making. *BMJ Global Health, 4*, e000899–e000899. https://doi.org/10.1136/bmjgh-2018-000899 (accessed on 13th June 2025).

25. Romieu, I., Dossus, L., Barquera, S., Blottière, H. M., Franks, P. W., Gunter, M. J., Hwalla, N., et al. (2017). Energy balance and obesity: What are the main drivers? *Cancer Causes & Control, 28*, 247–258. https://doi.org/10.1007/s10552-017-0869-z (accessed on 13th June 2025).

26. Tan, P. X., Tan, Y., Gong, Y., & Moore, J. B. (2024a). Overnutrition is a risk factor for iron deficiency in children and young people: A systematic review and meta-analysis of micronutrient deficiencies and the double burden of malnutrition. https://www.semanticscholar.org/paper/921ac2e8e674fe17fc7a04a27fafa8630b26ca8c (accessed on 13th June 2025).

27. Tan, X., Tan, P., Gong, Y., & Moore, J. B. (2024b). Overnutrition is a risk factor for iron, but not for zinc or vitamin A deficiency in children and young people: A systematic review and meta-analysis. *BMJ Global Health, 9.* https://www.semanticscholar.org/paper/f27416f3c67c3fb9bb2ed3b361516ba587167cda (accessed on 13th June 2025).

28. Tembo, P. (2024). Trends and inequalities in the nutritional status of females of reproductive age in Zambia from 2001 to 2014: A cross-sectional study. https://core.ac.uk/download/619652830.pdf (accessed on 13th June 2025).

29. Wong, V. W. S., Chan, W. K., Chitturi, S., Chawla, Y., Dan, Y. Y., Duseja, A., Fan, J. G., et al. (2017). Asia–Pacific Working Party on Non-alcoholic Fatty Liver Disease guidelines 2017—Part 1: Definition, risk factors and assessment. *Journal of Gastroenterology and Hepatology, 33*, 70–85. https://doi.org/10.1111/jgh.13857 (accessed on 13th June 2025).

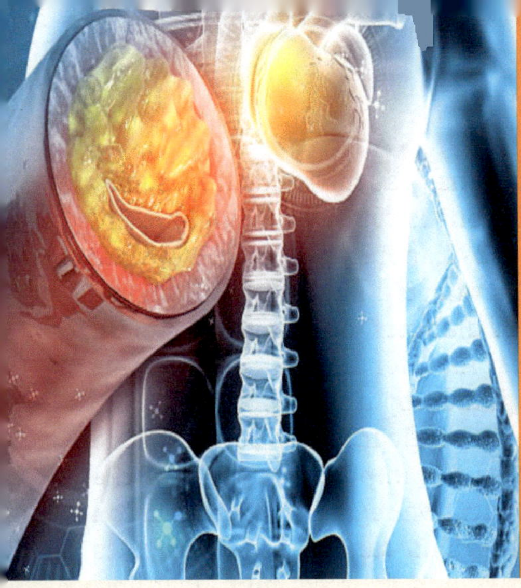

Chapter 7
DIABETES MELLITUS

Contents

Introduction....209
7.1. Types of Diabetes Mellitus....212
7.2. Causes and Risk Factors....216
7.3. Symptoms and Diagnosis....220
7.4. Complications of Diabetes....224
7.5. Management and Treatment....228
7.6. Prevention Strategies....232
Summary....238
References....240

Introduction

The prevalence of diabetes mellitus is a serious global health concern, with its various types, most notably Type 1 and Type 2 diabetes, having a wide coverage of millions of individuals across the globe. It disrupts the body's usual mechanism of glucose homeostasis, leading to hyperglycemia and a myriad of resultant complications. The increased prevalence is attributed to a myriad of causes, including sedentary lifestyles, dietary alterations, and increased rates of obesity. Furthermore, the impact of recent occurrences , such as the COVID-19 pandemic has brought to light other issues, as current studies report that the virus causes new-onset diabetes in apparently healthy individuals. These results point to the need for radical public health interventions with a focus on prevention, early diagnosis, and effective management of diabetes to enhance long-term outcomes, thus underscoring its significance in the context of chronic disease (Dubey et al., 2025). The polyvalent range of diabetes mellitus extends beyond mere hyperglycemia; it encompasses a range of dysregulations in the metabolic pathways that have the potential for causing significant complications, , such as cardiovascular disease, neuropathy, and renal damage. Recognition of these associations is required for healthcare providers who have to formulate intervention strategies. In Type 2 diabetes, for example, data indicate that lifestyle modifications and pharmacologic regimens can have a major impact on the course of patients. In addition, increased sensitivity to the causes of diabetes, both environmental and genetic, can encourage more effective preventive interventions. As interventions against this national health emergency take root in medicine, they need to be guided by a full appreciation of the pathophysiological pathways that underlie diabetes to create therapeutic interventions that are evidence-based as well as culturally appropriate (Ahsan et al., 2024). An important aspect of the management of diabetes mellitus is population-level awareness and education regarding identification of symptoms and life adjustment. Community public outreach programs can be powerful tools to empower people toward their health. In combination with dietary and exercise modifications, identification of the necessity for regular monitoring of blood glucose can lead to early intervention that can avert disastrous complications. Furthermore, the psychological dimensions cannot be ignored because the chronic nature of diabetes actually generates psychosocial stressors that affect self-management behaviors. By promoting resilience and flexibility for diabetic patients, health care systems can better equip patients to deal with the condition. Thus, an integrated approach through education, lifestyle changes, and psychological support is needed to address the complexities of diabetes mellitus and promote global quality of life (Dubey et al., 2025) (Figure 7.1).

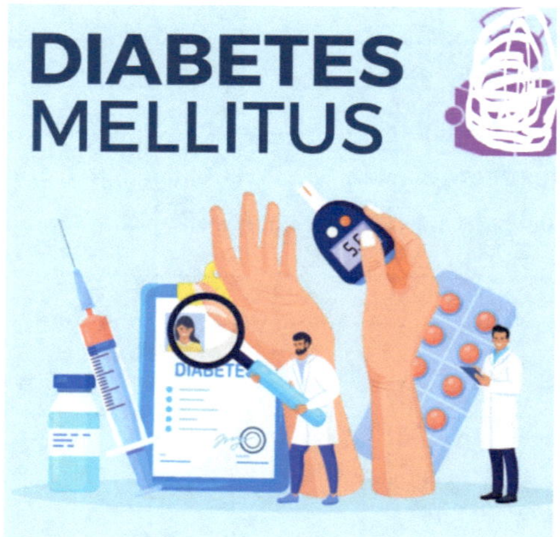

Figure 7.1. Overview of diabetes mellitus diagnosis and management.

Source: https://external-content.duckduckgo.com/iu/?u=https%3A%2F%2Fnursesrevisionuganda.com%2Fwp-content%2Fuploads%2F2023%2F01%2FPosterMaker_18012023_64407.jpg&f=1&nofb=1&ipt=758a414479c670ff37ce621e76fc5203a656cf28e3351913c9e175218798a3c9.

Definition of Diabetes Mellitus

Diabetes mellitus is a multifactorial metabolic disorder characterized by chronic hyperglycemia owing to a defect in insulin secretion, insulin action, or both. The World Health Organization (WHO) has highlighted the aspect that it involves millions of individuals worldwide and is going to be the seventh ranked cause of mortality in the year 2030. Diabetes pathophysiology is complex and is composed of multifactorial interactions between genetic predisposition and environmental factors, , such as lifestyle. In clinic, diabetes is essentially categorized under Type 1, Type 2, and gestational diabetes. The categorization enables clinicians to appropriately manage the strategies for treatment, addressing not only the regulation of glycemia but also prevention of associated complications. Diabetes management also includes drug treatment, dietary intervention, exercise, and regular checks, reflecting the multidisciplinary approach needed for proper care (Thenmozhi et al., 2021). Type 2 diabetes mellitus (T2DM) has become of particular interest with its widespread prevalence, particularly in the context of mounting globalization-related increases in obesity rates. But recently, the trend is also to see an increase in non-obese patients diagnosed with T2DM, particularly in various populations of Asians, as such a percentage is estimated at 60-80% or even more. This group represents unique difficulties in the treatment and diagnosis of diabetes, as the traditional definitions based on body mass index (BMI) are not always adequate to determine the health risks for these patients.

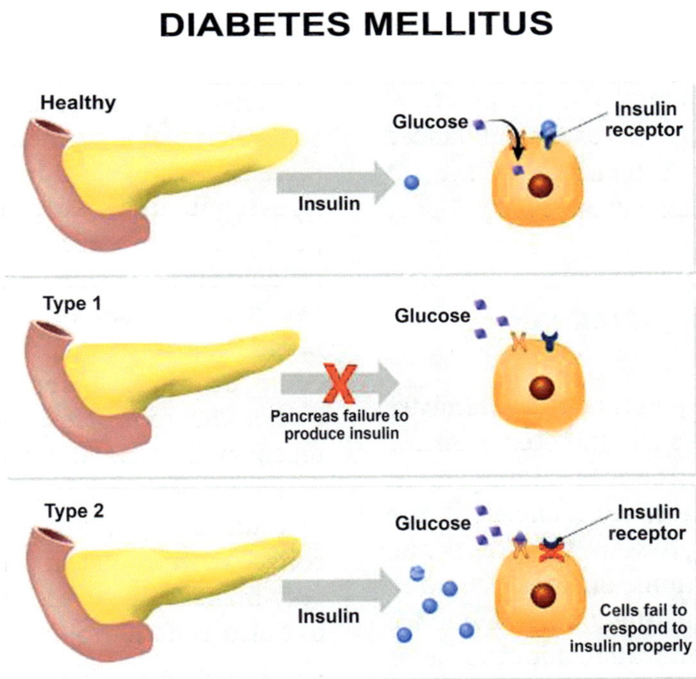

Figure 7.2. Insulin and glucose function healthy, Type 1, and Type 2 diabetes.

Source: https://external-content.duckduckgo.com/iu/?u=https%3A%2F%2Fthumbs.dreamstime.com%2Fz%2Fdiabetes-mellitus-53461273.jpg&f=1&nofb=1&ipt=bec97fdad9e0903b21c82136463fcf376709b7a11e77b39b6a81c02f596c2d94.

The traditional view associating diabetes primarily with obesity is now being challenged, as non-obese individuals can have similar metabolic dysregulations that lead to hyperglycemia. Hence, there is an urgent need for additional research to distinguish between the characteristics of T2DM in non-obese individuals, which can affect patterns of clinical management (Olaogun et al., 2020). Diabetes mellitus treatment is more than glycemic control; it also requires consideration of patient's lifestyle and risk factors for illness. The recognition of a diverse array of treatment modalities, the majority of which are traditional medicine modalities, indicates the need for an overall management of diabetes. Diabetes in the Siddha system, for instance, are treated by diet, lifestyle modification, and certain herbal preparations with established hypoglycemic activity. The traditional approach indicates that the definition of diabetes is not merely the clinical predictors but also the cultural and holistic paradigms of care that prescribe treatment modalities. Successful diabetes control therefore necessitates a thoughtful understanding of certain patient requirements, potential complications, and the sociocultural context in which they live to create an enhanced level of health result and quality of life for affected people (Thenmozhi et al., 2021) (Figure 7.2).

Importance of Understanding Diabetes

It is essential that both patients and healthcare practitioners are aware of diabetes mellitus because it greatly influences management protocols and outcomes. Awareness of the disease, including its types, its symptoms and signs, and its complications, enables people to take a proactive role in their care. Evidence indicates that effective education about diabetes can significantly enhance self-care behavior, which enhances blood glucose control and reduces the rate of complications. Better self-management of their conditions and early detection of signs of complications are facilitated by informed patients, which can ultimately lead to better health outcomes and lower healthcare costs, as evidence supports diabetes education programs (Borg et al., 2016). Implementation of such educational programs should start once a diagnosis of diabetes has been made since this initial knowledge forms a strong foundation to enable effective self-management. It has been found through research that specially developed educational programs that target specific segments and individual risk factors can significantly enhance the effectiveness of treatment plans. When patients possess overall awareness of diabetes care guidelines, as evidenced from studies that ensure knowledge assessment tools (Akrom et al., 2019), they are likely to adhere to prescribed medical treatment regimens, including medication management and lifestyle modification. Not only will this adherence translate into improved health outcomes, but it also plays a crucial role in the avoidance of diabetes mellitus long-term complications. Also, the significance of diabetes education extends beyond patient care at a person-specific level to impact public health in general. A well-educated population can lead to increased awareness and advocacy for diabetes issues, potentially influencing better healthcare policy and research allocations as well as funding for associated initiatives. As populations become educated regarding the etiology and prevention of diabetes, the disease potentially could be reduced overall. Multilateral action by healthcare professionals, policymakers, and teachers is crucial in providing a platform upon which diabetes education receives precedence in establishing increased health literacy. Such collective information can enable people to not only manage diabetes effectively in themselves but also contribute in some way to the overall struggle against this chronic disease, underlining the importance of know-how about diabetes in the world today.

7.1. Types of Diabetes Mellitus

The diabetes mellitus has been known to include a combination of a number of various forms, all of which are distinguished by varying pathophysiological mechanisms and clinical presentation. Type 1 diabetes mellitus (T1DM), also referred to as insulin-dependent diabetes mellitus, is largely an autoimmune condition characterized by the immune system of the body destroying and targeting the pancreatic beta cells that secrete insulin. T1DM commonly develops in children or adolescents and is therefore also fondly referred to as juvenile diabetes. T1DM patients must be treated with insulin lifelong in order to manage their blood glucose levels, as their bodies are unable to produce insulin. With its onset age and autoimmune causality, T1DM often co-exists with other autoimmune diseases, highlighting the complex relationship between genetics and environmental factors that contribute to the etiology of this disease. On the other hand, type 2 diabetes mellitus (T2DM) is the most prevalent form of diabetes and accounts for over 85% of all cases globally (et al., 2024). T2DM is an insulin-resistant condition in which the body's cells cannot respond appropriately to insulin, in addition to a relative reduction in insulin secretion through time. Risk factors for T2DM include obesity, physically inactive lifestyles, and genetics and therefore T2DM as a public health problem since it is associated with metabolic syndrome.

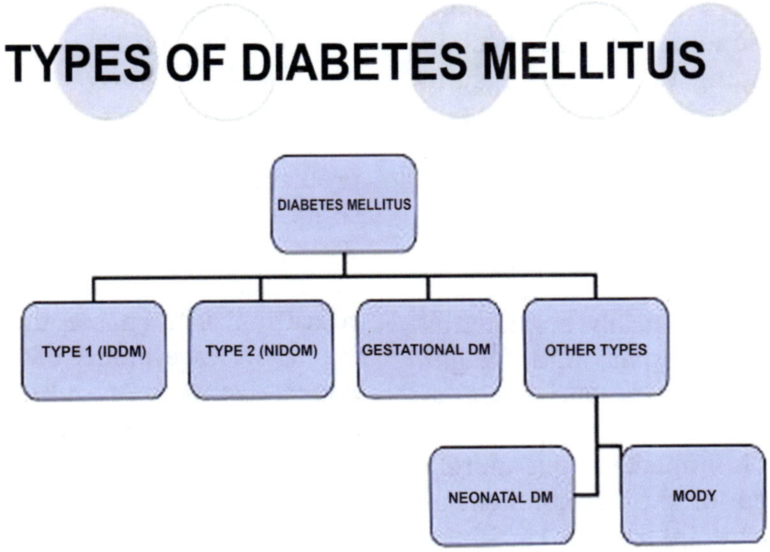

Figure 7.3. Types of diabetes mellitus and their classification.

Source: https://external-content.duckduckgo.com/iu/?u=https%3A%2F%2Fimage.slidesharecdn.com%2Fdiabetesmellitusppt-181120152616%2F95%2Fdiabetes-mellitus-introductiontypes-of-diabetes-mellitus-3-638.jpg%3Fcb%3D1542727994&f=1&nofb=1&ipt=cff048ec44a57720eb0c524e0686f6ff74f975797e30ee84394b02508980e8d7.

T2DM usually develops over time and therefore can lead to late diagnosis, with resultant complications of cardiovascular disease, neuropathy, and nephropathy if not managed. Lifestyle interventions, oral medications, and insulin treatment, in advanced cases, are all key components of the management strategy for T2DM, highlighting the significance of early intervention and prevention. Gestational diabetes mellitus (GDM) is another significant category falling under the general classification of diabetes. It manifests during pregnancy in women who have not previously been diagnosed with diabetes. GDM is primarily caused by hormonal changes that lead to insulin resistance, and it typically resolves after delivery; however, it also increases the risk for subsequent development of T2DM. GDM in pregnant women must have their blood glucose carefully monitored and regulated to minimize risks to both mother and fetus, including those related to macrosomia and preeclampsia (et al., 2024). The classification of GDM underscores the heterogeneity of diabetes mellitus and the necessity for targeted strategies to address the unique challenges of each type, showing a clearer understanding of this multifaceted disease landscape (Figure 7.3).

7.1.1. Type 1 Diabetes

Type 1 diabetes mellitus (T1DM) pathophysiology is based on autoimmune beta-cell destruction of the pancreas, leading to absolute insulin deficiency. Unlike Type 2 Diabetes, where disease directly correlates with insulin resistance and lifestyle, T1DM could possibly occur in children or adolescents. The immune attack against cells that secrete insulin could result in hyperglycemia, an imbalance which plays key roles in metabolic function. The symptoms typically manifest as frequent urination, polydipsia, and weight loss, which are alarming to the patients and caregivers. An understanding of this autoimmune nature is important not merely for diagnosis, but also for the development of targeted therapies and interventions which can manage blood glucose levels well and improve patient outcomes, particularly as patients move through childhood and into adulthood, where long-term complication risk can become enormously increased (Iughetti et al., 2016). T1DM management entails an all-inclusive approach with the use of insulin therapy, ongoing blood glucose monitoring, and education of diet practices. Insulin replacement remains the cornerstone of therapy, allowing the patient to maintain glycemic control and avoid acute complications , such as diabetic ketoacidosis. The use of advanced technologies, including continuous glucose monitoring systems and insulin pumps, has changed the way diabetes is managed, enabling the patient to receive real-time information and a better quality of life. Yet, with all these progresses, optimal glycemic control remains challenging to attain. The importance of personalized care that takes into consideration a patient's lifestyle, age, and own needs cannot be overstated, hence the importance of multidisciplinary management with families, healthcare providers, and the patients themselves (Iughetti et al., 2016). The recent studies also underscore the complex relationship between diabetes management and psychosocial factors of T1DM living. Psychosocial problems , such as anxiety, depression, and diabetes distress can exacerbate the complexity of day-to-day management and bad glycemic control. Moreover, the perpetual need for self-monitoring and a fear of acute complications exerts a tremendous workload on the patients. Treating these psychosocial problems is imperative in optimizing treatment compliance and overall health outcomes. Thus, the strategies that incorporate mental health care, along with the traditional diabetes education, can enable the patients to adopt the whole care model of T1DM. Through this integrative strategy, ultimately the patients are empowered with improved resilience and adaptive coping mechanisms while dealing with the burden of diabetes care and its long-term effects (Iughetti et al., 2016).

7.1.2. Type 2 Diabetes

The prevalence of Type 2 Diabetes Mellitus (T2DM) has reached epidemic proportions globally, just like the rise in other lifestyle chronic diseases. T2DM is characterized by insulin resistance and relative deficiency of insulin, typically due to physical inactivity, poor diet, and genetics. A key aspect of the management of T2DM is lifestyle modification, which engages the patient in dietary management, exercise, and weight control. These treatments not only improve glycemic control but also lower the risk of associated complications , such as cardiovascular disease and fatty liver disease.

Evidence suggests that even minimal weight reductions correlate with improved blood glucose and lower HbA1c, indicating the importance of an aggressive prevention and treatment approach. In the past years, new therapeutic drugs have been discovered, coupled with traditional management strategies, which have made great strides in T2DM treatment. Fecal microbiota transplantation (FMT) is one of the new therapies that draw attention due to its promising outcomes. Research has indicated that FMT can lead to a decrease in major parameters, including blood glucose concentration and body mass index, thereby improving the overall health status of patients with T2DM. As evident in the literature, FMT could also ensure cost-effectiveness of diabetes treatment, providing an option for health systems with escalating treatment costs. Even though the advantages are compelling, the application of FMT, especially in low-resource settings, remains a problem, and local healthcare capabilities and facilities should be considered while adapting (Ca KJAñar et al., 2025). Moreover, the relationship between Type 2 Diabetes and diseases , such as non-alcoholic fatty liver disease (NAFLD) demonstrates the complexity behind the management of this chronic condition. NAFLD, impacting a significant proportion of the global population, is inextricably linked with T2DM through shared risk factors , such as obesity and metabolic syndrome. Inflammation and liver injury are characteristics of NAFLD can exacerbate insulin resistance, complicating the management of diabetes. Current treatment guidelines require lifestyle interventions and targeted pharmacological treatment to address both diseases. Research is progressing towards novel drugs and their potential action in lowering T2DM and NAFLD simultaneously, paving the way towards combined treatment guidelines addressing multiple metabolic disturbances (Śliz et al., 2024) (Figure 7.4).

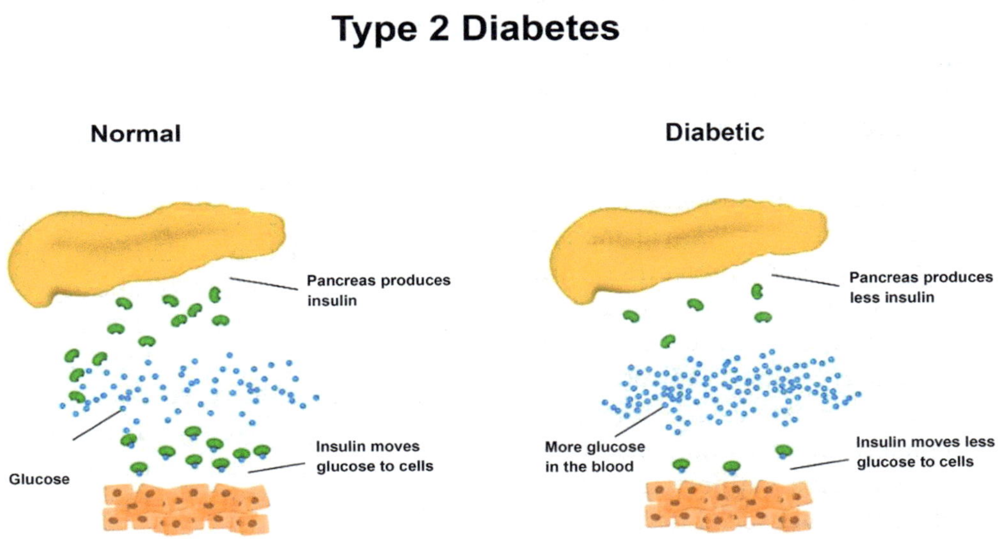

Figure 7.4. Glucose and insulin activity in normal vs. type 2 diabetes.

Source:https://images.ctfassets.net/4w8qvp17lo47/1VUR6nE10I07UIaZ1ARB0o/649f1d00c9ee90046eede057d786288e/in_type_2_diabetes__the_pancreas_produces_less_insulin_which_results_in_less_glucose_moving_from_the_blood_stream_into_the_c.jpg

7.1.3. Gestational Diabetes

Gestational diabetes mellitus (GDM) is a dangerous form of diabetes that occurs during pregnancy and is characterized by glucose intolerance that is first evident or found to exist during the gestational period. The condition not only endangers both maternal and fetal health immediately with issues , such as preeclampsia, macrosomia, and the increased risk of cesarean section, but it also lays the foundation for long-term health challenges. Women with GDM also have an increased risk of type 2 diabetes mellitus after delivery, making it critical to be properly managed and followed up. The pathogenesis of GDM remains a complex issue where various factors, ranging from genetic susceptibility to environmental elements, have an essential role in the generation of GDM. Hence, identification of GDM as a multifaceted disorder is necessary to prevent and manage it successfully and minimize its potential effect on both mother and child (Edwards et al., 2022). To control the growing prevalence of GDM, various interventions have been implemented to manage and minimize its effects. Mobile health (mHealth) technologies have been recognized as promising tools in the management of women with GDM by providing self-management materials. Devices utilized to monitor blood glucose levels, give instant feedback, and facilitate communication with health professionals are central in enhancing maternal participation in their own care. A review of mHealth interventions indicated that even though these technologies are primarily designed to augment clinical outcomes, they can incorporate extensive support features , such as peer interaction via social networking, which would also address the emotional and psychological problems of women with GDM (Edwards et al., 2022). Nevertheless, the field still requires comprehensive reviews to optimize these devices for better long-term health outcomes. The long-term consequences of GDM extend well past the initial post-pregnancy state, affecting both maternal and fetal health profoundly. Individuals with a history of GDM in the past continue to experience heightened cardiovascular disease and metabolic syndrome risk factors years following delivery. This persistent vulnerability underscores the importance of initiating preventive interventions following pregnancy, in addition to constant monitoring for the development of type 2 diabetes. Successful GDM care also needs an integrated approach, including educational interventions for lifestyle modification and control of weight as a means of decreasing recurrence risk. As knowledge on GDM continues to grow, the health care community must enact policies that effectively transition women from pregnancy to preventive services, improving long-term health outcomes for this group afflicted by complex physiological changes and health behaviors (Edwards et al., 2022).

7.2. Causes and Risk Factors

Diabetes mellitus onset, particularly type II, is due to a combination of genetic factors and style issues that synergistically contribute to raising the risk of an individual. One of the most common risk factors is obesity, were excess adipose tissue results in insulin resistance, the hallmark of type II diabetes. As incidence rises in children's obesity, so does the incidence of diabetes in younger groups. Even individuals with a regular body mass index (BMI) can be at risk, pointing to the impact of family history and genetics on the development and occurrence of diabetes. Early identification and intervention can be crucial, in this instance, in children who present such risk factors, as prevention measures can significantly reduce potential complications in health further down the line in life, which is why early proactive healthcare interventions are important in the control of diabetes mellitus (Puzianti et al.,

2020). In addition to heredity and obesity, environmental factors are also a significant cause of diabetes mellitus. Lack of exercise with minimal physical activity exacerbates the issue of insulin sensitivity, resulting in a higher vulnerability to type II diabetes. Poor food consumption in the form of excess consumption of processed carbohydrates and sugar speeds up the pace, allowing room for metabolic imbalance. An extensive strategy of preventing diabetes should include education regarding proper eating habits and keeping oneself physically active. Families must take supportive roles in influencing children and youths toward healthier lifestyles, hence ensuring long-term well-being and a decreased risk of diabetes mellitus (Edwards et al., 2022).

Psychosocial influences should also be regarded in managing diabetes risk. Mental illness, depression, and anxiety have previously been identified to influence diabetes self-management, such that it is hard to attain glycemic control. Family or community social support has a major influence on one's compliance and motivation to diabetes control regimes. Disease knowledge and disease management are key to empowering individuals since health patient education leads to healthy lifestyle adoption. Therefore, controlling these psychosocial determinants is not only significant in diabetes mellitus prevention but also enhancing the quality of life in people who are already afflicted by the disease, and this is a sign of multi-dimensional intervention in the management of diabetes (Edwards et al., 2022) (Figure 7.5).

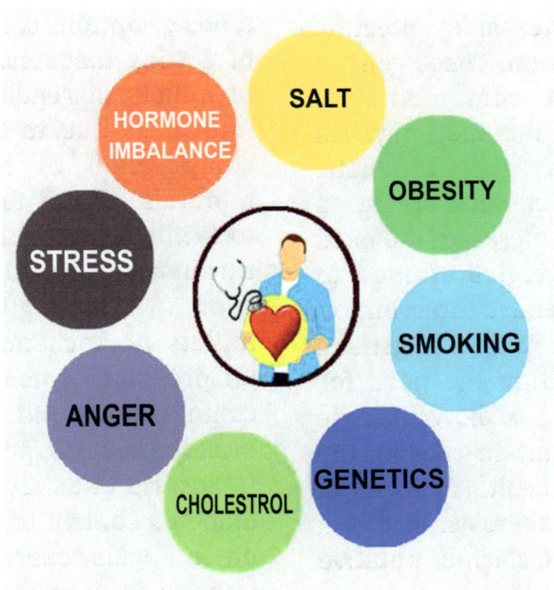

Figure 7.5. Common causes of hypertension.

Source: https://external-content.duckduckgo.com/iu/?u=https%3A%2F%2Fmantracare.org%2Fwp-content%2Fuploads%2F2021%2F08%2Fhypertension-causes.png&f=1&nofb=1&ipt=482be4c447be35d983c89192eadf79d2776c6d6e12fe443f0f2bb3eedca03d71.

7.2.1. Genetic Predisposition

Genetic predisposition is one key concept to understand regarding the causation and etiology of Diabetes Mellitus, particularly its type 1. Genetic predisposition is a critical risk factor for the etiology of type 1 diabetes (T1D), such that individuals with a family history of the disease are likely to get the disease. Despite this inherited relationship, it is noteworthy to note that genetic susceptibility does not necessarily translate into disease expression, as the observation that only half of those with familial history ends up developing T1D illustrations. This observation points towards the role of environmental in addition to genetic contribution to developing the autoimmune process underlying T1D. The subtleties of this interaction need to be investigated in more detail to understand better the involved mechanisms and to inform prevention and early intervention programs. In type 2 diabetes (T2D), genetic susceptibility also determines likelihood of disease, with differing mechanisms possibly than those in T1D. Several genes have been identified in T2D that have been implicated in a range of studies, many affecting insulin sensitivity and secretion. These genetic factors, however, are often combined with lifestyle characteristics , such as diet, physical activity, and obesity. The convergence of genetic susceptibility and lifestyle choices creates a complicated risk context that increases the need for tailored prevention strategies attuned to an individual's genotype. Effective intervention has the ability to reduce risk related to genetic susceptibility, thus emphasizing the need for an integrative understanding of how lifestyle and genetics act synergistically in causing the diabetes that threaten public health. Realization of the genetic etiology of diabetes transcends discovering risk factors; it also clarifies putative pathways involved in disease development and complications. For instance, genetic variations that are associated with cardiovascular diseases are most relevant because diabetic patients have a higher risk for these diseases owing to their disease condition. Facts indicate that genetic variation in ion channels, i.e., ATP-dependent potassium channels, may be involved in the response of the coronary system to diabetic status and hence lead to ischemic heart disease. Hence, intervention against genetic predisposition not only aids in recognizing persons at heightened risk but also aids in the creation of specific therapeutic approaches. Additional research is required, with an aim to elucidate the interactions of genetic predisposition, environmental factors, and pathophysiological mechanisms of complications , such as cardiovascular disease in diabetic patients, ultimately resulting in better management and treatment regimens (Marchis et al., 2018; Korneva et al., 2022).

7.2.2. Lifestyle Factors

The influence of lifestyle factors on diabetes mellitus onset and management is enormous, with lifestyle affecting significantly the glycemic control and well-being. Diet is arguably the most crucial factor, with studies showing that some foods or options can increase or reduce the risk of getting diabetes. Particularly, the inclusion of millets in regular diets has been brought into focus due to their extremely nutritional composition of high fiber and essential minerals. These features have the potential to facilitate better blood glucose management through enhanced feelings of fullness and evoking lesser glycemic effects. Moreover, millets phytochemical profile is accountable for potential protective action against diabetes complications and thus is a potential dietary intervention for prevention and management (Mansoria et al., 2023). Lifestyle modulator of diabetes control of physical importance is the other. Regular exercise has a twofold beneficial impact: it contributes to enhancing insulin sensitivity and aids in the regulation of body weight, both of which are critical in controlling blood glucose levels. Studies have revealed that diabetic patients with an active lifestyle not only have healthier outcomes but also possess superior metabolic markers compared to their sedentary counterparts. The lifestyle habit difference is particularly important between various population groups; for instance, a study among Polish patients highlighted that diabetic patients were less successful in attaining normal weight and normal physical activity than their non-diabetic counterparts (Czarnecka et al., 2021). This highlights the importance of highly targeted interventions in promoting physical activity as the core of diabetes management. Moreover, the synergy between diabetic conditions, such as smoking and diabetes, cannot be understated. It has been noted that smoking tends to exacerbate complications of diabetes, including cardiovascular diseases. Despite the much-publicized risks, prevalence among diabetic patients is just as high as among non-diabetic patients, which suggests the need for specialty smoking cessation programs. The programs will need to consider the unique incentives and challenges the diabetic patients might face. The inclusion of such comprehensive lifestyle modifications like the avoidance of smoking, dietary improvement, and physical exercise is necessary for enhancing health outcomes in diabetic patients. Comprehensive measures toward these lifestyle components can minimize complications and promote long-term health in diabetic patients (Figure 7.6).

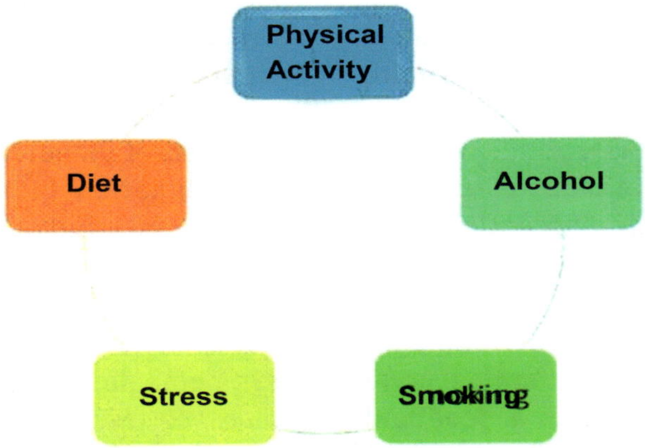

Figure 7.6. Major lifestyle factors influencing health.

Source: https://external-content.duckduckgo.com/iu/?u=https%3A%2F%2Fimage1.slideserve.com%2F1561021%2Flifestyle-factors-l.jpg&f=1&nofb=1&ipt=923cf1ea1263e52e1c756f451fecf21515f92541efd6309103089ffde4b0e62d.

7.2.3. Environmental Influences

In the study of environmental determinants for diabetes mellitus, it is evident that numerous factors, , such as lifestyle and biological factors, contribute significantly to the onset and development of the disease. Among the subjects of much interest is the role played by obesity, particularly body mass index (BMI). Research has shown that patients with a BMI of 30.0–34.9 kg/m^2 are at higher risk of developing associated conditions, , such as Fuchs endothelial corneal dystrophy, than those with less than 30.0 BMI score. This observation points to the importance of weight management for diabetes and its complications prevention, with the necessity that environmental determinants , such as diet and physical activity, have direct influences on body weight and glucose metabolism. Further, diabetes mellitus has been linked with increasing severity of age-adjusted conditions, complicating the management of diabetes and highlighting the extreme necessity for public health intervention in obesity reduction strategies (Zwingelberg, 2024). Exposure to various chemical substances, particularly perfluoroalkyl substances (PFAS), is another key environmental risk factor for diabetes. Recent studies indicate that prenatal exposure to PFAS, , such as perfluorooctanoic acid (PFOA), is associated with a higher risk of gestational diabetes mellitus (GDM). This is attributed to changes in glucose and thyroid function in pregnant women, indicating that while traditional risk factors like diet and lack of exercise prevail, environmental toxins play an important role in determining diabetes risk (Zang et al., 2023). The complexity of such interactions necessitates an improved understanding of how chemical exposure contributes to the augmentation of metabolic abnormalities and, therefore, underscores the essential necessity for effective control over industrial pollutants that could jeopardize public health. Moreover, the interplay between environmental determinants and genetic susceptibility further exacerbates the condition in diabetes mellitus. An individual with genetic susceptibility to diabetes may also develop enhanced risks if exposed to adverse environmental stimuli, , such as high levels of stress or city environmental conditions promoting a sedentary lifestyle. These interactions can create a feedback mechanism that accelerates the onset of diabetes and its related complications. For instance, individuals with underlying metabolic derangements exacerbated by environmental insults can increasingly struggle with keeping their health in optimal condition. Thus, public health policy will have to account for these complex environmental determinants and integrate them into comprehensive diabetes prevention and management approaches to offset the increasing prevalence of this chronic disease.

7.3. Symptoms and Diagnosis

Recognition of Diabetes Mellitus symptoms plays a vital role in facilitating early diagnosis and treatment. Classical symptoms are increased thirst, polyuria, and unwanted weight loss, which are manifestations of hyperglycemia. The patient can also present with weakness, visual symptoms, and delayed healing of cuts, which all contribute to lowering the quality of life. Public education regarding the symptoms is still low, and this can lead to late attendance at health facilities. As highlighted by studies, there is a need for general awareness regarding such symptoms to avert serious complications arising from undiagnosed diabetes, , such as cardiovascular disease and neuropathy, which are prevalent in type 1 and type 2 diabetes patients (Nawangnugraeni et al., 2021). Increased awareness campaigns can significantly improve patient outcomes by calling for higher awareness among individuals towards their health. In the diagnosis of Diabetes Mellitus, physicians utilize a combination of laboratory tests, physical assessment, and patient history. Diabetes is most often diagnosed using laboratory tests that give value for the level of glucose in blood, including the fasting plasma glucose test, hemoglobin A1c test, and the oral glucose tolerance test. Diagnosis criteria in this sense are required when there is a requirement to distinguish between type 1 and type 2 diabetes because they have different pathophysiological mechanisms. Type 2 diabetes, caused by insulin resistance, often needs additional tests for underlying conditions , such as hypertension and dyslipidemia, considering its widespread impact on metabolic status (Siegle et al., 2012). Accurate diagnosis is not only vital for the initial management protocol but also for long-term management protocols to prevent complications of established diabetes. Technology integration in the diagnosis process is revolutionizing the care of Diabetes Mellitus. New programs, , such as expert systems, are also being developed to assist healthcare professionals and patients in diagnosis from symptoms presented with diabetes. These programs employ methodologies like forward chaining to examine symptoms and produce an estimate of diabetes incidence, widening access to diagnostic technology that is critical (Nawangnugraeni et al., 2021). The use of mobile apps for diabetes management also reflects a general shift toward individualized care. These technologies allow patients to actively track their symptoms and receive immediate feedback, eventually leading to better disease control and healthier status. Technology implementation allows the healthcare system to improve the diagnostic speed and accuracy of Diabetes Mellitus, thus leading to timely intervention and better preventive measures (Figure 7.7).

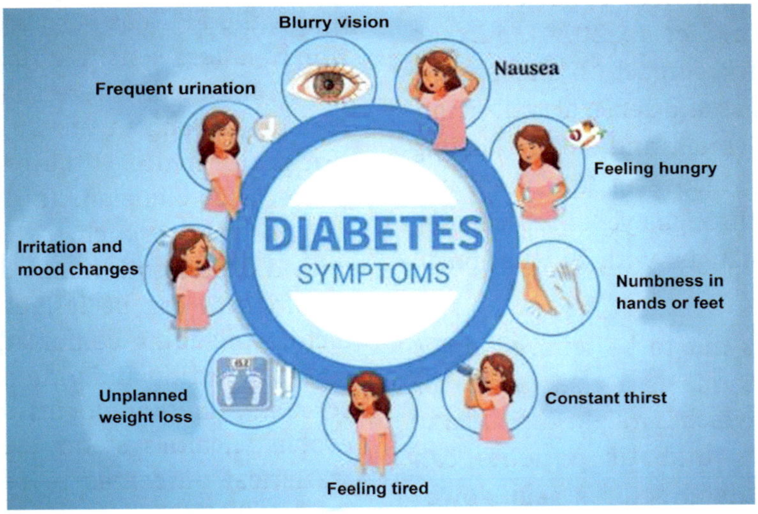

Figure 7.7. Key symptoms are associated with diabetes.

Source: https://external-content.duckduckgo.com/iu/?u=https%3A%2F%2Fblog.thyrocare.com%2Fwp-content%2Fuploads%2F2021%2F10%2FSigns-and-Symptoms-of-Diabetes.jpg&f=1&nofb=1&ipt=f4f4c01b19179b0aaa9094b86aff9c0efe312227c6d06ac29b04621b3cffd40f.

7.3.1. Common Symptoms of Diabetes

The overall symptoms of diabetes mellitus develop slowly and therefore remain undetected or overlooked initially. Excessive thirst (polydipsia) and urination (polyuria) are among the most common symptoms. As blood glucose rises, the kidneys need to work harder to remove and reabsorb surplus glucose, producing more urine.

This process can cause dehydration, which further produces a massive craving for thirst. People might discover themselves consuming a lot more water than normally would be needed, just to develop an immediate thirst once again soon after. Early identification of these symptoms is important since they can point towards the body's struggle to cope with unbalanced glucose levels, which could signify the onset of type 2 diabetes, an illness associated with insulin resistance and a failure to produce enough insulin (Xiao et al., 2024).

Another significant sign of diabetes is increased hunger, or polyphagia. Individuals feel an insatiable hunger even after eating normal meals, basically due to the inability of glucose to enter the cells where it can be utilized as energy. This insatiable appetite usually translates into overeating or eating high-calorie food, in a contra-intuitive manner influencing blood sugar levels in an unfavorable manner, creating a vicious cycle of worsening signs. Furthermore, out-of-control blood sugar can cause symptoms , such as weakness and fatigue because the body's cells are deprived of the energy that they require. The hypoglycemic symptoms significantly affect an individual's quality of life and impair both their day-to-day functioning and mental clarity, revealing the debilitating consequences of uncontrolled diabetes mellitus (Hoek et al., 2024). Further, diabetes has a physical impact on altering the individual's appearance and sense of well-being, causing visual impairment and slowly healing wounds. Storage of glucose in the blood can lead to loss of fluids through eye lenses, causing blurry vision that changes with fluctuation in blood sugar levels.

This symptom is not to be ignored, since prolonged hyperglycemia is a risk factor for diabetic retinopathy, which is a sight-threatening condition. Moreover, diabetic patients can observe that their cuts and sores heal slower due to the impaired circulation and the effect of high blood glucose on immunity. These are indicators of diabetes' impact on a wider scale, and by maintaining glucose levels normal, one prevents serious repercussions in the future (Xiao et al., 2024).

7.3.2. Diagnostic Tests and Criteria

Diabetes mellitus diagnosis employs a series of tests and criteria to definitively identify the disease. Centered among these tests are fasting plasma glucose (FPG), hemoglobin A1c (HbA1c), and the oral glucose tolerance test (OGTT). Each has its advantages; FPG is most commonly used for its simplicity and direct measurement of blood sugar after a fast, whereas HbA1c provides information about long-term glycemic control. The proposed diagnostic cut-off for FPG is ≥ 126 mg/dl, and that for HbA1c is ≥ 6.5%. These criteria allow clinicians to accurately classify patients and offer interventions that have the potential to prevent complications arising from uncontrolled glycemia. Increased awareness of testing practice is essential because early diagnosis will revolutionize the clinical course of diabetes and improve outcomes among patients. More contemporary studies, , such as a systematic review, highlight the comparative diagnostic accuracy of these tests in diabetes diagnosis. It is discovered that while FPG has very high specificity (0.98), HbA1c is less sensitive (0.51) than using both tests combined, where sensitivity is enhanced to 0.64 (Duong et al., 2023). This nuance of test performance is the province of particular concern for clinicians in determining the best diagnostic approach for patients presenting with diabetes symptoms. Secondly, both tests' sensitivities can be influenced by a variety of factors including comorbidities, ethnicity, and age, suggesting individualized application of screening methodologies to populations. With evolving health systems, the application of these statistical outcomes to routine practice will render diagnoses more accurate and enhance prevention methods against diabetes. For gestational diabetes mellitus (GDM), diagnostic tests have a greater role to play beyond the usual practice.

The evolving situation of maternal health is of critical significance, with differential screening practices across countries. A study revealed that most clinicians follow national standards for the selection of women to be screened for GDM, while others utilized risk-factor-based strategies to screen those at high risk in the first trimester (Davies et al., 2023). As GDM impacts not only maternal health but also neonatal outcomes, it becomes crucial to follow uniform diagnostic criteria. This heterogeneity underscores the need for standardized guidelines aligned with global best practices to ensure appropriate screening and care pathways for all pregnant women based on their needs, particularly in the wake of the impact of the COVID-19 pandemic on healthcare systems (Figure 7.8).

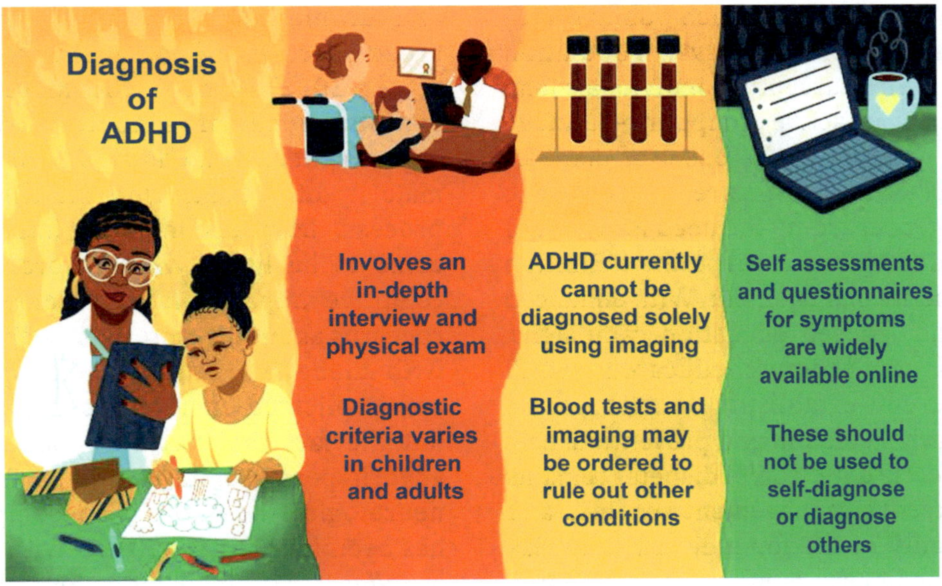

Figure 7.8. Key methods and limitations in diagnosing ADHD.

Source: https://external-content.duckduckgo.com/iu/?u=https%3A%2F%2Fwww.verywellhealth.com%2Fthmb%2FHaY6REXERNFcHTasAsi3xwiNxvg%3D%2F1500x1000%2Ffilters%3Ano_upscale()%3Amax_bytes(150000)%3Astrip_icc()%2Fadhd-diagnosis-5111350_final-2cf441f1d4334b12a73e6d52cd1ba3eb.jpg&f=1&nofb=1&ipt=791e758e2538d4dd0459a62da838fb66d247a62399be2e49da9be7ce2f348525.

7.3.3. Importance of Early Detection

Early detection of Diabetes Mellitus is core in avoiding potential complications of the illness. Regular screening for glycemia levels is crucial in avoiding, early identification, and management of early states of type 2 diabetes mellitus. Early detection of hyperglycemia forms a key part of reduced danger for long-term complications like cardiovascular illness, neuropathy, and nephropathy. In addition, greater understanding of the risk that comes with diabetes promotes awareness in communities about healthy living through appropriate nutrition and regular exercise. Through focus on risks of diabetes and effects of unhealthy lifestyles, health programs can promote informed health behavior among the public, thereby promoting frequent glucose monitoring as a preventive measure against contracting diabetes (Liashko et al., 2025). The rationale behind early detection is also supported by the ability it has to improve dramatically the outcomes of patients. A classic example is presented by the case of a 40-year-old male who developed nonspecific symptoms of tiredness and blurred vision, which were not initially recognized as presenting signs of type 2 diabetes mellitus. His case showed how atypical presentations threatened to make diagnosis more difficult, underlining the importance for practitioners of maintaining a high index of suspicion. Chief risk factors , such as obesity, physical inactivity, and family history were instrumental in making the correct identification and thus the subsequent management. With an approach of early intervention through lifestyle modification and pharmacotherapy, the patient demonstrated spectacular gains in health within a short time, highlighting the possible outcome that early detection and treatment can have on the condition's course (Ballmick, 2025). Furthermore, the impact of early detection transcends the individual patient result to reach public health interventions at a broader level. Population screening identifies susceptible individuals long before the onset of active symptoms—a move that not only postpones the onset of diabetes but also decreases healthcare costs. Public health messages regarding the need for ongoing glucose monitoring can reshape the definition of diabetes and its management. With enhanced awareness and focused education campaigns, communities can promote educated health practices, thereby establishing environments that enable early detection and prevention. Last but not least, early detection of diabetes remains the ace to effective management schemes and improved quality of life for individuals at risk for this chronic illness, reinforcing its essential relevance to modern practice (Liashko et al., 2025).

7.4. Complications of Diabetes

Diabetic complications of diabetes mellitus extend far beyond the classically recognized issues of macrovascular and microvascular disease. A major paradigm shift in the perception of diabetes has appreciated a continuum of poorly defined complications that occur as a consequence of the chronic status of hyperglycemia and associated metabolic disturbances. With better diabetes care contributing to increased life expectancy, cancer and dementia are now presenting a huge risk to diabetes patients. This comes as a chilling reminder of how crucial it is to have whole-person care systems to address not only the conventional cardiovascular risks but also such recently discovered complications. The accumulating evidence now suggests that diabetes mellitus must be dealt with from an ever more holistic perspective, considering the complex intertwined relation among diabetes, cancer risk, and neurocognitive compromise, and ultimately re-targeting care toward a broad spectrum of potential outcomes (Tomic et al., 2022). Among the more frightening complications of diabetes are cognitive impairment and functional disability in the vast majority of patients with the chronic disease process. Diabetes mellitus has increasingly come to be linked with disorders , such as cognitive impairment and dementia, raising concerns about their prevalence among patients with diabetes. Multiple metabolic pathways are implicated in this association, pointing out the fact that not only blood vessels are adverhyperglycemia, by hyperglycemia but neurological health is also compromised. It has been found that patients with diabetes are at higher risk for memory loss as well as for diseases , such as obstructive sleep apnea and depression, all of which worsen their overall health condition as well as their quality of life. Therefore, the inclusion of routine screening for cognitive impairment in diabetes care can be used as an essential part of routine diabetes care guidelines, being adapted to meet the increasing needs of this group (Ohiagu et al., 2021). Furthermore, complications of diabetes mellitus also comprise other infectious diseases affecting disproportionately this patient population. Diabetic patients are more vulnerable to infections , such as pneumonia, foot ulcers, and even lethal diseases like COVID-19. The reason behind such vulnerabilities is a combination of immune suppression and vascular complications in diabetes. For example, neuropathy and peripheral vascular disease conditions cause loss of healing potential and higher infection risks. Hence, infection treatment in diabetes cannot be overlooked. Instead, it must be included in healthcare plans in a way that lowers hospitalization and mortality rates because of infection among diabetic individuals. Enhanced screening and preventative care practices are necessary in treating diabetes in a global sense as in factoring its complex complications (Tomic et al., 2022) (Figure 7.9).

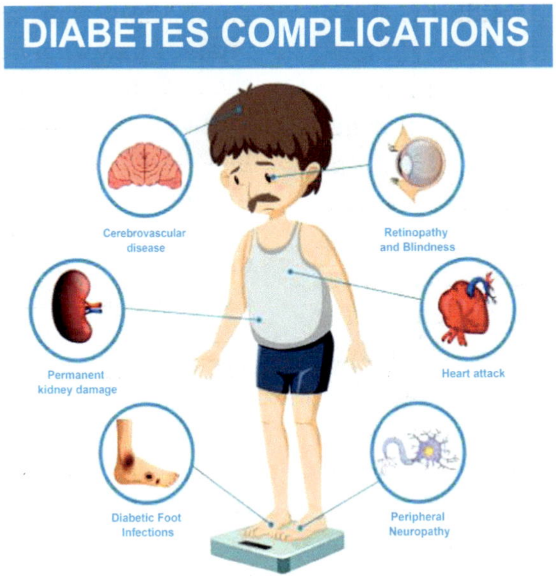

Figure 7.9. Common health complications caused by diabetes.

Source: https://external-content.duckduckgo.com/iu/?u=https%3A%2F%2Fcdn2.vectorstock.com%2Fi%2F1000x1000%2F29%2F36%2Fdiabetes-complications-information-infographic-vector-33352936.jpg&f=1&nofb=1&ipt=bee42bf3adc17dd19b163d920542dfb77e0e9ec4916b3895b4027e2e59fe31e5.

7.4.1. Short-Term Complications

Management of diabetes mellitus is crucial since disease patients are severely threatened by short-term complications, particularly during and after surgery. As per research, diabetes is not good for surgical outcomes since it possesses multiple factors that can impact it, including decreased healing of wounds and increased susceptibility to infection.

For example, a study on diabetic patients who underwent radical cystectomy indicated how robot-assisted procedures easily halve complications compared to traditional open surgery. Evidence suggested reduced chances of longer length of stay and fewer urinary complications in patients who underwent robot-assisted radical cystectomy, supporting the significance of surgical technique in minimizing risks of diabetes (Chung et al., 2025). It is thus crucial that healthcare professionals become aware of these dynamics in preparation to address diabetic patients who require surgery, providing the optimal outcomes within clinical settings.

T2DM patients are most vulnerable to short-term complications, which can be noted within the postoperative period in the context of various surgeries. In a recent study in patients administered semaglutide, a GLP-1 receptor agonist, its impact on short-term surgery-related complications after cervical spine decompression and fusion was examined. Despite the optimistic hopes for semaglutide, results showed that there was no variation in surgical site infection, wound complication, or reoperation rates within six months of surgery versus none." This highlights the complexity of managing short-term diabetic patient complications, and that glycemic control and comorbidities can be significant variables outside the realm of pharmacologic intervention alone (Tao et al., 2024). Such knowledge is valuable for both clinicians and patients, supporting informed decisions regarding surgical management. Managing short-term diabetes mellitus complications is a multi-variable process that focuses on prioritizing preoperative management and postoperative monitoring. Early detection of likely complications, like infections or delayed healing, is important in enhancing the outcome of the patient. Successful measures can involve the optimization of glycemic control before surgical intervention and the use of advanced surgery to avoid trauma and resulting complications. The results of the studies above attest to the necessity of tailoring surgical operations for diabetics according to their condition, as well as the nature of the surgery being performed. Greater awareness and intervention will not only lower the immediate danger of surgical procedures but also provide insight into how diabetes impacts the success of surgery as a whole, potentially to improve standards of care (Tao et al., 2024; Chung et al., 2025).

7.4.2. Long-Term Health Risks

The long-term health risks of diabetes mellitus extend far beyond immediate physiological damage, affecting not only the afflicted individuals themselves but also their own offspring. Pregnant women with gestational diabetes mellitus (GDM) are more likely to carry risks that will affect their children in the future. Genetically predicted GDM has been found to be linked with greater risk for most of the offspring's future illness, including neonatal complications and developmental abnormalities. As an example, increased risk of preterm delivery and placental pathologies has been observed, which could lead to significant short- and long-term adverse health outcomes in neonates (Yan et al., 2025). Such a scenario emphasizes the extensive implication of maternal health care, emphasizing that treatment for GDM is not just vital for maternal health but also for maximizing the health and well-being of future generations. The effects of maternal diabetes are later over into later neurological and cognitive health in children. Studies have shown that children born to diabetic mothers are at higher risk of exhibiting neurodevelopmental disorders (NDDs) , such as autism spectrum disorder (ASD) and attention deficit hyperactivity disorder (ADHD).

In fact, the incidence rates for these disorders are significantly higher among children exposed to maternal diabetes compared to their unexposed counterparts. For example, intellectual disability (ID) and cognitive disabilities have occurred at alarming rates among children whose mothers were diabetic in pregnancy (Bajaj and Davu, 2024). The connection highlights the imperative necessity for early intervention strategies that can reverse these long-term cognitive deficits associated with maternal diabetes. Also, the long-term health risk of diabetes mellitus includes an enhanced risk of metabolic syndromes and cardiovascular disease in offspring and mothers. Individuals with a history of diabetes are more susceptible to developing hypertension, dyslipidemia, and other metabolic abnormalities that will lead to cardiovascular disease in adulthood. This is particularly relevant to maternal diabetes, which has also been linked to future long-term risks of these diseases in offspring (Yan et al., 2025). Hence, the focus on controlling diabetes holistically has to encompass not only acute glycemic control but also preventive measures to reduce the overall risk of chronic diseases. Awareness of such long-term complications is significant in preparing effective healthcare strategies to promote the health of both the children and mothers in diabetes management (Figure 7.10).

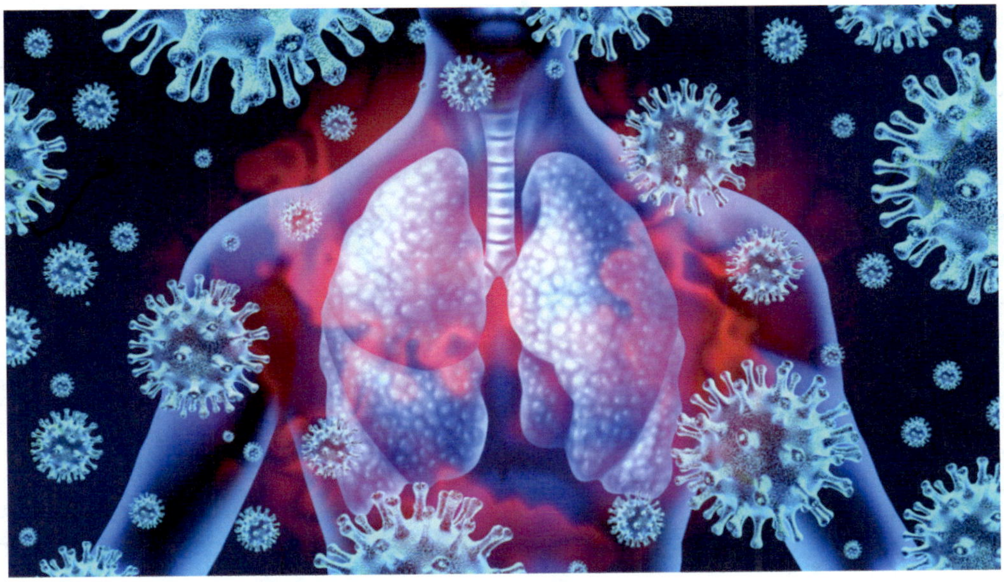

Figure 7.10. Viral infection affects the human respiratory system.

Source: https://external-content.duckduckgo.com/iu/?u=https%3A%2F%2Fpenntoday.upenn.edu%2Fsites%2Fdefault%2Ffiles%2F2020-09%2FiStock-1205199983.jpg&f=1&nofb=1&ipt=51fff57cf19171de4600ea73a5d2878100ea3f6da5fcdf1b8bc94ec5e42006a2.

7.4.3. Impact on Quality of Life

The impact of diabetes mellitus on quality of life does not go as far as the physical effects of the disease but extends to touch deep into emotional and social dimensions. The patients will also struggle with psychological issues , such as depression and anxiety because of the chronic nature of the condition. The impact of diabetes also comes out in bad sexual health, which significantly affects interpersonal relationships as well as individuals' self-esteem. One study cites that 57.7% of diabetic patients had unsatisfied sexual needs, indicating a direct relationship between sexual satisfaction and the overall quality of life. This emotional and situational stress is one way diabetes mellitus not only presents itself as a health concern but also compromises the overall wellness of its victims. An awareness of such multi-dimensional impacts is important in the development of patient-focused interventions that recognize and address the full spectrum of diabetes mellitus quality of life concerns (Malik et al., 2021). Also, the impact of support systems at the family level is an important variable that determines the quality of life in diabetic patients. Those patients who are nurtured emotionally and practically at home will be more likely to have good medication compliance and thereby improved health outcomes. Specifically, it has been demonstrated in studies that there is strong correlation between family support and quality of life and that as families become increasingly active, patients' outcomes get better with a p-value of 0.008. This association underlines the importance of educating family members about diabetes in order to provide them with information that promotes increased support. The convergence of disease control and family dynamics points out that by addressing the social issues of diabetes, patients' quality of life can be enhanced, thereby modifying their healthcare experience (et al., 2018). Moreover, diabetes patients who are aware of the condition exert a significant influence on their quality of life. Educated patients who understand the pathophysiology of diabetes and its complications are likely to make healthier lifestyle choices, which lead to better control of the disease.

This is crucial because it does not only empower the patient but also induce healthy behavior where complications of diabetes are minimized. Critical research indicates a p-value of 0.017 regarding the correlation between awareness and quality of life, indicating in favor of the argument that increased awareness leads to positive outcomes. Through focusing on patient education and patient advocacy, healthcare providers can achieve a scenario where the patient can cope with his or her condition better, thereby improving the overall quality of their life and reducing the burden of diabetes mellitus (et al., 2018).

7.5. Management and Treatment

Effective management and treatment of diabetes mellitus are essential in reducing the morbidity and mortality of this condition. The key to this is the coordination of lifestyle changes, medication, and serial glycemic monitoring. Among the most vital parts are diet changes resulting in a balanced intake of carbohydrates capable of stabilizing blood glucose levels significantly. Further, exercise is a key factor in raising insulin sensitivity and aiding weight control.

Both of these factors, combined with providing control of blood glucose, counteract cardiovascular risk factors and therefore promote overall health. The inclusion of individualized care plans adds the feature of tailoring approaches to meet specific patient needs, promoting compliance and maximizing health results for patients with diabetes mellitus. With growing incidences of diabetes, particularly in high-risk categories, the importance of early diagnosis and early intervention cannot be overstressed. Screening for type 2 diabetes should be a matter of routine in patients with risk factors , such as obesity or previous history of diabetes in first-degree relatives. Moreover, it is crucial to organize awareness-raising efforts about gestational diabetes because its occurrence is on the increase globally and it presents enormous dangers both to the mothers and the offspring. According to Galasińska et al. (2024), the management of gestational diabetes should involve a regimen of lifestyle modification as well as medicine where necessary, underscoring the significance of blood glucose monitoring during pregnancy.

By including education about risk factors and lifestyle change, health care systems can effectively decrease the long-term consequences of diabetes. As there has been a significant improvement in diabetes control due to pharmacologic interventions and clinical trials, the disease remains a dominant public health concern. The unprecedented prevalence of diabetes makes current interventions insufficient to prevent its worsening; therefore, a paradigm shift in treatment is essential. As pointed out in Rampal et al. (2010), there is a pressing need to bring to the forefront the promotion of prevention as a first-line strategy, targeting modifiable risk factors for the aim of preventing the onset of diabetes. Public policy must focus on the promotion of healthy lifestyles and access to resources facilitating permanent change to be implemented. Both policymakers and clinicians must join hands to establish systems that prioritize not only the management of diabetes but also prevention as their main agenda, hopefully reducing the disease burden on the individual as well as the population (Figure 7.11).

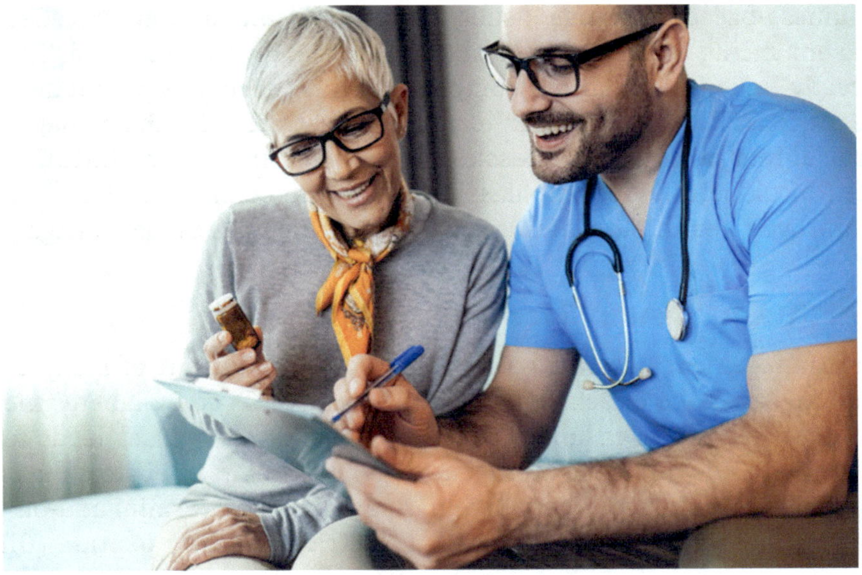

Figure 7.11. Doctor guiding patients on medication and care plan.

Source: https://external-content.duckduckgo.com/iu/?u=https%3A%2F%2Fpalliativedoctors.org%2Fuploads%2Fstarting-a-conversation%2Fdoctor-and-patient-medicine.jpg&f=1&nofb=1&ipt=77d69cd440a6bc4ebdefec7c8dc6af95472fffa28eea2b388b94a4588864d353.

7.5.1. Lifestyle Modifications

The role of lifestyle changes in Diabetes Mellitus management cannot be overemphasized, given that they are central in prevention as well as in the management of the disease. Successful dietary measures rank among the top approaches suggested for patients with diabetes. Through the emphasis on the balanced consumption of macronutrients in addition to correct portion control, the patients will be able to manage their blood glucose levels more effectively. For instance, consumption of a high whole grain, fruit, vegetables, and lean protein diet instead of extremely processed meals can significantly improve overall metabolic status. Additionally, weight management, as highlighted in the study of gestational diabetes, also helps improve glycemic control and the prevention of complications. People who embarked on lifestyle changes, including diet changes, fared better than those who declined to adopt these habits, showing the practical benefits of these interventions (Agarwal et al., 2025). Regular physical exercise is another cornerstone of effective lifestyle changes for Diabetes Mellitus control. Regular exercise not only reduces weight but also enhances insulin sensitivity. Thus, this double action is accountable for improved blood sugar control, thus minimizing the risk of long-term diabetic complications. Physical activities , such as walking, swimming, and cycling have been shown to be advantageous in diabetic individuals, with improvement in physical as well as mental health. On top of this, yoga has also established itself as an effective complementary practice in diabetes management, as it promotes relaxation and lowers stress levels. Because stress can significantly impact glycemic control by causing the secretion of hormones like cortisol, incorporating mindfulness practices like yoga emphasizes the place of holistic interventions in the management of diabetes (Sharma et al., 2025). Just as important is the place of stress management in the general treatment regimen for Diabetes Mellitus. Chronic stress can lead to hormonal imbalances that adversely affect blood sugar control, calling for effective coping strategies. Mindfulness-based therapies, , such as yoga and meditation, are effective in lowering stress levels, thus enhancing the individual's ability to attain glycemic control. The management of stress is also directly linked to enhanced compliance with other lifestyle modifications, , such as diet and exercise, since it allows for a longer-term lifestyle strategy for the management of diabetes. It is therefore crucial that healthcare professionals highlight lifestyle modification counseling as a crucial component of diabetes care. Emphasizing these interconnected lifestyle changes can lead to significantly improved health outcomes among individuals with diabetes (Agarwal et al., 2025).

7.5.2. Medication and Insulin Treatment

Diabetes Mellitus management has come a long way with the advent of many drugs and insulin therapy that form the backbone of achieving glycemic control. Type 2 diabetes mellitus (T2DM) is especially noted for its feature of insulin resistance, which in most cases leads to hyperglycemia. Metformin has emerged as the first-line therapeutic agent due to its effect to enhance the sensitivity of insulin and inhibit hepatic glucose production. Apart from metformin, add-on therapies , such as glucagon-like peptide 1 (GLP-1) and dual GLP-1/gastric inhibitory peptide (GIP) agonists play a central role by sustaining blood glucose control while further aiding in weight loss and lowering cardiovascular risks. Such drugs signify a change in treatment models, aiming not only at the metabolic and hormonal aspects of the disease but also at improving the management of T2DM as an overarching entity (Ponce et al., 2025). Insulin therapy remains paramount for patients with type 1 or well-established type 2 diabetes: its dose being modified to the individual needs of the patient. Insulins vary widely in their pharmacokinetic profiles, and thus the choice of regimen is based on the particular preparation. Blood glucose at meals is typically managed with short-acting insulins, while basal supply is provided by long-acting insulins.

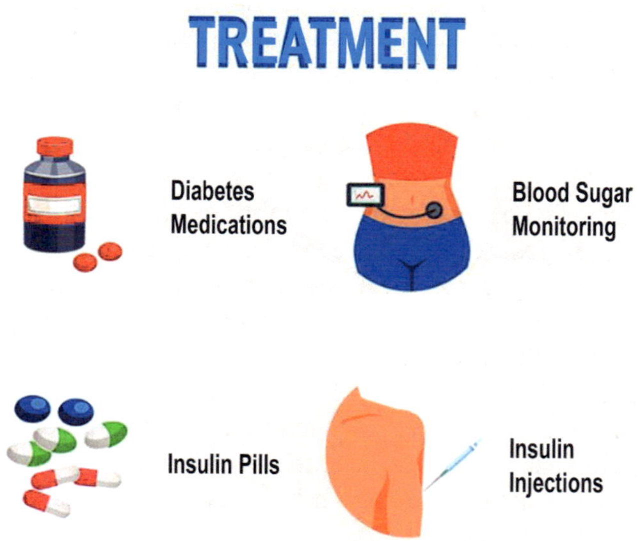

Figure 7.12. Common treatment methods for diabetes management.

Source: https://external-content.duckduckgo.com/iu/?u=https%3A%2F%2Fhoustonendocrinecenter.com%2Fwp-content%2Fuploads%2F2022%2F09%2FMicrosoftTeams-image-23.jpg&f=1&nofb=1&ipt=5b211c1c488f830f6ed19455bd5c408525baa0ebaf3459f07c4a03a53dd75069.

Advanced technologies like insulin analogs and inhaled insulin have enhanced patient compliance as well as outcome. Nevertheless, insulin therapy is typically accompanied by the risk of side effects like hypoglycemia and weight gain, which may dissuade patients from adhering to treatment. Therefore, continuous education of patients and regular monitoring are fundamental components of successful insulin treatment, with prevention of the complications and modification of the treatment protocols to ensure the optimization of quality of life in the patient (George et al., 2024). Apart from the difficulties presented by diabetes itself, even though drug and insulin treatment have succeeded well in managing diabetes, drug side effects create critical issues in treatment. For instance, oral hypoglycemic agents and insulin could lead to cutaneous side effects ranging from a mild rash to anaphylactic episodes. Since most patients with diabetes are under multiple drugs for related ailments, identifying a particular cause for an adverse effect can become extremely complicated. These are situations that need vast information on drug side effects and drug interactions among health practitioners to make quick decisions. Doctors ought to be vigilant in identifying side effects, adjusting therapeutic maneuvers as needed, and educating patients on potential reactions to enable an interactive approach in the treatment of diabetes (George et al., 2024) (Figure 7.12).

7.5.3. Monitoring Blood Sugar Levels

Maintaining adequate blood sugar control is a cornerstone of diabetes mellitus management, a lifetime illness brought on by a deficiency in insulin secretion or abnormal insulin function. Blood sugar testing relies on a series of significant biomarkers: fasting blood glucose (FBG), postprandial blood glucose (PPBG), and glycated hemoglobin (HbA1c). FBG represents the fasting blood glucose level after an overnight fast, and it serves as a significant indicator of metabolic status and liver function. On the other hand, PPBG reflects the body's efficacy in coping with glucose following food and is further connected to cardiovascular risk. Synergy between these parameters provides the most critical information about an individual's glycemic control, thus facilitating healthcare practitioners in designing individualized therapeutic strategies that prevent complications of diabetes, , such as retinopathy and nephropathy (Raghuvanshi et al., 2025). Understanding these parameters is essential for both patients and doctors to maintain optimal diabetes control. Technology application in blood glucose monitoring has changed the way diabetes is managed. Continuous glucose monitoring (CGM) devices offer real-time data, and patients can check their glucose levels throughout the day. This new approach saves time from traditional fingerstick glucose testing but provides a clearer view of glycemic patterns. By providing hypo- or hyperglycemic alert, CGMs allow patients to take immediate action regarding diet, exercise, and medication, thus improving overall glycemic control. Furthermore, data collected from CGMs can also help provide insight into personal glucose variability, which is essential when developing individualized treatment plans according to specific needs and lifestyles. This three-dimensional method of looking at blood sugar levels enhances patients' involvement in their own care, providing active involvement in effectively managing diabetes mellitus. Nutrition is also as important in monitoring and controlling the blood sugar level of diabetic mellitus patients. Dietary management can lead to significant improvement in glycemic control through health education. For instance, a study at the Gribig Community Health Center demonstrated that diabetes education in nutritional management showed a measurable impact on blood glucose. Those participants who received individualized dietary advice demonstrated statistically significant differences in their glucose levels, lending credence to the relationship between diet and blood sugar management (Widara et al., 2024). This identifies the importance of integrating nutrition education into diabetes care programs, enabling the population with knowledge and skills to promote improved eating habits. Such interdisciplinary programs are able to optimize control of diabetes, reduce complications, and maximize the overall quality of life of diabetes patients (Figure 7.13).

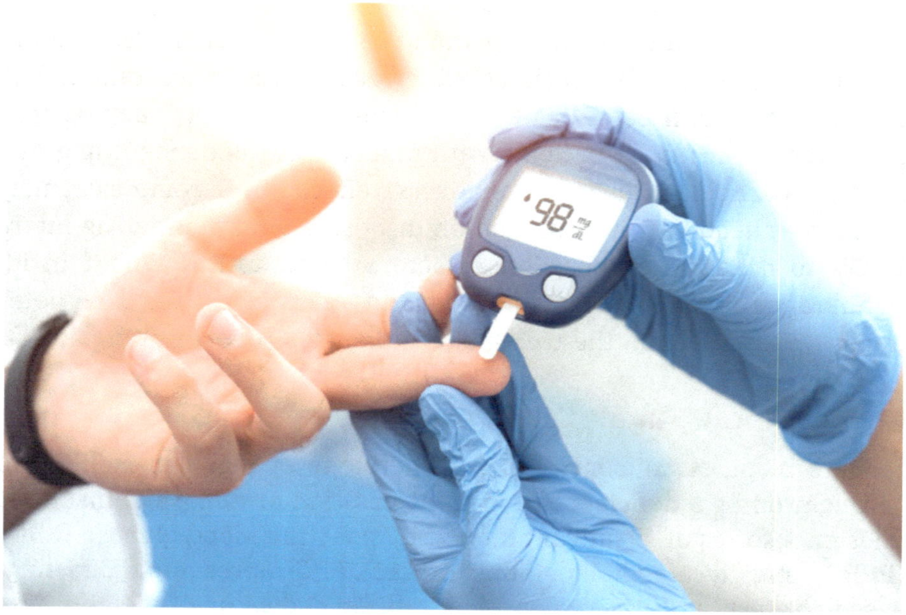

Figure 7.13. Healthcare professionals checking a patient's blood glucose level using a glucometer.

Source: https://external-content.duckduckgo.com/iu/?u=https%3A%2F%2Fbloodsugareasy.com%2Fwp-content%2Fuploads%2F2020%2F01%2FDoctor-checking-blood-sugar-level-with-glucometer-Proxima-Studio--scaled.jpeg&f=1&nofb=1&ipt=bbc332bf66e367b599c69decc611eab0a03e6f685efc823146c01156f3b7baca.

7.6. Prevention Strategies

Effective prevention strategies for diabetes mellitus are crucial in curbing the disease's prevalence and its associated complications. Primary prevention seeks to enlighten people at risk of developing diabetes concerning aspects of lifestyle contributing to the disease. They involve the promotion of good food choices, exercise, and control of body weight. Awareness of the risks associated with obesity, and a lack of physical activity can be used to make people change for the best. Furthermore, community initiatives that foster healthful food access and physical activity promotion can have a role in the battle against such risk factors. Emphasis on such measures indicates their efficacy in reducing the incidences of diabetes and its complications, , such as diabetic retinopathy, which can evolve as a result of prolonged hyperglycemic conditions (Afifah et al., 2024). Second, secondary prevention interventions are also essential in the early detection and management of diabetes mellitus. Routine screening of individuals with risk factors , such as family history of diabetes, obesity, and older age can detect prediabetic conditions and hence allow for early treatment. Early intervention is essential because it allows health professionals to implement individualized management programs, which can comprise lifestyle modification, pharmacological intervention, or a combination of both. The linkage of school and community health education programs is most likely to increase people's awareness of diabetes symptoms and risk factors and, therefore, lead to proactive management of health. It has been shown through studies that effective disease management is likely to enhance outcomes and slow the development of diabetes-related complications (Banda et al., 2020). For specific populations, like children, targeted prevention interventions are able to have lasting impacts in reducing type 2 diabetes mellitus occurrences. Nutrition education and physical exercise interventions within school settings have been accorded with priority as they have proven to be beneficial. Besides providing education on healthy eating habits, the interventions also encourage children to embrace an active lifestyle by engaging in related activities. Parental involvement and community activation are particularly critical in building these habits outside of school. Significantly, studies have validated that early intervention and habit formation determine the future for a lifetime, which can make people extremely unlikely to have diabetes in later years. Thus, these multi-dimensional approaches point towards the importance of collective action by schools, family, and local communities in fostering a health- and well-being-focused culture (Banda et al., 2020).

7.6.1. Healthy Eating Habits

Among the fundamental components of Diabetes Mellitus control is the ingestion of healthy foods, the function of which is most central to the normalization of blood glucose values and overall health. Healthy nutrition is premised on balanced eating composed of whole foods , such as fruits, vegetables, lean proteins, and whole grains in predominance, with minor inclusions of processed and sugary food. Diabetes patients are in a complex state of food choice, where nutritional value is the primary source of comprehension. It has been discovered that patients who choose to diet according to healthful eating habits not only exhibit better blood glucose control but also have favorable attitudes towards the disease. This adherence and engagement in eating changes lead to more consistent eating patterns that foster long-term health resilience and disease management (Amorim et al., 2016). Besides the individual dietary change, the social environment has a major influence on diabetic individuals' eating behavior. Social networks of family, friends, and community services assist in the success of nutritional interventions. Social involvement in healthy eating or cooking meal activities can facilitate positive behaviors and encourage adherence to dietary advice. Studies have shown that participants who are within supportive networks not only endorse healthier consumption practices but also show greater levels of self-efficacy for diabetes control. Furthermore, nutrition education and awareness significantly contribute to minimizing the stigma, which is most often associated with dietary limitation, hence making adoption and maintenance of healthier eating habits easier. In this context, combining social support and personal commitment creates a firm foundation to guarantee diabetes management (Jones, 2006).

Moreover, education for healthy eating makes a critical contribution. Nutrition programs in schools and the community have a key role in inculcating long-term dietary practices for healthy eating, particularly in high-risk groups. Research with inner-city minority adolescents has indicated extreme differences in diet, with the majority eating insufficient servings of fruits and vegetables despite reporting a desire to lose weight. By filling these gaps with systematic educational programs, we can promote a culture of health that gives high priority to healthy diets and physical activity. School nurses and community health workers are particularly well-positioned to lead these interventions, allowing at-risk populations to establish healthy eating habits that are specifically tailored to counteract the complicating agents of Diabetes Mellitus (Jones, 2006). Collectively, these educational interventions have the potential to trigger lifestyle changes with positive health outcomes (Figure 7.14).

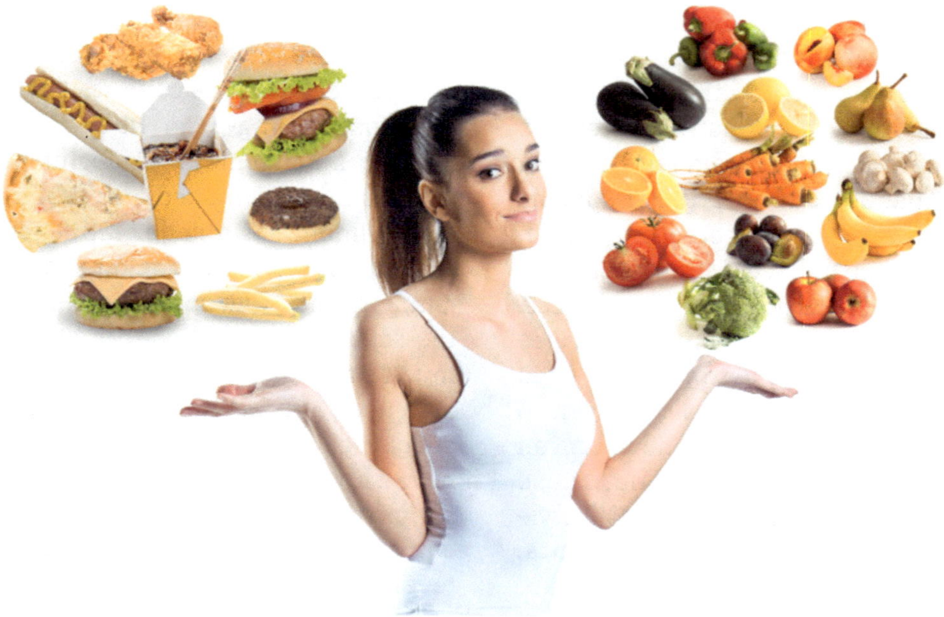

Figure 7.14. Choosing between unhealthy fast food and healthy nutrition.

Source: https://external-content.duckduckgo.com/iu/?u=https%3A%2F%2Fhealthonomic.com%2Fwp-content%2Fuploads%2FAdobeStock_79730894-1536x1019.jpeg&f=1&nofb=1&ipt=aaf95d71996d349f950e071e1175f809dfa825e57c6374f9303870856cfe943f.

7.6.2. Regular Physical Activity

Regular exercise is a cornerstone in the prevention and control of Diabetes Mellitus, particularly Type 2 diabetes. Regular exercise not only helps with body weight management, a key aspect for those dealing with insulin resistance—but also with metabolic health through the optimization of glucose metabolism. Moderately intense physical exercise activities , such as walking and cycling, have, according to research, been discovered to have profound effects on glycemic control and insulin sensitivity. This is particularly pertinent for individuals with poorly controlled diabetes, as exercise can enable dramatic reductions in fasting glucose levels and overall metabolic parameters, supporting the findings of studies on the therapeutic potential of organized exercise in the management of diabetes (Chinnawong et al., 2015). By introducing regular exercise into daily routine, therefore, individuals with diabetes are able to improve their ability to control the condition and be healthier in general. The diverse benefits of regular exercise extend far beyond the simple metabolic gain; they also contribute significantly to mental wellness. Diabetic patients are known to have psychiatric symptoms, , such as depression and anxiety, that tend to exacerbate their conditions. Regular physical activity has been shown to release endorphins, which translate to improved mood and reduced depression. Besides this, group exercise or group exercise programs provide social interaction that reverses the loneliness that often goes hand in hand with chronic disease. Among a study of exercise self-management programs, patients reported high confidence in managing food and physical activity behaviors, which in turn positively impacted their mental health and overall quality of life (Chinnawong et al., 2015). Thus, promoting an active physical life is a double benefit—both treating the physiological and psychological aspects of diabetic life. The contribution of technology cannot be overestimated in motivating regular physical activity among patients of Diabetes Mellitus. Technology , such as mobile apps, e.g., Glucose Buddy, has been developed to assist patients in monitoring physical activity habits and dietary behaviors for improved glycemic control. A quality improvement project illustrated the way a tool like this can lead to meaningful clinical outcomes, delivering patients with structured assistance to achieve their health goals. While the findings may require larger studies to be significant statistically, clinical conclusions are evident because participants' hemoglobin A1c levels were lower following the intervention. By uniting technology with regular exercise, individuals can take advantage of tailored resources that not only keep them in check but also enhance their understanding of the interplay between exercise and diabetic management, encouraging long-term commitment to active lifestyles (Figure 7.15).

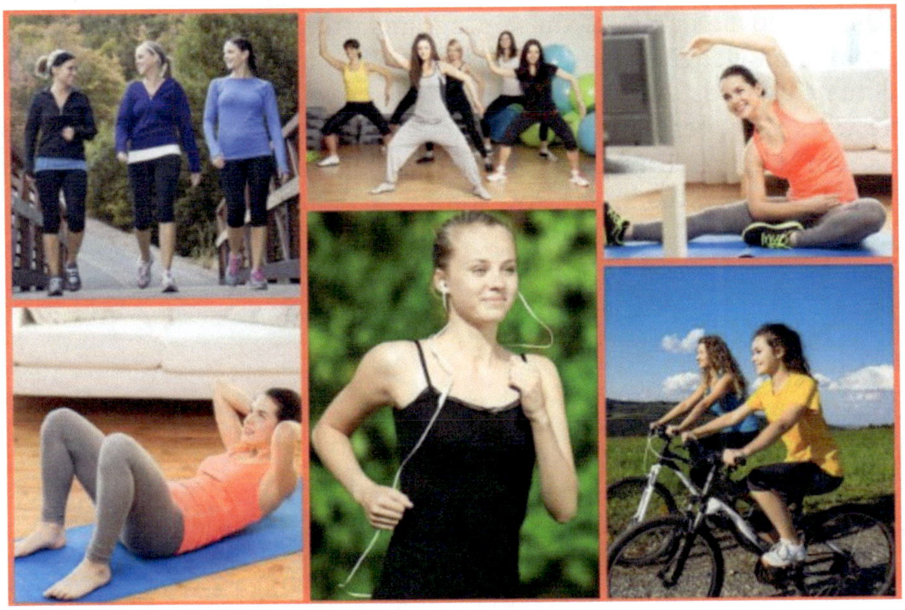

Figure 7.15. Different types of physical exercises for teens.

Source: https://external-content.duckduckgo.com/iu/?u=https%3A%2F%2Fwww.momjunction.com%2Fwp-content%2Fuploads%2F2014%2F07%2FRegular-Exercises-For-Your-Teens.jpg&f=1&nofb=1&ipt=dc737ecbadbdfd937a8499d0e2be3869e9c006f70ef1fd5f9a56e34a7eb78744.

7.6.3. Education and Awareness Programs

Implementation of education and awareness programs is an essential tool in the management of diabetes mellitus, particularly in high-risk groups , such as adolescents. Research has indicated that such programs significantly enhance self-perception and knowledge of type 2 diabetes, leading to better lifestyle choices. For instance, a research study employed an audio-visual-based educational intervention in at-risk adolescents with type 2 diabetes. The intervention group presented an improved self-knowledge compared to the control group, as evidenced by a highly significant p-value of <0.001 through Paired Sample T-test analysis. This demonstrates that systematic education programs can successfully transfer information and modify behavior patterns engaged in diabetes prevention and management, particularly in vulnerable adolescents (Puspasari et al., 2025). Additionally, focused interventions with an emphasis on nutrition education have demonstrated significant benefits in enhancing food habits among diabetics. Structured nutrition education programmers were reported by one study to impact knowledge and compliance with diet therapy, which is critical for type 2 diabetes management. The intervention included multimedia resources, including animation and video, for three months and produced statistically significant reductions in fasting blood glucose, hemoglobin A1c, body mass index, and lipid profiles among the participants. The above evidence brings out the fundamental role played by diabetes education and awareness programs in equipping patients with the knowledge and skills necessary to successfully manage diabetes, ultimately enhancing the health outcomes and reducing complications (Ameen et al., 2024). The final objective of diabetes education and awareness programs is to establish a preventive strategy towards health management. By equipping individuals with trustworthy information, these types of programs can de-stigmatize diabetes, thereby reducing stigma and misinformation associated with the condition. Moreover, access to these programs can contribute significantly to community health. By enhancing knowledge and attitude changes towards caring for diabetes, the programs encourage individuals towards adopting preventive behaviors as well as treatment adherence. As evident from the tests that were carried out, the efficacy of these interventions speaks to their capacity to transform diabetes care and ought to be part of public health planning as a way of stemming rising diabetes mellitus in society.

CLOSER LOOK

DIABETES

Diabetes is a chronic metabolic condition that is characterized by an excess level of glucose (sugar) in the blood as a result of the inability of the body to produce or use insulin—a hormone required for maintaining normal blood sugar. There are three types of diabetes: Type 1, Type 2, and gestational diabetes. Type 1 diabetes is an autoimmune disorder in which the body's immune system mistakenly attacks insulin-producing cells in the pancreas. It usually appears in children or young adults and requires a daily insulin shot. The most common form, Type 2 diabetes, occurs in adults and is commonly linked with obesity, lack of exercise, and familial risk factors. In Type 2 diabetes, the body resists insulin or produces inadequate amounts. Gestational diabetes occurs during pregnancy and is usually resolved after childbirth, although it increases the risk of developing Type 2 diabetes later in life.

Symptoms of diabetes include frequent urination, thirst, weight loss, fatigue, blurry vision, and slow healing of wounds. Diabetes, if not treated, can cause severe complications , such as heart disease, kidney disease, damage to nerves, blindness, and bad circulation, which can lead to amputation of limbs. Early diagnosis and proper management are crucial. Treatment varies according to the type of diabetes but typically involves a combination of blood glucose testing, balanced diet, exercise, and medication or insulin shots as needed. In people who have Type 2 diabetes, there are lifestyle changes that can control or even reverse the disease in some cases. Education and support are essential components of diabetes therapy. With proper control, individuals with diabetes can lead active, normal lives. Active research still explores further treatment, glucose monitoring technology, and potential cures, all of which give one hope for better outcomes in the future.

SUMMARY

Lastly, the multifactorial etiology of diabetes mellitus necessitates the right understanding of its various presentations, epidemiology, and complications. This chronic disease with dysregulation of blood glucose imposes significant health risks not only to patients with the disease but also to the general public health systems. The commonality of complications, i.e., neuropathy and cardiovascular disease, underscores the importance of early detection and effective management strategies. In light of evidence regarding associated disorders, , such as gestational diabetes and gastric adenocarcinoma, an expansive understanding of diabetes' far-reaching effect is vital to formulate focused treatment plans and education programs that can reverse damaging health effects (Alorabi et al., 2025; Seema et al., 2025). Moreover, the importance of lifestyle factors , such as diet, physical exercise, and adherence to regimens in the control of diabetes mellitus cannot be overemphasized. Effective interventions are vital, underlining the need for patient education and support structures that allow individuals to become active participants in their health care. By means of improved knowledge about the disease and its potential complications, medical professionals can encourage the patient to change lifestyle and treatment habits. Furthermore, multi-professional intervention involving healthcare professionals, patients, and families can enhance treatment compliance, with the end result being improved health outcome and quality of life for diabetes mellitus patients. Lastly, dealing with the challenges of diabetes mellitus requires a concerted effort through research, public health interventions, and active participation of the community. Ongoing research to explore the interplay of diabetes with other diseases is important in crafting future interventions. In light of the ever-changing health environment, the call for diabetes research will provide an impetus for coming up with new strategies towards prevention, early detection, and effective management of the condition. All these initiatives will not only improve the health condition of patients but also benefit the healthcare system as a whole in terms of addressing the burden of diabetes mellitus at the population level (Alorabi et al., 2025; Seema et al., 2025).

Diabetes mellitus is a cluster of metabolic conditions with the common characteristic of hyperglycemia resulting from abnormalities in insulin secretion, insulin action, or both. The condition is primarily classified into two categories: Type 1 diabetes mellitus (T1DM) and Type 2 diabetes mellitus (T2DM). In T1DM, there is an autoimmune destruction of pancreatic cells, and this results in absolute insulin deficiency. Conversely, T2DM is typically associated with insulin resistance with relative insulin deficiency, typically secondary to obesity and lifestyle. It is noteworthy to note the pathophysiology of the two so that one can develop focused treatment algorithms to control blood glucose and avoid complications. Successful management of diabetes highlights the importance of glycemic control, which is observed through HbA1c levels. Evidence has demonstrated that tight glycemic control greatly prevents long-term complications in T1DM patients (Calders et al., 2020). In addition, existing evidence also postulates that GV is a contributory factor to cardiovascular complications. Studies have proven an inverse relationship between GV and heart rate variability, highlighting that stable glucose levels play a significant role in preventing cardiovascular autonomic dysfunction. The association of GV with conditions , such as cardiovascular autonomic neuropathy (CAN) needs further study to ascertain whether GV has an independent role in disease onset. In T2DM, the introduction of sodium glucose co-transporter 2 (SGLT2) inhibitors has revolutionized the management of the condition, including its effects on the cardiovascular system. Clinical trials have proven that such medications, like canagliflozin, can significantly reduce the risk of cardiovascular and heart failure in older T2DM patients (Butler et al., 2017). Notably, studies have found that canagliflozin keeps cardiac biomarkers like NT-proBNP and hsTnI at stable levels for an extended treatment period. This result supports the hypothesis that SGLT2 inhibitors possess protective cardiovascular effects, hence being an essential component in diabetes mellitus treatment. With ongoing research, practitioners are sure to gain further insights into complicated interactions among glycemic control, cardiovascular condition, and patient outcome in diabetes treatment.

References

1. Agarwal, A., Dwivedi, S., Tyagi, P., & Dwivedi, D. (2025). Study the effect of lifestyle modifications on fetomaternal outcomes in gestational diabetes mellitus. International Journal of Reproduction, Contraception, Obstetrics and Gynecology, 14(2), 586–592. https://doi.org/10.18203/2320-1770.ijrcog20250198
2. (accessed on 13th June 2025).
3. Ahsan, E., Foo, F. F., Ravin, A., Akula, M., Hu, K., Ong, R., Holland, S., et al. (2024). 7725 Could COVID-19 be the trigger for type 1 diabetes? Journal of the Endocrine Society, 8. https://www.semanticscholar.org/paper/3e8ae71d7569a2303d3789ce8aab168d6d26d473 (accessed on 13th June 2025).
4. Amorim, M. M. A., Gazzinelli, M. F., & Ramos, N. (2016). Social representations of feeding people with type-2 diabetes mellitus. https://core.ac.uk/download/149226853.pdf (accessed on 13th June 2025).
5. Edwards, K. J., Maslin, K., Andrade, J., Jones, R. B., & Shawe, J. (2022). Mobile health as a primary mode of intervention for women at risk of or diagnosed with gestational diabetes mellitus: a scoping review. JBI evidence synthesis, 20(9), 2195–2243. https://doi.org/10.11124/JBIES-21-00294(accessed on 13th June 2025).
6. Bajaj, G., & Davu, G. (2024). The long-term impact of maternal diabetes on neonatal health and lifelong well-being. International Journal of Community Medicine and Public Health. https://www.semanticscholar.org/paper/e4e856010d5a55673bc0aa0cc0fa00582f2fb6bb (accessed on 13th June 2025).
7. Ballmick, A. K. (2025). Atypical onset of type 2 diabetes mellitus in a young male: Lessons for early detection in primary care. Journal of Diabetes Research Reviews & Reports. https://www.semanticscholar.org/paper/ef22b84be735a2b25ebea144a7c809c8935752cf (accessed on 13th June 2025).
8. Banda, M., Frantz, J., Himalowa, S., Kunda, M., et al. (2020). Strategies to prevent type 2 diabetes mellitus among school children: A systematic review. https://core.ac.uk/download/327125128.pdf (accessed on 13th June 2025).
9. Borg, D., Camilleri, F., Cuschieri, S., Pace, N., et al. (2016). A review of diabetic patients' knowledge in a high prevalent European country: Malta. https://core.ac.uk/download/46604043.pdf (accessed on 13th June 2025).
10. Butler, J., Davies, M. J., Desai, M., Januzzi, J., et al. (2017). Effects of canagliflozin on cardiovascular biomarkers in older adults with type 2 diabetes. https://core.ac.uk/download/84148409.pdf (accessed on 13th June 2025).
11. Calders, P., Celie, B., De Backer, T., Helleputte, N., et al. (2020). The relationship between glycemic variability and cardiovascular autonomic dysfunction in patients with type 1 diabetes: A systematic review. https://core.ac.uk/download/287940619.pdf (accessed on 13th June 2025).
12. Chinnawong, T., Kritpracha, C., & Pamungkas, R. A. (2015). The effect of dietary and exercise self-management support program on dietary behavior, exercise behavior and clinical outcomes in Muslim patients with poorly controlled type 2 DM in a community setting in Indonesia.

https://media.neliti.com/media/publications/154630-EN-the-effect-of-dietary-and-exercise-self.pdf (accessed on 13th June 2025).

13. Chung, C. H., Huang, I. S., & Kao, W. T. (2025). Short-term outcomes after robot-assisted versus open radical cystectomy for bladder cancer in patients with diabetes mellitus: An analysis of the United States Nationwide Inpatient Sample of 2005–2018. International Journal of Medical Sciences, 22, 409–416. https://www.semanticscholar.org/paper/6f5a55bec04e22638cc1fbaae86d79e8c1954182 (accessed on 13th June 2025).

14. Davies, A., Howell, A., Geraghty, S., O'Reilly, C., & Burden, C. (2023). An international cross-sectional survey to compare gestational diabetes mellitus diagnosis and management in antenatal care across the UK, Ireland, and Australia during the COVID-19 pandemic. Proceedings of the Nutrition Society, 82. https://www.semanticscholar.org/paper/61aabf990958f913c1f4677115489c38c3adeedb (accessed on 13th June 2025).

15. De Marchis, M., D'Amato, A., Fedele, F., & Mancone, M., et al. (2018). Diabetes mellitus and ischemic heart disease: The role of ion channels. https://core.ac.uk/download/159269109.pdf (accessed on 13th June 2025).

16. Duong, K., Tan, C. J., Rattanasiri, S., Thakkinstian, A., Anothaisintawee, T., & Chaiyakunapruk, N. (2023). Comparison of diagnostic accuracy for diabetes diagnosis: A systematic review and network meta-analysis. Frontiers in Medicine, 10. https://www.semanticscholar.org/paper/49955f2dcf1bf71c357aa7e37b10d86939922f8d (accessed on 13th June 2025).

17. Galasińska, I., Hajduk-Maślak, K., Michalik, B., Skóra, M., et al. (2024). Gestational diabetes–Management strategies including pharmacological treatment and lifestyle interventions. https://core.ac.uk/download/613192903.pdf (accessed on 13th June 2025).

18. Hoek, E., Dal Canto, E., Wenker, N., Bindraban, N., Handoko, M. L., Elders, P., & Beulens, J. (2024). Epidemiology of heart failure in diabetes: A disease in disguise. Diabetology, 67, 574–601. https://www.semanticscholar.org/paper/d7383f59ce5af0e28c9e2c834190b98981f586e9 (accessed on 13th June 2025).

19. Iughetti, L., & Lucaccioni, L. (2016). Issues in diagnosis and treatment of type 1 diabetes mellitus in childhood. https://core.ac.uk/download/54012618.pdf (accessed on 13th June 2025).

20. Jones, L. D. (2006). Minority adolescents are at risk for obesity: Health behaviors and perceptions. https://core.ac.uk/download/223074309.pdf (accessed on 13th June 2025).

21. Korneva, K. G., Nazarova, K. Y., Strongin, L. G., & Zagainov, V. E. (2022). Potential risk factors for diabetes mellitus type 1. https://core.ac.uk/download/547682306.pdf (accessed on 13th June 2025).

22. Malik, M. Z., Mikawati., & Purnamasari, D. (2021). Relationship between sexual needs and the quality of life of diabetes mellitus patients. https://core.ac.uk/download/417403527.pdf (accessed on 13th June 2025).

23. Mansoria, P., & Singh, S. B. (2023). Unlocking the therapeutic potential of millets: A path to diabetes control. https://core.ac.uk/download/617189540.pdf (accessed on 13th June 2025).

24. Martin, B., & Duggan, A. (2024). An exploration of gut hormone therapy to treat infertility caused by type 2 diabetes. https://core.ac.uk/download/628753436.pdf (accessed on 13th June 2025).

25. Ohiagu, F. O., Chikezie, P. C., & Chikezie, C. (2021). Pathophysiology of diabetes mellitus complications: Metabolic events and control. Biomedical Research and Therapy, 8, 4243–4257. https://www.semanticscholar.org/paper/58c962f7a419811c1c69347eb08474585b07c195 (accessed on 13th June 2025).

26. Olaogun, I., Farag, M., & Pousette Hamid, H. (2020). The pathophysiology of type 2 diabetes mellitus in non-obese individuals: An overview of the current understanding. Cureus, 12. https://www.semanticscholar.org/paper/3574981c9bd423acef9df10cd5d53bbaeac366f9 (accessed on 13th June 2025).

27. Patil, S. R., Chavan, A. B., Patel, A., Chavan, P. D., & Bhopale, J. V. (2023). A review on diabetes mellitus, its types, pathophysiology, epidemiology and its global burden. Journal for Research in Applied Sciences and Biotechnology. https://www.semanticscholar.org/paper/5b125d054b21b0ae2e7b505b55bc8386fff2c87c (accessed on 13th June 2025).

28. Rampal, G., Rampal, L., Rampal, L., Rampal, S., Loong, Y. Y., Md Zain, A., et al. (2010). Enhancing diabetic care in the community in Malaysia: Need for a paradigm shift. https://core.ac.uk/download/42995611.pdf (accessed on 13th June 2025).

29. Randall, A. (2016). Integrating technology to support and maintain glycemic control in people with diabetes. https://core.ac.uk/download/162578693.pdf (accessed on 13th June 2025).

30. Siegle, K., Stoltzfus, C., & Trainer, L. (2012). Health maintenance regarding carbohydrate counting and calorie restricted diets in diabetes mellitus type 2 patients. https://core.ac.uk/download/301474143.pdf (accessed on 13th June 2025).

31. Śliz, J., Popławska, N. A., Skorupska, M., Czeczotka, M., Woźniak, K., & Martka, M. M. (2024). Treatment of NAFLD: Diet, physical activity, and potential pharmacological options. Quality in Sport. https://www.semanticscholar.org/paper/d0877b0c030bd2917c055750b4dbb2e1528f7b20 (accessed on 13th June 2025).

32. Tao, X., Ranganathan, S., Van Halm-Lutterodt, N., Garcia-Vargas, J., Wu, A., Karnati, J., Shankar, S., et al. (2024). No difference in short-term surgical outcomes from semaglutide treatment for type 2 diabetes mellitus after cervical decompression and fusion: A propensity score-matched analysis. Spine. https://www.semanticscholar.org/paper/456fc44531c61943df70f11b5991d59b0014c9ce (accessed on 13th June 2025).

33. Thenmozhi, P., Lavanya, A., Kannan, M., Shyamala, R., & Sathiyarajeswaran, P. (2021). An overview of the Siddha treatment guideline for diabetes mellitus: A non-communicable disease. Journal of Research in Siddha Medicine, 4, 46–53. https://www.semanticscholar.org/paper/a89dfb89ec3ca1b1bf5f12e276bd3e27d29c4445 (accessed on 13th June 2025).

34. Widara, J. Z., Sukesih, S., & Jauhar, M. (2024). Health education on nutrition management reduces blood sugar levels in diabetes mellitus clients. Indonesian Journal of Health Research and Development. https://www.semanticscholar.org/paper/46a501dd8b72a96dc907cc6a4fde41d77f22ced9 (accessed on 13th June 2025).

35. Yan, M., Chen, Z., Tang, J., Duan, X., Peng, W., Liu, R., Li, W., et al. (2025). Association between gestational diabetes mellitus and offspring health: A two-sample mendelian randomization study. BMC Pregnancy and Childbirth, 25. https://www.semanticscholar.org/paper/d0b3d81ca13eadbece93a9ea3f225cd4bb173fcf (accessed on 13th June 2025).

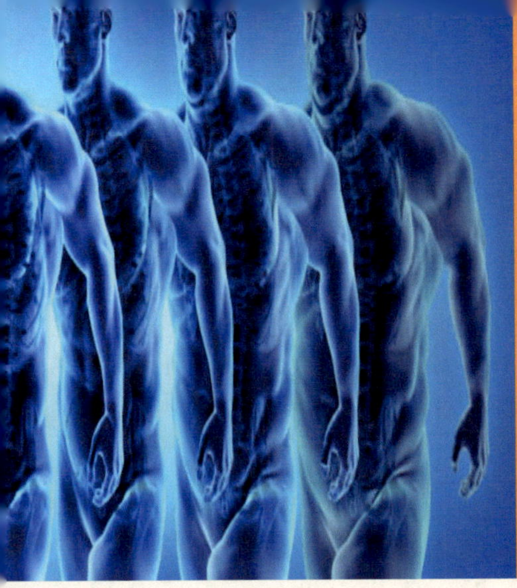

Chapter 8

METABOLIC BONE DISORDERS

Contents

Introduction 243

8.1. Types of Metabolic Bone Disorders 246

8.2. Causes of Metabolic Bone Disorders 251

8.3. Risk Factors 254

8.4. Symptoms and Diagnosis 258

8.5. Treatment Options 262

8.6. Prevention Strategies 266

Summary 271

References 273

Introduction

Metabolic bone disorders are a collection of diseases that adversely affect the structural and functional properties of bone, leading to severe health consequences in patients. The disorders can manifest as soft bones, abnormal bone development, and interferences with mineralization processes, most frequently resulting in concerns, such as fractures and deformities. Identification of the causative causes of metabolic bone diseases is crucial as it helps in the planning of appropriate diagnostic and therapeutic strategies. In the last few decades, the genetic and environmental origins of such conditions as osteoporosis and Paget's disease have become increasingly well understood, allowing interventions to be directed at particular causative causes and improving patient outcome. Moreover, the presence of sophisticated diagnostic equipment facilitates easier detection of these disorders at an earlier stage, which is extremely important in order to preventive interventions and introduce effective treatments to enhance the quality of life of the patients. The difficulties in the diagnosis of metabolic bone disorders are typically founded on their multifactorial etiology. For instance, manifestations of diseases, such as Osteomalacia or Paget's disease may overlap, and therefore, it is challenging to diagnose them accurately. This is compounded in regions where there is inadequate access to sophisticated diagnostic evaluation. In Mexico, for example, physicians are faced with difficulties in diagnosing inherited bone marrow failure syndromes, which clinically overlap with other metabolic bone disorders. To combat the impediments, initiatives, such as the Mexican Registry of IBMFS have been instituted in a bid to increase awareness and encourage the use of genetic testing by physicians. These initiatives highlight the necessity for continued education and partnership among healthcare professionals in further delineating diagnostic criteria and our knowledge of these disorders. More awareness can eventually translate into more individualized treatment approaches, strongly affecting patient care. With the frequency of metabolic bone disorders, the necessity for thorough management guidelines is more vital than ever before. Expert panels have begun to make recommendations for improving the clinical management of disease conditions like Paget's disease, given the nature of urgency involved. Although there is substantial evidence for the use of antiresorptive medications, particularly bisphosphonates, treatment is complex, and particularly for asymptomatic patients, the therapeutic situation is complicated. Thus, a prudent evaluation of treatment risk versus benefit is critical. By focusing heavily on early diagnosis and adhering to standardized treatment regimens, healthcare providers can minimize complications from metabolic bone diseases. Continued investigation of the genetic causes of these disorders will be expected to yield more information, leading to future practice that will foster better patient health outcomes with these common disorders (Gomez et al., 2024; Rendina et al., 2024) (Figure 8.1).

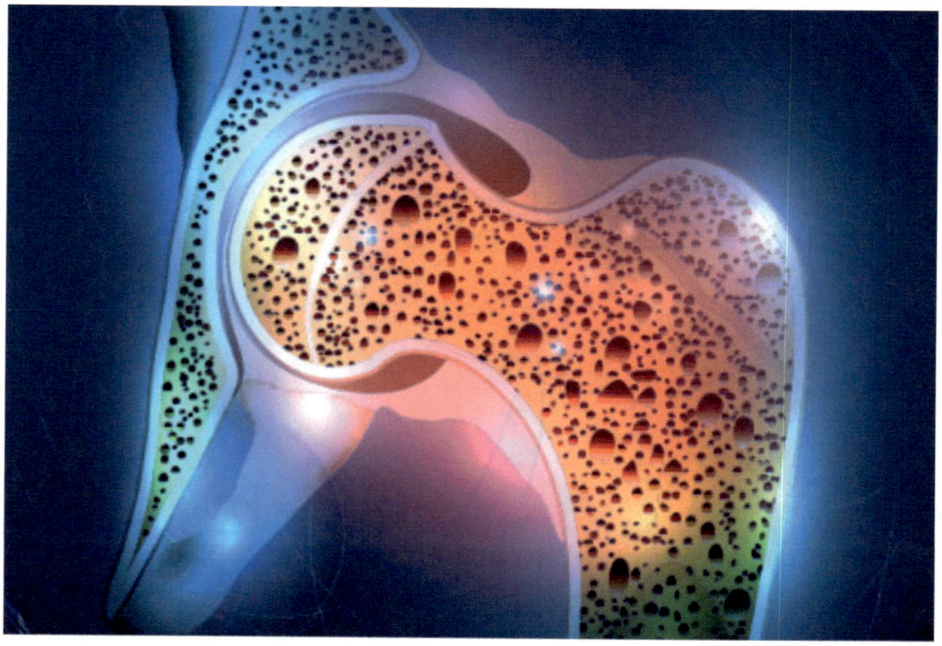

Figure 8.1. Visual representation of osteoporotic bone structure.

Source: https://external-content.duckduckgo.com/iu/?u=https%3A%2F%2Fashe-endo.com%2Fimages%2Fcta-bone-rollover.jpg&f=1&nofb=1&ipt=96267ab7092c5cf5a4922782ba585af8f908d3aa2d653b1bd47ec7fbda2d9932.

Definition of Metabolic Bone Disorders

Metabolic bone diseases are a collection of disorders that disrupt the normal metabolism of bone tissue, resulting in alterations in bone structure, function, and density. The disorders are characterized by a disturbance of the balance between bone apposition and resorption, which is predominantly brought about by hormonal, nutritional, and genetic factors. For example, osteoporosis, a very common metabolic bone disease, is characterized by decreased bone mass and augmented fracture risk with aging, hormonal alterations, and deficiencies in essential nutrients like calcium and vitamin D. Defining metabolic bone diseases requires intimate knowledge of these physiological mechanisms because they have an overwhelming influence on bone health and well-being. Central to the etiology of metabolic bone disease is the function of mineral metabolism, specifically that of calcium and phosphorus. These minerals are tasked with maintaining the strength of bone and are regulated by hormones , such as parathyroid hormone and calcitonin. Disturbances in these minerals typically manifest in conditions like osteomalacia, where bone softening occurs due to inadequate mineralization, which is typically secondary to vitamin D deficiency. Furthermore, research indicates that vitamin D's function extends beyond the simple absorption of calcium; it impacts bone remodeling, as well as cellular functions within the bone microenvironment. Therefore, the interaction among nutrient availability, hormonal control, and genetic susceptibility becomes central to comprehending the range of metabolic bone disorders and their influence on skeletal health (Thacher and Oberhelman, 2013). Clinical presentation of the metabolic bone disease can vary greatly, ranging from asymptomatic to painful bone fractures and deformities. Paget's disease of bone is one such disease where there is increased and uncontrolled bone remodeling resulting in larger and therefore weaker bones. Diagnosis is normally by imaging methods and biochemical markers for assessing the turnover of bone along with mineral status. Efficient management regimens, including dietary modification, nutritional supplementation of deficient nutrients in the diet, and, in some cases, pharmacologic treatment, treat the fundamental metabolic disorder. With research ongoing, there is increasing recognition of the importance attached to treatment protocols individualized to the specific needs of the patients, particularly as more new information emerges on the place of vitamin D and other biomarkers in bone metabolism (N/A, 2012) (Figure 8.2).

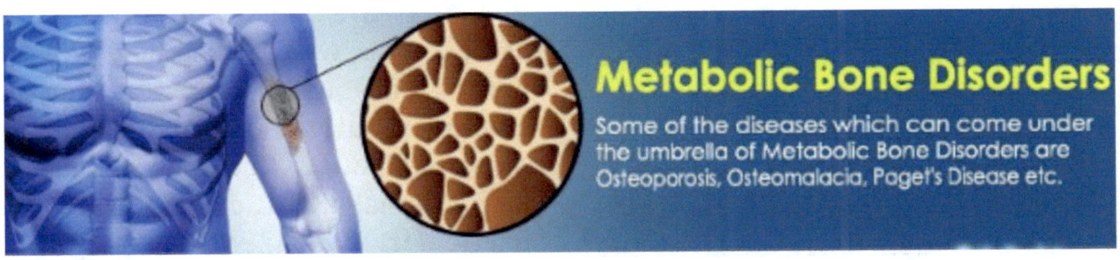

Figure 8.2. Metabolic bone disorders affect bone strength and structure.

Source: https://external-content.duckduckgo.com/iu/?u=https%3A%2F%2Fi.pinimg.com%2Foriginals%2F30%2F63%2Fe2%2F3063e2fb7012a49aee3b3050d09aeded.jpg&f=1&nofb=1&ipt=69c949925c91165568a4539493f2d1d198f2feed076ca3846a8af8cbf5439574.

Importance of Bone Health

The significance of possessing robust bone health cannot be overemphasized, particularly in metabolic bone disease. Bones are not mere passive structures; they play an active role in the body's metabolism, serving as reservoirs for minerals and housing bone marrow to produce blood cells. Physically stable bone density is important for conferring support and rendering the skeletal system resistant to mechanical stress. Decreased bone density, commonly resulting from an absence of vital nutrients , such as calcium and vitamin D, may lead to serious health issues like osteoporosis, which greatly increases the risk of fractures. Familiarity with the biochemical mechanisms that regulate bone status is of primary importance for the implementation of preventive practice and treatment against metabolic bone diseases. With emerging evidence in the spotlight about the multifunctional roles of vitamins and minerals in bone metabolism, the need for proactive intervention to promote bone health over a lifetime is more evident now than ever before. Vitamin D is a prominent nutrient in the maintenance of good bone health and prevention of metabolic bone diseases. Valued over history for its role in the metabolism of calcium and phosphate, vitamin D has been discovered to influence other physiological functions, including bone remodeling and muscle power. Scientific research has established that a deficiency in vitamin D results in diseases of the skeleton like rickets and Osteomalacia with potentially far-reaching, long-term effects on overall health. In addition, low vitamin D status has also been associated with increased risks of non-chronic diseases, which underscores the nutrients far-reaching physiological importance. As evidence continues to illustrate the broad effects of vitamin D deficiency, such as the association with diseases like type 2 diabetes as well as cardiovascular illness, the need for addressing deficiencies becomes a matter of urgency not just for bone, but overall well-being. Therefore, adequate availability of vitamin D through sunlight exposure, diet, and supplement is crucial for effective prevention of metabolic bone diseases. Childhood obesity is also a major determinant of bone health, with the paradoxical relationship to be resolved. While increased body mass can be related to greater bone mineral density, it will ultimately enhance fracture risks through impaired bone quality and deformed mechanical loading patterns. Of the most concern is that patients with syndromic obesity or atypical patterns of nutrition are especially at risk of bone fragility, suggesting subtle endocrine and metabolic dysfunction. Increasing evidence has pointed to the negative impact of pharmacological intervention for severe obesity on the skeleton, questioning its long-term implications. Given the increasing incidence of obese children, it is essential that these patterns are appreciated and particular prevention measures are formulated. Multidimensional approaches that treat weight control alongside retention of bone architecture are crucial in averting complications of metabolic bone illnesses in a manner that all aspects of children's health remain intact while they grow.

8.1. Types of Metabolic Bone Disorders

The morphology of metabolic bone disease is a spectrum of disease entities, each with distinct etiologies and resultant clinical implications. Perhaps the most obvious category is osteoporosis, which is characterized by reduced density and quality of bone tissue, and hence an increased risk of fracture, particularly in older individuals. Osteoporosis may be caused by hormonal alterations associated with aging, particularly declines in estrogen following menopause, which have a significant impact on bone remodeling. Additionally, secondary osteoporosis may also be caused by metabolic derangements, such as chronic kidney disease where disruptions in calcium and phosphate metabolism are of crucial significance. Findings suggest that bone mineral disorders are prevalent among end-stage renal disease patients, indicating that there is a wide interrelationship between metabolic dysfunctions and skeletal health (Fadel et al., 2024). It is crucial to understand the differences and similarities among such conditions for effective diagnosis and customized therapeutic interventions. Osteomalacia, another significant metabolic bone disease, consists of inappropriate mineralization of the bone, leading to soft and weakened bones. It normally occurs because of a deficiency of proper nutrients for normal bone metabolism, i.e., vitamin D, calcium, and phosphate. Lack of sunlight exposure, particularly in populations with limited outdoor activity, has a higher risk of Osteomalacia development, particularly where sunlight is scarce.

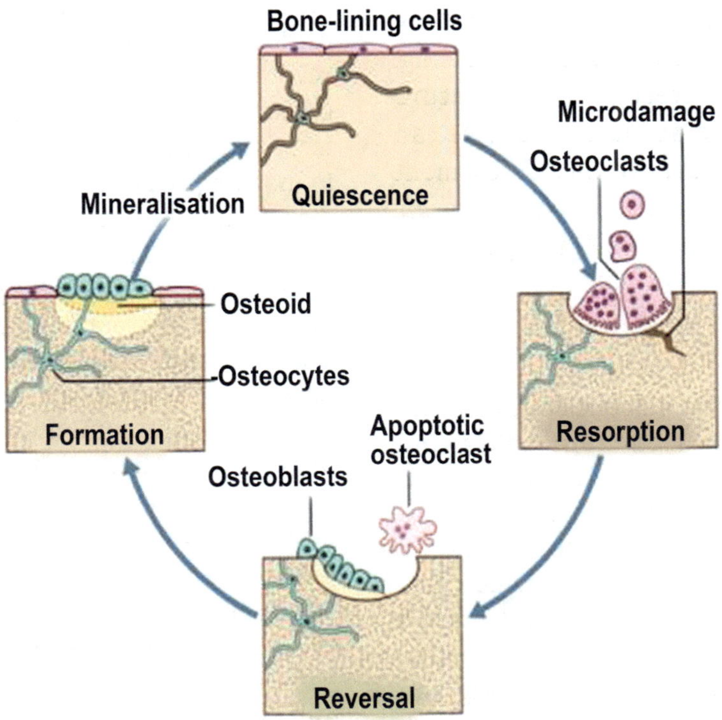

Figure 8.3. Bone remodeling cycle shows key cellular processes.

Source: https://external-content.duckduckgo.com/iu/?u=https%3A%2F%2Fo.quizlet.com%2FT1J76ry9dnsrSrg43ZDhoA.png&f=1&nofb=1&ipt=92942e8fe1049c49d578070ea888ad6d441601b5289b94cede1debc50e7c6faa.

Moreover, certain medical conditions like malabsorption syndromes exacerbate vitamin D deficiency, making the importance of interdisciplinary treatment paramount. Osteomalacia outcomes may significantly impair functional mobility and quality of life, underlining the importance of early diagnosis and management. In addition, since phosphate metabolism is also disrupted in other metabolic conditions, understanding its relationship with Osteomalacia is important to develop optimal management plans (Fadel et al., 2024). Paget's disease of bone is another significant metabolic bone disease, characterized by defective bone remodeling that leads to enlarged and deformed bones. The pathophysiology of Paget's disease involves heightened osteoclast activity with resultant hyperactivity and compensation of the osteoblasts, resulting in an abnormal and weakened bone structure. Etiology is unclear but genetic predispositions and environmental exposures like viral infections have been implicated. Bone pain, deformity, and heightened risk for fracture are possible in these patients, and hence, close monitoring and management are indicated. Management involves bisphosphonates, which are useful in inhibiting osteoclast activity and rebuilding bone density. This singular disorder underscores the value of a complete understanding of bone biology, particularly the cellular mechanisms of bone remodeling. Furthermore, the heterogeneous nature of metabolic bone disorders requires an interdisciplinary approach to their assessment and treatment, based on the pleiotropic interactions among various biological pathways (Figure 8.3).

8.1.1. Osteoporosis

Osteoporosis is a severe metabolic bone disorder that results from reduced bone mass and disturbed bone tissue structure, finally leading to a greater risk of fractures and enhanced fragility. The majority of individuals are not diagnosed until the development of a fracture, which may have a very significant impact on the individual's quality of life. Risk factors include age, gender, family history, lifestyle , such as smoking and heavy alcohol consumption, and dietary lack of calcium and vitamin D. Women, particularly following menopause, are most at risk due to hormonal changes that accelerate the loss of bone mass. Early diagnosis is made effective through bone mineral density tests, which are typically quantified in terms of dual-energy X-ray absorptiometry (DEXA) scans, which are capable of detecting decreased bone mass even before a fracture. As the global population ages, osteoporosis is expected to become more prevalent, necessitating more effective prevention and management through public health interventions. Lifestyle interventions like weight-bearing exercise and dietary changes can be especially crucial for maintaining bone health. Pharmacologic treatments including bisphosphonates, selective estrogen receptor modulators, and parathyroid hormone analogs have also become available to prevent bone loss and reduce fracture. The efficacy of the treatments depends on the patient's risk factor and extent of bone loss, underscoring the significance of individualized treatment plans. Education of patients and physicians on osteoporosis, risk factors, and treatment is critical in preventing and encouraging an active response to bone health. Differentiation between osteoporosis and other metabolic bone diseases is critical in ensuring correct diagnosis and management. For instance, diseases like Paget's disease and hypophosphatasia can have similar signs of bone pain and fractures (Rendina et al., 2024; Moro, 2024). Misdiagnosis and subsequent inappropriate treatment can occur due to this, thus the importance of careful clinical evaluation. Laboratory testing and radiological evaluation must be complemented by careful patient history and physical examination to make a correct diagnosis. This enhancement of clinical practice not only enhances the effectiveness of treatment but also allows for more effective use of healthcare resources, particularly among the elderly with increased risk of metabolic bone disease. The integration of evidence-based guidelines into practice can ultimately enhance osteoporosis and related disease management.

8.1.2. Osteomalacia

Osteomalacia is an important metabolic bone disorder characterized by bone softening primarily due to the ineffectiveness in mineralization of the bone matrix due to vitamin D deficiency, metabolic derangement, or abnormal phosphorus levels. The peculiar challenge in the diagnosis of Osteomalaciaoarthritis is that it may be imitated by other skeletal disorders. There is a typical clinical syndrome that is characterized by skeletal pain, tenderness, and increased susceptibility to fracture, especially in older adults. Besides, it may lead to deformities, making it a preventable but highly incapacitating disease. With the worsening of the intrinsic deficiencies, patients will be prone to the development of an increase in fragility fractures, thus an urgent need for effective monitoring and management schemes to prevent further complications resulting from Osteomalacia. The pathophysiology of Osteomalacia is directly linked to nutritional as well as genetic factors. In cases of nutritional Osteomalacia, dietary deficiencies of vitamin D, calcium, and phosphate are the prevailing causes, leading to the interference with mineralization of the bone. Genetic influences, , such as those involving phosphate-regulating genes, play a part in the impact by hampering the body's regulation of phosphate. A corollary case was that of a 43-year-old woman presenting with multiple fragility fractures secondary to undiagnosed X-linked hypophosphatemia Osteomalacia, showing the need for early diagnosis in the prevention of long-term disability. This adds to the need for comprehensive clinical examinations in uncovering patients at risk and facilitating appropriate therapeutic interventions that cover both nutritional needs and genetic propensity (Zehra et al., 2021). Other recent studies have also defined the overall implications of Osteomalacia, particularly how it relates to other serious illnesses , such as osteonecrosis of the jaw (ONJ). ONJ is an illness in which there are non-healing uncovered bones within the facial structures, more often seen in patients who are taking bisphosphonate treatment for illnesses , such as osteoporosis and cancer treatment. It has been observed that conditions like Osteomalacia and deficiencies in vitamin D are likely to be a major causative factor in the development of ONJ, thereby indicating the importance of adequate management of bone health in individuals receiving such treatments. This observation warrants reassessment of the treatment protocols, suggesting the addition of a holistic framework to the management of metabolic bone diseases involving both nutritional supplementation and strict surveillance of potential complications (Carbonare et al., 2021). Elucidating the interconnectedness of Osteomalacia with other conditions not only enhances patient outcomes but also informs future research regarding effective therapeutic strategies (Figure 8.4).

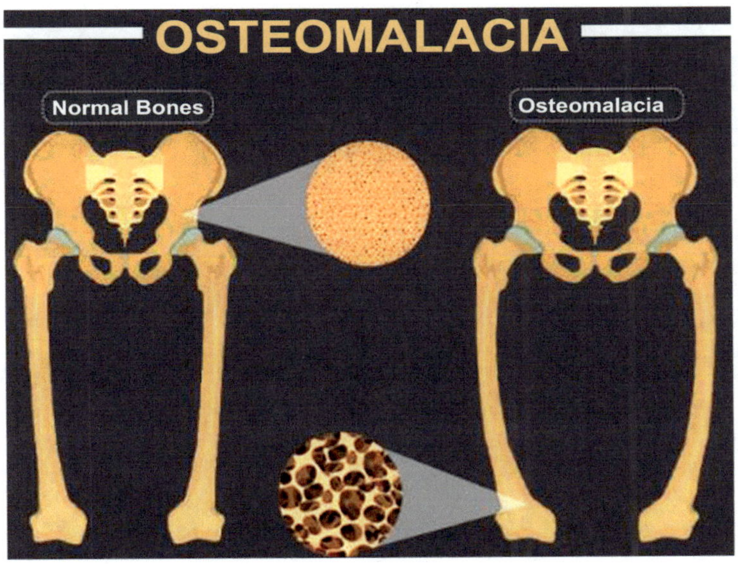

Figure 8.4. Bone density comparison: normal vs. Osteomalacia.

Source: https://external-content.duckduckgo.com/iu/?u=https%3A%2F%2Fwww.boldsky.com%2Fimg%2F2019%2F12%2FxOsteomalacia-1576837676.jpg.pagespeed.ic.T9eAzq9gX6.jpg&f=1&nofb=1&ipt=00ef9718aede01922a64cbd9d91a498d1fdc85512d1e70952cb9bc3c2ea329b9.

8.1.3. Paget's Disease

Paget's disease of bone is a systemic metabolic disorder characterized by disturbed bone remodeling, resulting in enlarged and weakened bones. It predominantly occurs in elderly individuals and leads to bone pain, deformity, and a raised risk of fracture. Ultimately, with advancing disease, the architecture of normal bone is destroyed and remodeled by excessive osteoclastic activity followed by adaptive osteoblastic overactivity that results in abnormal bone formation. Importantly, the disease can go undetected initially as it is asymptomatic in the majority of individuals until complications arise. Also, osteoarthritis risk for involved joints in Paget's disease is substantial, and it requires prompt intervention and control to prevent further morbidity and associated health outcomes. More recent evidence indicates that the geographical occurrence of Paget's disease is more extensive in some regions of the world, , such as the United Kingdom and some parts of Europe.

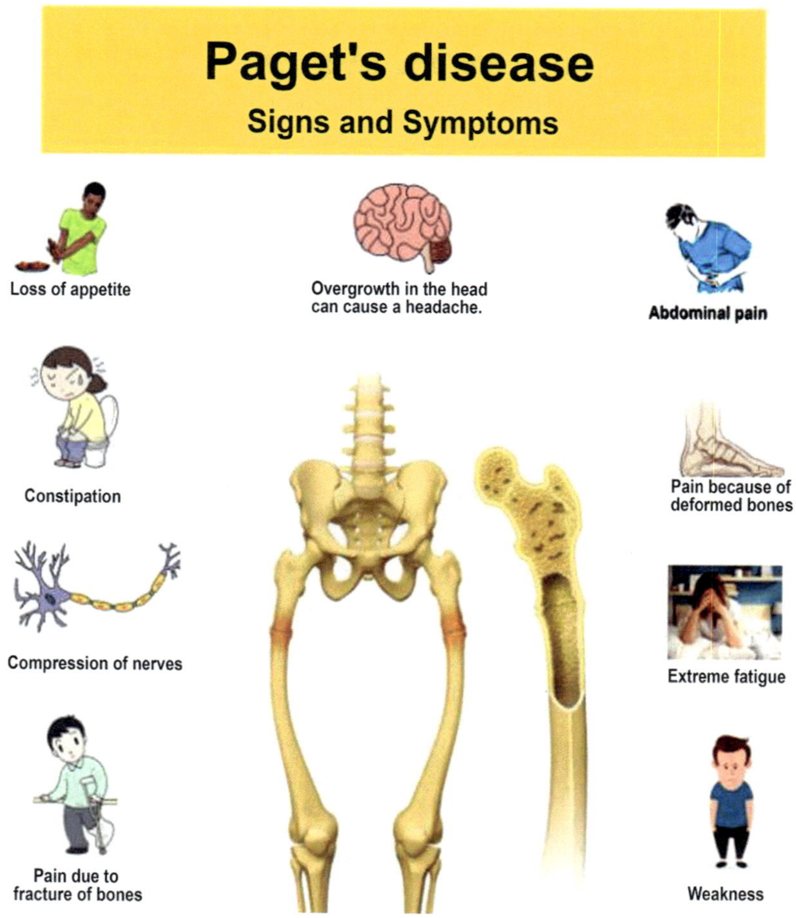

Figure 8.5. Common signs and symptoms of Paget's disease.

Source: https://www.nirujahealthtech.com/wp-content/uploads/2020/04/Paget%E2%80%99s-disease-Signs-and-Symptoms-1.png.

The pathophysiology of the disease remains poorly understood, though it is believed that both environmental and genetic factors are responsible for causing and progressing the disease. Secondly, the disease has also been associated with an increased risk for osteosarcoma, a malignant bone tumor, particularly in patients with extensive disease. These associations necessitate aggressive screening and bone health assessment of affected patients. Due to these complexities, clinicians need to adopt a multi-dimensional approach involving diagnostic imaging, clinical examination, and, if needed, biochemistry markers to treat effectively patients diagnosed with Paget's disease. Treatment of Paget's disease is predominantly pharmacological and is aimed at controlling bone remodeling, with bisphosphonates being the cornerstone of treatment. The medications markedly inhibit osteoclastic activity and thereby prevent resulting complications of bone integrity. Calcitonin has also been added to the therapeutic regimen of some patients, although its efficacy is not as dramatic as that of bisphosphonates. Current studies highlight the importance of understanding systemic changes in bone density in the context of Paget's disease. Considering that metabolic bone disorders like osteoporosis are sometimes combined with Paget's disease, histological assessment of bone mineral density is pertinent because increased resorption levels can pose problems relevant to both (Sumathy, 2007). Therefore, developing individualized treatment plans is critical in managing this complex disorder effectively as well as safeguarding the overall skeletal integrity of the patients (Figure 8.5).

8.2. Causes of Metabolic Bone Disorders

Metabolic bone diseases arise from a variety of factors that often reflect underlying systemic imbalances in factors , such as phosphorus, calcium, and vitamin D metabolism. Metabolic bone diseases include diseases like Osteomalacia, osteoporosis, and hyperparathyroidism, all of which can result from nutritional deficiency, endocrine disturbances, or genetic predispositions. For example, the primary cause of Osteomalacia is deficiency of intake of vitamin D, which plays a crucial role in calcium absorption. In the presence of low levels of vitamin D, calcium absorption from the intestines is decreased, leading to impaired bone mineralization and, hence, metabolic bone disease. Compounding this scenario is the presence of hormones , such as parathyroid hormone and calcitonin in bone metabolism, and dysregulation of which contributes to exacerbation of the condition and leads to increased bone resorption and loss in structural integrity. Another significant cause of the formation of metabolic bone diseases is the presence of underlying ailments, , such as kidney disease, that disrupt usual mineral metabolism. CKD can result in hyperphosphatemia and decreased calcitriol production, which can cause secondary hyperparathyroidism and bone disease. Moreover, conditions , such as hypercalciuria, which is prevalent in children and has a direct effect on bone quality, can predispose to urinary tract infection and cause low bone mineral content (Khawajah et al., 2024). Biochemical derangements in CKD have the propensity to set off a cascade of metabolic imbalances, which can lead to various disorders, including renal osteodystrophy. Thus, any disorder in the renal system can severely affect the health of bones by disrupting calcium and phosphate regulation. Lifestyle, i.e., diet and activity, can also significantly affect the prevalence of metabolic bone disorders. Poor nutrient intake, particularly deficiencies in calcium and vitamin D, does not support normal bone density and well-being. Lack of physical exercise, which stimulates bone remodeling and fortification, also aggravates the risk of metabolic bone diseases. The interplay between such life habits and genetic predispositions underlines the intricacies involved in metabolic bone diseases. Kids, for example, with hypercalciuria due to dietary imbalance are at increased risk of related complications , such as reduced bone mineral density (Khawajah et al., 2024). Conversely, interventions focusing on lifestyle modification , such as improved dietary intake and greater exercise can alleviate some of the risks of metabolic bone disease, demonstrating the promise of prevention in high-risk populations.

8.2.1. Nutritional Deficiencies

Deficiencies in nutrients play a central role in metabolic bone disease etiology, and they have an immense impact on the health of bones. Micronutrients are needed for a variety of biochemical reactions, like bone remodeling and mineralization. Compromised bone structure occurs due to a diet lacking important nutrients like calcium, vitamin D, and magnesium, which predisposes individuals to disorders like osteoporosis. The complexity of the diagnosis of nutritional deficiency calls for intensive evaluations, , such as dietary intake assessment and biochemistry testing. The association of the deficiencies with metabolic bone disorders underscores the importance of effective nutritional interventions as preventive measures. Despite the heavy emphasis on supplements, evidence proves that an optimal diet offers a more effective and safer method of achieving sufficiency of needed vitamins and minerals, resulting in better bone health and overall health (Combet & Buckton, 2014). In addition, the role of diet in metabolic bone diseases is more recognized in practice, particularly in patients with malabsorption issues following interventions , such as bariatric surgery. Patients who have undergone such operations are often presented with special nutritional problems that necessitate targeted interventions to prevent the hazards of deficiency. Poor nutrition or nutrient absorption can reduce bone density and accelerate the onset of osteoporosis or other conditions. It is therefore crucial for healthcare professionals to possess expertise in the care of the nutritional needs of post-bariatric surgery patients. By considering better-rounded dietary regimens with an emphasis on major nutrients, clinicians are able to significantly impact on the long-term metabolic health of such patients, with the capacity to directly correct deficiencies to prevent adverse outcomes concerning bone health (Busetto et al., 2017). In correcting nutritional deficiencies as a root cause of metabolic bone disorders, consideration of the broader public health significance is at issue. As conditions, such as obesity and malnutrition become more common, it is critical to be aware of the significance of micronutrient adequacy. Knowledge of the role of a well-balanced diet containing crucial vitamins and minerals is not only important for preventing metabolic bone diseases but can also have significant implications on the bone health of populations. As nutritional interventions show promise regarding disease prevention, identifying the relationship between dietary patterns and metabolic bone diseases can influence public health policy. By encouraging programs that support nutrient-dense diets, it is achievable to reduce the prevalence of metabolic bone diseases, emphasizing the need for ongoing research and public health interventions to offset nutritional deficiencies at a population level (Combet & Buckton, 2014) (Figure 8.6).

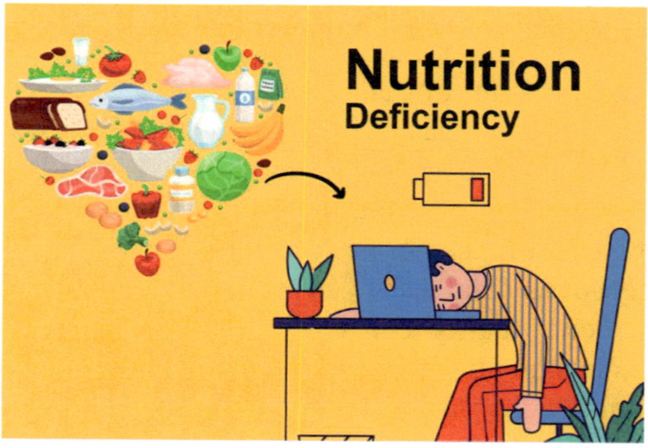

Figure 8.6. Effects of nutritional deficiency on energy and health.

Source:https://www.eggoz.com/blogs/lifestyle/nutrition-deficiency-prevention-cause-treatment

8.2.2. Hormonal Imbalances

Hormonal imbalances are mostly to blame for the etiology and pathogenesis of metabolic bone disease. Of special significance are fluctuations in primary hormones , such as parathyroid hormone (PTH), vitamin D, and sex hormones, which significantly affect bone health. For example, hyperparathyroidism may result in enhanced bone resorption, thereby decreasing bone density and increasing risk of osteoporosis. Furthermore, sex hormones , such as estrogen and testosterone are also crucial for maintaining bone mass, and their deficiency, particularly at menopause or in response to therapeutic maneuvers, can cause loss of bone at an accelerated rate. Additionally, the interaction of these hormones with other metabolic processes indicates the complex nature of hormonal regulation in the skeletal system and emphasizes the need for an integrated approach towards understanding and managing metabolic bone diseases. The connection between endocrine imbalance and metabolic bone disorders is better established with diseases , such as the polycystic ovary syndrome (PCOS), found in 5-10% of reproductive age women. PCOS is characterized by a syndrome complex consisting of insulin resistance and abnormal menses that are directly traceable to hormonal dysfunction.

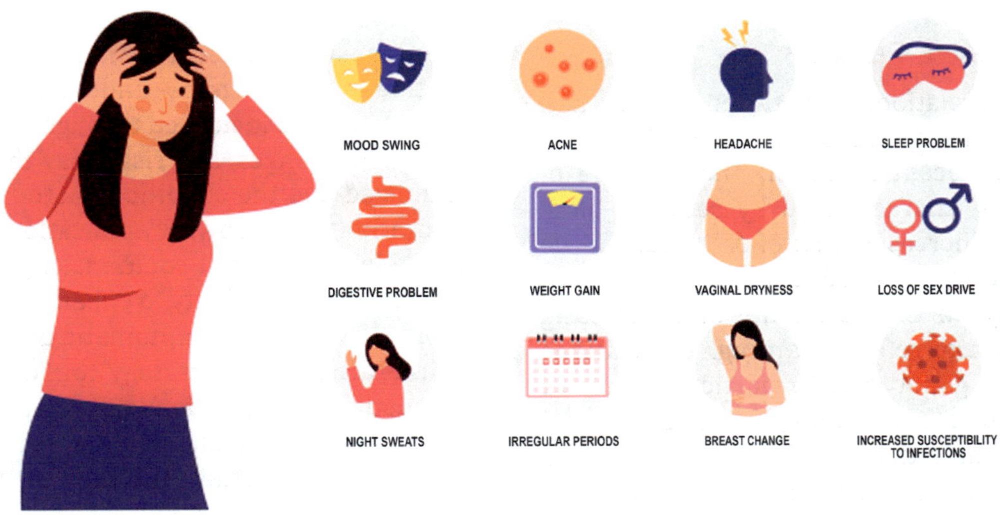

Figure 8.7. Common symptoms of hormonal imbalance.

Source: https://www.manipalhospitals.com/uploads/image_gallery/hormonal-imbalance-infographics-1.png.

The endocrine alterations in PCOS may lead to complications , such as decreased bone mineral density, which is rarely assessed in the clinical setting. Surprisingly, subjects may have long-term effects, , such as increased susceptibility to fractures. As PCOS usually co-exists with obesity, it is important to investigate the reciprocal relationship between obesity, hormonal imbalance, and metabolic bone disease, while pointing out the importance of integrated therapeutic regimens addressing all the relevant aspects of the disease (Khatun et al., 2022). Understanding the mechanisms by which hormonal imbalance causes metabolic bone diseases helps in identifying therapeutic alternatives. Interventions , such as hormone replacement therapy have been successful in the attenuation of hormonal deficiency impacts on the bone, particularly in postmenopausal women. Additionally, dietary and exercise lifestyle changes may also play significant roles in hormone regulation as well as bone fortification. Current findings also suggest that bariatric surgery may bring about significant hormonal changes that, while beneficial in inducing weight reduction, may be responsible for unfavorable effects on bone turnover. The complex interplay between improved metabolic control and possible endocrine dysfunctions highlights the significance of increased vigilance and research into the long-term consequences of these treatments for skeletal health, highlighting the necessity for continual improvement of clinical practice to maximize patient benefit (Tanweer et al., 2025) (Figure 8.7).

8.2.3. Genetic Factors

The complex relationship between genetics and metabolic bone diseases has drawn immense attention in recent research. The example of osteoporosis, characterized by reduced bone density and increased risk of fracture, can be a good illustration. Hereditary inclination could bear heavily on the possibility of contracting this condition, as reflected through correlations with certain genotypes. In particular, the GG genotype or the G allele of the 283 A> G polymorphism in the VDR gene has been found to predict osteoporosis in lumbar vertebrae L1-L4. This genetic marker points to the extent to which variations in specific genes affect bone health and the overall integrity of the skeletal system, suggesting that genetic screening may be a crucial asset in early diagnosis and treatment planning for individuals at higher risk of metabolic bone diseases (Vasilyeva et al., 2021). Beyond classical genetic factors, epigenetic processes have emerged to be noted as significant modulators of bone health. Unlike genetic mutations, in which permanent changes in the DNA sequence are involved, epigenetic changes are reversible and subject to the control of environmental factors , such as diet and lifestyle. For instance, the function of dietary phytochemicals resveratrol and pterostilbene has been established for their potential to regulate gene expression through epigenetic mechanisms. These compounds can regulate DNA methylation and histone structure and hence impact gene transcription involved in bone metabolism and density. This draws attention to the dynamic function of gene expression in relation to outside factors, illustrating how genetics and the environment collaborate to yield metabolic bone disorders (Pei-Lee et al., 2018). Being aware of the genetic origin of metabolic bone disorders not only improves our knowledge of these disorders but also offers windows for targeted therapies. Genetic research will be expected to elucidate the disease pathways in diseases , such as osteoporosis and osteogenesis imperfecta so that a more specific treatment plan can be undertaken. Specific markers may be identified through genetics and epigenetic changes, and risks may therefore be minimized and the conditions better managed. In addition, with growing application of genetic testing in the clinic, it could make pre-emptive intervention a possibility to enhance bone health before the onset of symptomatic disease. Thus, an interdisciplinary strategy founded on both epigenetic and genetic foundations is imperative in preventing and managing metabolic bone disease in the future (Pei-Lee et al., 2018; Vasilyeva et al., 2021).

8.3. Risk Factors

It is the knowledge of the risk factors for metabolic bone disorders (MBD) that is crucial for successful control and prevention. Foremost among these are age, sex, and heredity, with postmenopausal women, for example, being at higher risk because they have lower estrogen levels that influence bone mineral density. In addition, patients with a family history of osteoporosis or other such conditions are at a greater risk and hence genetic screening in high-risk groups gains relevance. Behavioral risk factors for low activity, inadequate diet, most importantly, insufficient calcium and vitamin D, by smoking trigger the risk of MBD. Complete assessment and review of intrinsic and extrinsic variables are required to determine people at risk so that early intervention and site-specific preventive treatment can be initiated so that early intervention and site-specific preventive treatment can be initiated. Another significant risk factor in metabolic bone disease is obesity, and more specifically so in the case of children. Obesity in children imposes complex challenges on bones with endocrine and mechanical influences that may lead to detrimental effects. Increased body fat is associated with increased bone mineral density but intriguingly increases the susceptibility to fractures due to compromised bone quality. Children who are obese are exposed to abnormal loads on the skeletal system, which can lead to abnormal loading and, with potential dysregulations of hormones, to bone weakness. Moreover, individuals undergoing syndromic obesity or following abnormal models of nutrition, e.g., eating disorders, are exposed to particular risks. These findings indicate the importance of complete measures to assess and deal with bone health among child populations, emphasizing dietary modification and lifestyle change in the avoidance of risk issues associated with obesity and bone disease (Farella et al., 2025). Ultimately, drug and surgical treatments for severe obesity present additional risk issues concerning bone health. Treatment modalities , such as glucagon-like peptide-1 (GLP-1) receptor agonists and bariatric surgery have been promising in the management of weight but may have harmful effects on bone strength. Emerging evidence suggests that while these treatment modalities cause weight loss, their impact on bone strength and structure in the short term and long term is not well studied. Thus, careful observation and research are needed to establish how such new interventions form a part of the greater paradigm of treating metabolic bone disorders. By comprehending the complex mechanisms of such risk factors, medical professionals are now able to design complex treatment protocols that not only cure obesity but also target the upkeep of bone health, illustrating the fine balancing act of metabolic mechanisms and bone health (Farella et al., 2025) (Figure 8.8).

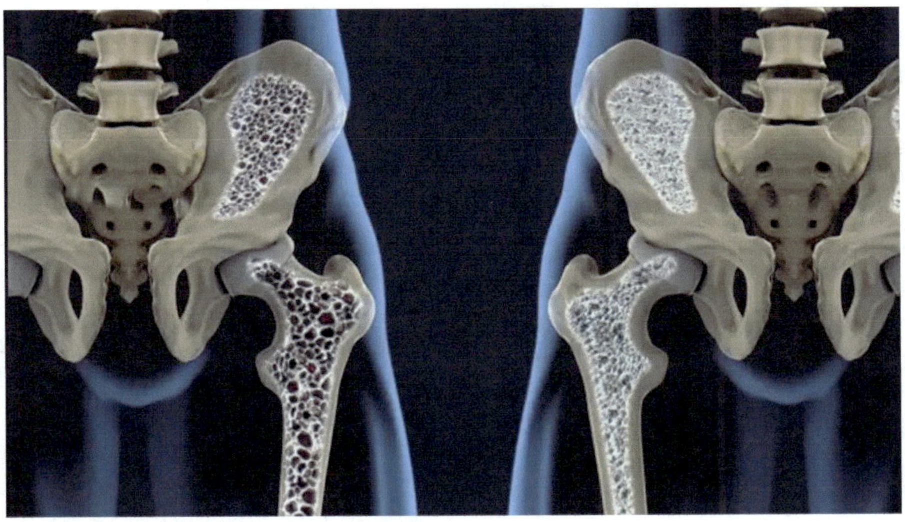

Figure 8.8. Healthy bone vs. osteoporotic bone comparison.

Source: https://thumbnails.icloudhospital.com/tr:w-1536,f-webp,q-75/2-df73cedd-ea23-4c59-8db7-13731900b18f.webp.

8.3.1. Age and Gender

Metabolic bone diseases are strongly influenced by age and gender, two diseases responsible to their prevalence and occurrence. With advancing age, physiological changes lead to bone weakening and susceptibility to fractures. For instance, women after menopause experience enhanced bone loss because of the drop in estrogen levels, a factor in the preservation of bone density. This condition is further exacerbated in the elderly, for whom they have a reduction of osteoblast function—the cells responsible for bone formation. Consequently, the process of aging can result in such diseases as osteoporosis, which largely impacts elderly women compared to men, showing the crucial juncture of gender and age in affecting metabolic bone health. Although bone loss with aging occurs in all individuals, gender also specifies the rate and extent of these metabolic bone diseases. Men tend to maintain higher peak bone mass than women, which typically offers a measure of protection against osteoporosis until much later in life. However, when men age, they also acquire a potential for metabolic bone loss, particularly if they have some underlying disease or lifestyle concerns on the bone health, , such as low testosterone levels. This change means that, in addition to biological factors, environmental factors also come into play, and interventions aimed at attempting to prevent these risks have to be age- and gender-specific. Understanding these nuances is vital to medical workers in creating fruitful prevention and treatment strategies for metabolic bone disease in patients of mixed populations. Furthermore, the interdynamics of age, sex, and metabolic bone disease call for the incorporation of preventive strategies aimed at lifestyle and dietary care. Nutritional factors, specifically calcium and vitamin D intake, are key factors in maintaining dense bones in men and women of all ages. Steady exercise can also play an important role in enhancing skeletal strength and integrity. Evidence has shown that resistance training could be responsible for the improvement in bone density, particularly in postmenopausal women with a potential osteoporosis risk. Health professionals need to consider these aspects in making efficient use of guidelines based on patients' individual profiles. Besides, the gender and age contribution to metabolic bone disorders needs ongoing work to demystify the complex mechanisms involved to ensure that evidence-based recommendations evolve as new data emerge, reflecting the evolving nature of practice in healthcare management of bone disease (Balali-Mood et al., 2021; Mach et al., 2019).

8.3.2. Lifestyle Choices

Lifestyle factors are the primary determinants of metabolic bone disorders, particularly regarding nutritional status and physical activity level. Diet, a fundamental lifestyle factor, has a direct impact on bone density, and nutrients , such as calcium and vitamin D have a unique role in maintaining dense bones. Lack of these nutrients can result in conditions , such as osteoporosis, where bones become brittle and more susceptible to fractures. Moreover, the overall context of consumption is viewed in a wide range of dietary lifestyles that are capable of structuring or destroying bone health in the long run. Identification of these dietary contributions forms the key for developing population-specific interventions for combating the menace of metabolic bone diseases (Kibler, 2025). Outside of nutrition, regular exercise also plays a crucial role in healthy bones. Weight-bearing resistance exercises stimulate bone growth and increase peak bone mass, which is particularly important in youth and adolescence. Lack of physical activity, on the other hand, is associated with bone loss and heightened susceptibility to fractures in the future. The Women's Sports Foundation supports the benefits of sports and physical activity participation, especially among women who are at specific risk for bone diseases. Physical activity and sports not only make bones stronger, but they also maximize an individual's general physical fitness, improving the prevention of metabolic bone diseases (Sabo et al., 2015). Other than diet and physical activity, lifestyle choices extend to other areas , such as smoking, alcohol consumption, and overall well-being routines. Smoking has been shown to have adverse effects on bone health by disrupting the body's ability to absorb essential nutrients and hormones that are required for maintaining bone. Consuming too much alcohol is also linked with increased osteoporosis risk. Addressing these lifestyle risk factors is central to developing successful prevention regimens for metabolic bone diseases. Encouraging healthier lifestyles, health professionals can guide individuals toward lifestyles that support more desirable bone and overall health, thereby reducing the incidence of such diseases and enhancing the well-being in at-risk populations (Figure 8.9).

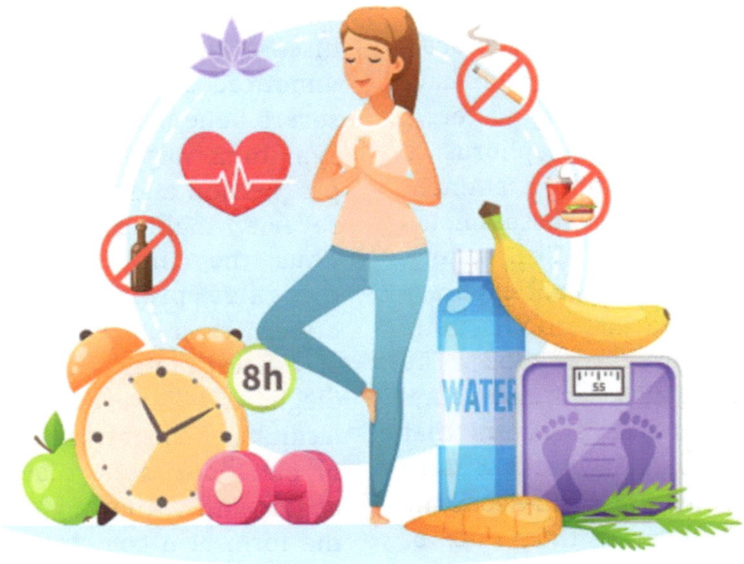

Figure 8.9. Healthy lifestyle habits for overall well-being.

Source: https://i0.wp.com/curaadvancedphysiotherapy.in/wp-content/uploads/2023/06/screenshot-2023-06-07-4.32.50-pm.png?resize=474%2C402&ssl=1.

8.3.3. Medical History

The investigation of metabolic bone disease demands a practical grasp of medical history, particularly in the context of established therapy and diagnostic techniques. By way of historical records, it appears that diseases , such as Osteomalacia and osteoporosis were well known for centuries and often misdiagnosed in terms of alternative dominant medical paradigms. Ancient knowledge of bones was poor, and ancient cultures explained brittle bones primarily in terms of aging or trauma. As medical science evolved, so did our knowledge of the metabolic pathways that controlled bone density and strength. This shift was brought about by developments in the fields of biochemistry and endocrinology, which unraveled the significant roles of hormones , such as vitamin D, parathyroid hormone, and calcitonin in bone metabolism. Thus, these historical developments illuminate current practice in the prevention and management of metabolic bone disorder and aim at physiological balance as central to healthy bones (Rinella et al., 2023). Metabolic bone disorder awareness in the medical past highlights ongoing diagnostic approaches that elucidate these disorders. The introduction of radiographic imaging in the 20th century was a paradigm shift, allowing clinicians to visualize changes in bone structure previously invisible. The invention of dual-energy X-ray absorptiometry (DEXA) scans allowed clinicians to quantify bone mineral density, which permitted earlier and more sensitive diagnosis of osteoporosis and other conditions. This imaging diagnostic advance has, in its turn, affected treatment protocols and follow-up care. Over time, researchers have also determined the role of dietary factors, , such as intake of calcium and phosphorus, in affecting bone health, fine-tuning treatment models to incorporate nutritional assessments alongside medical treatment. Medical history, then, is a foundation upon which contemporary approaches to managing metabolic bone diseases are built (Murray et al., 2022). The history of metabolic bone disorders also points to socio-economic and cultural factors that govern their incidence and management. History reveals the trend of dominant socio-economic and cultural factors influencing their rates of occurrence in various populations differently. For instance, urbanization and lifestyle changes have been linked to rising cases of osteoporosis as individuals have become sedentary and habituated to a poor lifestyle. Furthermore, historical health care disparities have long-lasting effects on the diagnosis and treatment of such disorders, particularly in low-resource settings. A review of these aspects of medical history will enable health care providers to create prevention programs and interventions that are tailored to the local needs, fostering an all-encompassing approach to addressing the global burden of metabolic bone disorders. By this, fusion of historic viewpoints with contemporary practice is essential to advance public health programs in bone health (Rinella et al., 2023).

8.4. Symptoms and Diagnosis

Metabolic bone diseases are a cluster of diseases characterized by structural defects and mineralization defects in the bone, and they can lead to symptoms that can severely compromise a patient's quality of life. Some of the symptoms include bone pain, deformity, fractures, and alterations in mobility, all of which are significant factors for the diagnosis of the diseases. For instance, in Paget's bone disease, the slow onset of symptoms may go unnoticed until complications arise, , such as severe bone pain or orthopedic complications. Symptoms vary based on the extent of disease progression and therefore, can be of different severity, making early detection important. Thus, the clinical approach must not only recognize presenting symptoms but also discern their meaning within the framework of general metabolic bone health, since early diagnosis will prevent future complications and facilitate efficient treatment planning. Diagnosis of metabolic bone diseases would typically begin with a thorough clinical evaluation in the form of a comprehensive medical history and physical examination. Individual laboratory tests, for instance, serum phosphate, alkaline phosphatase, and calcium, are important in validating the diagnosis. Radiography also plays an essential role in imaging procedures like bone scans or X-rays, revealing characteristic changes of diseases like Paget's disease. According to Rendina et al. (2024), the diagnosis should be made primarily based on symptoms and also biochemical and radiological findings, giving a firm understanding of the disorder. In addition, consideration of risk factors , such as family history or prior fracture history contributes to an individualized diagnostic approach that is critical for the direction of future treatment decisions and improved outcomes in patients. Application of international diagnostic standards as defined by Arai et al. (2023) directs the assessment process for metabolic bone disorders, particularly in the conduct of comprehensive evaluations among diverse populations. These criteria tend to ask for the inclusion of both subjective and objective measures in determining the complex state of disorders like cachexia, which may complicate metabolic bone health. Determining key clinical outcomes, , such as mortality rates and quality of life, aligns with the necessity of ongoing research on diagnosis and management strategies. By adopting a multidisciplinary framework that takes comprehensive diagnostic models into consideration, healthcare practitioners can gain a better understanding of metabolic bone disease, thus making diagnoses more accurate and treatment plans more effective. This dedication to keeping pace with changing diagnostic standards ultimately serves to tackle the distinct issues of patients with metabolic bone disease (Figure 8.10).

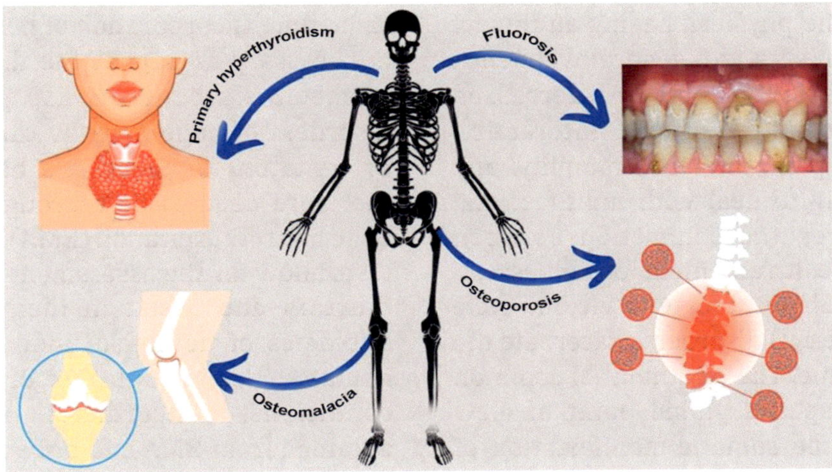

Figure 8.10. Bone disorders linked to systemic conditions.

Source: https://image.oaes.cc/ebedc12b-14af-4b7e-9c28-3d619e5bb933/mtod4038.fig.1.jpg.

8.4.1. Common Symptoms

Metabolic bone diseases, characterized by abnormalities of mineral and skeletal homeostasis, have numerous common symptoms that immediately impact the quality of life of patients. A common symptom is bone pain, typically chronic and incapacitating. It may cause focal or generalized pain, often impairing range of motion and activities of daily living. This symptom is frequently correlated with lowered bone mineral density (BMD) and also with a risk for fractures, most prominently in conditions like osteoporosis and Osteomalacia. In addition to this, musculoskeletal symptoms are also exacerbated by accompanying diseases like metabolic syndrome, which involve inflammation and obesity and can also contribute to joint stiffness and pain. It is very important to determine the interrelation between these symptoms and concealed metabolic derangement for effective management and treatment planning. The second most common symptom of metabolic bone diseases is the development of fractures in patients, particularly older adults. These fractures can even be seen with minimal trauma, indicative of underlying bone structural impairments due to lower mineralization or alterations in bone quality. Advanced age increases the risk of fractures, as comorbidities , such as diabetes mellitus, bring along the added burden of bone health. Recent studies have established the presence of a link between metabolic syndrome and increased prevalence of fractures, and there is evidence that insulin resistance is one of the systemic conditions contributing to bone loss. In Kearns-Sayre Syndrome patients, as with other metabolic abnormalities , such as impaired glucose tolerance, other metabolic abnormalities are likely to predispose to fractures and accelerate overall worsening of health, and hence utmost vigilance in monitoring and control of symptoms under this setting is warranted. The clinical presentation of metabolic bone disease also extends beyond the physical, having an impact on psychological health and general wellbeing. Patients often report fatigue and decreased quality of life because of the interaction between chronic pain, impaired mobility, and stress from having to deal with multifactorial diseases. Moreover, the connection between musculoskeletal health and metabolic illnesses, , such as Type 2 diabetes, creates a vicious cycle where musculoskeletal disorders exacerbate the metabolic syndrome. The treatment of common symptoms must span a global point of view concerning both the somatic manifestation of the disease and its psychological aspect. By the inclusion of lifestyle interventions, nutritional support, and medications that will aid in bone density enhancement, clinicians can significantly enhance patient outcomes and quality of life, as exemplified by increased overall health following specific therapies in patients with metabolic bone diseases (Amergoolov et al., 2024; Vaish et al., 2024).

8.4.2. Diagnostic Tests

Diagnostic testing is a valuable aid to the diagnosis and treatment of metabolic bone disease, reporting on the structural and functional makeup of the skeletal system. Metabolic bone disease is generally manifest as a multifaceted interplay between biochemical derangements and altered bone density. Clinical assessment typically begins with routine imaging techniques, , such as X-rays and dual-energy X-ray absorptiometry (DEXA), providing essential information on bone density and potential fractures. However, in certain situations, these tests may not reflect minor metabolic changes. Therefore, more advanced techniques, , such as bone turnover markers and histological examination, are increasingly being utilized to detect the underlying pathophysiology so that the full picture of each patient's status is obtained. Such diagnostic tests are essential while planning effective treatment regimens and monitoring therapeutic outcomes. At the same time, incorporation of hematologic studies is necessary as part of the diagnostic workup in metabolic bone disease patients. Certain disorders of bone marrow can be the etiology or imitators of metabolic bone disease and therefore need to be thoroughly evaluated by bone marrow aspiration (BMA) and biopsy. These tests allow for the assessment of hematopoietic function and assist in identifying potential etiologies of deranged bone metabolism, i.e., hematological neoplasms or other systemic conditions. Concordance between results obtained from BMA and bone marrow trephine biopsy (BMB) is considered to be very high, making it a useful diagnostic tool (Verma et al., 2024). These tests not only yield informative cytological data but also enhance the sensitivity of detection of concomitant diseases that can complicate the management of bone health. Additionally, molecular and genetic analysis have transformed the world of diagnostic assessment for metabolic bone disease. As more information becomes known about genetic susceptibility to most bone diseases, directed testing can illuminate us regarding risk factors and potential interventions. For example, with diabetic mellitus, there are particular metabolic alterations that are capable of influencing hematological performance substantially, with clear changes in blood cell circulation having a direct influence on bone integrity (Onishchenko et al., 2024). Consequently, the practitioner can take a more targeted approach to patient management, combining treatments in line with specific genetic and metabolic dispositions. This forward-thinking method underscores the necessity for using a multidisciplinary diagnostic strategy to guarantee that all aspects of metabolic bone health are evaluated and treated effectively (Figure 8.11).

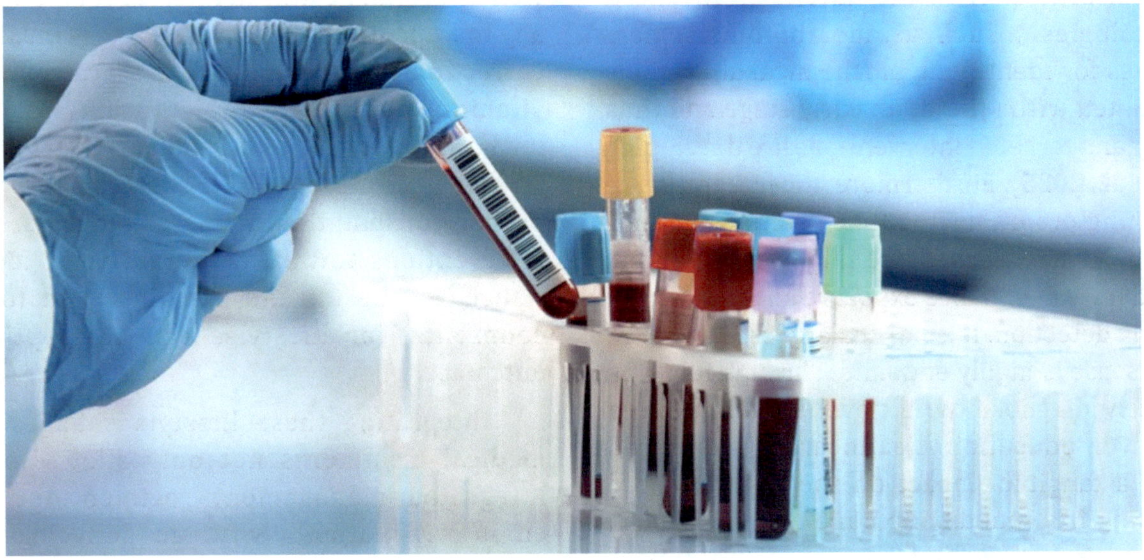

Figure 8.11. Blood samples prepared for laboratory testing.

Source: https://images.apollo247.in/pd-cms/cms/2023-10/Shutterstock_1114244621.jpg.

8.4.3. Importance of Early Detection

The significance of early detection, though, when it relates to metabolic bone disorders (MBD), cannot be emphasized enough. The diseases typically manifest as complications of chronic illnesses , such as chronic kidney disease (CKD) can have serious consequences if detected too late. Early detection of the initial signs and symptoms of MBD is achievable, allowing prompt interventions that will forestall the progression of the disease. For instance, metabolic bone changes can start in the later stages of CKD, whereas disturbances of mineral and bone metabolism can be detected as early as stage 3a CKD (Isa et al., 2025).

The earlier identification through routine monitoring and screening of at-risk populations can enable more favorable management strategies, eventually leading to reduced morbidity and improved patient outcomes, and thus reducing the burden on healthcare systems to some extent. Moreover, early detection prevents substantial amounts of healthcare spending on advanced metabolic bone disorders. With the progression of diseases, they would require more advanced and expensive treatments, more hospitalizations, and, ultimately, surgery. By identifying the patients that are at increased risk for MBD through precise screening procedures, medical professionals can perform preventive measures, , such as food modification or drug therapies, much earlier. According to newer research, utilization of novel biomarkers to enhance diagnostic sensitivity has the potential to lead to enhanced risk stratification for CKD-MBD patients (Isa et al., 2025). In this manner, preventive treatment can be targeted with a view towards preventing complications and conserving health care resources in a significant manner, reflecting the economic rationale of investing in early detection strategies. The area of early detection techniques is evolving, with the potential for improved outcomes in those with metabolic bone disorders. With the advent of advanced technologies , such as metabolomics, new avenues for identifying biochemical alterations associated with MBD at an early stage and thus timely and targeted interventions are developing (Isa et al., 2025). Furthermore, the integration of screening programs in public health programs, , such as newborn screening for metabolic disorders, can enhance exposure and availability of early detection. It is particularly crucial where the disease is highly endemic. Through focusing on early diagnosis with novel techniques and caregiver education, healthcare systems can make a tangible impact on the lives of those suffering from metabolic bone disorders, such that interventions may be initiated before damage is permanent.

8.5. Treatment Options

Effective management of metabolic bone diseases is often a multidisciplinary process, typically tailored to the patient's unique disease process and overall medical picture. Treatment for these diseases frequently involves pharmacologic treatments, including bisphosphonates and hormone replacement therapy, that have been successful in increasing bone density and decreasing fracture risk in patients with osteoporosis and other metabolic bone diseases.

Additionally, vitamin D and calcium supplementation are crucial for prevention and therapy of these disorders, particularly in those at heightened risk for deficiency. Advances in our understanding of metabolic processes have also led investigators to explore new therapies that act specifically on a biochemical process used by bone metabolism and could provide new avenues for more successful treatments in the future. Aside from pharmacologic treatment, changing lifestyle helps in the treatment of metabolic bone diseases. Regular weight-bearing exercise has been shown to strengthen bones as well as overall health, an integral component of any therapeutic management. Dietary measures correcting low dietary intake of calcium and vitamin D also have a significant influence on bone strength, and studies have focused on the key role of a well-balanced diet with proper consumption of these nutrients. Also, interventions toward modifiable risk factors , such as obesity and smoking with longer counseling for lifestyles can also optimize outcomes.

Integrating these lifestyle changes into medical treatments not only allows for an integrated management regimen but also empowers patients with an active role in their own health. New treatments are under development to expand the repertoire of existing treatments for metabolic bone diseases because, with a better understanding of their multifactorial etiology, there is more to treat.

New medications, , such as monoclonal antibodies against certain proteins involved in bone resorption, are in ongoing research; these medications can be more targeted and efficient in bone density growth than previous medications. In addition, regenerative medicine interventions, , such as stem cell therapy, hold potential in the treatment of inherent problems in bone remodeling. The increasing knowledge of metabolic factors, , such as obesity, has evolved inter-disciplinary interventions involving both surgical and non-surgical interventions further reiterating the need for a prolonged strategy in treatment of these disorders (Christy et al., 2024; Luca et al., 2024). This evolving arena of treatment options holds much to improve the quality of life for those afflicted with metabolic bone disease (Figure 8.12).

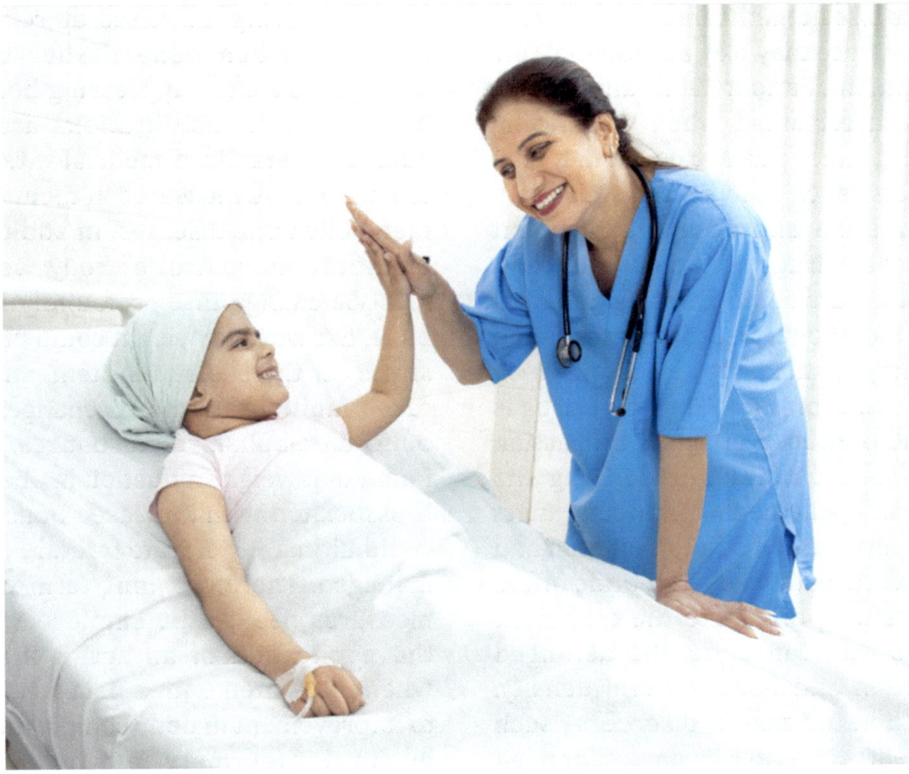

Figure 8.12. A nurse supporting a young cancer patient during recovery.

Source: https://hinduja-prod-assets.s3.ap-south-1.amazonaws.com/s3fs-public/2023-11/Cancer%20 treatment%20options.jpg.

8.5.1. Medications

The management of metabolic bone disease most frequently calls for multidimensional treatment, and drugs are the focal point of treatment modalities. Among the most commonly employed categories of medications are the bisphosphonates, which have been determined to effectively inhibit bone resorption by osteoclasts and thereby reduce fracture hazards in patients with osteoporosis. These drugs work through the mechanism of imitating the effect of pyrophosphate, a naturally occurring body substance that regulates bone metabolism. In addition, the discovery of denosumab, a monoclonal antibody against the receptor activator of nuclear factor-kappa B ligand (RANKL), has unveiled a novel approach to osteoporosis therapy. By inhibiting RANKL, denosumab strongly reduces osteoclast development and activity, further inhibiting bone loss. As more research is being carried out, it is important to evaluate the long-term outcomes of these medications on bone mineral density and overall skeletal health in various patient populations. Vitamin D analogues constitute another group of drugs that play a vital role in the treatment of metabolic bone disease. These are drugs that promote intestinal calcium absorption, which is necessary for normal maintenance of bones as well as to prevent conditions like Osteomalacia and rickets. In particular, calcitriol, the biologically active metabolite of vitamin D, has been found to be therapeutically useful in the management of secondary hyperparathyroidism in patients suffering from chronic kidney disease. This will improve bone mineralization and general skeletal health. In addition to vitamin D, calcium supplements are also administered to patients at risk of deficiency since they play an essential role in bone development. Patient needs and dietary intake must be ascertained when prescribing these supplements since excess calcium may lead to harmful effects , such as hypercalcemia, with stringent observation and dosage adjustment being required. New drugs used therapeutically, , such as tripeptide, are demonstrating potential in controlling metabolic disorders associated with bone health, particularly in persons with weight-related comorbidities. The novel drug is a dual GLP-1 and GIP receptor agonist, an action targeting metabolic pathways underlying the disorders , such as lipedema that indirectly affect bone health. By modulation of inflammation and inhibition of fibrotic pathways, tripeptide offers a potentially useful approach to the treatment of fat disorders that can underline deranged metabolic function and bone mineral density. Clinical research in the case of disorders , such as lipedema, is early and reveals an urgent need for clinical trials with rigorous investigation of safety and efficacy. With advancing therapy, the medical community must pace to achieve developments and integrate recent findings into best practice for proper treatment of metabolic bone disorders (Viana et al., 2025; Wasim et al., 2023).

8.5.2. Lifestyle Modifications

Lifestyle changes are critical in both the prevention and management of metabolic bone diseases since these are typically subject to diet patterns, exercise, and overall health practices. Inclusion of an adequate diet with vitamin D and calcium is needed to preserve bones, particularly as people age. Dietary items like milk, green leafy vegetables, and food fortified with nutrients like calcium, vitamin D, and magnesium are extremely helpful in ensuring the required amount of nutrients to preserve bone density. Reducing excessive consumption of sodium and caffeine, which can have negative effects on the absorption of calcium, is also advised. Weight-bearing exercises at regular intervals also strengthen bone tissues by promoting osteogenesis and suppressing bone resorption. Thus, lifestyle modifications are not only an adjunct to standard medical interventions but are preventive measures in themselves towards metabolic bone diseases. In addition to dietary modification, control of body weight is also a lifestyle change that profoundly influences the bone. Excess body weight could place additional stress on the skeletal system, and obesity can cause multiple hormonal changes, resulting in bone metabolism disturbances. Studies have found that weight reduction in obese individuals is associated with increased bone turnover and could ultimately elevate fracture risk if not well managed. Therefore, long-term weight control measures need to be employed. This includes the application of an active lifestyle, which, when integrated with a balanced diet, can lead to improvement in body composition and overall health. Furthermore, psychological problems being treated by counseling or support groups can assist in helping people overcome barriers to healthy weight, contributing to an integrated strategy to combat metabolic bone disease. Psychosocial problems also play an essential role in lifestyle modification compliance, indicating the need for individualized intervention methods. For instance, individuals who are not as wealthy and do not have access to resources , such as healthy food options or safe areas for exercise may become increasingly burdened with such adaptations. In addition, mental health plays a role; if an individual suffers from depression or anxiety, he or she may not be able to exercise adequately or maintain a healthy diet. Because behavioral health actually gets in the way of lifestyle change, the incorporation of mental health support into treatment strategies becomes vital. Effective intervention programs usually apply the multidisciplinary approach in a manner that ensures coordination among providers of health, nutritionists, and mental health workers towards establishing an environment that is maximized for sustainable improvement in health. By addressing the multi-faceted aspect of lifestyle modification, we are able to develop broad strategies to maximize bone health and minimize the danger posed by metabolic bone diseases, as revealed from research in this area (Figure 8.13).

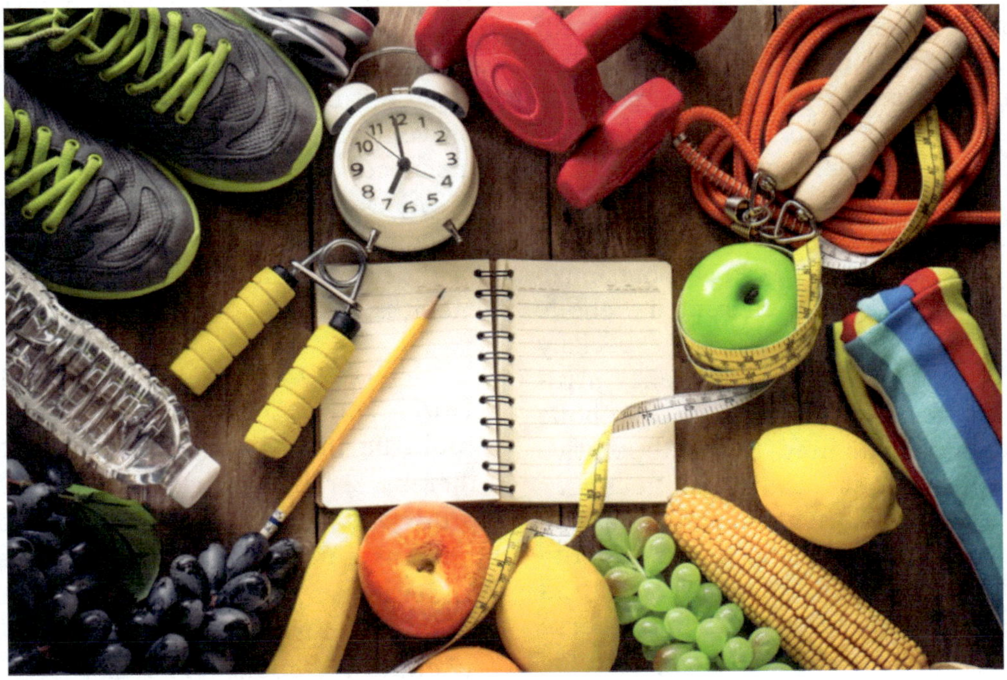

Figure 8.13. Healthy lifestyle tools for fitness and wellness.

Source: https://www.clinicaladvisor.com/wp-content/uploads/sites/11/2020/03/healthy.lifestyle.diet_.exercise_G_1084671586-1.jpg.

8.5.3. Surgical Interventions

Surgical interventions form a mandatory part of the treatment of metabolic bone diseases, particularly when the implementation of conservative modalities of care is not acceptable. In the majority of instances, the diseases result in structural weakening and deformity of the bones and require surgical treatment in the form of anatomical and functional correction. For instance, the treatments include fracture fixation or the correction of osteoporotic deformities via vertebroplasty or kyphoplasty. These operations not only alleviate the pain but also improve the overall structural stability of the bone system, and thus the quality of life of the patient. The efficiency of such surgical interventions is often supplemented by concomitant management strategies, , such as adequate nutritional supplementation and pharmacotherapy to maximize bone metabolism. Surgical intervention may also be advisable in some endocrine-related metabolic bone diseases, , such as primary hyperparathyroidism or thyroid-related bone loss. In cases where parathyroid adenomas are removed surgically, patients improve significantly in bone density post-surgery. An excellent example is the use of surgery in treatment of differentiated thyroid cancer (DTC), where local and regional recurrence can be treated efficiently by surgical resection followed by radioiodine ablation. While it is impossible in some cases to offer surgical treatment to all patients, particularly with widespread disease or comorbidity, an awareness of surgical options is important to maximize patient care and outcome, and any hope for recovery optimized by multidisciplinary therapy. Rehabilitation and care postoperatively are integral components of the surgical treatment process, particularly in surgical patients with metabolic bone disorders. Following surgery, the patients may require a customized rehabilitation program to regain mobility and strength while minimizing the risk of further fracture. The incorporation of infusion-detoxification and nutritional care post-surgery can also maximize recovery by resolving any current metabolic discrepancies. Such procedures are especially crucial in patients with concurrent intra-abdominal infections or comorbidities in bone metabolism, as highlighted by postoperative metabolic corrections studies. Collectively, effective surgical treatment, augmented by a comprehensive care program, has the ability to significantly maximize the treatment and outcome of patients suffering from diverse metabolic bone disorders, eventually leading to enhanced functional ability and quality of life.

8.6. Prevention Strategies

In the management of the increasing prevalence of diseases , such as osteoporosis, proper prevention practices for metabolic bone disorders are crucial. The approach must be holistic, incorporating lifestyle modifications that strengthen bones. Regular weight-bearing exercises are crucial in enhancing bone densification since they stimulate the activity of osteoblasts and suppress the development of osteoclasts. Furthermore, adequate consumption of vitamin D and calcium is also important, as these are crucial in maintaining bone form and function. Large-scale public health campaigns informing the population about nutrition and exercise would reduce the incidence of these disorders significantly. Through education empowerment and accessible resources, individuals can make evidence-based decisions that benefit their bone density and health, which is important for long-term prevention of metabolic bone disease (Ye et al., 2024). In addition to lifestyle modifications, medical interventions provide a critical option for prevention of metabolic bone disease. For instance, certain anti-diabetic medicines (ADA) were found to potentially be effective in maintaining bone structure during the treatment of underlying disorders , such as type 2 diabetes mellitus (T2DM).

Shared pathophysiological processes for T2DM and osteoporosis suggest that ADA could be involved in reducing fracture risk, thereby serving a dual function in treatment protocols. While ADA's impact on bone health remains to be definitively established, this underscores the necessity of conducting additional research elucidating their role in avoiding metabolic bone disease. Creating a plan that integrates pharmaceutical care and lifestyle change not only improves overall health care but also strengthens the skeletal system, which is particularly vital for patients with a tendency to fracture (Lee et al., 2022). Moreover, health practitioners have to take the initiative to screen and examine patients for risk factors of metabolic bone diseases. Subsequently identifying patient populations at risk based on comprehensive analyses, including family background and lifestyle factors, enables prevention through targeted means. Regular bone density screening enables early diagnosis and prompt intervention, with treatment programs tailored based on individual needs. In addition, backed by educational programs, these screening measures can empower patients to manage their bone health. By encouraging a culture of prevention and awareness, the healthcare systems can reduce the risks of metabolic bone disorders efficiently, leading to an improved population in the long run. The combination of lifestyle interventions, medical interventions, and preventive healthcare practices is an integrated approach to the prevention of metabolic bone disorders in contemporary society (Ye et al., 2024).

8.6.1. Nutritional Guidelines

Nutritional guidelines play a critical role in the management and prevention of metabolic bone disorders, particularly in individuals prone to conditions , such as osteoporosis and osteopenia. A balanced diet rich in essential nutrients is paramount for maintaining optimal bone health and density. Key dietary components include calcium and vitamin D, both of which are vital for bone formation and remodeling. Calcium supports bone structure, while vitamin D facilitates calcium absorption in the gut. Health organizations often recommend dietary sources , such as dairy products, green leafy vegetables, and fortified foods to meet these nutritional needs. Moreover, recent studies suggest that specific dietary patterns, , such as those that emphasize whole foods and minimize processed items, may further enhance bone health.

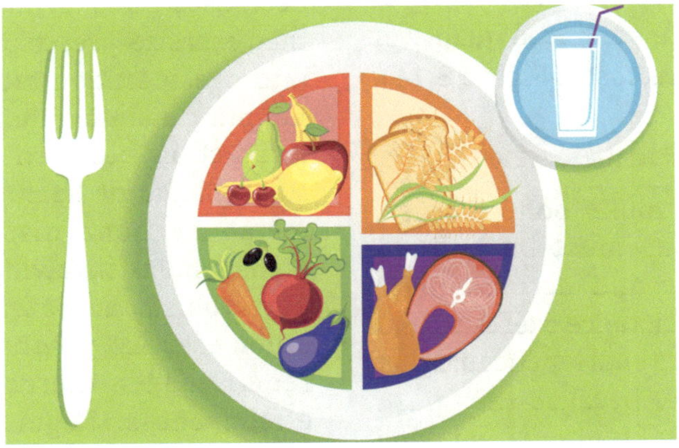

Figure 8.14. Balanced diet plate illustrating key food groups.

Source: https://communitycare.com/wp-content/uploads/2022/01/DietaryGuidelines.jpg.

Therefore, adhering to recommended nutritional guidelines can significantly impact the prevention and management of metabolic bone disorders. In addition to calcium and vitamin D, other micronutrients, including magnesium, potassium, and phosphorus, contribute to skeletal integrity. These minerals work synergistically to support bone metabolism and could mitigate the risk of metabolic bone disorders. For instance, magnesium has been found to influence osteoblast function, pivotal for bone formation. Likewise, potassium helps neutralize metabolic acids, which may otherwise lead to calcium loss and bone demineralization. Aside from individual nutrients, the overall dietary pattern, such as,, such as a Mediterranean or DASH diet—has been associated with improved bone health due to their anti-inflammatory properties and high antioxidant content, promoting systemic health. Public health initiatives should, therefore, emphasize comprehensive nutritional guidelines that include a broad spectrum of macro and micronutrients essential for bone maintenance and repair. Moreover, the influence of dietary habits on metabolic bone disorders is intertwined with lifestyle factors, , such as physical activity and body weight management. Nutritional guidelines often advocate for a combined approach that incorporates a healthy diet with regular exercise. Weight-bearing activities, in conjunction with a nutrient-dense diet, have been shown to enhance peak bone mass and reduce the risk of fractures in later life. Individuals suffering from obesity or metabolic syndrome are at increased risk for developing conditions like osteoporosis, which can be exacerbated by poor dietary choices and sedentary lifestyles. Therefore, intertwining nutritional guidelines with lifestyle modifications, such as,, such as promoting active living and encouraging healthy eating—can create a robust framework for the prevention and management of metabolic bone disorders. Implementing these holistic strategies can significantly improve health outcomes for at-risk populations, leading to enhanced quality of life and reduced healthcare costs (Figure 8.14).

8.6.2. Exercise Recommendations

In the treatment of metabolic bone disease, exercise recommendations must be tailored to make bones stronger and accommodate individual restrictions. Resistance exercises and weight-bearing activities are vital for encouraging bone strength and density because they push osteoblasts into more activity, stimulating bone formation. Moderate-level exercise, , such as walking, jogging, or resistance exercises, can enhance bone density and general physical function significantly. In particular, the Womens Sports Foundations report, Her Life Depends on It III, indicates the importance of exercise for promoting wholesome results for individuals, generally for women who tend to weather particular challenges for their bone strength as they age. An organized exercise program has the potential to decrease the risk posed by metabolic bone disorders by focusing on both physical capacity and social determinants of health to promote increased participation in active living. Flexibility and balance exercises are paramount among individuals with metabolic bone disorders because they can reduce the occurrence of falls and associated fractures. Exercise programs , such as tai chi and yoga enhance not only coordination but also general well-being. Moreover, muscle strength significantly influences the functional capability of patients with compromised bone health. The contribution of vitamin D to muscle function also reinforces the use of exercise as a management strategy for metabolic bone disease. Available evidence suggests that adequate vitamin D levels correlate with improved muscle function, highlighting the symbiotic relationship between bone and muscle health. As highlighted in a number of studies, , such as (Bover et al., 2017), an inadequate vitamin D status could aggravate conditions , such as weakness in muscles and decreased bone formation rates, thus requiring that exercise prescriptions be designed taking into consideration the nutrient aspect as well. Adopting an integrated approach which stresses interaction between exercise, nutrition, and surveillance of health is critical in managing metabolic bone disorders. Interdisciplinary management involving health care providers, nutritionists, and exercise specialists can help tailor exercise programs to individual patient requirements, thereby enhancing safety and effectiveness. Regular education about the benefits of exercise needs to be emphasized to overcome the sedentary lifestyle that is prevalent in high-risk populations. Frequent assessment and modification of exercise regimens also need to be done to adjust to changes in health status and functional capacity. Greater adherence to these exercise recommendations can play a notable part in improving the quality of life of patients with metabolic bone disease, and this is according to the evidence given by Sabo et al. (2015) of the vital role sport and physical exercise play in creating a healthier society overall.

8.6.3. Regular Health Screenings

Regular health screening is a cornerstone in the diagnosis and treatment of metabolic bone disorders , such as osteoporosis. Screening, sometimes involving bone mineral density (BMD) scans, enables clinicians to assess the quality and health of an individual's bones. Screening of high-risk patients prior to the development of clinical symptoms can enable timely intervention, either by modifying lifestyle or through medication. Given the severe impact of osteoporosis on the aged population, especially among women, continuance of routine screening is necessary to maintain bone health and minimize the risk of fractures. Finally, an informed habit of routine screening enables individuals to take charge of their health and makes them aware of their bones. This proactive behavior is fundamental to combat so-called silent onset of metabolic bone diseases. Besides, gaps in the access to health service between groups highlight the need for regular health screening. Osteoporosis has been found through studies to be handicapped in minority groups by barriers of limited access to health care providers and reduced health insurance coverage, thereby limiting their screening efforts and awareness regarding osteoporosis risk. For instance, a study of Korean American women noted that although bone health and awareness of screening was heightened among peri-menopausal women, significant gaps in knowledge existed in access to healthcare services across different ages. Specifically, 61.9% of the study population's BMD were below normal, indicating a critical requirement for health education and screening interventions in risk groups, with top priority to be given to those in the post-menopausal age group. Bridging these gaps is essential to improving health outcomes for metabolic bone disease. To achieve the optimum gain from regular health screening, concerted efforts must be directed towards ensuring that the health provider is in a position to effectively communicate the value of screening to their patient. Professional guidance plays a pivotal role in bridging the gap between perceived patient attitudes and recommended health behavior, particularly in relation to bone health. As indicated in previous research, there is often a gap between patient awareness of the risk and medical practitioners' recommendations. Accordingly, ongoing education and counseling need to be performed to enhance patients' knowledge regarding their osteoporosis risk factors, screening behavior, and treatment. Having a supportive healthcare environment that is focused on routine screening will maximize patient outcomes and ensure increased more active involvement in preventive health measures, leading ultimately to healthier aging and decreased fracture rates attributable to metabolic bone disease (Figure 8.15).

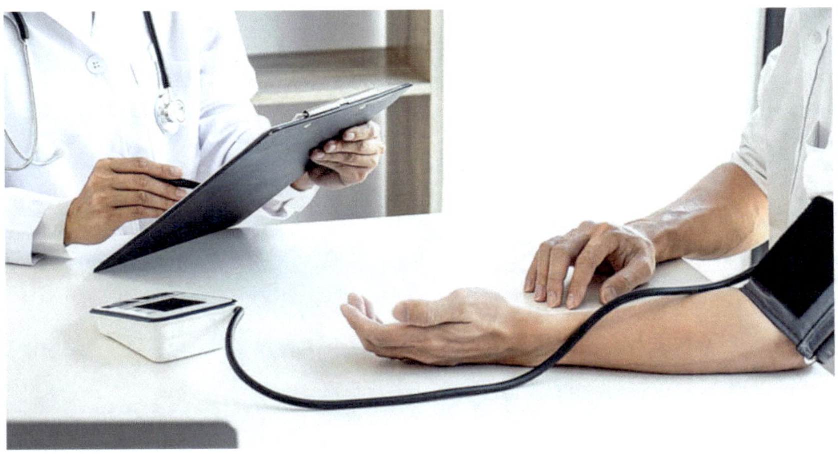

Figure 8.15. Routine health check-up for early disease detection.

Source: https://myclnq.co/wp-content/uploads/2020/12/why-regular-health-screening-is-important-for-everyone.jpg.

CLOSER LOOK

BONE DISORDERS

Bone disorders refer to a wide range of conditions that affect the strength, structure, and function of bones in the human body. These disorders can result from genetic factors, nutritional deficiencies, hormonal imbalances, aging, or other underlying diseases. Healthy bones require a proper balance of calcium, vitamin D, phosphorus, and hormonal regulation to maintain their density and strength. When this balance is disrupted, bone disorders can occur, leading to pain, deformity, and increased risk of fractures. One of the most common bone disorders is osteoporosis, a condition characterized by low bone mass and deterioration of bone tissue, making bones brittle and prone to fractures—especially in the hips, spine, and wrists. It is most prevalent among postmenopausal women due to decreased estrogen levels. Osteomalacia (in adults) and rickets (in children) are caused by vitamin D deficiency, leading to soft and weak bones. These conditions are often linked to poor dietary intake or limited sun exposure.

Paget's disease of bone is another chronic disorder that disrupts normal bone remodeling, causing bones to become enlarged and misshapen. Osteogenesis imperfecta, a genetic disorder, results in extremely fragile bones due to defective collagen production. Bone infections like osteomyelitis, and bone cancers such as osteosarcoma, also fall under the category of bone disorders. Preventing and managing bone disorders involves ensuring adequate intake of calcium and vitamin D, regular weight-bearing exercise, avoiding smoking and excessive alcohol, and, in some cases, medication or hormone therapy. Early diagnosis and lifestyle modifications play a crucial role in minimizing complications and maintaining bone health. The bone disorders can significantly impact mobility and quality of life. Awareness, proper nutrition, and preventive care are essential to support lifelong skeletal health.

SUMMARY

Metabolic bone disease research highlights the complexity and multidimensionality of these conditions, their significance in public health. An understanding of the mechanisms by which various metabolic conditions, , such as obesity and diabetes, can affect bone health is central to the development of effective treatments and prevention protocols. Research illuminated the necessity for precise methodologies, , such as the identification of stable housekeeping genes for gene expression analysis in bone. Such detail not only enhances the precision of outcomes in biological research but also provides important insight into metabolic bone diseases' mechanisms, fostering advances in clinical practice and therapeutic approaches (Ai et al., 2024). Furthermore, CKD implications are a key aspect of metabolic bone diseases where mineral and bone changes come together to form an individual clinical syndrome known as CKD-MBD. Patient CKD bone frailty is additionally complicated by mineral metabolism derangements, including phosphorus and calcium balance derangements, and also disturbances in hormone status. Findings of the most recent studies indicate a highly prevalent rate of secondary hyperparathyroidism and vitamin D deficiency among affected individuals, with likely resultant severe complications. Thus, early diagnosis and specific management strategies are necessary to reverse the long-term consequences of CKD-MBD and improve patient outcomes (Dod et al., 2024). Finally, treating metabolic bone disorders must follow an integrated strategy that includes research, medical practice, and public health actions. For the future, interdisciplinary cooperation between researchers, clinicians, and policymakers must be encouraged in order to respond appropriately to the challenges presented by these diseases. With further advances in scientific knowledge, it also becomes more evident that integrative strategies cutting across both preventive and treatment interventions will be vital for meeting the challenge of metabolic bone disease burden. Public education and healthcare provider education will also play a key role in the promotion of bone health in at-risk populations. Lastly, synthesizing these perspectives can guide future prevention and management of metabolic bone diseases that can contribute important quality of life for those affected.

A sound understanding of metabolic bone diseases (MBD) is crucial in determining effective treatment avenues and improved patient outcomes. Central to MBD is the dynamic between vascular health and bone metabolism, and most notably between CKD populations. The bone-vascular axis is a new paradigm that elucidates how interruptions in bone metabolism can lead to pathological vascular changes, , such as vascular calcification (VC) in patients with CKD. This occurrence is particularly notable due to the commonality of VC within this population, wherein vascular smooth muscle cells transform into osteoblastic cells, prompted by uremic toxins. Patient care will have to be improved by putting more emphasis on understanding the complex interactions as well as the drug targets that can avert undesirable bone and vascular consequences (Shen et al., 2024). Yet another key topic under the general rubric of metabolic bone disease is hormonal regulation of the condition of bone. For instance, the ovarian function dynamics in dairy cattle, more precisely the incidence of ovarian follicular cysts, yield valuable information on the endocrine and metabolic derangements that can potentially impact overall reproductive and bone health. It has been demonstrated through various studies that such cysts are associated with defects in hormonal secretion and receptor expression. Hormones , such as progesterone, estrogen, and insulin exhibit altered levels in cystic follicles compared to their normal counterparts, which reflect a delicate interaction between metabolic pathways and bone remodeling processes. Such findings point toward the significance of an in-depth inquiry of hormonal pathways towards the pathophysiology of MBD and underscores potential directions for therapeutic interventions (Xu et al., 2023). Lastly, a comprehensive framework for metabolic bone diseases ought to unite both systemic metabolic determinants and local mechanisms at the skeletal level. It should be mentioned that circulating factors and skeletal tissues secretory mechanisms influence bone strength and mineralization. Notably, sclerostin, a protein factor of bone remodeling, is significant to mediate between bone health and vascular calcification. By reducing the production of sclerostin, it is possible to treat the osteogenic trans differentiation of vascular smooth muscle cells and hence oppose VC. Consequently, targeting such molecular pathways presents a promising strategy towards maximizing the prognosis of patients at risk of developing metabolic bone disease and associated cardiovascular complications (Shen et al., 2024).

References

1. Agarwal, A., Dwivedi, S., Tyagi, P., & Dwivedi, D. (2025). Study the effect of lifestyle modifications on fetomaternal outcomes in gestational diabetes mellitus. *International Journal of Reproduction, Contraception, Obstetrics and Gynecology, 14*(2), 586–592. https://doi.org/10.18203/2320-1770.ijrcog20250198 (accessed on 13th June 2025).
2. Ai, Y., Peng, K., Li, C., Zhang, J., Wang, G., Wang, B., & Huang, E. (2024). Assessment of reference genes stability in cortical bone of obese and diabetic mice. *Diabetes, Metabolic Syndrome and Obesity, 17*, 1081–1091. https://www.semanticscholar.org/paper/c5cb3c4f598e5fd60a8d698299b03f6007acc601 (accessed on 13th June 2025).
3. Arai, H., Maeda, K., Wakabayashi, H., Naito, T., Konishi, M., Assantachai, P., Auyeung, W. T., et al. (2023). Diagnosis and outcomes of cachexia in Asia: Working consensus report from the Asian Working Group for Cachexia. *Journal of Cachexia, Sarcopenia and Muscle, 14*, 1949–1958. https://www.semanticscholar.org/paper/ce0f441bd2d89af4eba9dbb704cb2e13295556c4 (accessed on 13th June 2025).
4. Aron, C., & Ramya, A. (2024). Clinical insights into movement disorders in children: A review of etiology, diagnosis, and treatment options. *IP International Journal of Medical Pediatrics and Oncology.* https://www.semanticscholar.org/paper/892427a3ac85cee5e2177d05a943cbeb68d0f248 (accessed on 13th June 2025).
5. Busetto, L., Dicker, D., Azran, C., Batterham, R. L., Farpour-Lambert, N., Fried, M., Hjelmesæth, J., Kinzl, J., Leitner, D. R., Makaronidis, J. M., Schindler, K., Toplak, H., & Yumuk, V. (2017). Practical Recommendations of the Obesity Management Task Force of the European Association for the Study of Obesity for Post-Bariatric Surgery Medical Management. *Obesity facts, 10*(6), 597–632. https://doi.org/10.1159/000481825(accessed on 13th June 2025).
6. Balali-Mood, M., Naseri, K., Tahergorabi, Z., Khazdair, M. R., & Sadeghi, M. (2021). Toxic mechanisms of five heavy metals: Mercury, lead, chromium, cadmium, and arsenic. *Frontiers in Pharmacology, 12.* https://doi.org/10.3389/fphar.2021.643972 (accessed on 13th June 2025).
7. Bover, J., Carrero, J. J., Molina, P., Ureña Torres, P., Chauveau, P., & Mazzaferro, S. (2017). Vitamin D, a modulator of musculoskeletal health in chronic kidney disease. https://core.ac.uk/download/153367338.pdf (accessed on 13th June 2025).
8. Combet, Emilie and Buckton, Christina (2014) Micronutrient deficiencies, vitamin pills and nutritional supplements. Medicine, 14(2), pp. 66-72. (doi: 10.1016/j.mpmed.2014.11.002) (accessed on 13th June 2025).
9. Dalle Carbonare, L., Mottes, M., & Valenti, M. T. (2021). Medication-related osteonecrosis of the jaw (MRONJ): Are antiresorptive drugs the main culprits or only accomplices? The triggering role of vitamin D deficiency. https://core.ac.uk/download/388583943.pdf (accessed on 13th June 2025).
10. Fadel, N., Elsayed, I. A., Mostafa, D., & Morsi, F. T. (2024). Prevalence and pattern of mineral bone disorders in patients with end-stage renal disease and the impact of diabetic status and type of phosphate binders on these disorders. *Medicine Updates.* https://www.semanticscholar.org/paper/e3da1e469466c81b44b20cea0080d15b34ccbb42 (accessed on 13th June 2025).
11. Gopalakrishnan, R., Vijayakumar, P. G., Seethalakshmi, S., & Jeris, L. W. (2025). Early detection and management of glucose-6-phosphate dehydrogenase deficiency through newborn

screening: A case study and public health perspective. *Asian Journal of Biochemistry, Genetics and Molecular Biology.* https://www.semanticscholar.org/paper/9b0cd231c3ca705e1225907dd135d538cb405d55 (accessed on 13th June 2025).

12. Zehra, N., Jafri, L., Kirmani, S., & Khan, A. H. (2021). X-linked hypophosphatemic osteomalacia with PHEX mutation presenting late in Pakistan. *Annals of medicine and surgery (2012), 62,* 244–248. https://doi.org/10.1016/j.amsu.2021.01.067(accessed on 13th June 2025).
13. Kibler, M. (2025). Self-reported dietary behavior and its effects on healthcare expenditures for wellness participants at the University of Kentucky. https://core.ac.uk/download/pdf/6551308.pdf (accessed on 13th June 2025).
14. Lee, W. L., Wang, P. H., Yang, S. T., Liu, C. H., Chang, W. H., & Lee, F. (2022). To do one and to get more: Part I. Diabetes and bone. *Journal of the Chinese Medical Association: JCMA.* https://www.semanticscholar.org/paper/465285466da0b8d4917889120847e65fa39dd7c5 (accessed on 13th June 2025).
15. Mach, F., Baigent, C., Catapano, A. L., Koskinas, K. C., Casula, M., Badimón, L., Chapman, M. J., et al. (2019). 2019 ESC/EAS guidelines for the management of dyslipidemias: Lipid modification to reduce cardiovascular risk. *European Heart Journal, 41*, 111–188. https://doi.org/10.1093/eurheartj/ehz455 (accessed on 13th June 2025).
16. Maj, A., & Warno, M. (2024). Obesity as a civilization threat of the XXI century. The impact of obesity on individual functions of human organ systems. https://core.ac.uk/download/613694732.pdf (accessed on 13th June 2025).
17. Moro, L. (2024). A case study of hypophosphatasia: An underdiagnosed bone disorder characterized by low alkaline phosphatase. *Journal of the American Association of Nurse Practitioners.* https://www.semanticscholar.org/paper/6751aa328155bb09df6d170ec85ddecacb7461a2 (accessed on 13th June 2025).
18. Murray, C. J. L., Ikuta, K. S., Sharara, F., Swetschinski, L. R., Robles Aguilar, G., Gray, A. P., Han, C., et al. (2022). Global burden of bacterial antimicrobial resistance in 2019: A systematic analysis. *The Lancet, 399*, 629–655. https://doi.org/10.1016/s0140-6736(21)02724-0 (accessed on 13th June 2025).
19. Onishchenko, N., Karganov, M., Alchinova, I., Cherepov, A., Stepanova, O. I., Metelkin, A. A., Nikolskaya, A., et al. (2024). Blood and bone marrow cell disorders in the stages of progressive diabetes in mice. *Russian Journal of Transplantology and Artificial Organs.* https://www.semanticscholar.org/paper/1b5e6273adaef5fa7225349aaae72ca3665d8051 (accessed on 13th June 2025).
20. Rinella, M. E., Neuschwander-Tetri, B. A., Siddiqui, M. S., Abdelmalek, M. F., Caldwell, S. H., Barb, D., Kleiner, D. E., et al. (2023). AASLD practice guidance on the clinical assessment and management of nonalcoholic fatty liver disease. *Hepatology, 77*, 1797–1835. https://doi.org/10.1097/hep.0000000000000323 (accessed on 13th June 2025).
21. Sumathy, S. (2007). A study on serum prolactin in reduced bone mineral density. https://core.ac.uk/download/235653526.pdf (accessed on 13th June 2025).
22. Thacher, T., & Oberhelman, S. (2013). Vitamin D deficiency in the 21st century: An overview. https://www.semanticscholar.org/paper/ce4b5a201972dc7a3dcebca5e202913062ac09fc (accessed on 13th June 2025).

23. Vaish, R., Vaishya, K., & Iyengar, K. (2024). Metabolic syndrome and its impact on bone and joint health: A comprehensive review. *Apollo Medicine.* https://www.semanticscholar.org/paper/993898cff4a8b8d19bcbd02f5ebf81e49db0961f (accessed on 13th June 2025).
24. Wasim, M., Musani, M., Siddiqi, H. S., Muddasir, S., Amin, B. K., & Arain, F. (2023). Temporal lobe epilepsy with hippocampus sclerosis: Prevalence, etiology, and treatment options with herbal medicines. *Pakistan Journal of Neurological Sciences.* https://www.semanticscholar.org/paper/b812b990d99a934de9765448eecafb0332d575a5 (accessed on 13th June 2025).
25. Xu, X., Bai, J., Liu, K., Xiao, L., Qin, Y., Gao, M., & Liu, Y. (2023). Association of metabolic and endocrine disorders with bovine ovarian follicular cysts. *Animals, 13.* https://www.semanticscholar.org/paper/c17f08cbd85cd528be6f6fc94b0201813f8f5d97 (accessed on 13th June 2025).

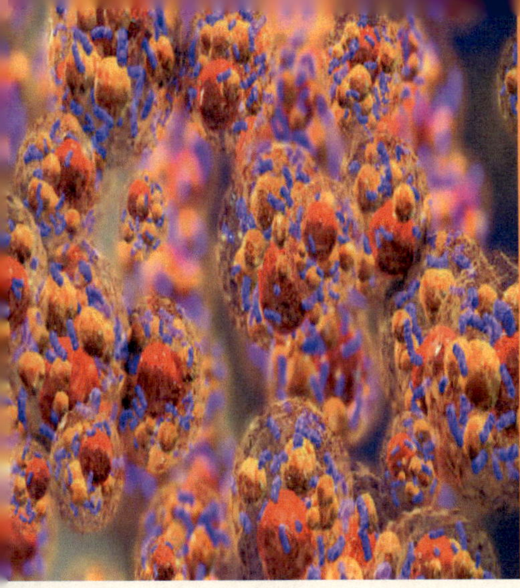

Chapter 9

LIPID METABOLISM DISORDERS

Contents

Introduction..........277
9.1. Types of Lipid Metabolism Disorders..........281
9.2. Causes of Lipid Metabolism Disorders..........285
9.3. Symptoms and Diagnosis..........289
9.4. Impact on Health..........294
9.5. Treatment Alternatives..........298
9.6. Research and Advances..........302
Summary..........308
References..........310

Introduction

Lipid metabolism disorders are a polyphyletic collection of conditions characterized by aberrant metabolism of lipids, which are essential molecules involved in numerous physiological processes. Lipid metabolism disorders may be either genetic defects in lipid metabolism enzymes or secondary phenomena secondary to other diseases, , such as diabetes or obesity. It is essential to identify the complex biochemical pathways that regulate lipid metabolism to understand the effects of disruption so that severe health complications like cardiovascular diseases, fatty liver disease, and metabolic syndrome can be identified to develop them. In addition, enhanced research has also revealed the multifactorial etiology of such disorders and has underscored the contribution of genetic, environmental, and lifestyle factors towards their pathogenesis. Healthcare providers' awareness of lipid metabolism disorders is extremely important as it informs their clinical acumen and response to the diagnosis and treatment of the same in the patient group (François et al., 2019). The consequences of lipid metabolism disorders extend beyond individual health risk and spill over into public health concerns on a broader scale. As the level of obesity increases globally, levels of associated lipid disturbances also increase, and therefore a multidisciplinary approach to prevention and management is required. Developments in metabolic science have shed more light on the role of gut microbiota in lipid metabolism, offering new insights into how dietary maneuvers might prevent or aggravate these conditions. The microbiota-gut-brain axis has also been found to be an extremely promising field of study, linking microbial regulation of lipid metabolism with genetic and environmental psychiatric and neurodegenerative effects (Cryan et al., 2019).

Thus, prevention methods targeting healthy lifestyle choices as well as intestinal health become increasingly vital in combating or regulating lipid metabolism disorders, highlighting the merits of a holistic regime for wellness. Educational and behavioral therapy for lipid metabolism disorders plays a key role in improving patient outcomes and reducing the economic cost of such disorders. Public health interventions must emphasize the importance of diet, physical activity, and regular health checks to detect and regulate risk factors at an early stage. Further, progress in genetics and biochemistry research is bringing with it the promise of personalized medicine approaches, tailoring the therapy depending on individual lipid profiles as well as genetic susceptibility. This demands ongoing interdisciplinarity among clinicians, researchers, and public health experts to ensure that improving knowledge is translated into effective preventive care and therapeutic treatments. As our understanding of lipid metabolism increases, so too must the training systems, prevention, and treatment systems for these diseases to achieve an active healthcare modus operandi instead of a passive (François et al., 2019).

Definition of Lipid Metabolism

Lipid metabolism is the biochemical process through which lipids, fats, and steroids are synthesized and degraded in the body. The complex system encompasses several pathways, like degradation of fatty acids by β-oxidation and synthesis of lipids by lipogenesis. The functions are required for energy production, cellular activity, and metabolic homeostasis. Lipid metabolism upsets could lead to a variety of disorders, including type 2 diabetes and obesity, and hence it is essential to research these processes at the cellular and molecular levels. Notably, recent evidence shows that a group of lipid metabolites including oxysterols is intimately connected with metabolic disease, impacting both health and disease conditions of individuals, particularly those with obesity and metabolic syndrome, as revealed in recent studies (et al., 2015). Moreover, lipid metabolism is controlled by numerous hormonal cues and transcription factors, which regulate the function of critical metabolic enzymes. Insulin, for instance, plays a crucial role in stimulating lipogenesis while inhibiting lipolysis to permit storage of fat within adipose tissue. Glucagon, by contrast, stimulates the breakdown of stored lipids with the release of fatty acids into the circulation for energy utilization. The balance between these two opposing mechanisms is extremely critical; its disruption can lead to fat deposition and metabolic dysregulation. An understanding of these hormonal pathways sheds light on the complex system of interactions that define lipid metabolisms function to maintain energy balance, thereby shedding light on potential therapeutic interventions to manage lipid metabolism disorders (Borro et al., 2017). Beyond energy balance, the importance of lipid metabolism affects various physiological systems including cardiovascular function and inflammatory processes. Dyslipidemia conditions have the ability to cause atherosclerosis and other cardiovascular diseases because high levels of certain lipids might be used for plaque formation within the arterial walls. Moreover, inflammation typically occurs along with deranged lipid metabolism, whose synergistic effect makes metabolic syndrome worse. Some lipid species, for instance, oxysterols, have been identified as major biomarkers and mediators of these pathological processes by several studies. Characterization of such lipid metabolites not only assists in unraveling the lipid metabolism disorder processes but also signifies their potential utility for clinical diagnostics as well as therapeutic follow-up (et al., 2015). Thus, full comprehension of lipid metabolism induces advancements in personalized medicine approaches to fight metabolic disease (Borro et al., 2017) (Figure 9.1).

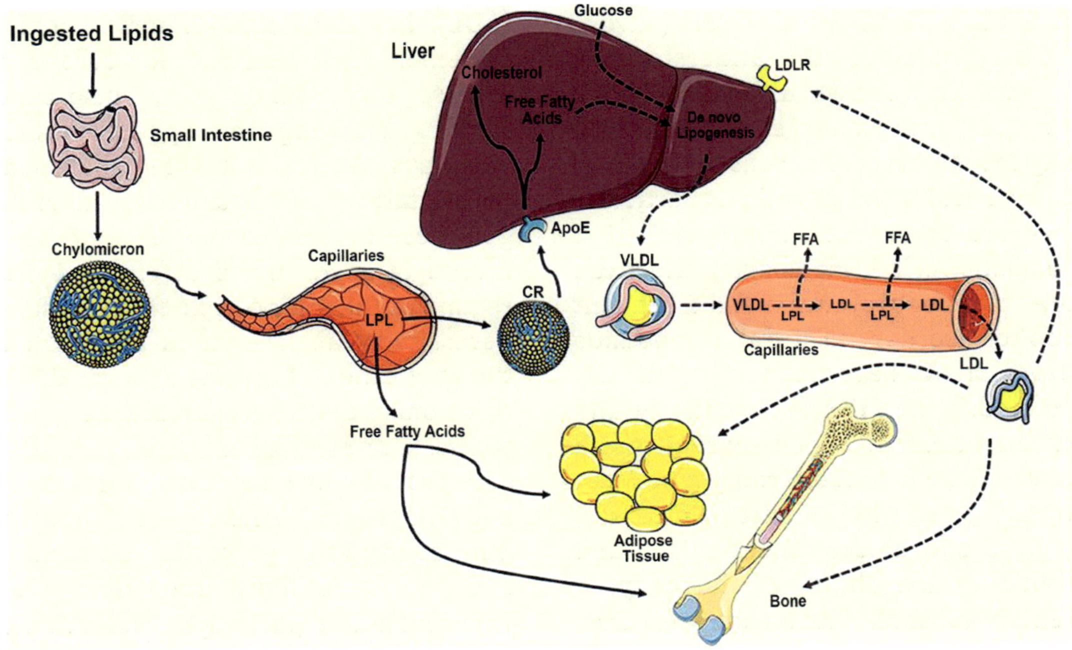

Figure 9.1. Overview of lipid metabolism and tissue distribution.

Source: lekos NS, Moorer MC and Riddle RC (2020) Dual Effects of Lipid Metabolism on Osteoblast Function. Front. Endocrinol. 11:578194. doi: 10.3389/fendo.2020.578194

Importance of Lipid Metabolism in Human Health

Metabolism of lipids plays a vital role in maintaining human well-being, influencing numerous biological processes and cellular functions. Triglycerides, phospholipids, and cholesterol constitute the bulk of fat, which is not only a store of energy but also a key structural cell membrane material that lends strength and fluidity. Lipids are also signaling molecules that mediate important physiological responses, including hormone release and inflammation modulation. Regulated lipid metabolism is required for optimal metabolic health because there is a disturbance in this process that leads to unprecedented health issues like obesity and cardiovascular disease complications. For instance, the interaction between gut microbiota and lipid metabolism exhibits the complexity of these relationships, where dietary lipids are able to influence microbial diversity and the production of bioactive lipids, which in turn regulate metabolic processes and well-being (Bourdeau-Julien et al., 2023). The function of lipid metabolism has also increased in obesity, now a global health crisis with extensive impacts. Obesity triggers a cascade of metabolic dysregulations, particularly in the phosphatidylinositol 3-kinases (PI3K)/protein kinase B (AKT) signaling pathway. The pathway heavily controls the metabolism of glucose and lipids by mediating insulin's effect on target tissues. When lipid metabolism is disrupted, it can potentially lead to insulin resistance, which contributes to the establishment of type 2 diabetes and other metabolic disorders (Savova et al., 2023). Therefore, the understanding of lipid complexity allows us to determine probable targets for the management of obesity, underlining the importance of considering lipid homeostasis in health and disease. Of particular significance are therapeutic approaches that involve modulation of lipid metabolism, which can lead to new forms of prevention and treatment for metabolic disorders. Natural compounds derived from plants have been of significant interest to modify the PI3K/AKT pathway, and their implications extend to obesity control and metabolic regulation. Natural compounds can modify a variety of physiological processes, including lipid and glucose metabolism, and thereby enhance the ability of the body to maintain energy balance. With ongoing research, the understanding of how lipid metabolism overlaps with dietary habits, gut microbiota, and metabolic signaling pathways will facilitate the development of targeted interventions that promote healthier lipid profiles and minimize the hazards associated with lipid metabolism disorders (Bourdeau-Julien et al., 2023; Savova et al., 2023). Thus, the multi-dimensional approach illustrates the central position of lipid metabolism in maintaining human health and preventing chronic diseases.

Overview of Lipid Metabolism Disorders

Lipid metabolism disorders are a general class of diseases disabling the body's function of metabolizing fats, and their effects can be most harmful to overall health in the form of cardiovascular disease, diabetes, and obesity. The human body relies on a complex system of enzymes, hormones, and metabolic pathways to regulate lipid levels. If any component of these fails, it can cause an imbalance either in the form of more lipid deposition or inadequate breakdown. For example, familial hypercholesterolemia is an inherited lipid abnormality caused by an elevation of the level of low-density lipoprotein (LDL) cholesterol that renders an individual at extremely increased risk for coronary artery disease. Understanding such disorders would involve studying the specific biochemical pathways involved in lipid metabolism and thus necessitate a multidisciplinary effort including genetics, biochemistry, as well as clinical investigation to arrive at effective treatment regimens. Disorder of lipid metabolism analysis necessitates an integrated approach through the application of diverse analysis devices, e.g., multi-omics tools. Recent research indicates that biomarkers of cardiometabolic disease (CMD) can provide insights into lipid metabolism and disorders. These biomarkers derived from sources like genomics and metabolomics can provide insights into lipid processing and regulation pathways. The complexity of lipid metabolism is such that examination of individual omics sequentially will often give only a limited picture, but by integrating these data types, a more comprehensive understanding of metabolic interactions with the potential to identify CMD biomarkers is obtained. Therefore, continued research on lipid metabolism in an integrative approach has the potential to better diagnose and treat patients suffering from such conditions (Argano et al., 2019). Moreover, the implications of gender differences in lipid metabolism disorders are being put forward and are worthy of more research. Research has shown that the effect of lipid imbalance can differ markedly according to gender, perhaps due to the interaction of biological, psychological, and sociocultural factors. An understanding of how lipid metabolism may differ not only between individuals but also between the two sexes can render prevention and therapeutic interventions more effective. For instance, women may acquire lipid disorders in a different way, particularly at the time of the menstrual cycle or menopause, and this points to the need for gender-sensitive research techniques when studying lipid metabolism disorders. Revisiting these differences is crucial as it can lead to gender-sensitive interventions that are more attuned to the biological realities of each sex, which in turn can lead to improved clinical outcomes and quality of care (Buxton et al., 2011) (Figure 9.2).

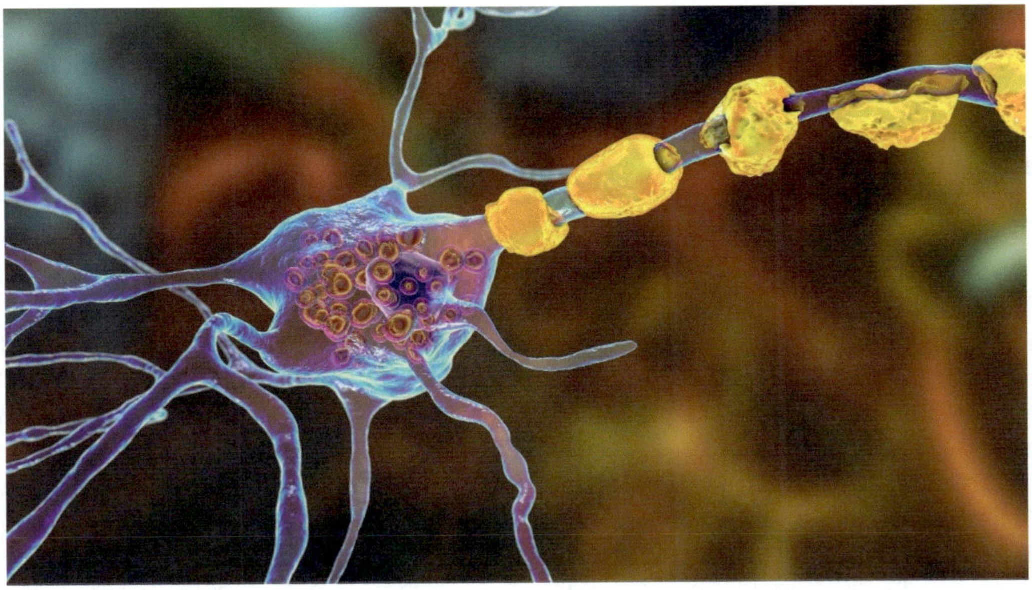

Figure 9.2. A neuron affected by lipid metabolism disorder.

Source: https://medlineplus.gov/images/LipidMetabolismDisorders_share.jpg.

9.1. Types of Lipid Metabolism Disorders

Lipid metabolism disorders form a collection of illnesses characterized by abnormal body lipid levels, leading to a number of illnesses. They are best reflected by dyslipidemia, lipidosis, and fatty liver disease. Dyslipidemia, a qualitative or quantitative deviation of lipids in blood circulation, typically manifests as elevated levels of low-density lipoprotein (LDL) cholesterol or triglycerides, which markedly enhances the chances of cardiovascular diseases. Diseases , such as familial hypercholesterolemia demonstrate genetic dyslipidemia where lipid processing is disrupted by genetic changes. Further, conditions , such as lipidosis, involve the abnormally stored lipids in tissues, leading to cellular dysfunction and organ damage. These include diseases , such as Gaucher's and Fabry disease, thereby emphasizing the importance of diagnosing lipid metabolism disorders to implement proper management strategies to prevent morbidity in such conditions. The second basic element of lipid metabolism disorders is the connection of these conditions with metabolic syndrome, i.e., a group of conditions including hypertension, glucose intolerance, and obesity. Their connection with obesity is particularly striking because excess fat accumulation can alter lipid metabolism to exacerbate underlying disorders. Clinically, obesity was identified as a significant risk factor for developing type II diabetes mellitus, which in turn is usually associated with dyslipidemia. Experimental studies have demonstrated that this relationship can also relate some genetic predispositions to lipid metabolism disturbances and atherosclerosis and thus complicate the health picture. Moreover, increased adiposity can impact circulating lipids through several hormonal mechanisms and illustrate the interdependence of lipid metabolism and regulation of body weight. Consequently, understanding the fundamental mechanisms is necessary for the treatment of the broader implications of lipid derangements in treating metabolic syndrome. Additionally, more recent research shows potential relationships between abnormalities of lipid metabolism and neurologic disorders. New data indicate that primary headache, particularly migraine, may be an initial symptom of lipid metabolism disturbance and atherosclerosis. With the rising prevalence of obesity, the prevalence of headache disorders, particularly in children, also rises, building a close relationship between adiposity, lipid imbalance, and headache development. Investigation into the biochemical pathways in migraines has identified a number of suspected risk factors related to lipid metabolism, including abnormal adiponectin levels and the presence of inflammatory markers. These findings remind us of the complex interaction between neurological health and lipid metabolism and suggest that the management of lipid disorders may have implications for preventing or treating chronic pain disease. Ultimately, continued research into these connections might reveal novel insights into the complicated nature of lipid metabolism disorder and its larger impact on health, which would necessitate multidisciplinary intervention and prevention (Bakshtanovskaya et al., 2024; Sordyl et al., 2020).

9.1.1. Hyperlipidemia

Hyperlipidemia is a critical metabolic disorder characterized by elevated blood levels of lipids, usually in the form of increased cholesterol and triglycerides. As a disease, hyperlipidemia is increasingly common in contemporary society, where unfit diets and a sedentary lifestyle are common. The association with cardiovascular disease is well known; increased levels of low-density lipoprotein (LDL) cholesterol play a particular role in the pathogenesis of atherosclerosis. Atherosclerosis, arterial hardening due to lipid deposition, can potentially generate severe cardiovascular morbidities in the form of heart attacks and strokes. Hyperlipidemia control is thus not only significant for individual well-being but also for population-oriented public health interventions aimed at reducing the burden of cardiovascular disease." In addition to its cardiovascular effects, hyperlipidemia is causally linked to many metabolic dysfunctions, , such as Type II Diabetes Mellitus. The rising prevalence of Type II Diabetes among children and young people highlights the complex association of lipid metabolism with insulin resistance. Modifiable risk factors associated with hyperlipidemia, , such as obesity and inappropriate diet, predisposed to Type II Diabetes and increase lipid derangements. Risk factors. Diabetic individuals are more susceptible to developing further complications, particularly cardiovascular complications. Based on recent findings, the chronic diabetic status could potentially cause significant morbidity; hence important that healthcare systems prioritize lipid screening and lipid control in high-risk groups to prevent such risks (Kapke et al., 2015). The treatment and management of hyperlipidemia include the use of pharmacologic drugs , such as statins that have been shown to cause a remarkable decrease in LDL cholesterol levels and consequently reduce cardiovascular events. However, a comprehensive approach with lifestyle modification is required in the long term. Dietary changes to reduce saturated fat intake, increase the amount of omega-3 fatty acids, and regular exercise are important parts of hyperlipidemia control. Moreover, education and knowledge of the implications of dyslipidemia are needed because many individuals do not know their lipid profile and the resulting health consequences. Taking into consideration that lipid disorders in metabolism are prevalent, medical professionals have to emphasize interventional management practices that not only cure hyperlipidemia but also consolidate associated health conditions in a bid to improve patient outcomes (Khalimovich et al., 2023) (Figure 9.3).

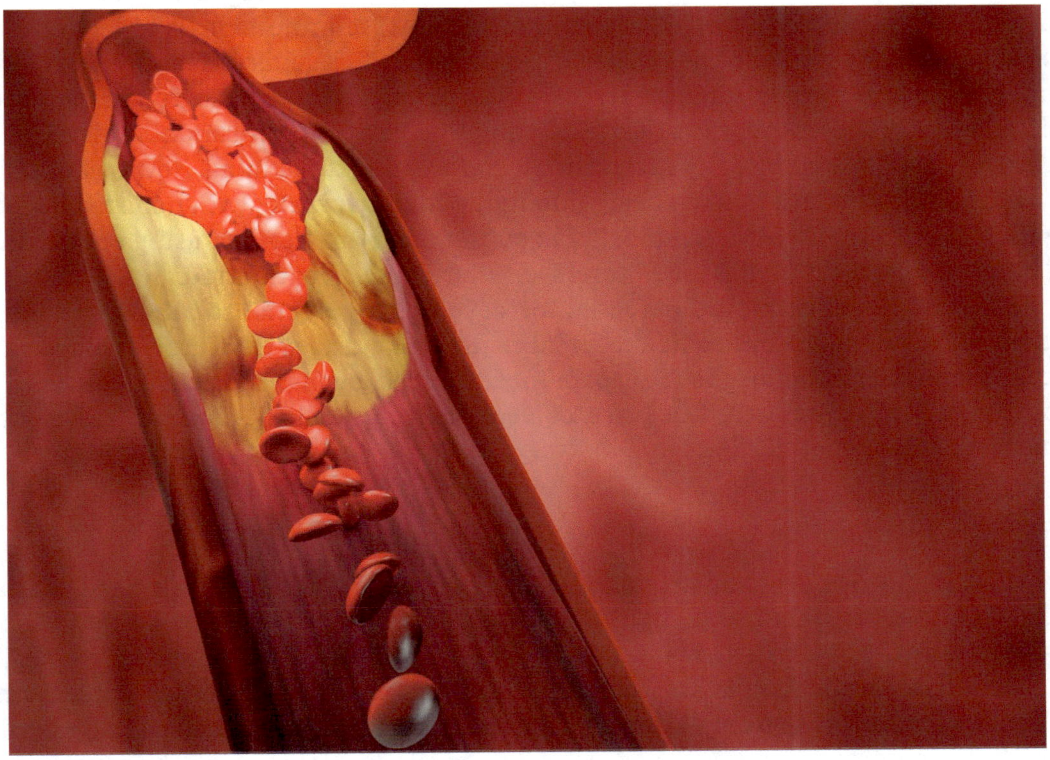

Figure 9.3. Arterial plaque buildup due to hyperlipidemia.

Source: https://lifecarehospital.ae/wp-content/uploads/2023/10/Hyperlipidemia.jpg.

9.1.2. Lipid Storage Diseases

Lipid storage diseases represent a category of genetic metabolic disorders in which there is abnormal lipid deposition in the cells of various tissues. The conditions arise due to enzyme deficiencies interfering with the normal metabolism of lipids, leading to their abnormal storage in cells, particularly in the liver, muscle, and nervous tissue. One of the prominent disorders in this group is the lysosomal storage disorders (LSDs), which are due to defective lysosomal enzymes that are responsible for lipid catabolism. The deficiencies of these enzymes can cause severe clinical manifestations, as the lipid storage impedes cell function, leading to organ dysfunction and complex symptoms ranging from physical weakness to neurological decay. Specifically, identification of a patient's lipid storage disease may significantly impact management and treatment planning for the patient. A classic example of such a lipid storage myopathy is multiple acyl-coenzyme A dehydrogenase deficiency (MADD), which most aptly represents the inconstancy of diagnosing lipid metabolism disorders. This specific disorder is the result of mutations in the ETFDH gene, leading to lipids accumulating in the muscle fibers and causing such symptoms as intolerance to exercise, muscle weakness, and pain. Clinical misdiagnosis is common, as such presentations can be mistaken for other disorders like polymyositis. However, with the progress in genetic analysis, the diagnostic accuracy has improved, and MADD has been diagnosed early, and accordingly, treated. Treatment could involve modulation of diet and vitamin supplementation, which, as seen in some cases, could lead to improvement of symptoms and an increase in quality of life. The case of a 14-year-old girl illustrates the requirement for genetic testing in the diagnosis of rare forms of lipid storage diseases and illustrates the requirement for healthcare professionals to be knowledgeable about this aspect (Ou et al., 2025). Furthermore, lysosomal storage disorders are being diagnosed with greater frequency through newer screening techniques that measure lysosphingolipids as diagnostic markers. These novel first-tier tests allow the early identification of elevated levels of lipids, which can be followed by early intervention and treatment planning. New evidence indicates that this method was effective in diagnosing different patients initially with nonspecific symptoms, referring to lipid storage diseases. Diagnosis can subsequently be verified using enzymatic activity tests and molecular genetic studies, and therefore, tailored therapeutic strategies. Through ongoing research into these biomarkers, the potential for developing personalized interventions expands exponentially throughout the entire field of lipid metabolism disorders. Future prospects indicate that increased knowledge and diagnostic capabilities will reshape management procedures, improve patient outcomes, and emphasize the place of personalized medicine for the treatment of lipid storage diseases (Civelek et al., 2024).

9.1.3. Fatty Liver Disease

Fatty liver disease, particularly nonalcoholic fatty liver disease (NAFLD), has emerged as a critical public health issue directly linked to lipid metabolism disturbances. This condition occurs when fat accumulates in the liver in the absence of excessive alcohol consumption, typically in an environment of obesity, insulin resistance, and metabolic syndrome. NAFLD is a spectrum of liver diseases ranging in severity from steatosis to nonalcoholic steatohepatitis (NASH), which can evolve into hepatic fibrosis, cirrhosis, and even hepatocellular carcinoma. The initial mechanism is an excess of fat in the liver, with subsequent inflammation and further complications if left untreated. Therefore, understanding the pathophysiology of NAFLD is crucial in developing optimal management strategies that not just treat fatty liver but also associated metabolic illnesses (Anania et al., 2017). When investigating the relationship between liver fat and metabolic health, new imaging techniques , such as magnetic resonance imaging (MRI) have been employed in recent research to quantify liver fat content. For instance, a study on spinal cord injury patients showed that elevated liver adiposity, as measured by the fat signal fraction (FSF), was directly correlated with many metabolic markers , such as triglycerides, non-HD cholesterol, fasting blood glucose levels, and inflammatory markers like tumor necrosis factor alpha (TNF-). These findings provide insight into the complex relationship between generalized metabolic derangements and hepatic fat accumulation. Specifically, the study identified that increased liver fat may influence metabolic health beyond visceral adipose tissue, leading to the perception that measurements of liver adiposity could provide important insight into individualizing therapeutic approaches to lipid metabolism disease (Gorgey et al., 2017). Increasing recognition of fatty liver disease, particularly against the backdrop of the global obesity epidemic, is relevant to both health professionals and policymakers. Because NAFLD can potentially have a profound impact on liver function and overall metabolic health, there is an urgent need for effective screening and early intervention strategies. This is especially true in high-risk populations , such as obese patients and those who have type 2 diabetes, in which the prevalence of fatty liver disease is notably high. Interventions may be lifestyle modifications like diet and exercise, pharmacologic interventions that target lipid metabolism, or multidisciplinary interventions that integrate nutrition, endocrinology, and hepatology. Treatment of this silent epidemic is paramount because early treatment not only improves individual patient outcomes but also reduces the healthcare burden by arresting the progression of established liver disease and complications (Anania et al., 2017) (Figure 9.4).

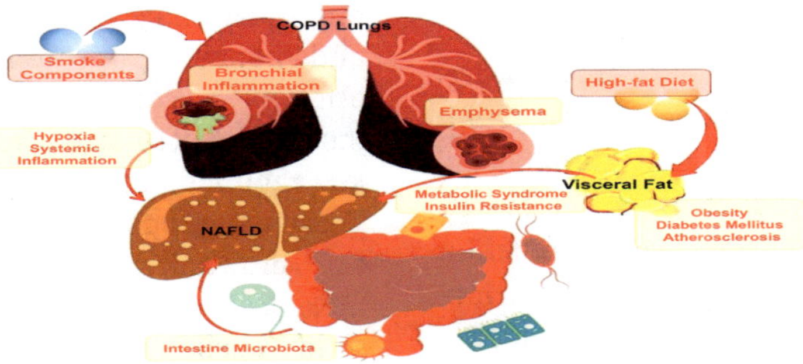

Figure 9.4. Healthy liver versus cirrhotic liver comparison.

Source: https://hospitalpharmacyeurope.com/wp-content/uploads/2004/03/Hepatic-disorders-1.jpg.

9.2. Causes of Lipid Metabolism Disorders

The cause of lipid metabolism disorders is multi-factorial and includes genetic, environmental, and lifestyle determinants. Genetic mutations can cause direct effects on lipid metabolism enzymes, leading to familial hypercholesterolemia or hyperlipidemia. These genetic predispositions are likely to cause dysregulation of lipid profiles, ultimately leading to elevated blood cholesterol and triglyceride levels. Environmental conditions, including dietary life, also significantly influence the development of lipid metabolism disorders.

High-saturated-fat diets and high-sugar diets are proven to cause the accumulation of lipids in the body, which can disrupt proper metabolic activities. In addition, sedentary lifestyles serve to worsen these conditions by weakening the body's capacity for the effective processing of lipids, opening the way for a range of metabolic syndromes with severe health consequences. Obesity is a leading risk factor that leads to lipid metabolism disorders because excess fat content can distort the function of lipid processing and storage.

Adipocytes are not merely passive lipid storage compartments; they actively secrete varying metabolites and cytokines that can influence lipid metabolism. Notably, overproduction of free fatty acids and inflammatory mediators is involved in insulin resistance, which is a component of the complexity of lipid homeostasis. This pernicious cycle allows for a climate in which the evolution of lipid metabolism disorders, type 2 diabetes, and cardiovascular disease is stimulated, hence facilitating the necessary relationship between obesity and lipid metabolism disorders. The disorders are also enhanced by the interaction between other aspects of metabolic syndrome, , such as hypertension and dysglycemia, increasing the threat to chronic diseases. Furthermore, some medications and underlying ailments have a pivotal role to play in lipid metabolism. Medications like corticosteroids and beta-blockers can induce dyslipidemia through alterations in lipid degradation and biosynthesis processes. Likewise, conditions like hypothyroidism and chronic liver disease can disrupt lipid metabolism through alterations in enzymatic processes and energy expenditure. For example, thyroid hormones are important in the modulation of lipoprotein metabolism, and their deficiency can contribute to elevated serum cholesterol. In addition, liver dysfunction suppresses lipid breakdown and excretion, causing disturbances in metabolism. Curing the underlying condition is pivotal in the management of lipid metabolism disorders and can direct treatments unique to the patient's condition, acknowledging the necessity for individualized therapeutic interventions (Mollinedo and Gajate, 2020; François et al., 2019).

9.2.1. Genetic Factors

The complex relationship between lipid metabolism disorders and hereditary factors makes insight into hereditary components responsible for susceptibility to such disorders essential. Hereditary differences in the form of single nucleotide polymorphisms (SNPs) have been found to influence lipid composition regulation and susceptibility to disorders , such as nonalcoholic fatty liver disease (NAFLD). There are numerous family studies, which have shown increased vulnerability of first-degree relatives among the affected individuals, manifestly demonstrating the strong hereditary component. With developments in Genome Wide Association Study (GWAS) technology, various genetic polymorphisms , such as PNPLA3 and MBOAT7 have been discovered, which have key functions in the progression of NAFLD, manifestly demonstrating the significant contribution of genetics to the pathogenesis of lipid-related diseases. This genetic susceptibility accentuates the utmost significance of early detection and treatment among susceptible populations to stem the impact of these diseases. In addition to genetic susceptibilities, epigenetic modifications, , such as DNA methylation and histone modification, are also a potent force in lipid metabolism disorders. Altered epigenetic modifications can influence gene expression and, hence, lipoprotein metabolism and the etiology of conditions , such as NAFLD. For instance, SIRT1 has also been recognized as a key regulator of these physiological pathways, presenting possible therapeutic targets for the modulation of NAFLD. Furthermore, measurement of circulating microRNA profiles is increasingly being viewed as a promising technique to non-invasively monitor disease severity and progression. These epigenetic observations provide more comprehensive perspectives on the interaction of genetic and non-genetic factors in exacerbating lipid metabolism disorders and present possibilities for targeted interventions and tailored approaches to individualized medicine in upcoming research. The identification of loci associated with plasma lipid levels has significant implications for the understanding of lipid metabolism disorders and their association with cardiovascular disease. A genome-wide screen of over 100,000 individuals of European ancestry was able to discover 95 major lipid trait loci that shed light on the genetic etiology of diseases , such as coronary artery disease (CAD). New associations near important lipid modulators , such as CYP7A1 and NPC1L1, as well as new loci previously unknown, shed light on lipid metabolism mechanisms. These findings not only emphasize the role of genetic contributions to normal and exaggerated lipid phenotypes but also express their expression in CAD risk in different ethnic groups, for example, East Asians, South Asians, and African Americans. By untangling these genetic effects, researchers can better understand the pathogenesis of lipid metabolism disorders and explore new therapeutic targets to forestall and treat CAD effectively (Figure 9.5).

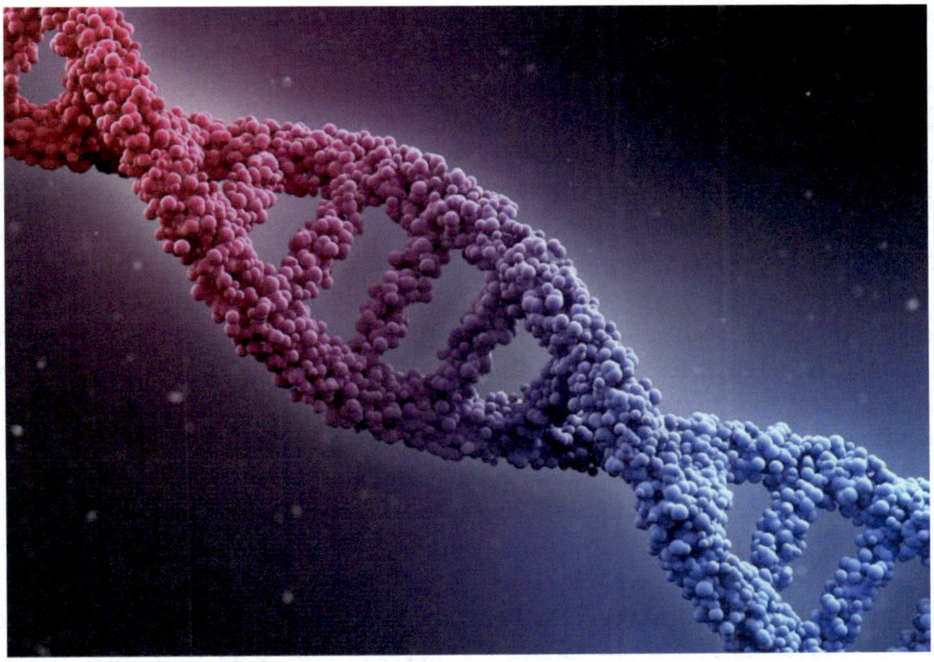

Figure 9.5. DNA double helix structure illustrating genetic material.

Source: https://depts.washington.edu/mbwc/content/adrc-page-img/238/19923051108_7dae5ecacb_o__full.jpg.

9.2.2. Dietary Influences

The relationship between nutrition and lipid metabolism disorders is complex and multifaceted. Diet plays a pivotal role in the regulation of lipid profiles and impacts processes like lipogenesis and lipolysis. The consumption of particular macronutrients will significantly influence the body's ability to metabolize lipids. Diets high in saturated fats, for example, have the potential to result in the accumulation of lipids within tissues, which has the potential to result in fatty liver disease and insulin resistance. Conversely, the addition of healthy fats, , such as the omega-3 fatty acids in fish and flaxseeds, has been associated with improved lipid metabolism and reduced inflammation. This balance of nutrients is important for the maintenance of metabolic health and for avoiding dysregulated lipid metabolism disorders caused by dietary behavior. An understanding of these dynamics serves to underscore the importance of education around diet in the prevention of lipid metabolism disorders. Antioxidants also contribute to the significance of dietary influences on lipid metabolism because they are able to oppose oxidative stress associated with lipid dysregulation. Oxidative stress happens when there's a disproportion in the production of reactive oxygen species (ROS) and the body's ability to fight against their harmful effects. Long-term oxidative stress can impair adipocyte function and cause Lipotoxicity, leading to insulin resistance. A diet full of antioxidants like fruits, vegetables, and whole grains can counteract these effects by salvaging cellular infrastructure and restoring redox equilibrium. Fu et al. (2025) discusses the role of endogenous and exogenous antioxidants in the regulation of oxidative stress and healthy adipogenesis, pointing to their importance in dietary interventions for enhancing metabolic well-being. Therefore, the consumption of food containing antioxidants could be a preventive measure to avoid lipid metabolism disorders. Intermittent fasting (IF) is also turning out to be a critical nutritional intervention with the potential to influence lipid metabolism and thyroid function. Fasting has been reported to favor metabolic flexibility, enhance lipid oxidation, and improve insulin sensitivity. Along with nutritional supplementation, , such as vitamin E, IF may have protective roles against thyroid dysfunction, a much-underemphasized consideration in lipid metabolism disorders. Kumar et al. (2025) document how IF, supplemented with antioxidants, not only rectifies thyroid homeostasis but also alleviates oxidative stress and related metabolic dysfunctions. This composite strategy of dietary effects explicates the promise of lifestyle interventions in reshaping our understanding and management of lipid metabolism diseases. Through changes in diet and incorporating specific nutrients, human beings are capable of transforming their metabolic outcomes drastically, highlighting the importance of dietary effects in long-term health situations.

9.2.3. Lifestyle Choices

Lifestyle determinants are of critical relevance to the cause and control of lipid metabolism disease, significantly determining the health status of an individual. The increase in the prevalence of obesity, particularly among children and adolescents, underscores the necessity for intervention in addressing lifestyle domains , such as physical activity and nutritional intake. Obesity, a chronic disease that perturbs energy homeostasis, has emerged as a major risk factor for most metabolic disorders, including type 2 diabetes and cardiovascular diseases. Severe obesity in US children above 120% of the 95th percentile of BMI-for-age indicates an ominous trend with attendant health consequences that increase in severity. This highlights the role of effective preventive measures over and above just dependence on therapeutic interventions, which usually meet with limited success in managing severe obesity and comorbid complications (Ameer and Weintraub, 2018). Dietary practices play a crucial role in lipid metabolism, thus influencing risk and disease treatment of conditions like non-alcoholic fatty liver disease (NAFLD). Recent evidence indicates that some food choices, most notably the adoption of a vegetable diet, can reverse epigenetic alterations related to lipid metabolism. The dietary regulation of liver gene expression with increased intake of high-fiber foods and healthy fats is pivotal in the battle against NAFLD. Reducing consumption of processed foods, sugars, and alcohol also works to prevent lipid storage in the liver significantly. Therefore, the inclusion of informed dietary recommendations in the public health agenda is in line with the incidence reduction of lipid metabolism disorder. Such trends highlight the interconnection of lifestyle behavior and genetics in the determinacy of metabolic well-being (Bars-Cortina and Martín, 2024). Moreover, the complexity of lifestyle choices necessitates multi-dimensional interventions to counter the rising obesity epidemic. Merely promoting eating healthfully and physical activity alone may not be sufficient without addressing the multifaceted psychological and social dilemmas that get in the way of an individual's behavior. Behavioral therapy, combined with tailored nutrition and exercise routines, has been limited in its capacity to create long-term change and suggests that more comprehensive solutions may be necessary. Clinicians must also exercise caution in adding pharmacologic interventions, weighing their potential complications against resorting to lifestyle modifications as central components of treatment. Thus, the creation of a comprehensive concept of health, encompassing lifestyle, nutrition, and behavior change, can help individuals make informed choices and lower lipid metabolism disorder risk factors (Ameer and Weintraub, 2018) (Figure 9.6).

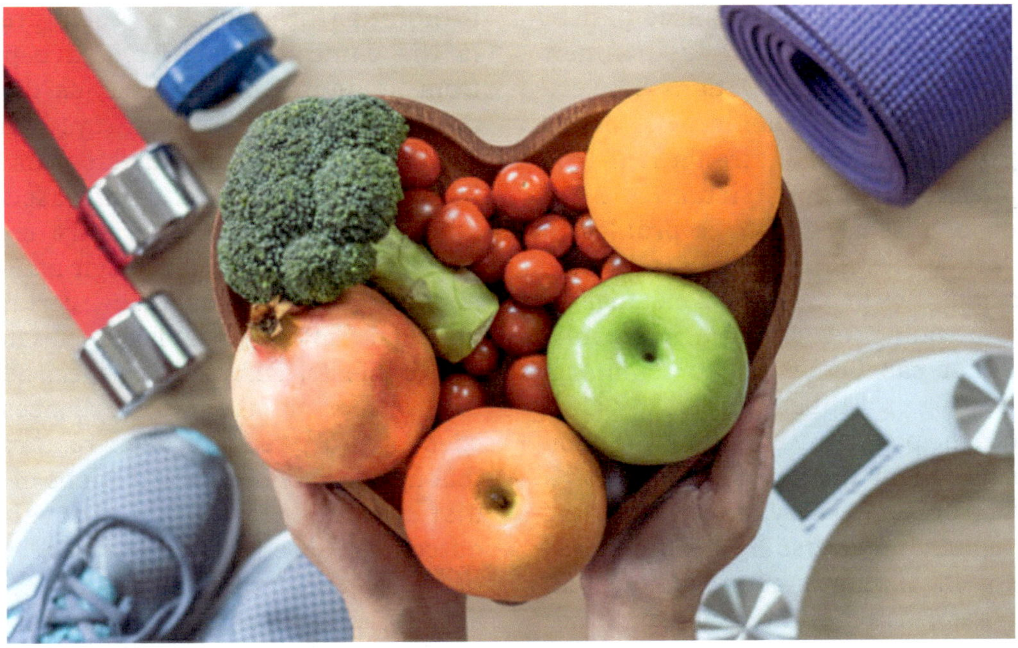

Figure 9.6. Balanced diet and regular exercise support heart health and overall well-being.

Source: https://www.nps.org.au/assets/_750x468_crop_center-center_75_none/GettyImages-953674568.jpg.

9.3. Symptoms and Diagnosis

Awareness of the symptoms of lipid metabolism disorders is crucial in diagnosing and managing the disorders early enough. Such disorders manifest themselves through a variety of clinical symptoms, including developmental delay, neurological impairment, and physical abnormality. For instance, the symptoms of inborn errors of metabolism overlap to a considerable degree, and therefore, it is difficult to diagnose them. In terms of lipid metabolism, the presentation can range from acute metabolic crises in infancy to chronic illness , such as cardiovascular disease in adulthood, depending on the nature of the disorder. This diversity underscores the importance of clinicians possessing a multifactorial high index of suspicion, particularly when presenting symptoms are not unmistakably suggestive of a single, more common condition. Early diagnosis can lead to timely interventions that have a tremendous impact on the long-term health outcome of patients. Biochemical analysis is the cornerstone in the diagnostic arsenal of lipid metabolism disorders. Classic targeted metabolic measurements have been the cornerstone of newborn screening programs, focusing on specific markers of well-established metabolic disease. Targeted approaches possess some limitations, including false-positive and false-negative results, which may lead to undue delay in appropriate treatment. A significant development in this area is the use of untargeted metabolomics, where it is possible to scan for a vast majority of metabolites found within biological samples without pre-specifying them. By increasing the metabolic profile that is being assessed, clinicians are able to reach a more integrated understanding of a person's metabolic status. This shift in approach not only improves the specificity and sensitivity of the diagnosis but also enables the identification of unidentified metabolic pathways that contribute to various lipid disorders, ultimately enabling more personalized patient care strategies (Sandlers, 2020). In addition, new evidence indicates close correlations between metabolic disturbances and neurodevelopmental disorders, which further strengthens the wider implications of lipid metabolism. An examination of plasma metabolic profiles in ASD and other developmental disabilities identified similarities in one-carbon metabolism pathways, including overlapping metabolic signatures that can be employed to inform diagnosis strategies (Abbeduto et al., 2019). This indicates the possibility of the identification of lipid metabolism disorders as part of a broader group of metabolic syndromes affecting neurodevelopment. By pursuing such research, clinicians not only better understand how lipid metabolism disorders may intersect with other conditions but also broaden the diagnostic framework to encompass a wider range of symptoms. By doing so, the understanding of patient health is made richer and more individualized, increasing the prospects for tailored therapies and interventions.

9.3.1. Common Lipid Metabolism Disorder Symptoms

Lipid metabolism disorders are a group of conditions characterized by the abnormal processing of lipids in the body, which can appear through an array of clinical features. In most cases, it is characterized by abnormal deposition of lipids in organs and tissues, manifesting as xanthomas or yellow, cholesterol-filled deposits on the skin. The patients can also present with hepatomegaly or liver enlargement secondary to fat overaccumulation. These diseases are likely to have cardiovascular comorbidities, as the impaired lipid metabolism is prone to generate elevated levels of low-density lipoprotein cholesterol (LDL-C). These dyslipidemias are highly risky for atherosclerosis and other cardiovascular diseases, bearing witness to the importance of early diagnosis and treatment. Lipid metabolism disorder management requires a thorough awareness of their presentation in the clinic to ensure effective prevention from long-term health risks, as discussed in research on metabolic pathways in the case of congenital errors of lipid metabolism (Sandlers, 2020). In addition to cardiovascular signs, lipid metabolism disorders are expected to present with various neurologic and endocrine manifestations. For instance, certain genetic disorders can lead to intellectual disabilities and developmental delays, and these can be explained in terms of metabolic disturbances of brain chemistry. There have been research studies that have established correlations of metabolic disturbances with neurodevelopmental outcomes based on convergent metabolic profiles between children with Down syndrome and autism spectrum disorder (Abbeduto et al., 2019). These observations bring out the complex relationship between lipid metabolism and neurodevelopment, suggesting that early metabolic assessment will be crucial in delivering important information on atypical neurodevelopment. The appearance of overlapping symptoms across disorders has the consequence that lipid metabolism disorders will give rise to a wide array of conditions, and this underscores the necessity of vigilance during diagnosis and treatment. Besides this, gastrointestinal symptoms will also reflect underlying lipid metabolism disorders. Patients usually have symptoms of abdominal pain, diarrhea, and fat malabsorption, resulting from defective lipid absorption in the gastrointestinal tract. An elevated triglyceride level is likely to cause pancreatitis, which occurs as acute abdominal pain and necessitates prompt medical attention. Such gastrointestinal derangements can further complicate the presentation and cause delay in diagnosis owing to their nonspecific character. To properly address such issues, clinicians will be required to identify the potential of lipid metabolism disorders as the cause of many symptoms. With that knowledge, health professionals can transition towards a more thorough patient assessment process, ultimately leading to better diagnostic accuracy and optimized treatment plans according to patient needs (Sandlers, 2020) (Figure 9.7).

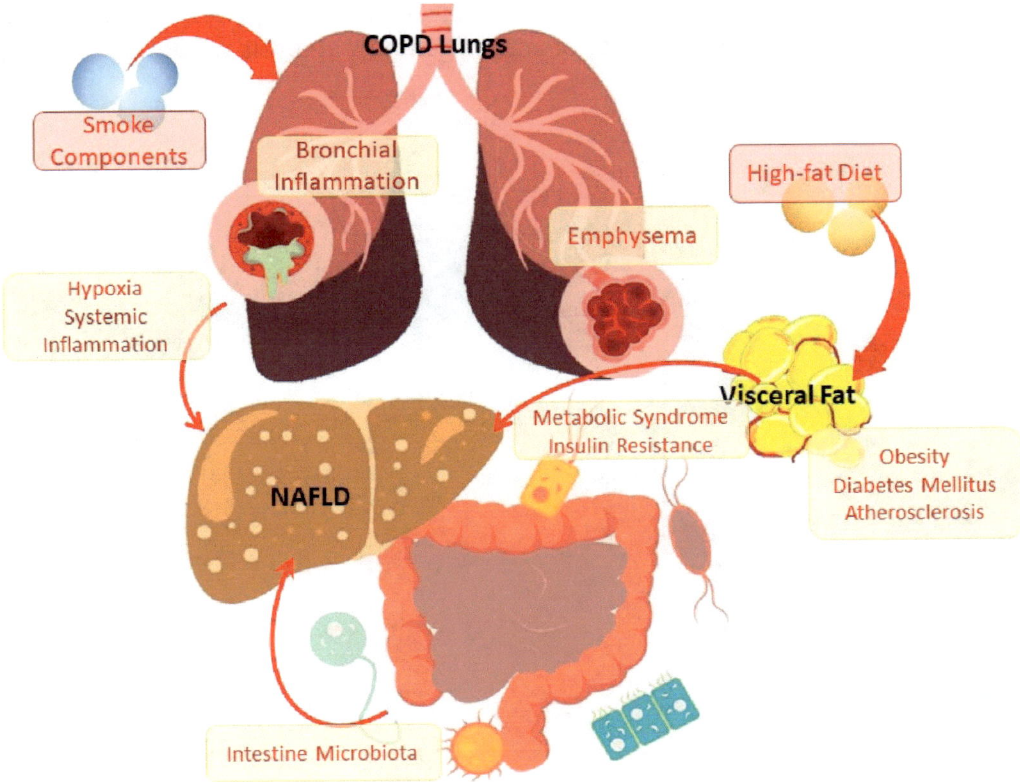

Figure 9.7. Impact of smoking and high-fat diet on lungs, liver, and gut health contributing to chronic inflammation and metabolic disorders.

Source: https://external-content.duckduckgo.com/iu/?u=https%3A%2F%2Fpub.mdpi-res.com%2Fcells%2Fcells-10-02978%2Farticle_deploy%2Fhtml%2Fimages%2Fcells-10-02978-g001.png%3F1635931240&f=1&nofb=1&ipt=8eeffc72b293d202a47572e66b65432c54a701ad3e1339f353b0bc02bc8b9694.

9.3.2. Diagnostic Tests and Procedures

Diagnostic procedures and processes are the main tools for the identification and treatment of lipid metabolism disturbances. Clinical evaluation often begins with a complete anamnesis of the patient and physical examination, which provides significant information on possible hereditary tendencies and symptomatology. Following this preliminary assessment, various biochemical analyses are employed to measure levels of lipids like cholesterol and triglycerides, which are of central importance in screening for hyperlipidemia and familial hypercholesterolemia. Higher-order lipid profiling is able to distinguish between heterogeneous lipoprotein subtypes and yield a comprehensive picture of lipid metabolism in an individual. These tests are necessary because, in addition to confirming a diagnosis, they also guide treatment strategies to reduce the long-term health risks associated with these diseases, including cardiovascular disease and pancreatitis, thus emphasizing the necessity for precise diagnostic testing. Further enhancing the diagnostic picture, genetic testing has proved itself a useful addition to the evaluation of lipid metabolism disorders. With the hereditary origins of diseases like familial dyslipidemias, the identification of individual mutations in genes for lipid metabolism enzymes can enhance diagnostic accuracy. Advances in personalized medicine indicate the relevance of adding genomic analysis to routine testing protocols.

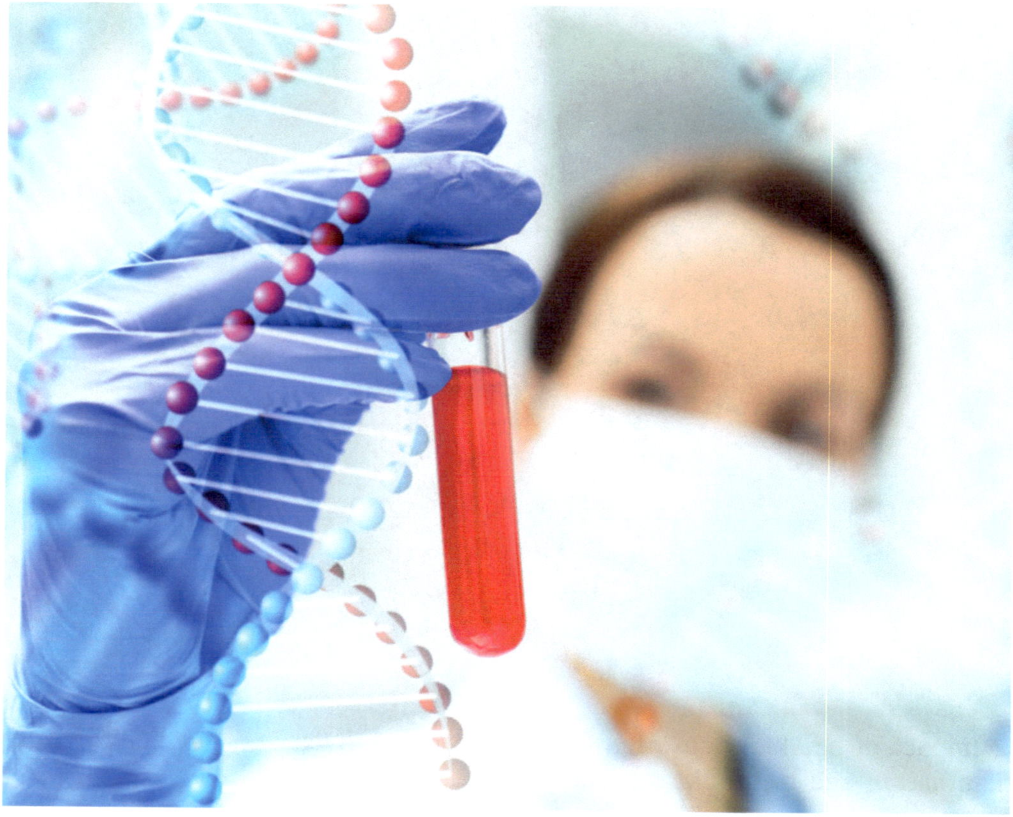

Figure 9.8. Genetic testing through blood analysis in a clinical laboratory setting.

Source: https://www.nchealthinfo.org/wp-content/uploads/2019/08/LabTestsAndDiagnostic.jpg.

This bears a direct relation to principles of precision medicine, where the physician can tailor interventions based on the patient's genetic makeup, which can significantly enhance results in the patient with the disease. Advancements in molecular diagnostics and genomics technology have provided new options for understanding how genetic variation affects lipid metabolism, opening the door to the potential development of targeted therapies that address the root cause of these disorders rather than their manifestations, as taught by Borro et al. (2017). In addition to biochemical and genetic testing, imaging techniques play a critical role in the evaluation of lipid metabolism disorders. Non-invasive modalities , such as ultrasound, computed tomography, and magnetic resonance imaging are able to delineate characteristics of lipid deposition and related complications and may aid in the comprehensive assessment of patients. Imaging modalities may help detect fat accumulation in the liver, a condition known as alcoholic non-alcoholic fatty liver disease, which is often associated with lipid metabolism disorders. Merging imaging outcomes with biochemistry and genetics creates a comprehensive image of the condition, which enhances clinicians to make better management planning. Furthermore, utilization of untargeted metabolomics for inborn errors of lipid disorders diagnosis is rapidly gaining popularity, since it could potentially detect more metabolites of various metabolic pathways, as elaborated by Fiehn et al. (2019). These extensive diagnostic strategies are important for the successful and timely management of lipid metabolism disorders (Figure 9.8).

9.3.3. Importance of Early Detection

The significance of early detection of lipid metabolism disorders cannot be overemphasized, as early detection of the disorders may completely transform the fate of patients. Lipid disorders are usually not diagnosed as they fail to present with apparent clinical symptoms, thereby leading to severe complications in the form of cardiovascular diseases and metabolic syndromes. The correlation between lipid levels and cardiovascular risk is established, but evidence indicates that a high percentage of patients are still below the target low-density lipoprotein cholesterol (LDL-C) goals. In Poland and the overwhelming majority of Central and Eastern European countries, just a quarter of individuals are appropriately screened for LDL-C level, showing the need to systematize screening and precise diagnostic criteria, as the Polish Society of Laboratory Diagnostics (PSLD) and the Polish Lipid Association (PoLA) recommend. Through early detection of lipid disorders, doctors are able to activate timely interventions that ultimately reduce the occurrence of adverse health events associated with dyslipidemia Early detection is also very crucial in light of the complex connection between lipid metabolism disorders and the development of a wide variety of cancers, including thyroid cancer. Recent studies have shown that lipid metabolic abnormalities are common in cancer cells, which enhance their growth and survival. Overproduction of some fatty acids (FA) has been associated with tumor development, showing that alterations in lipid profiles can be employed as a marker of malignant transformation.

Understanding these derangements in metabolism not only adds to the early diagnosis of lipid abnormalities but also opens the door for anticancer preventive therapy. By monitoring lipid levels and associated metabolic changes, healthcare providers can enhance their capacity to identify cancer-susceptible persons and initiate early treatments along with improved patient prognoses. The interconnectedness of lipid metabolism and carcinogenesis highlights the importance of early detection campaigns in the prevention of both diseases (Lukasiewicz et al., 2024). Lastly, the promotion of early detection for lipid metabolism disorders is essential in optimizing the total population's public health benefits. By integrating intensive screening programs into routine healthcare practice, practitioners can achieve significantly enhanced identification rates for at-risk individuals. This earlier detection allows for the implementation of lifestyle modification or pharmacologic therapy before the emergence of advanced complications, reducing the intensity of cardiovascular diseases and associated disorders. Furthermore, with the addition of a solid framework for earlier detection, ongoing patient monitoring and repeated assessment of lipid profiles can be guaranteed, thus ensuring sustained management of dyslipidemia. As evident from recent guidelines and results, , such as those supported by PSLD and PoLA, the establishment of early warning systems is an essential component in battling growing numbers of lipid-related disease and cascading effects on overall well-being (Solnica et al., 2024).

9.4. Impact on Health

The impact of lipid metabolism disorders on health is widespread and reaches not only physical but also psychological and social aspects of life. The deposition of lipids in the liver, a common effect of these disorders, may lead to non-alcoholic fatty liver disease (NAFLD), further disrupting metabolic processes and culminating in systemic inflammation. As highlighted in recent research, dietary elements , such as *Flammulina velutipes* mycorrhizae fiber content (Fv-DF) are in the limelight for their ability to reverse such health issues. Specifically, it has been established through studies that Fv-DF supplementation results in a significant reduction in weight gain and serum lipid levels, making it a potential remedy for lipid metabolism disorders (Jia et al., 2025).

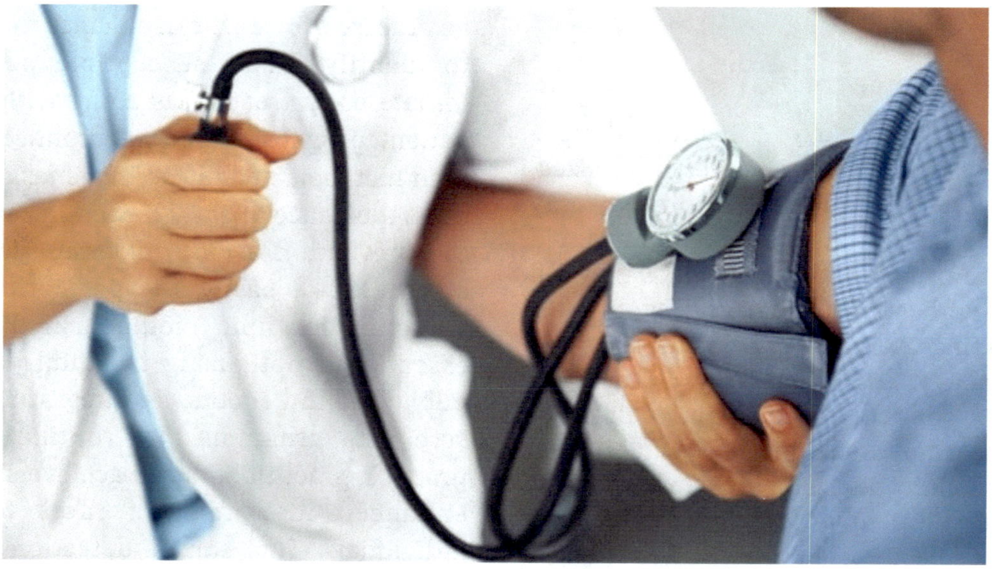

Figure 9.9. Blood pressure check for early detection of hypertension.

Source: https://images.hindustantimes.com/img/2024/07/24/550x309/Health-minister-Tanaji-Sawant-on-Tuesday-directed-_1691684369563_1721815629315.jpg.

This interaction of diet with lipid metabolism also holds promise for the development of interventions that can restore not only physical health but also psychological resilience in impacted individuals. Lastly, the link between substance uses disorders (SUDs) and lipid metabolism also reveals a rich interaction between lifestyle choices and health outcomes. Individuals with SUDs also typically have nutritional deficiencies that make lipid metabolism-related issues harder to overcome, creating a vicious cycle of poor health. Literature indicates that such individuals find the consumption of drugs more important than eating in healthy ways, resulting in immense metabolic disorders with alterations in the lipid profile and energy (Joaquín et al., 2025). In this context, correction of such nutritional imbalances becomes vital as part of a comprehensive program to treat individuals suffering from SUDs. With the application of targeted nutritional interventions in rehabilitation planning, clinical professionals can more effectively improve recovery outcomes, showing the need for a holistic strategy for addressing both metabolic and behavioral disorders. Moreover, understanding the role of separate nutrients in managing lipid metabolism disorders sets avenues for new treatment approaches. For instance, the intake of certain micronutrients may enhance lipid oxidation and decrease fat storage within the liver, thus promoting metabolic health. Studies on the effects of excessive consumption of foods high in sugar and suboptimal micronutrient intakes have indicated that such a food imbalance may lead to adverse health consequences, including susceptibility to obesity and associated metabolic disease (Joaquín et al., 2025). The findings point to the necessity of incorporating nutrition education and management into public health interventions for the prevention and management of lipid metabolism disorders. An integrated treatment could not only alleviate the load of these illnesses but also improve overall well-being and quality of life for individuals with lipid-associated conditions (Figure 9.9).

9.4.1. Cardiovascular Diseases

The complex relationship between lipid metabolism disorders and cardiovascular disease (CVD) indicates the significance of lipid profiles for the prediction of heart health risk factors. Dyslipidemia, the presence of an abnormal level of lipids—increased low-density lipoprotein cholesterol (LDL-C) and lowered high-density lipoprotein cholesterol (HDL-C)—is a known risk factor for atherosclerosis, a major underlying cause of CVD.

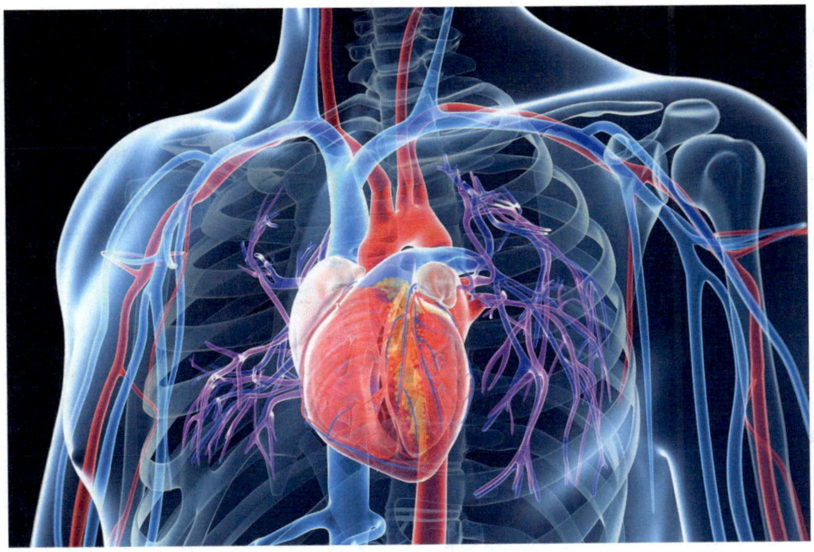

Figure 9.10. Illustration of the human cardiovascular system showing the heart, arteries, and veins.

Source: https://external-content.duckduckgo.com/iu/?u=https%3A%2F%2Fcvmedicalsoftware.com%2Fwp-content%2Fuploads%2F2016%2F06%2Fslider1.jpg&f=1&nofb=1&ipt=6e07f59151d1d273dcfe733a469d1309db819c3b00baafab5925681656e8cd2e.

This condition may be due to genetic factors, lifestyle, or effects of other metabolic illnesses , such as obesity and diabetes mellitus. Increased rates of obesity across the globe have been found to be parallel with increased CVD, particularly in populations at risk for metabolic illness, emphasizing the significance of certain interventions toward lipid control and modification of lifestyle to decrease cardiovascular risk (Rinella et al., 2023). Therefore, lipid metabolism is extremely important for the design of effective preventive strategies against cardiovascular diseases. Furthermore, the interconnection between non-alcoholic fatty liver disease (NAFLD) and cardiovascular events represents a classic example of the complicated interconnection between lipid metabolism disease and CVD. NAFLD usually leads to higher liver fibrosis, which has implications with respect to higher cardiovascular morbidity and mortality. Severe hepatic fibrosis, a common complication of NAFLD, occurs in patients with an augmented risk of non-hepatic mortality due to systemic cardiovascular disorders (Rinella et al., 2023). Studies show that while the liver lipids accumulate, so do systemic inflammation and insulin resistance, thus elevating cardiovascular risk factors , such as dyslipidemia and hypertension. Therefore, the treatment of NAFLD by lifestyle intervention and therapeutic regimens can potentially reduce cardiovascular risk, illustrating the interconnectedness of liver status, lipid metabolism, and cardiac disease. The potential interaction between HDL-C and cardiovascular status illustrates the multifaceted nature of lipid management interventions. Although low HDL-C levels typically indicate an increased risk of cardiovascular disease, recent evidence suggests that a single measurement of HDL cholesterol levels will not be sufficient due to the fine differences in the function of HDL. Specifically, high-density lipoproteins (HDLs) consist of heterogeneous subpopulations with differential contributions to cardiovascular protection, particularly with regard to their roles in reverse cholesterol transport and anti-inflammatory activities. Hence, there is an urgent need for interventions to alter HDL function rather than HDL-C levels. Investigation of HDL function can potentially bring about more impactful cardiovascular interventions by shifting the paradigm from raising HDL-C to maximizing the anti-atherosclerotic and other cardiovascular disease protective functions of HDLs. Clarification of these dynamics may be instrumental in devising integrated approaches to the prevention of cardiovascular disease in patients with lipid metabolism disorders (Figure 9.10).

9.4.2. Pancreatitis

Pancreatitis, which refers to inflammation of the pancreas, also tends to be linked with lipid metabolism disorders due to its effect on fat metabolism within the body. Either acute or chronic occurrence is possible for the disease, and acute pancreatitis is usually caused by such factors as gallstones, excessive alcohol intake, or hypertriglyceridemia. Elevated triglyceride levels are particularly important, as they can stimulate the release of toxic free fatty acids that cause damage to pancreatic cells. Understanding the influence of lipid metabolism on pancreatic function is significant, as disturbed metabolism not only exacerbates the severity of pancreatitis but also complicates its management. Therefore, treatments typically need to first address underlying lipid derangements to achieve proper treatment and improved patient outcomes. Diet plays a role in pancreatitis management, particularly in terms of dietary fiber consumption and its influence on lipid metabolism. Dietary fiber is suggested to have both protective and detrimental effects in patients with pancreatic disease. For instance, dietary fiber can stabilize the intestinal barrier and reduce the rate of infection in acute pancreatitis, as described in numerous studies. Conversely, excessive fiber content also blocks pancreatic enzyme activity, which is problematic for exocrine pancreatic insufficiency patients. Specifically, the intraoperative mechanisms of this blocking are not well understood but are believed to be related to the entrapment of enzymes by ingested fibers, resulting in increased fecal excretion of fat. These paradoxical findings highlight the value of individualized nutritional therapy that considers both pancreatic enzymes and lipid metabolism to facilitate recovery in pancreatitis patients (Badiali et al., 2019). Beyond this, the relationship between hyperlipidemia and pancreatitis is well recognized in veterinary practice, particularly in Miniature Schnauzers, where hypertriglyceridemia is prevalent. Research shows that an extremely high proportion of this breed has hypertriglyceridemia, which suggests an inherited predisposition that reflects the human disease. Hypertriglyceridemic dogs also show an association with increased serum liver enzyme activities, which suggests that lipid abnormality may compromise not only pancreatic inflammation but also overall hepatic function. Such findings in veterinary and pediatric medicine reaffirm that derangements in lipid metabolism can lead to systemic complications consistent with human pancreatitis. Therefore, regulation of lipid abnormalities becomes essential in the overall management of pancreatitis, and this points to the interdependent relationship between pancreatic function and lipid metabolism (Xenoulis, 2008) (Figure 9.11).

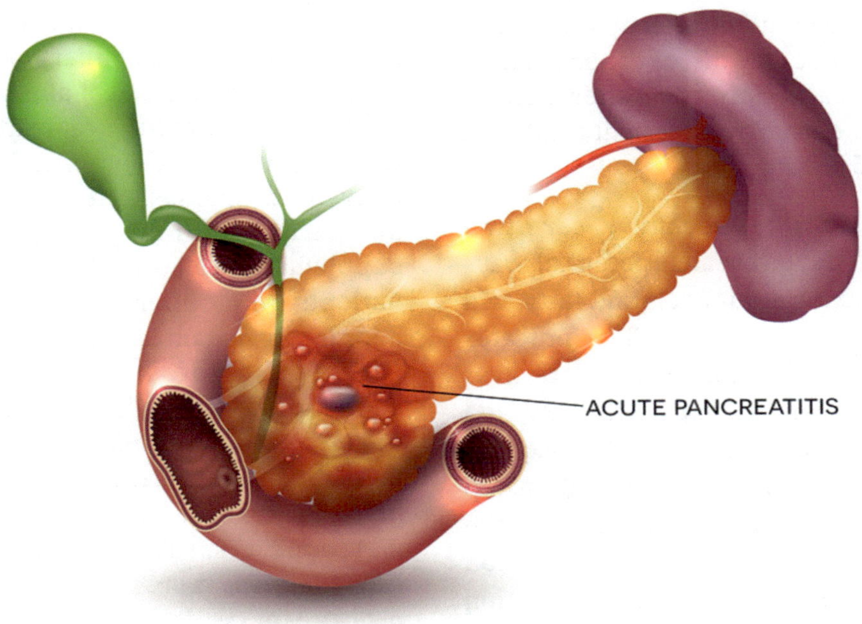

Figure 9.11. Acute inflammation of the pancreas and nearby digestive structures.

Source: https://excellaparoscopy.com/Admin/uploads/sub12_12_201711_480.jpg.

9.4.3. Liver Dysfunction

Liver impairment is increasingly being identified as a major cause of lipid metabolism disorders. With its roles as the main organ involved in lipid synthesis, storage, and degradation, the liver is instrumental in the upkeep of systemic lipid homeostasis. Disorders like non-alcoholic fatty liver disease (NAFLD) and metabolic dysfunction-associated steatosis liver disease (MASLD) are expressions of this impairment, accompanied by dysregulation of the fat content in hepatocytes. Interestingly, the link between chronic inflammation and such conditions cannot be overstressed. Studies found a higher neutrophil-to-high-density lipoprotein cholesterol ratio (NHR) to be positively correlated with NAFLD and MASLD risk development, with indicators demonstrating how inflammatory pathways integrate with derangement of lipid metabolism to further liver pathology

(Zhu et al., 2025). These results point to the complex interconnection between liver health and lipid metabolism, necessitating an urgent need for effective diagnostic and therapeutic methods. In addition, the function exhibited by infectious pathogens, , such as the Hepatitis B virus (HBV), further complicates the scenario of liver dysfunction and lipid metabolism. HBV infection has been shown to result in fatty acid β-oxidation disorder and mitochondrial damage in hepatocytes, which may increase the risk of lipid accumulation and downstream metabolic comorbidities. The pathophysiology involved is explained as HBV not only disrupts normal liver function but also causes profound alterations in lipid metabolism, such that treatment is difficult (Sun et al., 2025).

Interventions like decanoyl carnitine supplementation have revealed potential ways to regain mitochondrial function and fatty acid metabolism in HBV infection. This indicates a therapeutic line of action to alleviate liver dysfunction in persons infected with HBV, and as liver dysfunction becomes more prevalent in incidence, finding out the complex relationship between lipid metabolism and the health of the liver is necessary in order to enable prevention as well as intervention programs. Recognition of the pathogenic role of liver failure in lipid metabolism disorders is ever more vital for public health and clinical medicine. MASLD and NAFLD are more and more frequently seen, and recognition of the link between lifestyle factors, obesity, diabetes, and dietary habits, and liver well-being becomes an urgent imperative. Moreover, the addition of markers like NHR would enhance diagnostic precision and enable early intervention, potentially reducing the duration of liver disease. Subsequent research will require examining the mechanisms linking liver disease to lipid dysregulation, particularly in diverse populations. Implementation of personalized treatment regimens tied to the patient's metabolic profile and underlying liver disease could lead to better clinical outcomes and health-related quality of life. Treatment of liver disease in the context of overall lipid metabolism disorder will be pivotal in tackling this growing health problem.

9.5. Treatment Alternatives

The treatment of lipid metabolism disorders requires a multidisciplinary strategy, focusing on both pharmacological and lifestyle changes. Dietary adjustment is a central element in therapy, with the potential to profoundly alter lipid profiles. Saturated fat restriction and supplemental omega-3 fatty acid supplementation are key interventions for patients who suffer from hyperlipidemia. In addition, a sustained exercise routine has been proven to improve lipid metabolism as well as enhance the sensitivity of insulin, particularly beneficial for patients with symptoms of metabolic syndrome. Interventions of lifestyle must be tailored to the patient's individual metabolic disorder, as well as his overall health status, thereby establishing a baseline measure for treating lipid metabolism disorders effectively. Pharmacological management is also an extremely significant factor in the treatment of lipid metabolism disorders, particularly when lifestyle modifications are not good enough. Statins, ezetimibe, and fibrates are generally prescribed to lower increased levels of lipids. Statins, for instance, are effective in reducing low-density lipoprotein (LDL) cholesterol and have been associated with a decrease in cardiovascular risk. In addition, current studies have also emphasized the therapeutic role of insulin sensitizers in the regulation of lipid metabolism, particularly among individuals with chronic hepatitis C, where insulin resistance complicates treatment. Identification of the metabolic derangements that contribute to lipid disorders guides the selection of pharmacologic interventions to establish an individualized approach that reduces risks and enhances therapeutic benefit (Enjoji et al., 2012). Novel treatment strategies, including advanced metabolomics and lipidomics, have the potential to improve diagnostic and therapeutic interventions in lipid metabolic disorders. New methods enable close exploration of metabolic pathways and lipid profiles that may reveal unique metabolic patterns that could inform more focused treatment interventions. With the use of untargeted metabolomics, practitioners are able to gain knowledge on a greater number of metabolites, thereby expanding their understanding of each patient's profile. This strategy overcomes the limitations of traditional screening methods used for inborn errors in metabolism, and it is suggested that a shift towards untargeted analyses could further maximally improve treatment choices significantly for lipid metabolism disorders and allow for earlier intervention and improved patient outcomes (Sandlers, 2020) (Figure 9.12).

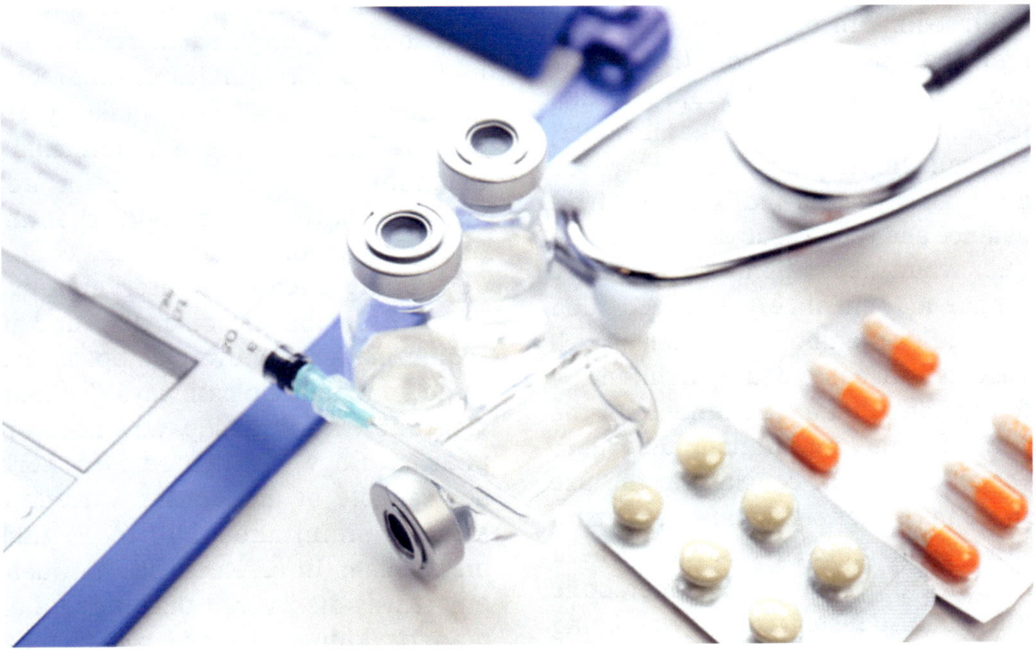

Figure 9.12. Essential medical tools and medications used in patient treatment and care.

Source: https://www.ibdrelief.com/uploads/files/adobestock_138698385_gallery_image_814_163.jpeg.

9.5.1. Dietary Modifications

In lipid metabolism diseases, nutritional management is vital in symptom control and overall health status improvement. Among the critical aspects of nutritional management is the application of high-fiber food, which exerts significant impacts on gut microbiota and, consequently, lipid metabolism. Short-chain fatty acids (SCFAs) that are produced upon fermentation of dietary fiber by gut microbiota have emerged as key metabolites to stimulate metabolic pathways associated with immune function and metabolic health. Research indicates that SCFAs , such as acetate, butyrate, and propionate not only influence lipid profiles but also reduce systemic inflammation, a prevalent underlying cause of diseases like cardiovascular disease and type II diabetes. Thus, the promotion of high-fiber intake is able to enhance SCFA production, justifying the merit of diet alteration in the management of lipid metabolism disease (Cadenhead et al., 2017). In particular, condition-specific dietary strategies are able to control lipid metabolism derangement. For example, for polycystic ovary syndrome (PCOS), females tend to have insulin resistance and elevated lipid levels, and well-formulated dietary management might be necessary. First-line interventions typically induce weight reduction on a low-fat, balanced, and fruit-, vegetable-, and whole-grain-rich diet and pushes unsaturated fats. Furthermore, carbohydrate consumption has to be controlled because the high glycemic index foods drive insulin resistance and type 2 diabetes risk. These diet changes, when accompanied by routine physical exercise, may enhance generalized PCOS symptoms, including metabolic disorder, as well as cardiovascular disease, again highlighting the need for specific dietary treatments in the management of lipid metabolism disorders (Ghazeeri et al., 2021). In conclusion, the use of diet changes may offer significant benefits to patients with lipid metabolism disorders. These modifications not only correct the metabolic abnormalities but also foster general well-being by treating the interconnected cause and effect of the health states, , such as inflammation, weight, and insulin resistance. By placing a strong focus on whole, high-density foods and limiting bad fats and processed sugars, people can achieve better metabolic health status. Also, the growing body of evidence regarding the role of gut health in lipid metabolism underlies the premise that specific dietary changes can aid in maintaining a healthier microbiome, opening up additional pathways by which risks from lipid disorder can be mitigated. In this way, dietary interventions will thus form part of any treatment protocol addressing lipid metabolism disorder, ultimately serving to enhance long-term health and lifestyle.

9.5.2. Pharmacological Interventions

Pharmacotherapies are of particular significance for the treatment of lipid metabolism disorders, which occur primarily due to an imbalance between lipid synthesis, utilization, and transportation mechanisms within the body. These disorders, , such as obesity-induced dyslipidemia and metabolic syndrome, may have extremely severe cardiovascular consequences unless addressed. Therapeutic properties of bioactive compounds, , such as bibenzyl derivatives, in ensuring normal lipid metabolism have been highlighted in recent reports. For instance, research indicates that molecules like gigantol enhance glucose uptake by a significant level, lending support to a multiaxial approach to modulate lipid storage in adipocytes. Such revelations highlight the importance of exploring pharmacological compounds in developing treatment interventions effective in lipid metabolism disorders and justify the requirement of innovative approaches through targeted metabolic pathways (Nuamnaichati et al., 2025). Additionally, advances in network pharmacology highlighted how herbal drugs are capable of modulating various biological targets simultaneously to regulate lipid metabolism. In research on the Gualou Qumai pill, it was discovered that it could ameliorate diabetic kidney disease renal complications by regulating peroxisome proliferator-activated receptors (PPARs), key regulators of lipid and homeostasis. Through a network analysis, researchers identified numerous active components in the herbal cocktail that participate in significant metabolic pathways (Liu et al., 2024). This highlights the application of integrating ancient medicinal concepts with modern pharmacological understanding in the management of lipid metabolism diseases more efficiently, presenting an exciting platform for future drug therapy. Besides, research into pharmacological treatments includes optimization of existing pharmaceutical medicines aimed at lipid control. Statins are widely employed to manage hyperlipidemia by inhibiting HMG-CoA reductase, thereby inhibiting liver cholesterol synthesis. However, research is unveiling that customized therapies, like a combination of statins with other bioactive compounds, may enhance efficacy while minimizing side effects. This pharmacological synergy is instrumental, as it not only treats the manifestations of lipid metabolism disease but also attacks the root pathophysiology. By examining the molecular mechanisms and interactions of pharmacological drugs, scientists can more precisely fine-tune treatments, eventually making clinical care for those affected by these multifactorial disorders better (Nuamnaichati et al., 2025) (Figure 9.13).

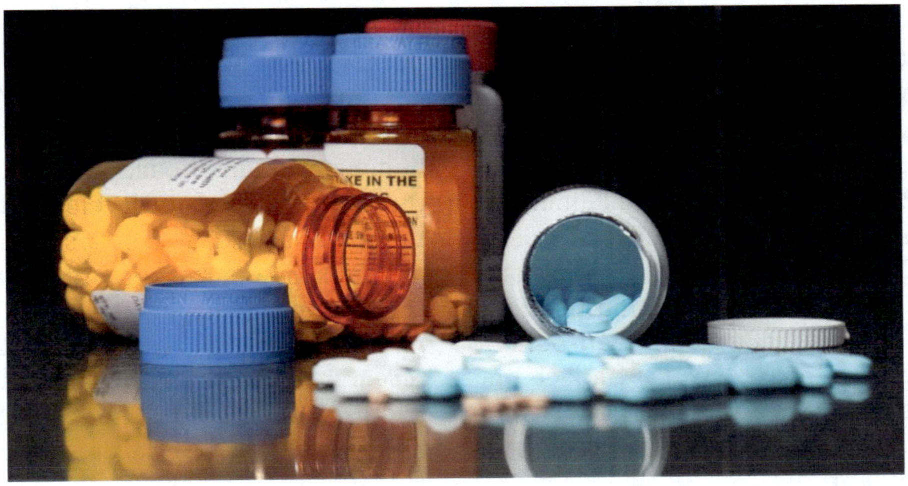

Figure 9.13. Various prescription medications are used in chronic disease management.

Source: https://external-content.duckduckgo.com/iu/?u=https%3A%2F%2Fwww.findatopdoc.com%2Fvar%2Ffatd%2Fstorage%2Fimages%2F_aliases%2Ffb_thumb%2Fhealthy-living%2Fmedical-advancements-new-treatments-and-perspectives-on-fibromyalgia%2Fpharmacological-treatments%2F3584078-1-eng-US%2FPharmacological-treatments.jpg&f=1&nofb=1&ipt=0d717e77b0b729ca71d55fba31cc1d85d6b3905f827c2d5bbd11a8a6f496e419.

9.5.3. Lifestyle Changes

Lifestyle change is a vital element in the treatment of lipid metabolism disorders since the majority of them are brought about by a combination of genetic susceptibility and environmental factors. A good lifestyle, which involves regular exercise and a balanced diet, has been shown to have positive effects on lipid profiles. For instance, reducing the intake of saturated fats and raising the ratio of unsaturated fats can lead to increased cholesterol levels. Studies have demonstrated that individually adopted dietary changes can curb the incidence of atherogenic disorders by modifying serum lipid profiles in the long term. In particular, people with certain genetic traits, , such as the ND2-237Met polymorphism, are bound to react variably to dietary lifestyle, highlighting the necessity for individualized approaches to lifestyle adjustment. Physical exercise is also essential since it promotes achieving and sustaining optimal weight and supports lipid metabolism, consequently reducing the risk of cardiovascular complications. Body weight management is also an essential part of lifestyle adjustment to improve lipid metabolism and health in general. Obesity, which is prevalent among patients with lipid disorders, enhances lipotoxicity and consequently insulin resistance and associated metabolic derangements. Therefore, intentional weight loss through caloric restriction and physical training can be quite helpful. For instance, individuals with polycystic ovary syndrome (PCOS) are encouraged to embark on a weight reduction regimen because it not only allows for weight management but also deals with the inherent hormonal imbalance behind lipid metabolism issues. Moreover, sustainable weight loss has also been linked with increased insulin sensitivity and better serum lipid control. Lifestyle treatment in the form of the maintenance of physical exercise for at least 30 minutes on the majority of days of the week can enhance lipid profiles and diminish the severity of accompanying disorders. Apart from diet modifications and weight reduction, a holistic approach to lifestyle modification involves mental and emotional well-being. Chronic stress also has a strong impact on lipid metabolism since, by affecting patterns of eating and activity, it can interfere with efforts at improving lipid profiles. Stress management, yoga, and mindfulness have been shown to reduce stress-related craving for fatty foods, which can counteract efforts at improving lipid profiles. Besides, with a supportive group or community exercise, motivation and adherence to lifestyle changes can be more easily instilled, such that the attainment of health goals is easier. Therefore, embracing integrative lifestyle changes, which consist of dietary, physical activity, and stress modifications, gives an overall more comprehensive mechanism for reducing risk for lipid metabolism disorder as well as improving overall metabolic health.

9.6. Research and Advances

Recent research has significantly enhanced our understanding of lipid metabolism disorders through the description of underlying biological mechanisms and potential therapeutic options. Lipid metabolism is not only responsible for maintaining cellular function but is also intimately related to various metabolic disorders, including obesity, diabetes, and cardiovascular disease. Current reports highlight complex regulatory networks that regulate lipid synthesis and breakdown, with a focus on the roles of particular enzymes and transcription factors in these functions. Recent developments in lipidomics and molecular biology have pointed to novel regulatory mechanisms encompassing non-coding RNAs, , such as microRNAs, which play critical roles in lipid homeostasis maintenance. These results open the avenues for the development of targeted therapies aimed at the dysregulation of lipid metabolism and thus provide new windows for the efficient management of lipid metabolism-related disorders (Titus et al., 2025). Moreover, research on the relationship between the gut microbiome and lipid metabolism has become the focal point in recent research studies. Evidence shows that microbial metabolites play a profound role in lipid metabolic pathways, revealing an underappreciated aspect of lipid regulation. The impact of gut microbiomes extend to inflammatory processes, insulin sensitivity, and lipid storage, suggesting it can be developed as a therapeutic target of metabolic disorders. This is addressing the requirement for a holistic perspective of how lifestyle, diet, and microbial communities contribute to lipid metabolism. Progress in genetic and genomics tools continues to facilitate this research, with scientists being able to decipher the complex host metabolism-microbial populations interactions, hence gaining information that could revolutionize therapy protocols in lipid pathologies (Titus et al., 2025). In dermal science, the role of lipids in skin health has been of concern, particularly with regard to the influence of fungal microbiomes on skin lipid metabolism. The Malassezia genus, a ubiquitous fungal inhabitant of human skin, has been linked to a variety of skin conditions through its lipid-dependent metabolic pathways. A wide range of studies has elucidated the mechanisms by which Malassezia induces disruption of the skin's lipid barrier, producing a range of dermatological syndromes. This interference not only emphasizes the complexity of skin lipid metabolism but also suggests that interfering with lipid or fungal balance repair could offer new therapeutic approaches to skin disorders. Continuous research expands the understanding of the correlation between microbial flora and skin lipids, particularly Malassezia, and opens up a new frontier of potential treatments, potentially enhancing skincare and skin health (Figure 9.14).

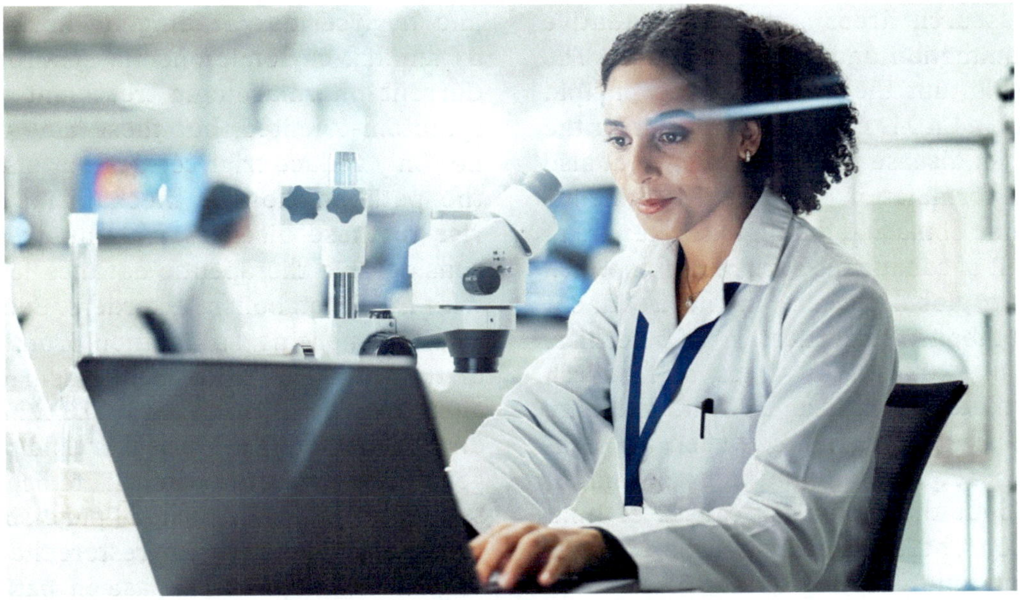

Figure 9.14. A medical researcher working with a microscope and computer in a laboratory setting.

Source: https://external-content.duckduckgo.com/iu/?u=https%3A%2F%2Flirp.cdn-website.com%2Fb2f6d08f%2Fdms3rep%2Fmulti%2Fopt%2F60166592_laptop-woman-and-scientist-with-research-in-laboratory-for-medical-innovation-with-biotechnology-science-computer-and-female-biologist-typing-online-for-pharmaceutical-experiment-in-office-1920w.jpg&f=1&nofb=1&ipt=fd43d157b3269e6f75c1c1996d5dcca45a6bfc6e6d32587f160ae732a7290df1.

9.6.1. Current Research Trends in Lipid Metabolism

Recent research into lipid metabolism has also increasingly emphasized its central role in various pathological conditions, , such as neurodegenerative diseases and chronic illnesses. Studies have interrogated the multifaceted relationship between lipid metabolism and cellular processes, , such as ferroptosis, to find new therapeutic targets. For instance, current research is focused on defining how lipid peroxidation, deranged antioxidant control, and iron disturbances may influence disease progression, particularly in Parkinson's disease (PD) models. The studies point to the potential of ferroptosis-directed therapies that might prevent disease worsening in PD through the regulation of lipid metabolic pathways. In particular, the cross-disciplinary collaboration between nations and institutions is stimulating the field, as part of a broader trend in solving difficult biological problems with cross-disciplinary approaches that focus on lipid metabolism (Chen et al., 2024). Further, the intersection between lipid metabolism and CKD has been specifically in the spotlight in the scholarly community. Research has indicated that derangement of lipid metabolism can exacerbate CKD to the point of leading to severe complications like cardiovascular disease and diabetic kidney disease. Bibliometric analyses have revealed a sharp increase in publications revolving around this intersection, thereby depicting popular research areas , such as oxidative stress, inflammation, and insulin resistance. The study reveals that the understanding of lipid metabolism in CKD is not only important for the elucidation of disease pathophysiology but also vital for the formulation of effective treatments. Countries like China and the United States are at the forefront of conducting such research, which represents a global concern in the treatment of lipid metabolism disorders in CKD settings (Wang et al., 2024). New lines of research for lipid metabolism are also introducing technological advancements, , such as high-throughput sequencing and metabolomics, to learn about the molecular causes of lipid dysregulation. These technologies enable further specificity in lipid profiling so that researchers can identify biomarkers that can predict the incidence of lipid metabolism diseases. This promises more precise diagnostic tools and more targeted therapies aimed at specific patient profiles. In addition, interdisciplinary research convergences are increasingly becoming essential, deriving power from biochemistry, molecular biology, and pharmacology to promote the understanding of lipid roles in disease and health. Synergism of advanced methodologies with integration showcases the changing nature of lipid metabolism studies to be a leading field in combating metabolic disorders and chronic diseases (Chen et al., 2024; Wang et al., 2024).

9.6.2. Emerging Therapies and Treatments

The identification of new therapies has been transforming the treatment process of lipid metabolism disorders. Among these new therapies, biological inhibitors have created a buzz for their ability to treat hyperlipidemia on a molecular level. Specifically, anti-apolipoprotein (apo) C-III and angiopoietin-like protein 3 (ANGPTL3)-based treatments have shown promise. These inhibitors are being developed to counteract the effects of genetic mutations that disrupt the metabolism of cholesterol and triglycerides, leading to diseases , such as familial chylomicronemia syndrome (FCS). Current pharmacologic treatment is disease symptom-oriented, but these new medicines not only reduce triglycerides but also address the pathophysiologic mechanisms that give rise to these diseases and thus represent a considerable therapeutic advance for patients with lipid metabolism disorders. Gene therapy is also emerging as another promising area of treatment for lipid metabolism disorders, alongside apo C-III and ANGPTL3 inhibitors. By directly modifying the genes for lipid processing, gene therapy has the potential to achieve long-term correction of inherited lipid disorders. For instance, gene therapy can restore the metabolic activity of lipoprotein lipase in patients with severe forms of hypertriglyceridemia, e.g., those diagnosed with FCS, for whom standard therapies have little to recommend. With continuous research, gene therapy techniques will need to address various challenges, including delivery strategies and potential off-target effects. However, the prospect of treating the etiology of lipid metabolism disorders rather than just suppressing their signs and symptoms may significantly influence patient prognosis and redesign the standard of care for this field (Shashikant et al., 2024). Furthermore, the addition of lifestyle interventions and complementary treatments to the therapeutic treatment for lipid metabolism disorders points to the strength of a multi-modal approach. Recent research suggests that nutritional treatments, including intense low-fat diets and customized dietary therapies, are capable of enhancing the effect of drug treatment. Along with dietary treatment, exercise and weight management also have prominent effects on lipid profiles. In addition to new drug treatments, these interventions could lead to more comprehensive management practices that address both the biological and behavioral aspects of lipid disorders. With the progress in the field, the combination of these new therapies with traditional lifestyle modification will most likely be an effective approach in the treatment of lipid metabolism disorders, pointing to the necessity of ongoing research and clinical trials to guarantee the implementation of these interventions (Shashikant et al., 2024) (Figure 9.15).

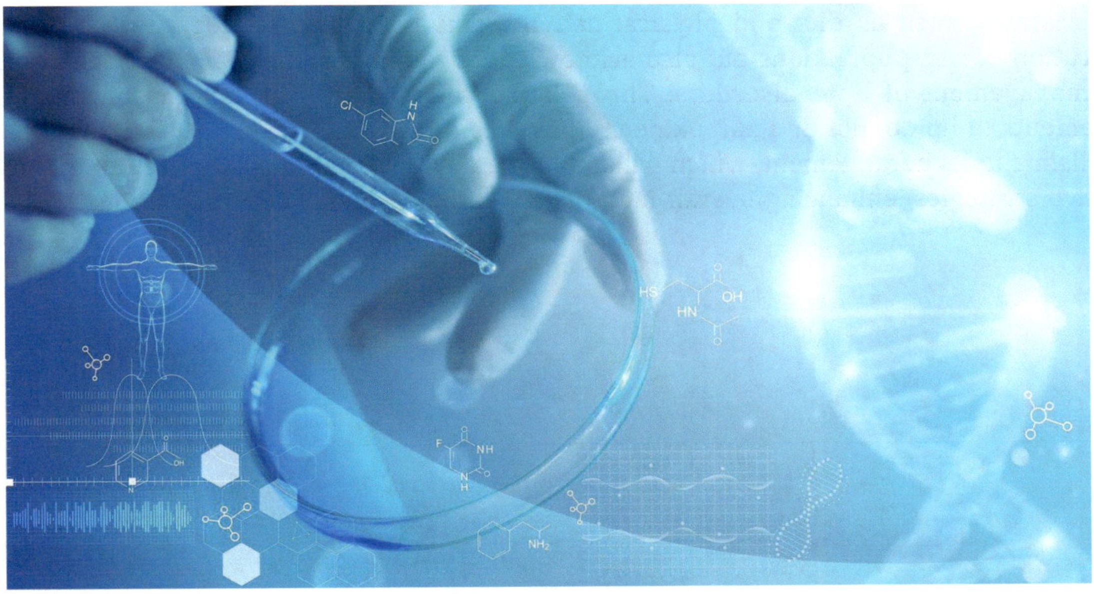

Figure 9.15. Advanced laboratory research exploring the human microbiome and genetic science.

Source: https://external-content.duckduckgo.com/iu/?u=https%3A%2F%2Fwww.aranca.com%2Fassets%2Fuploads%2Fspecial-reports%2Fmicrobiomeban.jpg&f=1&nofb=1&ipt=47fdc41106a0bed8a8678ee2073828aab162f7819532515948945566 16d95f10.

9.6.3. Future Directions in Lipid Metabolism Research

Current and ongoing future in lipid metabolic research trends lie in the inclusion of lipidomics technology, which has dramatically changed our understanding of metabolic pathologies , such as pre-diabetes and type 2 diabetes mellitus (T2DM). Using this new idea, researchers can now explore the complex alterations in plasma lipid profiles across changes from normal metabolic states to disease. For instance, more contemporary investigations have used lipidomics to identify distinct lipid signatures in pre-diabetes compared to T2DM and provided insight into the biochemical mechanisms that govern them. These advances not only allow for preclinical diagnosis of lipid metabolism disease but also provide information that can guide the development of targeted therapies, thereby expanding therapy and optimizing preventive interventions in the clinic (Gu et al., 2025). In addition, understanding the role of adipokines in lipid metabolism is an exciting avenue to explore. Among these, retinol-binding protein 4 (RBP4) has been interesting due to its multifunctional character in lipid metabolism as well as metabolic and cardiovascular disease pathophysiology. Levels of RBP4 have been linked to insulin resistance and inflammation, which makes it a useful biomarker for disease monitoring. Research on the molecular pathways through which RBP4 influences lipid metabolism can pave the way for novel therapeutic approaches, resulting in novel interventions with the hope of reversing or opposing lipid disorders. Hence, adipokine research like that on RBP4 in the coming years will be crucial in formulating novel means of effectively addressing metabolic diseases (Zhang et al., 2025). Lastly, understanding genetic and environmental determinants of lipid metabolism disorder remains a key research priority. With every new GWAS, more genetic variants associated with lipids are being identified, and follow-up studies can further define the interaction between genetic predisposition and lifestyle characteristics, , such as diet and physical activity. This concerted strategy not only facilitates identification of risk populations but also acknowledges the importance of personalized medicine in the management of lipid disorders. Through the consolidation of genetic information with advancements in lipidomics and adipokine studies, scientists can form a concerted picture of lipid metabolism and its derangement, which will aid in the development of customized therapeutic and preventive strategies, enhancing overall metabolic well-being in various populations.

CLOSER LOOK

POLYPHYLETIC COLLECTION

A polyphyletic collection refers to a group of organisms that are classified together but do not share an immediate common ancestor within that group. Instead, the similarities among the members arise independently, often due to convergent evolution—where different species evolve similar traits in response to similar environmental pressures. This differs from monophyletic groups, which include a common ancestor and all its descendants, and paraphyletic groups, which include a common ancestor and some, but not all, of its descendants.

Polyphyletic groupings are generally considered problematic in modern systematics and evolutionary biology because they do not accurately reflect evolutionary relationships. For instance, grouping bats and birds together because they both have wings would be polyphyletic; their common ancestor did not have wings, and each lineage evolved flight independently. As such, polyphyletic classifications can mislead our understanding of how traits evolved and how organisms are related. Historically, polyphyletic groups arose from classifications based on superficial traits, such as morphology or ecological role, before the advent of genetic and molecular analysis. With modern phylogenetics, scientists aim to revise these groupings to reflect true evolutionary lineages, favoring clades (monophyletic groups) instead.

Despite their flaws, polyphyletic groupings may still appear in informal contexts or transitional classifications where full phylogenetic information is lacking. They can also be useful in specific practical settings, such as in ecology or epidemiology, where function or phenotype may be more immediately relevant than ancestry. Ultimately, understanding and identifying polyphyletic groups is crucial in evolutionary studies. It highlights the importance of distinguishing between homology (shared traits due to common ancestry) and analogy (shared traits due to convergent evolution), thereby sharpening our view of the tree of life and improving the scientific classification of organisms.

SUMMARY

It is important to appreciate the complex interdependence of genetic, environmental, and physiological factors that are involved in such disorders. The pathophysiology of disorders like hypercholesterolemia and dyslipidemia underscores the complexity of lipid levels and overall well-being. New therapeutic approaches, particularly those using proprotein convertase subtilisin/Kewin type 9 (PCSK9), mark a breakthrough in the therapy of lipid metabolism disorders. The development of PCSK9 inhibitors not only enhanced the efficacy of cholesterol management but also highlighted the importance of personalized medicine in addressing the sophistication of lipid metabolism disorders, as exposed by recent clinical evidence and applications in therapeutic treatment (Bao et al., 2024). These developments pave the way for improved patient outcomes and demonstrate the importance of continually enhancing therapeutic strategies in cardiovascular medicine. As we synthesize the evidence on lipid metabolism disorders, it is evident that child health and malnutrition have a very large role in developing cardiovascular disease over the long-term. The connection between acute childhood malnutrition and subsequent cardiometabolic non-communicable diseases provides evidence that early interventions in nutrition could decrease future risks to health. Research indicates that individuals with a history of severe malnutrition are at higher risk for conditions like hypertension and deranged glucose metabolism, thereby establishing a link between early health adversity and future disorders (Grey et al., 2021). This fact is noteworthy, not only because it underlines the potential value of public health interventions to support nutritional improvement in target populations at risk, but also because it identifies one potential area to explore further. Determination of these associations may prove useful to inform prevention programs for lipid metabolism disorders through early intervention. Lastly, management of lipid metabolism disorders requires a multidimensional strategy that integrates preventive measures, therapeutic breakthroughs, and investigation of disease mechanisms. PCSK9's significant regulation of cholesterol homeostasis is a paradigm for how targeted solutions can make dramatic improvements in the health of individuals at risk for lipid disorders. Moreover, this conversation also brings forward the necessity for ongoing research on the long-term implications of early nutrition and its contribution to metabolic syndrome. While the medical fraternity continues to unravel the complexities of lipid metabolism, there is increasing interest in developing holistic prevention protocols and individualized treatment strategies. Lastly, a better comprehension of lipid metabolic disorders will be essential to the development of public health and for improving the lives of those afflicted by these widespread diseases.

The complexity of lipid disorders of metabolism is exemplified by the interplay between environmental and genetic influences. Recent genome-wide association studies have illustrated how gene polymorphisms, for example, those coding for the organic cation transporter OCT1, can have a major effect on body lipids. Such research has established an association between reduced-function alleles of OCT1 and elevated cholesterol, LDL cholesterol, and triglyceride concentrations. Notably, the functional implications of these results go beyond lipid profiles since such genetic differences have been postulated to also increase the risk for developing type 2 diabetes mellitus. This relationship underlines the metabolic relevance of OCT1 in the regulation of hepatic glucose as well as lipid, highlighting potential mechanisms by which lipid metabolism disorders lead to more extended cardiometabolic diseases (Abad et al., 2018). Apart from genetic predispositions, enzymatic deficiencies' effects, , such as that of glucose-6-phosphate dehydrogenase (G6PD) deficiency, provide another dimension to lipid metabolism disorders. As the most prevalent enzymopathy globally, G6PD deficiency leads to decreased enzymatic activity in major metabolic pathways, most significantly the pentose phosphate pathway. This disruption leads to impaired antioxidant defense and elevated oxidative stress, with the end result being cell injury and tumorigenic alterations. More recent investigations with patient-derived fibroblasts, a disease linked to oxidative stress in the chronic condition of pterygium, showed that G6PD-deficient cells contained more lipid deposits and higher growth rates typical of proliferative diseases. The finding supports the importance of G6PD deficiency as not only a disorder of metabolism but also an etiological event in the pathogenesis of severe ailments , such as atherosclerosis and cancer (Pani et al., 2009). Lastly, investigation of lipid metabolism disorders reveal an complex interaction among genetic, enzymatic, and environmental factors. Elucidation of these interactions is crucial in the development of preventive and therapeutic strategies to mitigate the risk associated with dyslipidemia and associated disease. Enhanced knowledge of the role of OCT1 in hepatic metabolism regulation and the role of G6PD deficiency in cellular oxidative stress reveals prime areas for further research. Such research can enable a more holistic strategy for lipid metabolism disorders, where individualized treatment and risk assessment protocols are emphasized to enhance patient outcomes in an environment characterized by widespread metabolic diseases. A consideration of both underlying and applied features of such disorders will be crucial to the overall aim of alleviating the burden of cardiovascular and metabolic diseases globally.

References

1. Abbeduto, L., Hertz-Picciotto, I., Orozco, J. S., Slupsky, C. M., et al. (2019). Metabolomics analysis of children with autism, idiopathic-developmental delays, and Down syndrome. https://core.ac.uk/download/323071890.pdf (accessed on 13th June 2025).
2. Ameer, B., & Weintraub, H. (2018). Pediatric obesity: Influence on drug dosing and therapeutics. https://core.ac.uk/download/155271623.pdf (accessed on 13th June 2025).
3. Argano, V., Balistreri, C. R., Giarratana, R. M., Lio, D., et al. (2019). On the road to accurate biomarkers for cardiometabolic diseases by integrating precision and gender medicine approaches. https://core.ac.uk/download/268910274.pdf (accessed on 13th June 2025).
4. Aulchenko, Y. S., Barbalic, M., Bis, J. C., Chambers, J. C., et al. (2010). Biological, clinical and population relevance of 95 loci for blood lipids. https://core.ac.uk/download/323079709.pdf (accessed on 13th June 2025).
5. Badiali, D., Bruno, G., Ribichini, E., Rossi, M., et al. (2019). Role of fiber in nutritional management of pancreatic diseases. https://core.ac.uk/download/231748461.pdf (accessed on 13th June 2025).
6. Bao, X., Liang, Y., Chang, H., Cai, T., Feng, B., Гордон, K., Zhu, Y., et al. (2024). Targeting proprotein convertase subtilisin/nexin type 9 (PCSK9): From bench to bedside. *Signal Transduction and Targeted Therapy, 9.* https://doi.org/10.1038/s41392-023-01690-3 (accessed on 13th June 2025).
7. Bars-Cortina, D., & Martín Barraza, J. I. (2024). Dietary pattern's role in hepatic epigenetic and dietary recommendations for the prevention of NAFLD. https://diposit.ub.edu/dspace/bitstream/2445/216596/1/nutrients-16-02956.pdf (accessed on 13th June 2025).
8. Bourdeau-Julien, I., Castonguay-Paradis, S., Rochefort, G., Perron, J., Lamarche, B., Flamand, N., Di Marzo, V., et al. (2023). The diet rapidly and differentially affects the gut microbiota and host lipid mediators in a healthy population. *Microbiome, 11.* https://doi.org/10.1186/s40168-023-01469-2 (accessed on 13th June 2025).
9. Buxton, M. J., Grant, J., Hanney, S., Pollitt, A., et al. (2011). Project Retro sight. Understanding the returns from cardiovascular and stroke research: Case studies. https://core.ac.uk/download/6113193.pdf (accessed on 13th June 2025).
10. Joseph, J., Depp, C., Shih, P. B., Cadenhead, K. S., & Schmid-Schönbein, G. (2017). Modified Mediterranean Diet for Enrichment of Short Chain Fatty Acids: Potential Adjunctive Therapeutic to Target Immune and Metabolic Dysfunction in Schizophrenia?. *Frontiers in neuroscience, 11,* 155. https://doi.org/10.3389/fnins.2017.00155Campo, J. A. del, Gallego, P., Gallego-Durán, R., Grande, L., et al. (2018). Genetic and epigenetic regulation in nonalcoholic fatty liver disease (NAFLD). https://core.ac.uk/download/161254838.pdf (accessed on 13th June 2025).
11. Cheng, Y., Cong, J., Xu, J., Tang, L., Zhou, Z., Yang, X., Hu, Y., et al. (2025). Research progress on the exacerbation of lipid metabolism by *Malassezia* and its impact on the skin barrier function. *Cosmetics.* https://www.semanticscholar.org/paper/4772315260b5a326996960843c4f1b413a217147 (accessed on 13th June 2025).
12. Cryan, J. F., O'Riordan, K. J., Cowan, C. S. M., Sandhu, K. V., Bastiaanssen, T. F. S., Boehme, M., Codagnone, M. G., et al. (2019). The microbiota-gut-brain axis. *Physiological Reviews, 99,* 1877–2013. https://doi.org/10.1152/physrev.00018.2018 (accessed on 13th June 2025).

13. Gorgey, A. S., Khan, M. R., O'Brien, L. C., Rankin, J. W., et al. (2017). Liver adiposity and metabolic profile in individuals with chronic spinal cord injury. https://core.ac.uk/download/215481810.pdf (accessed on 13th June 2025).

14. Gu, Y., Liu, X., & Gao, Z. (2025). To analyze the differences in plasma lipid composition among healthy, prediabetic and type 2 diabetic populations based on lipidomic. *International Journal of Biology and Life Sciences.* https://www.semanticscholar.org/paper/bf7c012acf631bfd17e24b4ecfa250fbf3020da6 (accessed on 13th June 2025).

15. Guillou, H., Iuliano, L., Lubrano, C., et al. (2015). Effect of obesity and metabolic syndrome on plasma oxysterols and fatty acids in humans. https://core.ac.uk/download/54518705.pdf (accessed on 13th June 2025).

16. Hayashi, J., Ishikawa, M., Karita, K., Kitamoto, A., et al. (2009). Longevity-associated NADH dehydrogenase subunit-2 237 Leu/Met polymorphism modulates the effects of daily alcohol drinking on yearly changes in serum total and LDL cholesterol in Japanese men. https://core.ac.uk/download/12548146.pdf (accessed on 13th June 2025).

17. Kapke, D. R. (2015). Childhood type II diabetes: The risks and complications. https://core.ac.uk/download/58826199.pdf (accessed on 13th June 2025).

18. Lukasiewicz, M., Zwara, A., Kowalski, J., Mika, A., & Hellmann, A. (2024). The role of lipid metabolism disorders in the development of thyroid cancer. *International Journal of Molecular Sciences, 25.* https://www.semanticscholar.org/paper/6073a7edda3ec20478bf60d8f1e46e2bc302c912 (accessed on 13th June 2025).

19. Mollinedo, F., & Gajate, C. (2020). Lipid rafts as signaling hubs in cancer cell survival/death and invasion: Implications in tumor progression and therapy. *Journal of Lipid Research, 61,* 611–635. https://doi.org/10.1194/jlr.tr119000439 (accessed on 13th June 2025).

20. Pani, A., Mandas, A., Abete, C., Norfo, C., Peiretti, E., Angius, F., Diaz, G., et al. (2009). Glucose-6-phosphate-dehydrogenase deficiency as a risk factor in proliferative disorder development. https://core.ac.uk/download/pdf/288358.pdf (accessed on 13th June 2025).

21. Rohatgi, A., Westerterp, M., von Eckardstein, A., Remaley, A. T., & Rye, K. A. (2021). HDL in the 21st century: A multifunctional roadmap for future HDL research. *Circulation, 143,* 2293–2309. https://doi.org/10.1161/circulationaha.120.044221 (accessed on 13th June 2025).

22. Sandlers, Y. (2020). Amino Acids Profiling for the Diagnosis of Metabolic Disorders. IntechOpen. doi: 10.5772/intechopen.84672

23. Sordyl, J., Malecka-Tendera, E., Sarecka-Hujar, B., & Kopyta, I. (2020). Headache in children: Selected factors of vascular changes involved in underlying processes of idiopathic headaches. *Children, 7.* https://www.semanticscholar.org/paper/0d03beb914be36dd5dd237e5c4ade3d0458358c3 (accessed on 13th June 2025).

24. Wang, Y., Liu, T., Liu, W., Zhao, H., & Li, P. (2024). Research hotspots and future trends in lipid metabolism in chronic kidney disease: A bibliometric and visualization analysis from 2004 to 2023. *Frontiers in Pharmacology, 15.* https://www.semanticscholar.org/paper/212edc3801db730c1e9b9fb0049f780f560f9497 (accessed on 13th June 2025).

25. Xenoulis, P. (2008). Investigations into idiopathic hypertriglyceridemia in the Miniature Schnauzer in North America. https://core.ac.uk/download/11030060.pdf (accessed on 13th June 2025).

26. Zhang, K., Wang, L., Gao, W., & Guo, R. (2025). Retinol-binding protein 4 in skeletal and cardiac muscle: Molecular mechanisms, clinical implications, and future perspectives. *Frontiers in Cell and Developmental Biology, 13.* https://www.semanticscholar.org/paper/a2a49eae85306b3bc9506b9a258f05e856d20e2b (accessed on 13th June 2025).

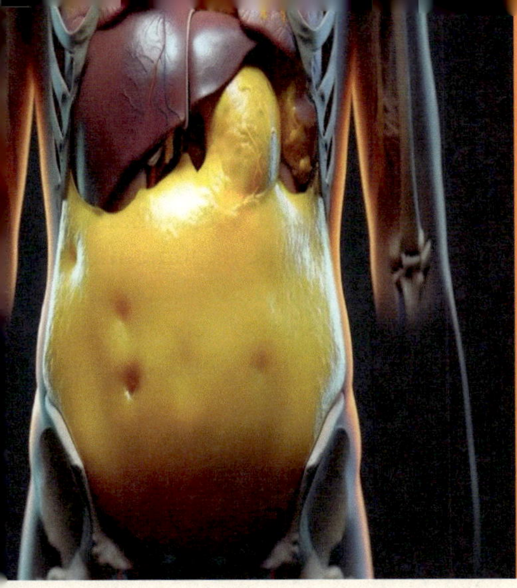

Chapter 10

INBORN ERRORS OF METABOLISM

Contents

Introduction....313
10.1. Types of Inborn Errors of Metabolism....317
10.2. Genetic Basis of Inborn Errors of Metabolism....321
10.3. Symptoms and Diagnosis....325
10.4. Treatment Options....329
10.5. Case Studies....333
10.6. Impact on Patients and Families....337
Summary....343
References....345

Introduction

The study of inborn errors of metabolism (IEMs) is a milestone towards the integration of genetics and clinical practice. The inherited metabolic disorders result from genetic mutations causing disruption of specific enzymatic activities, which result in the disorganization of metabolic processes. The significance of IEMs is not only because of their clinical relevance but also because of their wide-ranging presentation that can coincide with many other conditions, which makes diagnosis difficult. Hence, effective and early identification of IEMs is ever more critical because these conditions can significantly impact the long-term health and wellbeing of their victims. Prevalence heterogeneity of IEMs across different populations only compounds the necessity to develop population-specific strategies for diagnosis and screening, further emphasizing the imperative need to have an educated appreciation of such multivariate disorders (Sandlers, 2020). In modern clinical practice, the advent of newborn screening programs has made it possible early detect certain IEMs early with targeted metabolic tests.

However, the methods have limitations with their reliance on preselected panels and hence lead to false negatives and missed diagnoses. Thus, the application of untargeted metabolomics is now becoming a more comprehensive method for screening IEMs. This strategy allows for the analysis of additional metabolites, thereby supporting the concurrent assessment of multiple pathways and identification of yet untargeted disorders. The use of such sophisticated techniques by healthcare professionals will enhance the diagnostic efficacy for IEMs, thereby ensuring enhanced management (Sandlers, 2020). Increasing the breadth of metabolite analysis is highly promising for future IEM diagnosis. Moreover, awareness of IEMs in adult presentations is also important. While these disorders have traditionally been associated with children, new evidence suggests that IEMs present in adolescents and adults, often leading to misdiagnosis or delay. Neurodegenerative presentation, especially movement disorder, can be the precursor to underlying IEMs, but these are relatively underemphasized in neurologic training. Having a systematic approach to the identification of adult-onset IEMs would significantly improve diagnostic accuracy. The use of next generation sequencing along with detailed clinical phenotyping can facilitate the detection of subtle or atypical presentations, thereby optimizing care outcomes. Raising awareness and adding diagnostic protocols in this area will prevent clinicians from suffering further complications from IEMs due to delayed treatment.

Definition of Inborn Errors of Metabolism

Inborn errors of metabolism (IEM) represent a group of genetic diseases that disrupt normal metabolic processes. They are usually caused by mutations in some genes encoding enzymes important for biochemical reactions, resulting either in the accumulation of toxic metabolites or in the deficiency of necessary substances. IEM can manifest at any age of life and typically presents with heterogeneous and occasionally severe clinical features, including developmental delay, neurological abnormalities, and metabolic disturbances. The conditions are extremely varied in classification, with over 1,000 conditions, which include amino acidopathies, organic acidemias, and fatty acid oxidation disorders. This broad array of metabolic dysfunctions highlights the need for early diagnosis and treatment since prompt management of IEM can prevent irreversible complications and improve the quality of life in such patients. The pathophysiology of inborn errors of metabolism typically involves some metabolic pathways that become deranged due to genetic anomalies. For example, in phenylketonuria (PKU), the absence of the enzyme phenylalanine hydroxylase leads to an accumulation of phenylalanine, toxic at high levels and causes rapid neurological deterioration. Similarly, conditions, such as galactosemia disrupt carbohydrate metabolism, leading to a buildup of galactose and other substances, with liver damage and cataracts if not adequately treated. With the human genome increasingly being mapped and understood, equipment like the human genome-scale metabolic reconstruction has proved invaluable in describing such complex metabolic networks and predicting the effects of various metabolic disorders. Such baseline data is central in the planning of targeted treatment and personalized treatment regimens for patients afflicted with IEM (Ang et al., 2016). Advances in imaging, such as newborn screening programs and biomarker identification, have vastly improved the diagnosis and management of inborn errors of metabolism. Early discovery provides clinicians with the opportunity to institute required dietary restriction, enzyme replacement therapy, or gene therapy intended to correct the metabolic derangement. An example is the dietary management employed in PKU, which is a phenylalanine-restricted diet that allows affected individuals to live well but without adverse neurological effects. Furthermore, continuous research is necessary in the field of metabolic disorders, since greater understanding of metabolic processes and the development of novel treatments, , such as gene editing technologies, hold the promise of better intervention. Incorporation of elaborate metabolic annotations and balancing techniques (JA et al., 2001) ensures that ongoing research is directed towards advancing knowledge of the disorders, which consequently will be beneficial to the efforts put towards the control and potential cure of inborn errors of metabolism (Figure 10.1).

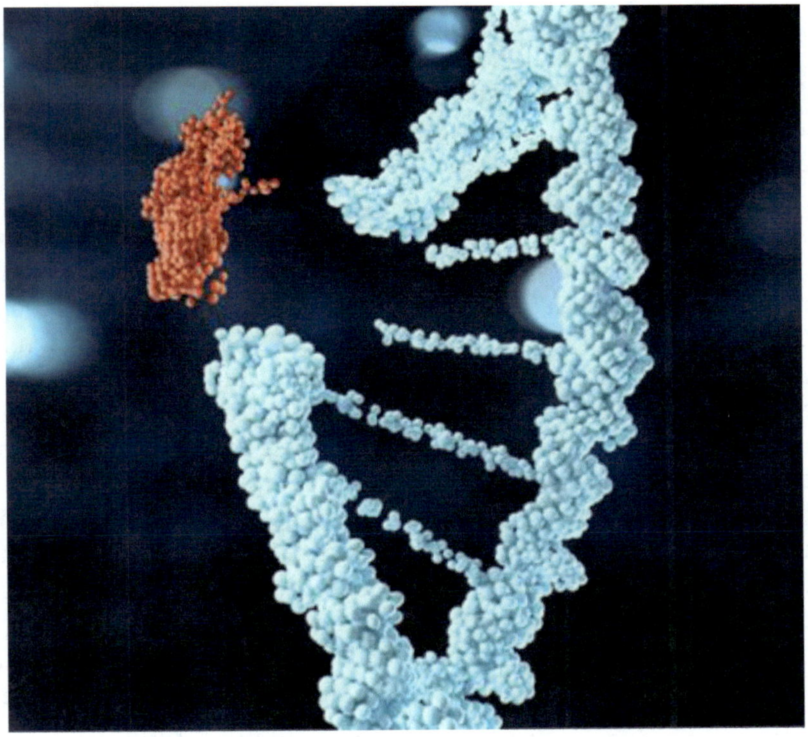

Figure 10.1. Illustration of gene editing showing targeted modification within a DNA strand.

Source: https://www.frontiersin.org/files/special%20topics/17463/thumb_400.jpg.

Historical Context and Discovery

The history behind the discovery of inborn errors of metabolism (IEMs) is one of significant progress both on the clinical and laboratory fronts. The term "inborn errors of metabolism" was coined during the early part of the 20th century, largely due to the pioneering work of Archibald Garrod, who suggested that metabolic diseases resulted from the absence of specific genes. Garrod's work laid the foundation for understanding the way in which one biochemical pathway can go wrong due to inherited causes and thereby lead to a variety of diseases. The impact of this concept on genetics has been immense, as it laid the path for further studies into the mechanisms behind these metabolic disorders. Consequently, IEMs not only became a clinical problem but also an important field of genetic counseling and disease management, which revolutionized diagnosis and treatment strategies during the following years. No less important has been the role played by advances in technology and methodology in the historical evolution of IEMs. After new techniques of molecular biology came into being, researchers began examining the genetic origins of these diseases in greater detail. High-throughput sequencing has particularly revolutionized the discipline of metabolic medicine with the potential to identify causative mutations in various IEMs. Moreover, new stem cell technologies, specifically induced pluripotent stem cells (iPSCs), have provided unparalleled toolkits for modeling these diseases. Use of patient-derived iPSCs for IEM modeling enhances researchers' knowledge of disease pathogenesis and the ability to test hypothesized therapeutic interventions. As a result, ongoing research continues to maximize our genetic insight and generate novel opportunities for successful therapeutic interventions in the treatment of IEMs, significantly altering the prognosis of metabolic disease research (Escribá et al., 2021). Notably, historical figures like Achille de Giovanni have contributed to the evolution of clinical practices that inform the understanding of IEMs today. De Giovanni's work in clinical anthropometry focused on correlating body morphology with metabolic function, underscoring the importance of individualized medical assessments. Although his ideas faded into relative obscurity shortly after his death, they emphasize a critical perspective on the complexities of human health. The relationship between metabolic processes, physical characteristics, and genetic differences highlights the intricacy involved in the IEMs study. While recent studies develop, integrating past findings as de Giovanni proposed may help explain the pathways in which the metabolic defects take place, connecting past concepts with today's science (Zampieri, 2018). Comprehension of this rich history of explorations dictates the present state of metabolic disorders, ultimately informing diagnostic and therapeutic endeavors.

Importance of Studying Metabolic Disorders

The significance of studying metabolic disorders, particularly under the topic of inborn errors of metabolism (IEMs), should not be overestimated because of their far-reaching consequences on individual health and the healthcare system as a whole. The disorders arise from genetic mutations leading to enzyme deficiencies that disrupt metabolic processes and result in the formation of toxic substrates. Understanding the biochemical and genetic foundations of such disorders enables early diagnosis and intervention, eventually resulting in better patient outcomes. By examining metabolic disorders, medical progress is encouraged in treatments, including new drugs and gene therapy methods. Through rigorous research, researchers can find candidate biomarkers for early detection, more critically in diseases where rapid treatment can prevent irreparable damage and enhance quality of life. In addition, the research on metabolic disorders holds broader significance for the field of personalized medicine. The identification of induced pluripotent stem cells (iPSCs) allows scientists to produce disease models that mirror the complexity of IEMs and demonstrate a valuable point of view regarding the underlying mechanisms of the disease. Patient-specific iPSC models of most IEMs have been produced, as detailed in recent reviews, which hold the potential for drug testing and experimental therapy guided by individual genotypes. This novel model system not only allows for the appreciation of human pathophysiological mechanisms but also enhances the likelihood of drug discovery, with likely acceleration of the delivery of effective therapeutic interventions to affected individuals. All these developments underscore the need for continued investigation of metabolic disorders, with a devotion to translating scientific information into practical healthcare solutions (Escribá et al., 2021). Finally, a closer examination of how metabolic disorders affect neurological and cognitive processes emphasizes the need to study these conditions further. For example, diseases , such as urea cycle disorders (UCD) may cause elevated levels of ammonia, which can cause extreme neurocognitive impairments if addressed late. It has been suggested that UCD patients are likely to have executive function problems critical to reasoning, problem-solving, and self-regulation. Understanding the interactions between metabolic imbalance, cognitive impairment, and effective management enables medical practitioners to implement comprehensive care plans that cover physical as well as mental health. The integration of neuroimaging with neuropsychological testing provides a robust foundation for managing these complex interactions, supporting the necessity for a multi-aspect treatment and research strategy in the case of metabolic disorders (Gropman, 2019) (Figure 10.2).

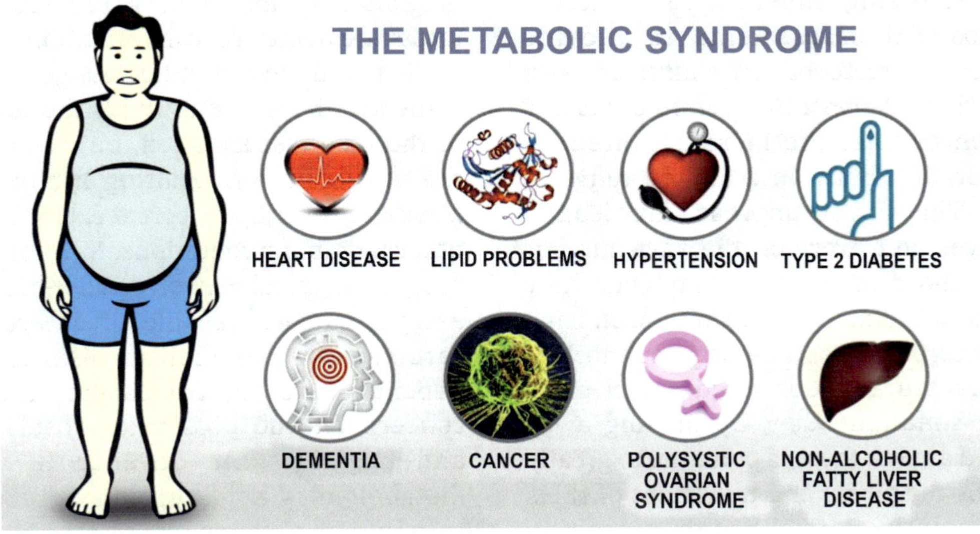

Figure 10.2. Complications associated with metabolic syndrome.

Source: https://external-content.duckduckgo.com/iu/?u=https%3A%2F%2Fhealthjade.com%2Fwp-content%2Fuploads%2F2016%2F12%2Fmetabolic-syndrome.jpg&f=1&nofb=1&ipt=b3f1b15172ac4203645db2db5c4d6a963d47b00979d4183925342f75e55bc708.

10.1. Types of Inborn Errors of Metabolism

IEMs are a diverse group of genetic disorders involving the body's normal biochemical pathways. Disorders have been classically divided based on the involved metabolic pathways; for instance, carbohydrate metabolism-associated disorders are galactosemia and glycogen storage diseases. While amino acid diseases , such as phenylketonuria and maple syrup urine disease, present unique challenges to management on a dietary basis and life-long health status, lipid metabolism disorders constitute a significant category as well, with such diseases as familial hypercholesterolemia and lysosomal storage diseases impairing lipid processing in complex ways. Classification of these disorders is critical, as this determines not only treatment strategies, but also nutritional care needed for management of symptoms and long-term health outcomes of the affected patients, enhancing quality of life and prognosis (Sandlers, 2020). Clinical presentation of IEMs can be heterogeneous, often overlapping with several clinical presentations depending on impaired enzymes or pathways. For example, while some of the patients may present with obvious neurological findings, others may have largely metabolic crises or developmental delays. This heterogeneity complicates clinical diagnosis and treatment. Of specific interest, IEM movement disorders also reflect this complexity, for example, in children, as revealed in research studies. Research suggests a radical reduction in HRQOL and adaptive functioning among the group, defining the margin to which movement disorders' severity is associated with overall health and well-being (Peall, 2014). Clinicians are hence in need of an integrated diagnostic approach, involving biochemical, genetic, and psychosocial assessments to provide comprehensive care to patients afflicted with these disorders. Screening technologies for the detection of IEMs are more advanced, as previous methods focus on a limited range of metabolites. This narrow approach may lead to false negatives and overlook the vast number of possible inborn errors that can occur. New technologies in metabolomics show promising lines for increasing screening capability, where untargeted analyses could detect more metabolites simultaneously. By moving away from targeted assays, there is potential to greatly advance early diagnosis and treatment of IEMs and, consequently, better health outcomes. As technology progresses, advanced studies comparing the effectiveness and durability of these new tools to existing targeted approaches will be crucial to refining our understanding of IEM diagnostics and enabling timely, effective management strategies (Sandlers, 2020).

10.1.1. Carbohydrate Metabolism Disorders

Carbohydrate disorders are a significant subgroup of the general category of IEMs. Carbohydrate disorders result when specific enzymes used to digest and utilize carbohydrates become dysfunctional due to genetic mutations. These dysfunctions may lead to the accumulation of toxic metabolites or a deficiency of essential metabolic products. For instance, disorders , such as Glycogen Storage Diseases (GSDs) demonstrate how enzymatic deficiencies interfere with normal glucose homeostasis and lead to manifestations ranging from hypoglycemia to muscle weakness and even life-threatening complications. Owing to the heterogeneity of such disorders and their consequences, the understanding of their biochemical background is crucial for accurate diagnosis and treatment, thereby underlining the importance of definitive metabolic assays in the clinical setting (Sandlers, 2019). Carbohydrate metabolism disease diagnosis is most often a process of multiple facets involving clinical evaluation, biochemical testing, and, where indicated, genetic analysis. Difficulty lies not only with the identification of the true disease itself, but with controlling the vast array of resulting symptoms, which frequently overlap to a great extent with those of other metabolic conditions. Newborn screening programs typically involve panel-based targeted assays that are capable of detecting certain carbohydrate metabolism disorders, but the dependence on restricted panels has been a concern for the possibility of false positives and negatives. An advance in untargeted metabolomics holds promising observations, as it offers a wider analytical view, allowing for complete detection of several metabolites participating in carbohydrate metabolism at one time. Such an integrated approach could significantly enhance early diagnosis and intervention processes, particularly in challenging scenarios where traditional methods will prove ineffective (Sandlers, 2020). Effective treatment of carbohydrate metabolism disturbances needs both dietary treatment and ongoing clinical follow-up. Treatment interventions usually concentrate on dietary adaptation to prevent the buildup of toxic substrates or to balance energy needs, treating the specific metabolic derangements of the disturbance. For example, patients with certain types of GSDs will require frequent meals of carbohydrate-containing or complex sugars to avoid oscillations in glucose levels. As for diet, meticulous observation of metabolic parameters should be conducted to avoid acute complications as well as to guide optimal fine-tuning of treatment regimens. Therefore, an integrated understanding of carbohydrate metabolism disorders and progress in diagnostic methods holds the potential to improve the quality of life and prognosis of patients tormented by such metabolic disorders (Sandlers, 2019) (Figure 10.3).

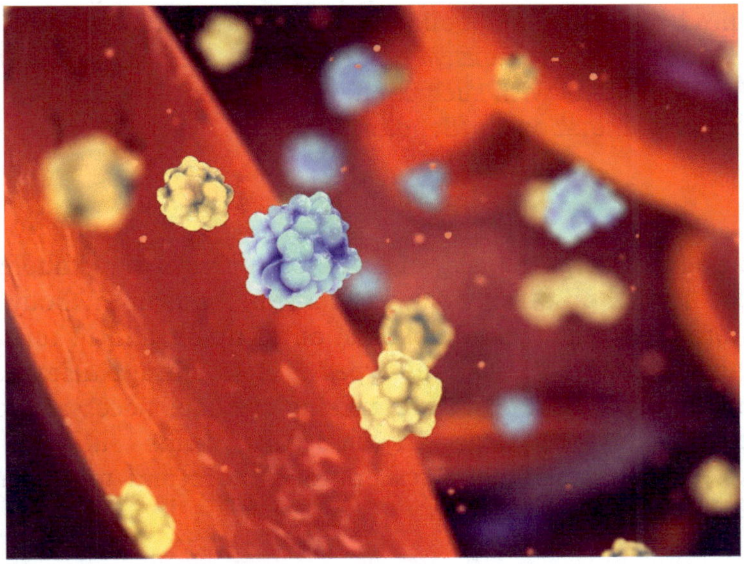

Figure 10.3. Visualization of carbohydrate metabolism with enzymes active in the bloodstream.

Source: https://external-content.duckduckgo.com/iu/?u=https%3A%2F%2Fmedlineplus.gov%2Fimages%2Fcarbohydratemetabolism_share.jpg&f=1&nofb=1&ipt=773dc72671103b9466e38b1f11e80baa44747587b36832a2da9be35e22536620.

10.1.2. Amino Acid Metabolism Disorders

Amino acid metabolism disorders are a significant group of inborn errors of metabolism caused by genetic mutation in genes encoding enzymes that are involved in amino acid metabolism. These disorders usually lead to the production of toxic metabolites, leading to more than one clinical presentation. Phenylketonuria (PKU), a well-known metabolic disorder, is made up of a deficiency of the enzyme phenylalanine hydroxylase, leading to the toxic build-up of phenylalanine. If not treated, PKU can lead to severe neurological impairment, emphasizing the need for early diagnosis and metabolic screening. The breakdown of amino acid diseases shows how crucial such metabolic pathways are to maintaining physiological balance and underscores the need for even minor enzymatic dysfunction within a child's health and development (Eldin et al., 2009). Recent research on amino acid metabolism disorders has highlighted their prevalence among some groups, , such as Egyptian children. A study of infants and children with intractable mental retardation found that 3.72% were suspected to have amino acid metabolism disorders, of which 40% were diagnosed by advanced diagnostic techniques, , such as amino acid analyzers. This highlights the effectiveness of current metabolic screening technologies in making precise diagnoses for such conditions. Such patients typically present with clinical manifestations of mental retardation, convulsions, and somatic abnormalities, and collectively increase the demand for public health awareness as well as for targeted genetic counseling among afflicted groups (Eldin et al., 2009). Treatment and diagnosis of amino acid metabolic disorders mandate an interdisciplinary approach involving pediatricians, geneticists, and metabolic specialists. The clinical dilemma is not only in the heterogeneous presentation of the disorders but also in the wide variety of potential underlying genetic mutations. Effective management requires precise interventions, i.e., dietary restrictions and supplements, tailored to the disorder. Additionally, periodic monitoring in the form of biochemical investigations is required to ensure metabolic control and avoidance of secondary complications. Through the implementation of comprehensive care strategies, medical practitioners can significantly improve the well-being of patients with such conditions, ultimately transforming the prognosis of debilitating inborn errors of metabolism (Sandlers, 2019).

10.1.3. Lipid Metabolism Disorders

Lipid metabolism disorders are a principal group of inborn errors of metabolism involving genetic defects that disrupt the normal processing and transport of lipids in the body. The conditions may result in abnormal storage or inadequate mobilization of lipids, and in turn produce a range of medical conditions. An example is the various types of lipid storage diseases, , such as Gaucher disease and Tay-Sachs disease, where there are missing enzymes necessary for lipid degradation. This leads to catastrophic outcomes, particularly on organ systems , such as the liver and nervous system. Early detection through newborn screening is more and more stressed with greater knowledge of these disorders.

Despite the fact that the current technique often employs certain metabolic assays, the addition of broader analytical approaches would ensure the early diagnosis and management of lipid metabolism disorders, hence improving patient outcomes (Sandlers, 2020). For adults and neonates, the effects of lipid metabolism disorders could emerge in varied clinical manifestations, from organ hypertrophy, neurological deficit, and even fetal death. One of the most recognized categories is the function of pulmonary surfactant, a lipoprotein complex that is crucial in reducing surface tension within the alveoli. Disorders of surfactant metabolism, , such as surfactant protein B (SP-B) deficiency, illustrate the way deficient lipid metabolism can lead to severe respiratory distress and secondary complications. Pathophysiology of these disorders may be complex and demand an interdisciplinary method of effective diagnosis and treatment. Genetic considerations are relevant, as mutations in the SFTPB gene have a direct relation to SP-B deficiency. Continued research on the disorders has relevance to targeted therapeutic treatment, demonstrating the necessity of complete screening to identify affected individuals at an early age (JA et al., 2001). Emerging techniques , such as untargeted metabolomics, are revolutionizing the diagnosis of lipid metabolism disorders. Unlike the traditional method involving targeting a limited panel of compounds, untargeted analyses will screen a wide array of metabolites, hence supporting the identification of more inborn errors of metabolism. Through this widely based approach, multiple metabolic pathways can be evaluated at once, improving the likelihood of identifying the underlying lipid metabolism disorders. Moreover, the ability to identify previously unexpected metabolic derangements has the potential to improve treatment and patient care regimens. Through the bridging of the gap between clinical utility and metabolic profiling, such newer methods can potentially revolutionize the quality and amount of care available to patients with lipid metabolism disorder, ultimately resulting in an improved long-term health outcome and quality of life (Sandlers, 2020) (Figure 9.4).

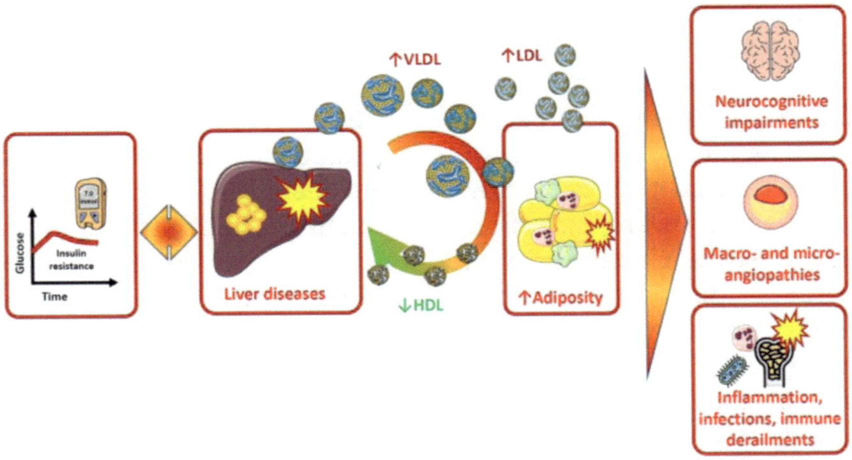

Figure 10.4. Overview of insulin resistance cascade: from liver disease and dyslipidemia to adiposity and systemic complications.

Source: https://external-content.duckduckgo.com/iu/?u=https%3A%2F%2Fmedia.springernature.com%2Flw725%2Fspringer-cms%2Frest%2Fv1%2Fcontent%2F25249610%2Fdata%2Fv4&f=1&nofb=1&ipt=1226512f5850300eda695d2447e42f334e6c784d0dc3e8c3ca77043149b145b1.

10.2. Genetic Basis of Inborn Errors of Metabolism

The genetic basis of the inborn errors of metabolism (IEMs) relies on the mutation that compromises the activity of enzymes to ensure proper metabolic pathway function. These inherited disorders lead to a variety of presentations of symptoms since they result in the accumulation of harmful metabolites or loss of necessary products. Research indicates that mutations occurring in genes taking part in enzyme genes can be caused by different mechanisms including nonsense mutations, frameshifts, and missense alterations resulting in decreased enzyme activity or loss of function. The phenotypic heterogeneity, normally the situation with patients, does not only result from the type of mutation present but also from environmental factors and interactions of other present genetic modifiers. Early diagnosis is crucial because it could influence treatment approaches and long-term well-being. To this end, the genetic etiology of such disorders has to be elucidated so effective treatment and screening programs can be developed (Sandlers, 2020). Of all the types of IEMs, erotic aciduria is a prime example that illustrates the intricacies of genetic imbalances in metabolic pathways. This condition is primarily caused by the mutation of the uridine monophosphate synthase (UMPS) gene, leading to extensive impairment in pyrimidine synthesis. This is an autosomal recessive disorder and commonly found with increased excretion of erotic acid in the urine along with megaloblastic anemia and developmental delay symptoms. The UMPS genetic variation might explain three forms of erotic aciduria, and thus proper diagnosis becomes essential to start with effective treatment. Newborn screening technologies that utilize cutting-edge metabolomics can potentially advance early detection capabilities further, reducing the likelihood of severe complications from untreated cases. Hence, understanding erotic aciduria's genetic pathology is symbolic of the broad concept of genetic influences on inborn errors in metabolism (Fonteh et al., 2018). The effects of genomics and metabolomics advancements play a critical role in determining inborn errors in metabolism. Recent studies suggest that untargeted metabolomics may provide a more comprehensive approach to screening for IEMs, one that prevents the pitfalls associated with traditional targeted approaches. Because a wide variety of metabolites are explored without preselected targets, doctors can identify anomalies in several metabolic pathways simultaneously. A global approach would provide greater diagnostic accuracy and prevent false positives and false negatives, ultimately translating to early treatment. With the advancements of technology, including genetic testing and metabolomic analysis, the inclusion of these within newborn screening programs can potentially boost the management of IEMs significantly. Thus, continued studies and dedicated research are needed to effectively take advantage of these technological advancements in providing better results to the affected population (Sandlers, 2020).

10.2.1. Function of Genes in Metabolic Pathways

The complex interplay between genes and metabolic pathways is the foundation for understanding inborn errors of metabolism. Genes hold the code for the manufacture of enzymes that catalyze the metabolic processes, and mutations, if any, can lead to dysfunctional pathways that constitute the spectrum of metabolic disorders. As an example, disruption of a single gene can stall the transformation of nutrients into energy so that harmful substrates accumulate. Inborn errors of metabolism encompass a variety of conditions, , such as phenylketonuria or maple syrup urine disease, where certain enzyme deficiency interferes with the integrity of metabolism. Genetic elements in these pathways not only have a role in diagnosis but also therapy, , such as gene therapy. These treatments aim at alleviating such metabolic shortcomings through the repair of genetic mutations, thus restoring normal enzymatic function and implementing metabolic pathways conducive to health and vitality (Vasconcelos and Lacerda, 2022). Furthermore, understanding gene-environment interactions enhances comprehension of inborn errors of metabolism-associated metabolic pathways. The phenotype manifesting as a consequence of genetic mutation not only relies on mutation but also on environmental factors, including dietary intake, exercise, and exposure to toxins. For example, individuals with metabolic disorders may display a set of symptoms based on variation in the intake of diet, which can vary through their metabolism and overall impact of their genetic status. Interventions that are based on both gene susceptibilities and environment can be more effective at symptom relief and quality of life enhancement. Hence, integrating metabolic pathways and gene function with environmental inputs is a balanced strategy for inborn errors in metabolism with a focus on the necessity of individualized measures in therapeutic approaches (Chiang and Ferrell, 2020). The significant advances in genetic research have introduced new therapeutic strategies toward the treatment of inborn errors of metabolism. Gene therapy, for instance, has the potential to rectify the root cause of the genetic defect itself, rather than symptomatically treating the defect. The technologies of CRISPR and other gene-editing technologies have the potential to provide long-term solutions toward metabolic disorders through targeted correction of defective genes. In addition, hematopoietic stem cell transplantation has also been explored as a novel approach for certain metabolic disorders, wherein the stem cell regenerative capacity is exploited to restore functional metabolic pathways (Vasconcelos and Lacerda, 2022). These developments pinpoint an exciting frontier in the treatment of inborn errors of metabolism, where insight into the action of genes in the metabolic pathway directly informs clinical use and new therapy, with the aim of improved prospects for those affected (Figure 10.5).

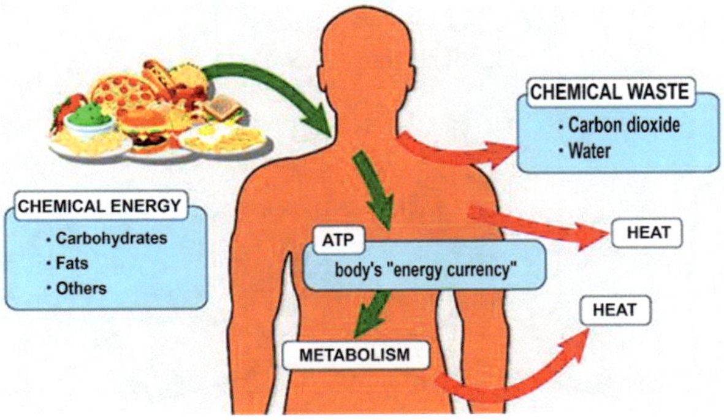

Figure 10.5. Conversion of food into ATP and heat through metabolic processes in the human body.

Source: https://cdn1.byjus.com/wp-content/uploads/2018/02/ENERGY-AND-HUMAN-LIFE-2.png.

10.2.2. Inheritance Patterns (Autosomal Recessive, Dominant, etc.)

Patterns of inheritance of IEM are relevant to the genetic nature of the diseases. Among these patterns, the most common is autosomal recessive, particularly for diseases , such as phenylketonuria and galactosemia. For autosomal recessive diseases, an individual must receive two copies of a gene that are mutated, one from each parent, to get the disease. This form of inheritance tends to cause carriers, individuals who have only one copy of the defective gene but otherwise remain unaffected. Frequency of such disorders is contingent upon factors like consanguinity, which incidentally occurs much more in certain population groups, ultimately leading to an increased rate of homozygous recessive genotypes in these groups. This genetic heterogeneity emphasizes the importance of information on ethnic and regional variation in the manifestation of IEMs. Autosomal dominant inheritance, although less frequent in inborn errors of metabolism, also has significant implications for families and patients. In this form, only one copy of the faulty gene is sufficient to lead to the disease, so transmission to offspring is more likely. Conditions like Huntington's disease and certain types of hypercholesterolemia are examples of this trend. Unlike other cases, dominant mutations can have incomplete penetrance, so that not everyone who carries the mutated gene will express the symptoms of the condition. This unpredictability makes it difficult for clinical management and genetic counseling because families might receive surprise diagnoses. Besides, sporadic mutations could happen, and this accounts for de novo instances where no family history exists, further complicating these patterns of inheritance and their clinical relevance. The addition of advances in genetic analysis has significantly enhanced the diagnosis and understanding of IEM patterns of inheritance. Techniques , such as next-generation sequencing (NGS) have made it possible to recognize mutations in both autosomal dominant and autosomal recessive IEM. As an example, research indicates that a considerable percentage of variants identified in the patients are in autosomal recessive mode, particularly in regions with high consanguinity, which reflects on the role played by genetic testing in such populations (Hawary et al., 2022). Additionally, as inborn errors of immunity (IEI) intersect with metabolic disorders, it becomes evident that the inheritance patterns can manifest differently within the immune system, leading to varied clinical outcomes. The recognition of these complex genetic interactions underscores the necessity of a tailored approach toward diagnosis and management, maximizing the potential for effective treatments and interventions tailored to individual genetic backgrounds (Bravo-Perez et al., 2023) (Figure 10.6).

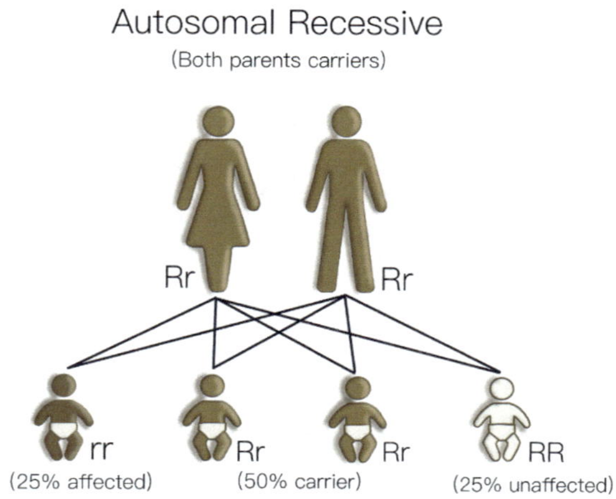

Figure 10.6. Autosomal recessive inheritance shows carrier parents and risk distribution in offspring.

Source: https://retinaaustralia.com.au/wp-content/uploads/2022/11/Autosomal-recessive-inheritance.png.

10.2.3. Genetic Mutations and Their Effects

Understanding genetic mutations is essential to understanding the pathogenesis of inborn errors of metabolism (IEMs). Mutations in significant metabolic pathways are responsible for these conditions, generally through enzymatic deficiencies. These deficiencies have the potential to lead to the accumulation of poisonous metabolites or to the inability to synthesize required compounds, and ultimately to manifest as a variety of phenotypic expressions. The genetic origin of IEMs is predominantly monogenic, i.e., alterations in a single gene can create heterogeneity in clinical presentation. Phenylketonuria and methylmalonic acidemia are some of the most prevalent IEMs that have varying mutations leading to variability in disease severity and response to treatment. This highlights the importance of genetic profiling in identifying those at risk and in directing therapy, allowing it to be possible to implement more tailored medicine approaches to these potentially disabling diseases, ultimately improving patient outcomes with metabolic disorders. The interaction between environmental factors and genetic mutations plays an important role in determining the expressivity of metabolic disorders. Research has shown that while certain genetic mutations predispose an individual to certain inborn errors of metabolism, in many cases, environmental factors can often significantly affect the phenotypic expression of the conditions. As an example, changing diet can minimize the role of mutations related to diseases , such as phenylketonuria, which is dependent on control of phenylalanine intake by diet. This is a holistic model that highlights the gene-environment interaction determining metabolic well-being, avoiding the oversimplification of thought that disease pathology is genetically determined. This interaction is vital for clinicians to implement effective intervention mechanisms, which can enhance patients' quality of life with IEMs, a shift towards holistic practice in treating metabolic disorders. Also, the research of personalized medicine and genetic research has great promise in advancing the treatment of inborn errors of metabolism. Advances like patient-derived intrahepatic cholangiocyte organoids (ICOs) are revolutionizing research into metabolic disorders. Using patient-specific cell models, researchers can investigate the function of multiple metabolic pathways and identify personalized treatment regimens. Recent research has demonstrated that ICOs can be employed successfully to replicate satisfactorily defects in major metabolic pathways, , such as Wilson disease and cystic fibrosis. However, issues exist, particularly with regard to issues of limitations of such models as well as their applicability to the large range of IEMs. More research into ICO functional assays is warranted, as it might make possible more targeted treatments and improved quality of life for patients with these diseases, which points to the critical overlap of genetic mutation and individual patient care within the context of metabolism (Lehmann et al., 2021).

10.3. Symptoms and Diagnosis

Symptom presentation in patients with inborn errors of metabolism (IEMs) is very heterogeneous, with a tendency to perplexing diagnosis. The disorders are present through genetic mutations that disrupt the functions of single enzymes and thereby form defective pathways of metabolism. Symptoms range from acute metabolic emergencies to chronic ailments based on the individual disorder and age of presentation. For instance, there are IEMs that will have presentations in early infancy with clinical features , such as developmental delay, failure to thrive, and dysfunction of organs, and there are those that will have presentation only in late childhood or adulthood, and at times with misdiagnosis or presentation being delayed.

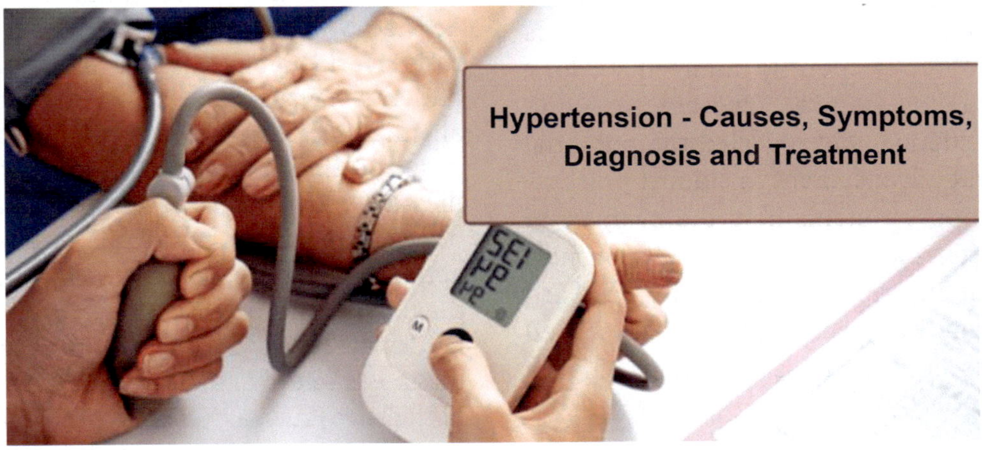

Figure 10.6. Monitoring blood pressure to manage and diagnose hypertension.

Source: https://possible.in/wp-content/uploads/2022/07/Hypertension-Causes-Symptoms-Diagnosis-Treatment.png.

The recognition of these signs early on is significant since early interventions can significantly affect patient outcomes and also stop irreversible complications of metabolic derangement (Sandlers, 2020). Diagnosis of inborn errors of metabolism is typically multifactorial, beginning with clinical suspicion based on the patient's presentation and family history. Health workers can subsequently employ biochemical screening methods, , such as blood samples and urinary analysis, to measure levels of particular metabolites involved in metabolic pathways. Developments in newborn screening in recent decades have greatly boosted the rate at which various IEMs are detected early in life and allowed early intervention and treatment. Yet, targeted metabolic essays have disadvantages, including the risk of false positives and false negatives, which can mislead clinical decision-making. Towards enhancing diagnostic precision for the sake of improving diagnostics, some researchers advocate the use of expanded fanning-out screening strategies, , such as untargeted metabolomics, with the capability of identifying a wider variety of metabolic disturbances without target lists (Sandlers, 2020). Decision support system advancements have also recently enhanced the diagnostic environment for inborn metabolic disorders. Such systems rely on machine learning algorithms that can process information from patients and construct decision trees that allow for enhanced diagnosis. In a patient study involving three specific IEMs, it was discovered that a classification algorithm was utilized effectively to review cases and deliver correct diagnostic outcomes. Such an approach made clinicians correctly identify many disorders, including galactosemia, fructosemia, and propionic acidemia, and revealed the potential for significant advancement in clinical practice. Decision support systems hold the promise to enhance better matching of metabolic profiles with clinical information, ultimately toward more efficient early screening and improved health status in individuals with IEMs (Figure 10.6).

10.3.1. Common Clinical Manifestations

Inborn errors in metabolism (IEMs) represent a diverse collection of genetic disorders that disrupt normal metabolism and result in a broad variety of clinical manifestations. Growth failure, neurological dysfunction, and metabolic crisis at any age are characteristic presentations. The specific clinical presentation is often unpredictable based on the specific metabolic pathway disrupted and the buildup or lack of metabolites. For instance, metabolic disorders of amino acids lead to encephalopathy and failure to thrive, while defects in carbohydrate metabolism led to ketoacidosis and hypoglycemia. Such pervasive clinical presentations are significant in initiating the right treatment and diagnosis at once, allowing clinicians to deploy effective interventions likely to significantly improve patient outcomes. The presentation heterogeneity of the symptoms also complicates the diagnostic process, and increased awareness and standardized screening processes should be utilized in healthcare centers (Sandlers, 2020). Numerous IEMs present with specific biochemical markers that are accountable for specific clinical presentations. For example, erotic aciduria, an autosomal recessive disease of low prevalence, is primarily defined by the occurrence of erotic acid due to a dysfunctional uridine monophosphate synthase (UMPS) enzyme. Clinically, the condition is typically defined by lethargy, failure to feed, and failure to thrive in neonates. Of a different kind, the patients may also have secondary megaloblastic anemia caused by defective pyrimidine synthesis required in DNA and RNA. Laboratory testing usually shows conspicuously elevated levels of urinary uric acid and reduced UMPS activity, which serve to establish the correct diagnosis. The occurrence of these indicators is underscored by the importance of early diagnosis and treatment, since early treatment with drugs , such as Xu Riden has been promising in reducing severe symptoms and improving quality of life (Fonteh et al., 2018). The clinical heterogeneity of the different IEMs reflects the complexity of treatment and diagnosis. Initial presentation with manifestations of failure to thrive, irritability, and fatigue can be deceptive, especially in neonates. Overlapping presentations of complex cases render it difficult to determine the metabolic disorder, necessitating intensive metabolic screening and diagnostic studies. Furthermore, the clinical misclassification of IEMs is further exaggerated by the utilization of targeted metabolic assays that may miss uncommon presentations and lead to false negative reports. With improved research in the area, there is a critical requirement to adopt untargeted metabolomic approaches to provide broader coverage of analyte detection in the diagnosis of IEM. Through optimized early recognition mechanisms for these congenital defects, clinicians can optimize treatment procedures and check for potential complications and, hence, enhance the prognosis of patients (Sandlers, 2020) (Figure 10.7).

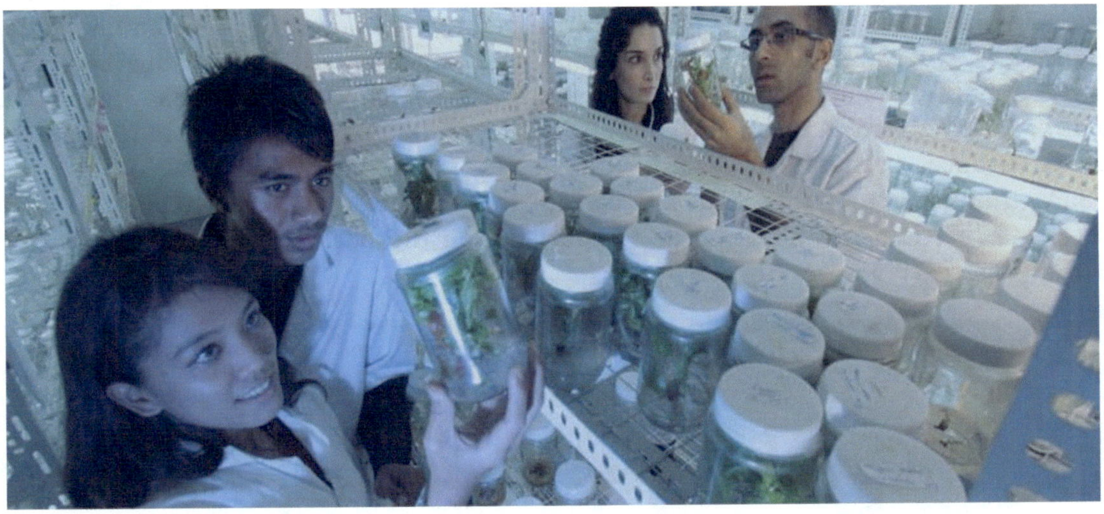

Figure 10.7. Plant researchers analyzing tissue culture samples in a laboratory setting.

Source: https://www.slideteam.net/media/catalog/product/cache/1280x720/c/l/clinical_manifestations_of_shigella_infection_shigella_boydii_ppt_example_st_ai_ss_slide01.jpg.

10.3.2. Diagnostic Tests and Procedures

The diagnostic pathway of IEMs is also multidisciplinary, combining clinical evaluation with a variety of diagnostic tests and investigations. Clinicians first utilize patient history and physical examination to narrow down a suspected metabolic disorder. These are critical, particularly because IEMs are clinically non-specific and tend to mimic other diseases. Following the initial workup, targeted metabolic assays become central to the diagnostic process. Newborn screening programs aim at these assays, designed to scan for individual metabolites associated with selected IEMs, to identify them early and treat them. The strategy is flawed, with potential false positives and negatives, posing as barriers to treatment in time. Thus, diagnostic criteria must continually be revised for them to become more accurate and valid in identifying metabolic disorders to bring to light the pathways towards effective patient treatment and care. As soon as more is known about the limitations of targeted metabolic testing, more availability has been demonstrated of untargeted metabolomics as an effective alternative for the diagnosis of IEMs. Untargeted approaches allow for the screening of a large number of metabolites in a single sample and thus provide a broader picture of the involved metabolic pathways. Compared with the traditional methods that target predefined lists of targets, untargeted metabolomics can identify multiple metabolites simultaneously and thereby greatly increase the chances of identifying abnormal or low-frequency metabolic states. Furthermore, it could possibly allow for a more nuanced biochemical understanding of individuals with the affected condition, thereby serving to guide treatment plans on an individual basis. Nevertheless, while the potential of untargeted metabolomics is intriguing, there are challenges in its standardization for application in the clinic, particularly in terms of sensitivity and specificity across different IEMs, necessitating further validation research. In addition to the technical advances in diagnostic methods, cooperative practice among medical professionals remains critical in the diagnosis and treatment of IEMs. As noted, effective treatment is dependent on early recognition of the relevant metabolic disorder, underscoring the importance of collaboration between experts. The cooperation ensures that proper diagnostic tests and procedures are selected, thereby enhancing the diagnostic process. Specialized laboratories assume a central position in this setup by combining advanced technologies and expert knowledge, which are downright necessities for amenable IEMs' diagnosis. Not only do they provide access to leading-edge diagnostic technologies, but they also establish a culture of constant improvement and refinement, allowing healthcare professionals to keep pace with recent advances in metabolic disorder diagnostics (Sandlers, 2020Bili et al., 2014; Sandlers, 2020). Such a multi-step approach ultimately equates to better patient outcomes, emphasizing the critical intersection of innovation and experience in the battle against congenital errors of metabolism (Figure 10.8).

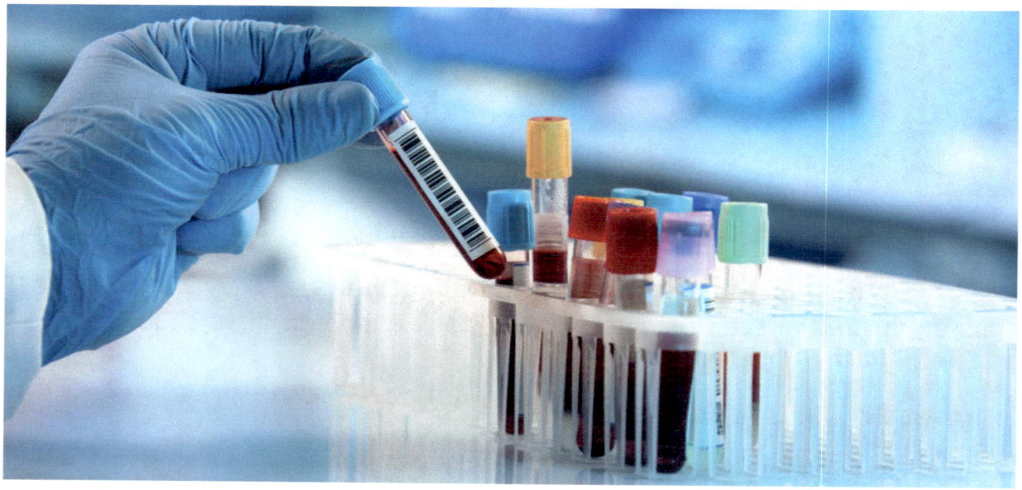

Figure 10.8. Laboratory technician handling blood samples for diagnostic testing and analysis.

Source: https://images.apollo247.in/pd-cms/cms/2023-10/Shutterstock_1114244621.jpg.

10.3.3. Importance of Early Detection

Early recognition of inborn errors of metabolism (IEM) is crucial for ideal management and optimal health outcomes. IEMs often reveal themselves during infancy, hence the importance of routine screening. The implementation of neonatal screening programs allows metabolic disorders , such as phenylketonuria (PKU) and medium-chain acyl-CoA dehydrogenase (MCAD) deficiency to be recognized early in life. Evidence suggests that screening using tandem mass spectrometry is very specific and sensitive, with more than 93% and 99% rates for PKU and MCAD deficiency (Beverley et al.). Early diagnosis of affected newborns enables health professionals to initiate dietary treatment or therapy to prevent devastating neurological damage or systemic disease and thus justify early intervention to maximize long-term outcomes. Furthermore, advancements in analytical techniques like liquid chromatography tandem mass spectrometry (LC-MS) enhance the effectiveness of early detection systems. The technique not only involves high specificity and sensitivity but also allows screening of a greater variety of metabolites to increase the possibilities of detecting various IEMs (RE F et al., 2003). The ability of LCTMS to perform high-throughput analysis with little human intervention makes it a critical tool for clinical labs. With more conditions being included in screening panels due to the assistance of these technologies, the horizon of managing metabolic disorders continues to shift, opening up prospects for an expansion of early identification of conditions which, if left untreated, can lead to life-altering consequences or even death. The implications of early detection extend beyond real-time clinical benefit, influencing public health policy and healthcare resource planning. With screening programs displaying efficacy in preventing severe health outcomes in children affected by IEM, there is an increasing push towards their applicability in various geographies, ensuring equity in healthcare access. Early detection not only saves the expense of chronic health complications but also enhances the well-being of impacted families (Beverley et al., 2025). By developing a culture that fosters early detection, communities are in a better position to direct healthcare funds and invest in education, care, and further research on metabolic disorders. This general appreciation of the importance of early diagnosis in IEMs highlights the demand for ongoing developments and overall promotion of screening programs.

10.4. Treatment Options

Within the framework of IEMs, therapy is increasingly diverse, as medical science and technology evolve. From the early days of treatment regimens based on diet modification and supplements, many disorders have been managed. Diet therapy, for instance, is often the basis of management of most of the metabolic disorders, , such as phenylketonuria (PKU), where a rigorously low-phenylalanine diet is needed to prevent neurotoxicity. The pharmacologic treatment advances have also transformed the treatment paradigm, with enzyme replacement therapies and small molecules being viable treatments for some of the metabolic deficiencies. According to recent studies, approximately 275 of the 1,564 known IEMs are treatable, demonstrating that findings , such as these radically expand the therapeutic realm of potential within the field of genetic illness, eventually leading to improved patient outcomes and quality of life (den Hollander et al., 2025). Apart from dietetic and pharmacologic management, another significant area of research is underway with gene therapy, holding promise to correct the genetic abnormalities responsible for IEMs. This technique treats the etiology of the disease per se rather than the manifestations, dramatically altering the therapeutic approach to IEM patients. Gene replacement therapies have shown promising results in the clinic, most famously for conditions , such as X-linked adrenoleukodystrophy and certain urea cycle disorders. The excitement surrounding these advances is tangible, as gene therapy could lead to a cure rather than lifelong treatment. Besides, database growth beyond IEMbase is essential, providing clinicians and researchers with vital information regarding potential treatments, thus facilitating early, effective intervention in affected patients (Byth et al., 2024). Finally, care of IEMs involves multidisciplinary treatment that not only includes medical care but also supportive care to address the inherent needs of the patients. This includes regular follow-up with metabolic specialists, nutritionists, and social workers for individualized care. Psychological support integration is furthermore universally recognized as necessary given the chronic nature of most IEMs and potential for concomitant disabilities. Specific mention can be given in the case of prolidase deficiency, where skin symptoms are sufficient to severely compromise quality of life, necessitating specialty dermatological therapy in addition to metabolic therapy. Since scientists learn to unravel the complexities of such disorders, an individualized treatment plan in line with every patient's specific needs turns out to be the solution to maximum health gain and well-being (Byth et al., 2024) (Figure 10.9).

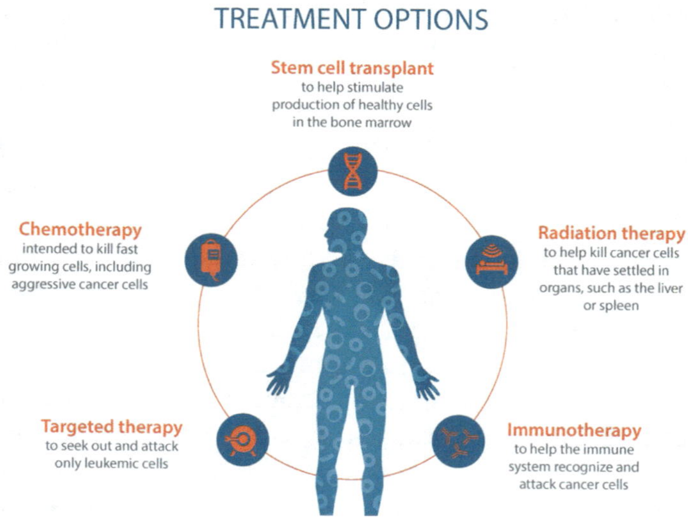

Figure 10.9. Overview of leukemia treatment options including chemotherapy, targeted therapy, stem cell transplant, radiation therapy, and immunotherapy.

Source: https://cdn.cancercenter.com/-/media/ctca/images/feature-block-images/medical-illustrations/coh-leukemia-treatment-dtm.jpg.

10.4.1. Dietary Management and Restrictions

Nutritional care is a key component in the prevention and control of metabolic disturbances because of IEM. The majority of these diseases necessitate extremely specialized diets so as to avoid the buildup of toxic metabolites, which can lead to severe health impairments. For instance, individuals with phenylketonuria (PKU) must drastically limit their dietary consumption of phenylalanine, an amino acid present in the majority of protein foods and must consume specially prepared low-protein diets. Adherence to these dietary requirements is paramount to facilitate metabolic normalcy as well as maximally favorable developmental experience, particularly among most compromised children. Successful dietary management not only requires delivery to be delivered under the care of a physician but also includes wise education of patients and their families regarding selection and preparation of appropriate foods, thereby maximizing compliance with the diet ordered and minimizing the risk of metabolic emergencies. The pragmatic issue of diet management in IEMs is commonly the unpalatability of diet preparations, and these factors heavily in noncompliance. Most of the therapeutic foods and supplements required to adhere to dietary limitations are unpleasant in flavor or texture and, therefore, create problems with compliance. For example, patients might have trouble ingesting certain mixtures of amino acids that are vital for their well-being but are not very palatable. As presented in recent studies, new technologies, including the development of semi-solid extrusion (SSE) technology, are being established in order to produce individualized chewable dosage forms of drugs with improved palatability. It not only eliminates the issue of taste, but it also supports the flexibility of dosing, which is a necessity because adjustment of dosing in relation to a patient's growth and metabolic needs must be achieved. These innovations are promised to bring about a better quality of life for patients with IEMs (Alvarez-Lorenzo et al., 2023; 2024). In addition, ongoing research and development efforts in this field are critical to determining the overall effectiveness of dietary treatment in the management of inborn errors of metabolism. Tailor-made dietary regimens designed following the individual metabolic requirements of each patient, foster a more personalized treatment approach. Additionally, there are regulatory concerns regarding the use of these newer dietary preparations that are crucial for their use in clinical practice. Ensuring that the products are safe, effective, and acceptable is highly essential to ensure that the patients will trust and comply with them. By the application of advances in technology and the overcoming of the very real challenges of dietary management, clinicians can effectively mitigate the impact of IEMs in people's lives, thus paving the way to improved long-term health in this at-risk population (Alvarez-Lorenzo et al., 2023; 2024).

10.4.2. Enzyme Replacement Therapy (ERT)

ERT is a valuable intervention for treating inborn errors of metabolism (IEM), particularly for those conditions where the metabolic defect is due to a deficiency in a single enzyme. Replacement of the deficient enzyme in the patient can be therapeutic and improve overall metabolic balance. This treatment has transformed the management of several lysosomal storage disorders, , such as mucopolysaccharidoses (MPS), to lengthen survival and enhance quality of life in patients. Advances in ERT preparations have optimized its efficacy, which now facilitates better delivery of the enzyme to tissues, including the central nervous system, proving the therapy's efficacy in reaching previously inaccessible sites in the body. Thus, ERT is an essential intervention in the treatment landscape for IEMs, providing a platform on which subsequent innovation in the management of metabolic disease occurs (Chról et al., 2025). For specific metabolic deficiencies, ERT has proven highly useful, yet it also has its disadvantages. As treatments fix metabolic profiles and reduce lysosomal storage, they can potentially have to be taken for life, as such genetic conditions constantly remain active. Therapeutic outcomes may be variable in patients, depending on the time of initiation of the treatment, the initial severity of the illness, and other comorbid conditions. Secondarily, access and cost may be limited in most instances, with socioeconomic considerations to be considered during treatment planning. ERT is now being used in combination with other newer methods, , such as substrate reduction therapy or gene therapy, in an attempt to further enhance the outcomes. These multiligand approaches have the potential to both correct enzymatic deficiency and its metabolic manifestations, resulting in synergy that may change treatment paradigms for IEMs in the future (Angarita et al., 2016). With continuous research on ERT, integration of emerging therapies holds the promise for additional innovation in managing metabolic disorders. Most promising is the development of blood-brain barrier-permeable enzymes, an area that has enormous promises for enhancing the efficacy of ERT for central nervous system-related symptoms that are seen with frequency in IEMs. Advances in the genetic editing technology , such as CRISPR/Cas9, may also see ERT being combined with cellular therapies, correcting enzymatic function at the cellular level. Such approaches can redefine the therapy by not only substituting enzyme deficits but also addressing the root cause of primary genetic defects. This integrated approach shows the efficacy of ERT not merely as a standalone therapy but as a tool in a grand, overall therapeutic model for adequately addressing the complexity of inborn errors of metabolism (Chról et al., 2025) (Figure 10.10).

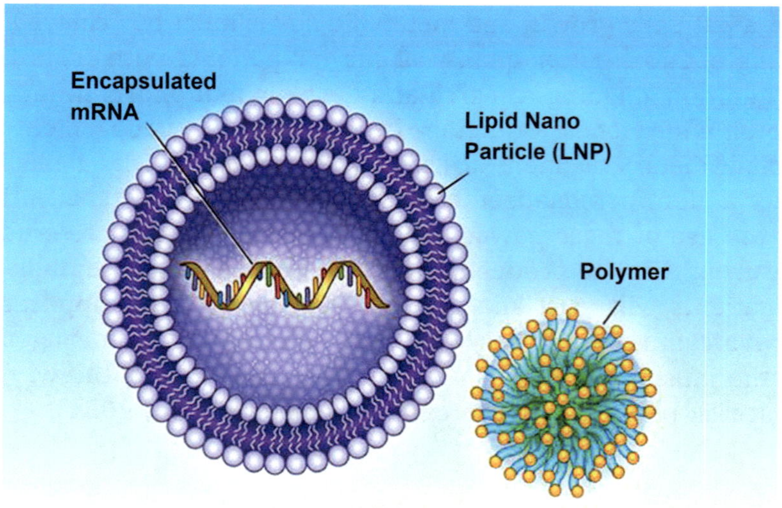

Figure 10.10. Illustration of i-ERT formulation using lipid nanoparticles and polymers to deliver encapsulated mRNA.

Source: https://www.genengnews.com/wp-content/uploads/2018/10/Dec19_2014_HeLaI_6002411142847.jpg.

10.4.3. Gene Therapy Advancements

The climate for the treatment of inborn errors of metabolism (IEMs) has experienced tremendous advances, particularly in gene therapy. Previously, the classical modalities for treatment of IEMs, , such as enzyme replacement therapy and hematopoietic stem cell transplantation, have been palliative measures but often cannot restore the underlying causes of the genetic defects. Gene therapy tries to restore the defects at their causative levels by providing functional copies of the causative gene responsible for the metabolic disorder. This has become increasingly possible with technological advancements in the creation of vectors, especially through the adeno-associated virus (AAV) vectors that allow for tissue-specific delivery. The production of such vectors marks a move towards the promotion of treating previously unconditioned patients with lesser therapeutic intervention, and they hold promise for significant improvement in the results of patients (Wanat et al., 2025). As there are further advancements with genetic therapies, various avenues are being explored to correct the different presentations of IEMs. Of particular interest are the growing uses of CRISPR/Cas9 technology and lentiviral vectors. Beyond maximizing the specificity of gene editing, these technologies enable modifications to the gene at more than one level of the genetic hierarchy, hence widening the range of diseases that can be treated. Of even newer interest are investigations into blood-brain barrier (BBB)-permeable enzyme replacement therapy as an adjunctive method. New treatment regimens, including substrate reduction and nonsense suppression, are also being explored, expanding the treatment horizon for conditions , such as mucopolysaccharidoses (MPS). This multi-faceted approach is indicative of the evolving nature of treatment models in IEMs and highlights the imperative for ongoing research to close the gap between laboratory findings and clinical use (Wanat et al., 2025). Despite the potential of gene therapy, several challenges are involved that must be taken seriously. Long-term safety and effectiveness of these new therapies must be thoroughly investigated, as must immune reactions to the vectors delivered. Regulatory pathways must keep pace with these new modalities in order that patients may be offered the safest and most advantageous therapies possible. Furthermore, the availability of these state-of-the-art treatments presents an additional quandary in that cost may render them unavailable to a vast majority of patients, especially in resource-poor environments. Evolving collaboration between policymakers, clinicians, and researchers is necessary to ensure that the benefit of gene therapy reaches everyone with inborn errors of metabolism. Field growth, as it continues, will have these challenges in the process to enable translation of the potential of gene therapy into clinical practice in general (Hergenrother et al., 2025).

10.5. Case Studies

Case study analysis in the context of inborn errors of metabolism (IEMs) provides critical information on the clinical presentation, management outcomes, and epidemiology of such rare genetic diseases. Case studies are a crucial tool for understanding the typical presentations of different IEMs, particularly witnessing the interplay of environmental influences and genetic susceptibility in a clinical setting. From the study of specific cases where patients exhibit IEMs, clinicians can gain a better understanding of the conditions. This qualitative approach not only describes the unique symptomatology and complications of each condition but also underscores the requirement for individualized treatment strategies that can adapt to the spectrum of presentation and severity of IEM patients, thus highlighting the role of case studies in enhancing clinical knowledge. Use of systematic reviews and case study assessments in low- and middle-income countries (LMICs) has played a critical role in understanding the broader public health implications of IEMs.

These reviews, as cited in Kachroo et al. (2024), define the prevalence and occurrence of IEMs, which subsequently enables the development of large-scale newborn screening programs. These studies' findings highlight the lack of diagnostic capacity and healthcare resources in LMICs, compelling policymakers to give impetus to metabolic screening programs. Since case studies tend to unveil the exclusive challenges of these populations, , such as genetic diversity and availability of care, they become critical in arguing the need for customized health solutions that cater to the particular needs of the affected individuals, hence leading to improved health outcomes among varied demographic segments. The collection of case study data, as presented in Wang et al. (2024), is conducive to enhanced understanding of IEM's clinical spectrum and diagnostic procedure efficacy. The analysis of large-scale hospital datasets is conducive to elaborate thought on IEM incidence rates, , such as the distinction between full-term and premature infants. These findings emphasize the critical need for special screening protocols, particularly in newborns who have an elevated risk of metabolic disorders. Through the identification of the incidence of specific IEMs, , such as organic acid metabolism disorders and amino acid metabolism disorders, case studies can guide clinical practice and advance increased understanding of genetic malformations. Ultimately, this collection of research confirms the ongoing development of more efficient and focused screening guidelines, providing a template for future clinical research and practice that will enhance the treatment of IEMs.

10.5.1. Phenylketonuria (PKU)

PKU is recognized as the most frequent congenital disorder of amino acid metabolism resulting from a deficiency of the enzyme phenylalanine hydroxylase. The enzyme is crucial in the conversion of phenylalanine—a ubiquitous amino acid in most protein-containing foods—into tyrosine, a critical amino acid. If this process is disrupted, phenylalanine accumulates to toxic levels within the body and, if left untreated, may lead to severe neurological impairment. The molecular etiology of PKU is mutations in the PAH gene that encode for the phenylalanine hydroxylase enzyme. Early diagnosis is crucial because timely interventions can substantially alter the life course of individuals affected with the disease, saving them from progressive mental deterioration and other destructive effects on development and overall well-being. The traditional treatment option for PKU is a rigorous diet restriction program that restricts phenylalanine intake throughout the individual's life.

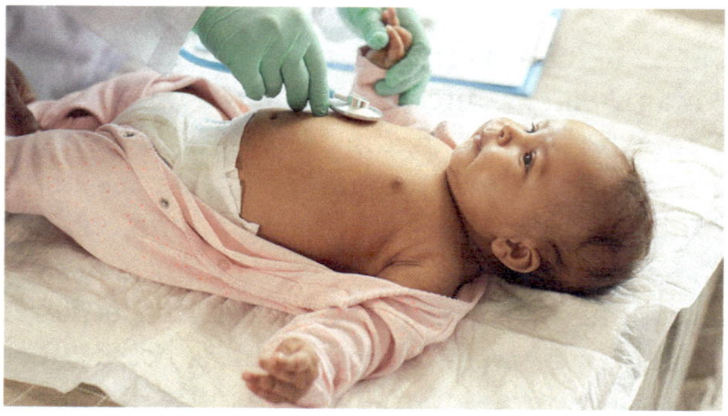

Figure 10.11. Infants undergo routine clinical examinations for early health assessment.

Source: https://hcpbreastfeeding.com/sites/default/files/2021-08/pku-iStock-1253264012.jpg.

This management involves the avoidance of high-protein foods, , such as meat, milk, and eggs, all of which are common sources of phenylalanine. Alternatively, patients typically subsist on specially prepared low-protein diets and amino acid supplements to offer needed nutrition. While this dietary management is beneficial in maintaining phenylalanine, it leads to nutritional deficiencies, particularly in polyunsaturated fatty acids like docosahexaenoic acid (DHA) and arachidonic acid (AA). These deficits are of concern given the important roles these fatty acids must play in brain development and function. Present research demonstrates that PKU patients have irregular lipid profiles, which have been attributed to the restrictive diets maintained by PKU patients (Sandlers, 2020). Further, current dietary restrictions impair PKU treatment in the short term but can affect long-term health, including an increased risk of developing other chronic diseases. There have also been reports of changes in lipid metabolism secondary to PKU, making it important to continue metabolic follow-up of such patients. Oxidative stress and peroxidation of lipids also occur, suggesting that PKU not only interferes with amino acid metabolism but also deranges lipid homeostasis. Consequently, new tools , such as mass spectrometry-based lipidomics are now gaining popularity in evaluating these metabolic disturbances. This approach has the potential for biomarker identification of risk and prognosis, which will pave the way to improved management for individuals with PKU and enhance disease knowledge in the broader context of inborn errors of metabolism (Sandlers, 2020) (Figure 10.11).

10.5.2. Maple Syrup Urine Disease (MSUD)

Inborn errors in metabolism are a series of inherited genetic diseases that disrupt normal biochemical mechanisms in the body. One such magnificent example is the maple syrup urine disease (MSUD), which occurs due to a deficiency in the branched-chain alpha-ketoacid dehydrogenase (BCKDH) complex, the key enzyme responsible for the metabolism of amino acids leucine, isoleucine, and valine. This metabolic disruption creates a toxic accumulation of these branched-chain amino acids (BCAAs) and their metabolites, with very severe health effects if left untreated. The patient can have neurological signs, growth retardation, and a distinctive sweet-smelling urine, reminiscent of maple syrup, after which the disease is named.

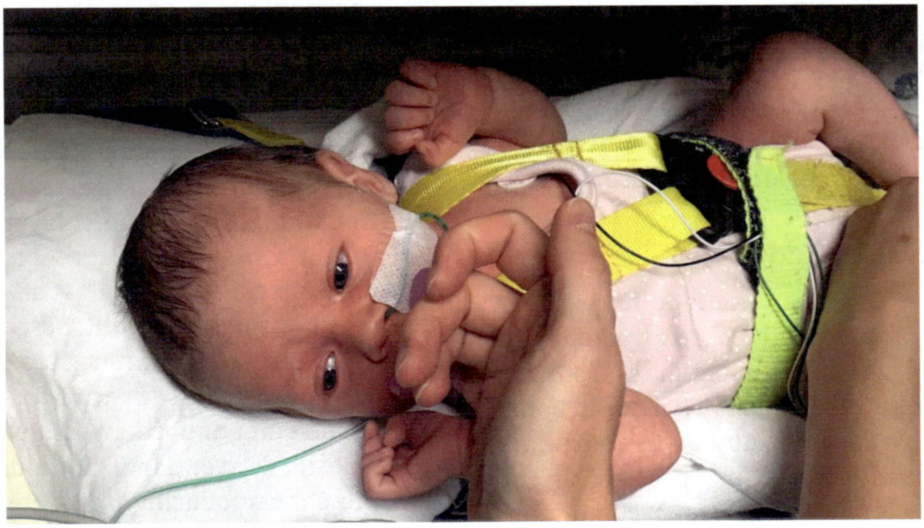

Figure 10.12. Newborn receive specialized monitoring and support in a clinical environment.

Source: https://content.api.news/v3/images/bin/8aa51b1d8203d9b0daf91734d6eac77c.

Early diagnosis and nutritional management, primarily by restricting BCAA intake, are crucial for enhanced clinical response and to prevent irreversible metabolic damage in the patient. Recent improvements in genetic and molecular research have unraveled the complex pathophysiology of MSUD. Multi-omics integration analysis illustrates the complicated interaction among genomic, epigenomic, and transcriptomic alterations in patients with MSUD. Specifically, the research has detected a robust episignature that reorganizes the world DNA methylation pattern. Most significantly, this alteration favors HOX cluster gene expression, simultaneously suppressing cell cycle gene-related signatures. In addition, transcription factors , such as AP1 and CEBPB facilitate the observed molecular reorganization, implicating MEIS1 as a candidate subject to epigenetic repression. With strict data integration, researchers began identifying underlying molecular networks rewired in MSUD, which directs to new diagnostic and treatment approaches for this rare metabolic disease (Alba-Linares et al., 2024). The neuropsychiatric manifestations of MSUD complicate clinical presentation, emphasizing the imperative for interdisciplinary care models. Research has also indicated that inborn errors of amino acid metabolism, , such as MSUD, are prevalent among patients who, even with excellent metabolic control, frequently have neurodevelopmental disturbances. Analysis of biomarkers , such as brain-derived neurotrophic factors (BDNF) and genes essential for normal brain functioning have been instrumental in defining the pathophysiologic pathways of neural dysfunction. Significantly, specific biomarkers have strongly correlated with impairment of executive attention and behavioral disorders. For instance, levels of mRNA and protein expression of CACNA2D2 and MECP2 have been reported to be potential biomarkers for the detection of MSUD-related neural dysfunction (Alcántara et al., 2020). In doing so, these findings pave the way for more research in biomarkers as critical tools for better patient management and quality of life for patients with MSUD (Figure 10.12).

10.5.3. Galactosemia

Galactosemia is a genetic metabolic disorder where one is unable to metabolize galactose, a form of sugar found in milk and milk products. This develops as a result of deficiencies in some enzymes, particularly galactose-1-phosphate uridyltransferase (GALT), required for converting galactose into glucose. Accumulation of galactose and its metabolites in the body can lead to severe complications, , such as liver damage, cataracts, and developmental delay, particularly if left untreated. Early diagnosis and dietary treatment are essential components of therapy due to the potentially life-threatening consequences associated with the disorder. Newborn screening programs are important in the early detection of galactosemia, enabling interventions that minimize long-term health consequences. The role of early intervention cannot be overstated as it paves the way for the development of tailored diet plans restricting the consumption of galactose, thus dramatically improving patient outcomes. The prevalence of galactosemia varies globally and is influenced by genetic determinants and levels of consanguineous marriages. For example, there are populations where this inborn error of metabolism has higher occurrences because it follows common genetic backgrounds, which sustain the prevalence of certain mutations within the GALT gene. From a large perspective study in Egypt, galactosemia was found to contribute to 1.6% of all diagnosed inborn errors of metabolism in the country, thus underscoring the need for specific screening programs. Before the development of diagnostic facilities, most of the conditions were undiagnosed or misdiagnosed, leading to poor patient outcomes. The organization of specialized metabolic units, like the Biochemical Genetics Unit in Egypt, is an example of how local expertise should be established for the diagnosis and management of inherited metabolic disorders. This development has led to more accurate identification of galactosemia and associated diseases in populations that otherwise may have gone undiagnosed (Abdallah et al., 2014). Recent developments in metabolic screening and the shift from targeted to untargeted metabolomics offer promising ways forward for the diagnosis of galactosemia and other congenital errors of metabolism. Conventional methods often rely on specific panels focusing on limited compounds and therefore yield false negatives and false negatives missed diagnoses. Metabolomics, on the other hand, allows global metabolite profiling of metabolites in biological samples without prior assumption of which metabolites might be present. It has the potential to strengthen the diagnostic process with less chance of conditions like galactosemia being missed due to inefficient screening protocols. With such advanced techniques widely employed, the stability and accuracy of IEM diagnostics improve, allowing more cases to be diagnosed at an earlier stage and therapeutic measures to be initiated sooner. Such technological developments promise a new era in the management of metabolic disorders, better ensuring the welfare of individuals with such disorders who must make lifetime dietary changes to combat the effects of their illness (Sandlers, 2020) (Figure 10.13).

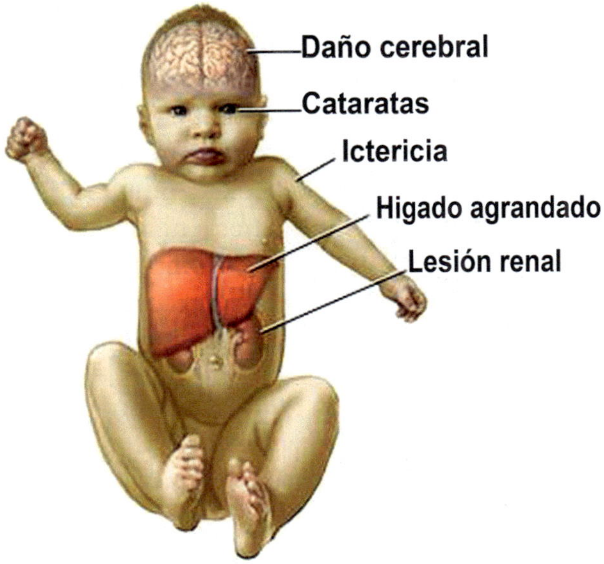

Figure 10.13. Symptoms of galactosemia in an infant, highlighting organ and neurological complications.

Source: https://upload.wikimedia.org/wikipedia/commons/f/fc/Bebe_Galactosemia.jpg.

10.6. Impact on Patients and Families

The impact of inherited errors of metabolism (IEMs) on families and patients is profound and complex. IEM patients tend to have a challenging medical background with uncertainty and emotional pain. The randomness of these conditions, resulting from genetic mutations that stop critical metabolic pathways, can lead to different clinical presentations. Early and accurate diagnosis becomes vital to prevent long-term health effects. Such families usually grapple with the burden of information regarding the genetic effects of such disorders on family planning and relationships. Furthermore, the psychological and emotional burden experienced by such families worsens when the affected individuals suffer from chronic health conditions requiring long-term medical care and interventions that tend to strain their emotional and financial resources (Sandlers, 2020). For parents, a diagnosis of an IEM can be particularly daunting due to the extreme lifestyle adjustments that usually accompany it. Caregivers must make new caregiver adjustments, often for extended amounts of time, and can lead to resentment, burnout, and feelings of isolation. Additionally, the necessity of incorporating specialized diets or routine medical visits into family life can disrupt family life and routines. Also, the unpredictability of certain IEMs adds to the stress, as families may find themselves having to negotiate complex healthcare systems to receive appropriate support and treatment. The emotional stress placed on family members can be further compounded by feelings of powerlessness or guilt in seeing their loved one struggle. In this regard, it is clear that IEMs impact not just the patient but resonate across the entire family, requiring holistic care strategies that integrate mental and emotional assistance (Ceci et al., 2015). The extended implications of IEMs are beyond short-term health factors, impacting educational and social environments in patients' lives. People with IEMs may experience developmental delays or problems in their ability to perform well academically and socially. These challenges will result in isolation for the individual, and this creates a lower quality of life in addition to exposing them to mental health issues. Families will often be confronted with the dilemma of negotiating proper educational services and support systems, further increasing their burden. Furthermore, the prevalence of stigma involving visible disabilities or unmet educational needs might compound the feelings of isolation among families and patients. Ensuring access to integral resources, including educational support and psychological guidance, becomes essential in countering some of the difficulties IEMs create for families and individuals and promoting overall well-being and resilience to adversity (Sandlers, 2020).

10.6.1. Psychological Effect on Patients

The psychiatric effect of congenital errors of metabolism (IEM) exceeds the physiological effect of the disorders themselves by far. The conditions are likely to impose significant emotional loads on patients and their families, affecting their everyday functioning and their quality of life. Patient- and observer-reported outcomes (PROs/ObsROs) were found to be essential to their insight into these psychological effects.

A consensus-based design has facilitated the establishment of key dimensions covering social participation, emotional well-being, and parents' feelings of stress regarding their children's IEM diagnosis. Prioritizing such factors ensures that medical professionals are able to better tailor interventions, so they address not just the physical needs but also the psychological health needs of patients and families. This focus on psychological impact is part of a comprehensive treatment process, emphasizing the importance of mental health as well as management techniques in clinical settings within IEM (Bösch et al., 2022). In addition, interventions that enhance psychological well-being can significantly improve patients with inborn errors of metabolism in quality of life. To illustrate, more recent studies have looked into the possibility of complementary interventions, including Internet-delivered yoga, to establish emotional stability and mental resilience among recovering IEM treatment patients. While directed towards physical well-being in the main, evidence suggests these interventions have been effective in reducing anxiety, improving social function, and reducing depression. Satisfactorily, participants spoke out about such interventions, which lends further credibility to a growing recognition of the mental health influence of chronic health conditions. Incorporating adjunctive therapeutic interventions into IEM treatment protocols can therefore assist in responding to the multi-dimensional aspect of health, corroborating the psychological components intertwined with physical conditions (Eckert et al., 2022).

The intersection of mental health and congenital metabolic errors cannot be bypassed because emotional pain will complicate medical outcomes. IEM families may experience loneliness, distress, and anxiety depending on the long duration and complex nature of their conditions. Interventions focused on the established PROs/ObsROs can alleviate this burden, fostering an empowering environment that prioritizes mental well-being. Regular evaluation and flexibility in patient-centered care approaches can facilitate enhanced communication among healthcare professionals and families. By identifying and meeting such psychological impacts, there will be better patient compliance with treatment protocols and enhanced overall health status for IEM patients, ultimately leading to a more knowledgeable consciousness of the quality of their life (Bösch et al., 2022) (Figure 10.14).

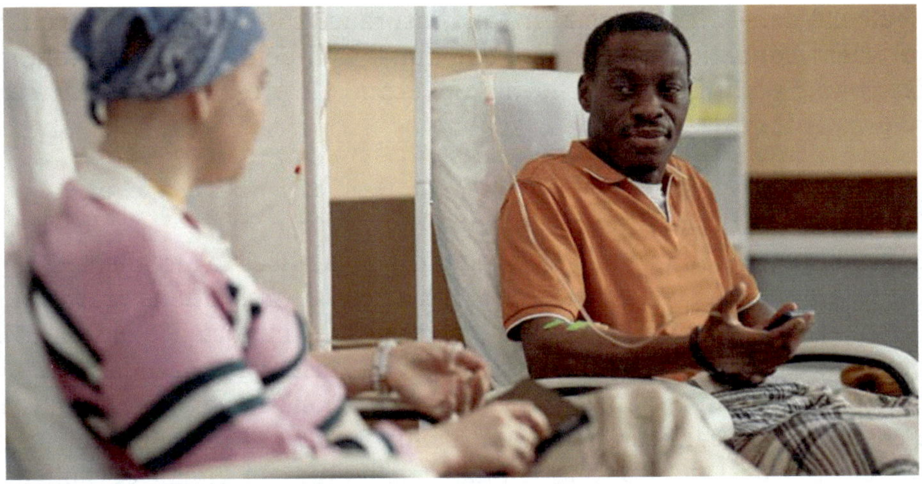

Figure 10.14. Chemotherapy patients sharing support during treatment.

Source: https://www.apa.org/images/cancer-younger-adults-tile_tcm7-332165.jpg.

10.6.2. Financial Burden of Treatment

The expense of inborn errors of metabolism (IEM) treatment is a significant concern for patients and families. Treatment for these disorders, , such as phenylketonuria (PKU), requires continuous diet adjustment and consumption of special medical foods required to avoid health complications. These treatments are not only expensive but also often outside the financial resources of most families. From existing literature, the two factors that are closely related and correlated with poor quality of life both for the patients and their families are the high caregiver burden and the perceived disease severity, which suggests that the burden of caring for these diseases extends beyond even health problems (Baumgartner et al., 2022). Consequently, the economic impact poses serious challenges, rendering proper treatment difficult and further reasons to adopt integrative healthcare policies aimed at IEM management's economic aspect. In addition, the limited insurance coverage of medical foods complicates the situation further, raising the economic load on IEM families. Conducting a survey of adult PKU patients, they indicated out-of-pocket expenses for dietary items ranging from $100 to $500, a financial blow to family budgets (Bernzen, 2017). The study results suggest that patients face significant economic barriers in accessing essential nutritional therapies. Inadequate insurance coverage not only prevents appropriate compliance with treatment but also raises concerns about the fairness of healthcare access among patients who have metabolic disorders. The resolution of these costs is critical because effective dietary management can save those neurological complications that could arise due to untreated PKU and other IEMs, thereby emphasizing the necessity of governmental and institutional support. The emotional and psychological burden of the costs of IEM treatment extends beyond the economic to caregivers' health and family dynamics. Parents, unlike other groups, bear the brunt of living under intense anxiety and stress concerning how they can facilitate their child's treatment. As indicated in caregiver burden studies, these emotional stressors can drain their care-giving capacity to the affected child, creating a cycle of deteriorating health-related quality of life (Baumgartner et al., 2022). Interventions to reduce such economic and emotional burdens have the potential to bolster family support systems and patient outcomes. Therefore, it becomes increasingly crucial for healthcare stakeholders like policymakers and insurance companies to determine the point of convergence between economic, physical, and emotional well-being while developing policies that support families coping with IEMs. By relieving the economic pressure, the treatment protocol as a whole can be greatly improved.

10.6.3. Support Systems and Resources Available

The intricacies of IEM require robust support systems and services to aid affected families. Parents of children with IEM often present a range of psychosocial complications that could significantly weigh against family welfare. A qualitative study highlights the importance of salient issues like the uncertainty of disease and family relationship alterations during pre-diagnosis and post-diagnosis. This identifies the important function that medical professionals can provide to assist families in navigating the complicated healthcare system. Providing personalized support and resources can alleviate emotional pressures confronting families, facilitating an enhanced holistic approach to IEM management. In dealing with these psychosocial factors, healthcare workers can empower families, enhancing coping mechanisms and overall resilience in coping with the effects of IEM on their lives (Gannavarapu et al., 2020).

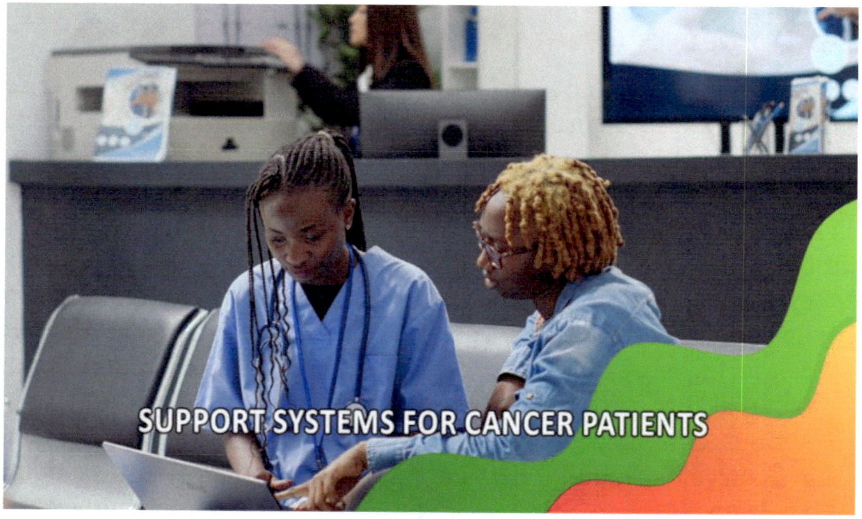

Figure 10.15. Support systems play a vital role in the care and recovery of cancer patients.

Source: https://besta.co.tz/wp-content/uploads/2024/10/Support-Systems-for-Cancer-Patients-1024x683.jpg.

Also, patient-centered care plays an essential role in helping families navigate the challenges posed by IEM. Patient organizations and self-advocacy groups for individual IEM disorders have emerged as essential champions, bringing concerns and voices of affected families to the fore. Thematic content from qualitative interviews with representatives of IEM patient groups reveals top themes to family experiences and priorities, e.g., managing uncertainty and supporting life transitions. These patient groups not only provide valuable information regarding treatment and services but also form a community of empathy among the families who share similar problems. When health care providers engage with such groups, they are well equipped to deliver individualized interventions that consider the unique challenges facing families. Through collaboration with patient advocates, healthcare providers can make a significant impact in the quality of care delivered to children with IEM (Chakraborty et al., 2016). Support systems for the family of IEM patients need to be beyond healthcare. Education and community services are a must. Schools and the education system play an extremely crucial role in the integration of special medical needs, ensuring learning and socialization settings that prove healthy for the child. Community organizations can also provide financial assistance, counseling, and social services, which collectively help contribute to the health and happiness of the family dealing with the issues of IEM. It is important that families are informed about available resources in this manner, as information and access can do much to diminish the burden that they carry. Equipped with a complete array of support that includes healthcare, education, and community resources, families can be supplied with the integrated care that is needed to address the complexities involved with being born with inborn errors of metabolism. This working framework is critical to enhancing outcomes as well as the quality of life for patients and their loved ones (Figure 10.15).

CLOSER LOOK

GALACTOSEMIA

Galactosemia is a rare inherited metabolic disorder that affects the body's ability to process galactose, a simple sugar found primarily in lactose, the sugar present in milk and dairy products. In healthy individuals, galactose is broken down into glucose and used for energy. However, in individuals with galactosemia, a genetic mutation leads to a deficiency or absence of the enzyme galactose-1-phosphate uridyltransferase (GALT), which is essential for properly metabolizing galactose. As a result, toxic levels of galactose and its byproducts accumulate in the body, causing serious complications. Galactosemia typically presents in newborns within the first few days after ingesting breast milk or formula. Symptoms may include jaundice, vomiting, poor feeding, lethargy, diarrhea, liver enlargement, and failure to thrive. If left untreated, it can lead to liver damage, cataracts, intellectual disability, sepsis, and even death. There are different types of galactosemia, with classic galactosemia (type I) being the most severe. Other forms, such as type II (galactokinase deficiency) and type III (epimerase deficiency), are typically milder but still require monitoring. Diagnosis is usually made through newborn screening programs, which test for elevated levels of galactose or low GALT enzyme activity. Early detection is crucial for preventing serious complications.

The primary treatment for galactosemia is the lifelong elimination of galactose from the diet, which means avoiding all milk and dairy products, as well as certain processed foods and medications that may contain lactose. Even with strict dietary control, some individuals may still experience long-term issues such as speech delays, learning difficulties, and reproductive problems. The galactosemia is a serious but manageable metabolic disorder. With early diagnosis and strict dietary management, many individuals can lead healthy lives, although ongoing medical supervision is essential.

SUMMARY

The clinical study of inborn errors of metabolism (IEMs) emphasizes the need for increased screening and diagnostic tests, particularly among diverse ethnic populations. The data from recent studies presented reveal extensive differences in the incidence of IEMs in different groups with a very high incidence rate among minority ethnic populations compared to the Han nationality in Huaihua, China (Xiao et al., 2024). These differences in prevalence also challenge the dimension of genetic susceptibility as well as emphasize the necessity of customized health interventions that are sensitive to the unique genetic landscapes of these populations. The identification of incidence differences can even guide clinicians and health professionals to implement more effective screening protocols in order to have at-risk infants offered appropriate and timely interventions. Furthermore, the innovation of metabolomic techniques enhanced effectiveness in the diagnosis of IEMs. Targeted metabolomic techniques certified by rigorous external quality assessment programs reveal that targeted techniques are crucial for accurate detection and treatment of metabolic disorders (Oliva et al., 2024). Early diagnosis is important since early medical intervention can significantly improve prognosis among those who are affected, transforming what was otherwise an untreatable condition into a manageable one. The integration of these newer diagnostic modalities into practice will not only improve rates of identification but also facilitate better management of those affected, ultimately lowering neonatal mortality from IEMs. Finally, the acquired knowledge gained through the research of IEMs is used as a foundation for further policymaking and research endeavors. With insight into the population-specific genetic variants that are present in the different populations, healthcare systems are better able to make an informed and equitable attempt at newborn screening. Enhancing education and clinician resources will bring greater awareness of IEMs, leading to improved outcomes for affected infants and families (Xiao et al., 2024). Addressing the challenge of enduring metabolic disorders will involve targeting research that addresses the different populations' differing genetic contexts to decrease health disparities and create a healthier environment in healthcare.

IEMs represent a heterogeneous group of genetic conditions that disrupt the metabolic pathway to produce a variety of clinical manifestations. IEMs often arise from disturbances in single enzymes critical to metabolism, impacting carbohydrate, protein, and lipid metabolism. Early diagnosis is a critical component of the management of IEMs as early intervention can alter the disease course and reduce morbidity and mortality. There is evidence to support that the ability to recognize early symptoms and perform targeted diagnostic tests is capable of facilitating timely referral to experts, , such as clinical immunologists. This is critically important in the MENA region, where congenital errors of immunity are unexpectedly common and therefore result in more complex disease phenotypes due to late diagnosis (Celik et al., 2024). Moreover, the differential diagnosis of IEMs comprises both acute and chronic diseases, a portion of which are present in infancy and others that can present later in life. This heterogeneity is one of the factors for which healthcare professionals must maintain a high index of suspicion and become familiar with the multitude of presentations of these illnesses. For instance, patients with IEMs may have presentations not only of metabolic crises but also of noninfectious presentation, and therefore, clinical presentation becomes of interest. A thorough understanding of the biochemical basis for these characteristics, as well as a wide-ranging family history, will enable clinicians to make rational diagnostic and therapeutic decisions. The advancement of MENA region practitioner-specific guidelines and protocols has been promising in enhancing the diagnosis and treatment of IEMs, thereby enhancing patient outcomes in various healthcare facilities (Celik et al., 2024). Moreover, the treatment of IEMs by multidisciplinary method includes treating acute complications and embracing long-term treatment patterns. Conditions , such as acute kidney injury caused by metabolic disorders may require continuous kidney replacement therapy, which is also riddled with challenges in pediatric intensive care. Successful anticoagulation during such treatments is essential because filter systems used in the treatment can clot, and therefore, a balance of the therapeutic benefit versus the probable adverse effects must be maintained. Incidental literature shows that different anticoagulant strategies can significantly affect the prognosis of patients with IEMs in critically ill children. As healthcare systems evolve and include advancements in targeted medicine and genetic screening, focus on the management of IEMs through multidisciplinary interaction continues to be important to improve treatment effectiveness and overall care.

References

1. Abdallah, Z. Y., Fateen, E. M., & Ibrahim, M. S. (2014). Fifteen years' experience: Egyptian metabolic lab. https://core.ac.uk/download/478418888.pdf (accessed on 13th June 2025).
2. Alcántara Horrillo, S., Armstrong, J., Artuch Iriberri, R., Balada Caballé, M., et al. (2020). Discovery of biomarker panels for neural dysfunction in inborn errors of amino acid metabolism. https://core.ac.uk/download/323328845.pdf (accessed on 13th June 2025).
3. Alvarez-Lorenzo, C., Awad, A., Basit, A. W., Carou-Senra, M., et al. (2024). 3D printing of dietary products for the management of inborn errors of intermediary metabolism in pediatric populations. https://core.ac.uk/download/597056679.pdf; https://core.ac.uk/download/595950851.pdf (accessed on 13th June 2025).
4. Ang, K. S., Borth, N., Brewer, J., Dobson, P., et al. (2016). Recon 2.2: From reconstruction to model of human metabolism. https://core.ac.uk/download/323064087.pdf (accessed on 13th June 2025).
5. Angarita, S. A., Byrne, J. A., Cederbaum, S. D., Chang, C. J., et al. (2016). Restoring ureagenesis in hepatocytes by CRISPR/Cas9-mediated genomic addition to arginase-deficient induced pluripotent stem cells. https://core.ac.uk/download/323079209.pdf (accessed on 13th June 2025).
6. Baumgartner, M. R., Bösch, F., Fernandez, S., Forny, P., et al. (2022). Caregiver burden, and parents' perception of disease severity determine health-related quality of life in pediatric patients with intoxication-type inborn errors of metabolism. https://core.ac.uk/download/527938080.pdf (accessed on 13th June 2025).
7. Bernzen, M. C. (2017). The financial burdens are associated with managing PKU dietary needs as an adult. https://core.ac.uk/download/154555246.pdf (accessed on 13th June 2025).
8. Beverley, C., Chilcott, J., Eastham, J., Paisley, S., et al. (2025). Newborn screening using tandem mass spectrometry: A systematic review. https://core.ac.uk/download/49665.pdf (accessed on 13th June 2025).
9. Bravo-Perez, C., Gurnari, C., Guarnera, L., Kawashima, N., Unlu, S., Mandala, A., Williams, N. D., et al. (2023). Bone marrow failure and inborn errors of immunity: An immunogenomic crossroad. *Blood.* https://www.semanticscholar.org/paper/5169b58e3ffde4e67876e35daa708da5dff35828 (accessed on 13th June 2025).
10. Ceci, R., Kisinovsky, I., Roa, N., Rozenfeld, P., et al. (2015). The continuous challenge of diagnosing patients with Fabry disease in Argentina: Genotype, experiences, anecdotes, and new learnings. https://core.ac.uk/download/161267105.pdf (accessed on 13th June 2025).
11. Celik, I. K., Azizi, G., & Artaç, H. (2024). Practical considerations in diagnosing inborn errors of immunity according to the Middle East and North Africa guidelines. *Current Opinion in Pediatrics.* https://www.semanticscholar.org/paper/ebbae84823ec6ef9b1f439f08aeecc5e1b6eb048 (accessed on 13th June 2025).
12. Chakraborty, P., Coyle, D., Khangura, S. D., Kronick, J. B., et al. (2016). Child and family experiences with inborn errors of metabolism: A qualitative interview study with representatives of patient groups. https://core.ac.uk/download/534388460.pdf (accessed on 13th June 2025).

13. Chiang, J. Y. L., & Ferrell, J. M. (2020). Bile acid biology, pathophysiology, and therapeutics. *Clinical Liver Disease, 15*, 91–94. https://doi.org/10.1002/cld.861 (accessed on 13th June 2025).

14. de Koning, T. J., de Vries, J. J., Koens, L. H., Tijssen, M. A., et al. (2021). How to detect late-onset inborn errors of metabolism in patients with movement disorders: A modern diagnostic approach. https://core.ac.uk/download/562034913.pdf (accessed on 13th June 2025).

15. Diogo, L. M., Domingues, M. R., Ferreira, H. B., Guerra, A., et al. (2021). Lipids and phenylketonuria: Current evidence pointed to the need for lipidomic studies. https://core.ac.uk/download/325954421.pdf (accessed on 13th June 2025).

16. Eldin, E. M. B., Elsedfy, H. H., Mahmoud, A. O., Rashad, M. H., et al. (2009). Study of amino acid disorders among a high-risk group of Egyptian infants and children. https://core.ac.uk/download/478418622.pdf (accessed on 13th June 2025).

17. Ford, R. E., Kushnir, M. M., Muck, W., Murdter, T. E., Rashed, M. S., Streit, F., et al. (2003). Liquid chromatography–tandem mass spectrometry–Application in the clinical laboratory. https://core.ac.uk/download/19418476.pdf (accessed on 13th June 2025).

18. Gannavarapu, S., Mantulak, A., Napier, M., Potter, B. K., et al. (2020). Parental psychosocial aspects and stressors involved in the management of inborn errors of metabolism. https://core.ac.uk/download/475152258.pdf (accessed on 13th June 2025).

19. Gropman, A. L. (2019). Emerging knowledge from noninvasive imaging studies: Is ammonia control enough? https://core.ac.uk/download/322445282.pdf (accessed on 13th June 2025).

20. Hergenrother, S., Husein, M., Thompson, C., Kalina, E., & Raina, R. (2025). Updated gene therapy for renal inborn errors of metabolism. *Genes.* https://www.semanticscholar.org/paper/65703bf5ca990d2c9bd30943874ce9c4e8496886 (accessed on 13th June 2025).

21. Peall, K. (2014). Rare inborn errors of metabolism with movement disorders: A case study to evaluate the impact upon quality of life and adaptive functioning. https://core.ac.uk/download/42532112.pdf (accessed on 13th June 2025).

22. Rao, N., Ananth, S. N., Sarbadhikari, S., & Kavitha, K. (2006). Automated screening for three inborn metabolic disorders: A pilot study. https://core.ac.uk/download/pdf/86755.pdf (accessed on 13th June 2025).

23. Sandlers, Y. (2020). Amino Acids Profiling for the Diagnosis of Metabolic Disorders. IntechOpen. doi: 10.5772/intechopen.84672Vasconcelos, P., & Lacerda, J. F. (2022). Hematopoietic stem cell transplantation for neurological disorders: A focus on inborn errors of metabolism. *Frontiers in Cellular Neuroscience, 16.* https://doi.org/10.3389/fncel.2022.895511 (accessed on 13th June 2025).

24. Zampieri, F. (2018). Rise and fall of Achille de Giovanni's clinical anthropometry. https://core.ac.uk/download/157767229.pdf (accessed on 13th June 2025).

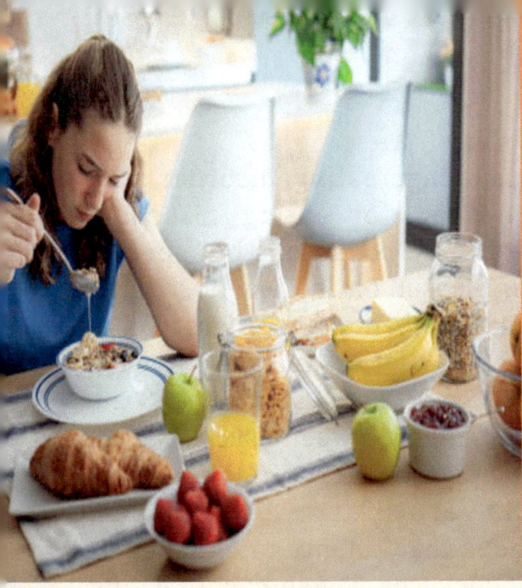

Chapter 11
EATING DISORDERS

Contents

Introduction....347
11.1. Types of Eating Disorders....351
11.2. Causes of Eating Disorders....355
11.3. Symptoms and Diagnosis....359
11.4. Consequences of Eating Disorders....363
11.5. Treatment Options....367
11.6. Prevention Strategies....371
Summary....377
References....379

Introduction

The increasing prevalence of eating disorders is a critical public health concern that affects individuals from diverse groups. These complex disorders, including anorexia nervosa, bulimia nervosa, and binge eating disorder, are usually the outcomes of an interaction of genetic, psychological, and sociocultural factors. The core of these conditions is an altered relationship with food and body image, wherein individuals might develop unhealthy eating habits to deal with emotional pain or social pressure. Learning about the complex nature of eating disorders is important to prepare successful prevention and treatment strategies. Studies determine the need for heightened awareness and education on such issues, as false information can continue to perpetuate stigma and prevent people from receiving the assistance they require (Xia et al., 2023). Furthermore, social media's idealization of thinness and incessant pursuit of the ideal body form can contribute to growing exposure to engaging in disordered eating patterns. Beauty images presented by the media promote unrealistic standards, and these may lead to body dissatisfaction and unhealthy behavior among susceptible groups. For example, with the advent of the internet and social media, such exposure has been greatly increased, particularly among adolescents and young adults. Through this exposure, such influences may lead a fight against self-esteem and eating disorders throughout the rest of their lives. This social pressure is seen to be related to increased incidence rates for eating disorders and underlines the need for programs capable of enhancing body positivity as well as positive self-esteem. Treatment of these cultural factors is required for the formation of an extensive understanding of eating disorder occurrence and continuance (Janmohammadi et al., 2017). Multilateral intervention and treatment practices require an extensive understanding of each person's experience with eating disorders. The treatment is typically in the form of cognitive-behavioral therapy, nutritional counseling, and medical care, depending upon the severity of the disorder and individual needs. Multi-disciplinary treatment is mandatory with psychologists, nutritionists, and medical professionals teaming up to develop treatment protocols according to individuals. There is also increasing emphasis on early intervention, as it can help increase recovery rates by offering timely advice and intervention. By establishing an environment that encourages conversation in terms of eating behavior and mental health, society is better able to counteract the negative impacts of eating disorders and help those afflicted with them down the road to recovery (Xia et al., 2023).

Definition of Eating Disorders

The term eating disorders is a general term to cover a range of psychological ailments with abnormal or disturbed food habits. Eating disorders are not weight or food problems, but they are serious mental illnesses that can have an impact on one's emotional and physical well-being in a serious way. The basic types of eating disorders include anorexia nervosa, bulimia nervosa, binge-eating disorder, and other specified foods or eating disorders (OSFED). Each of these conditions has specific diagnostic criteria based on the Diagnostic and Statistical Manual of Mental Disorders (DSM-5). An appreciation of the nuances of each condition relies on an understanding of the interlocking interaction between psychological, sociocultural, and physiological variables, which underscores the requirement for combined treatment methods that balance mental health with nutritional concerns. The impact of eating disorders is not only on the patient but also on communities, families, and the healthcare system due to the complexity involved in caring for and managing them. These patients typically have associated mental illnesses, , such as depression, anxiety, and substance abuse, which worsen their treatment and course of recovery. Moreover, the impacts of social determinants of health, social economic status, access to healthcare, and culture, must be addressed during eating disorder treatment and assessment. Empirical evidence suggests higher levels of acceptance of new treatment modalities, particularly hybrid models that integrate both in-person and telehealth treatment, which expand access and tailoring of care (Novack and Chadi, 2025). These approaches can be invaluable to addressing the issues of eating disorders, providing personalized solutions that consider the personal circumstances and needs of individuals. Sleep issues are another critical aspect in the research of eating disorders. A percentage as much as 50% of individuals experiencing eating disorders are purported to also have sleep disorders (Leah et al., 2024). This crossing raises critical questions about the causal relationships between disturbed sleep patterns and the development or activation of eating disorder symptoms. For instance, poor quality sleep can lead to impaired executive function and increased negative effects, which allows unhealthy eating habits to develop, creating a vicious cycle. As the research on sleep's role within eating disorders develops, it points towards highlighting the significance of convergent methodologies used in addressing both the sleeping characteristics and food behavior systematically. Through such broad-based examination, useful information could be accessed that can improve clinical practice and inform more efficient treatment options for individuals struggling with eating disorders (Figure 11.1).

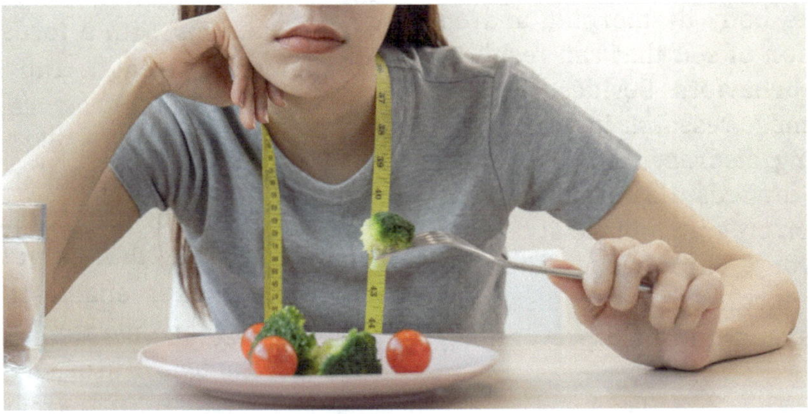

Figure 11.1. An individual exhibiting signs of restrictive eating behavior, commonly associated with eating disorders.

Source: https://cdn.rehabfiles.com/sites/oasisrehab/wp-content/uploads/2024/10/OR-eating-disorder.svg.

Prevalence and Statistics

Epidemiology of eating disorders has come into prominence as a significant public health concern, particularly among young participants in sport. Each of these disorders, , such as anorexia nervosa, bulimia nervosa, and binge eating disorder, has significantly affected males and females, though their rates can be exacerbated by competitive environments. Such a study with taekwondo athletes revealed that older athletes tended to have more eating disorders, stress, and social support compared to young athletes and presented a clear correlation between psychosocial variables and the prevalence of eating disorders (Apriady et al., 2024). The study revealed that senior athletes' mean scores were considerably higher than juniors,' which further suggests that experience and age can increase eating disorder risk factors. Thus, it is crucial to understand the particular pressures on different groups of athletes to formulate targeted preventative strategies. In addition to pressures within competitive sport, societal pressures , such as presentation by the media of ideal body images, significantly add to the prevalence of eating disorders among adolescents. There is growing evidence to suggest the impact of social media on body image and self-esteem, particularly in young people. Research indicates that such sites' notion of unattainable body shapes perpetuates body dissatisfaction, which in turn leads to greater frequencies of eating disorders (Kiley, 2023). While eating disorders are found in both men and women, there is a large disparity in that women are more likely to be forced to conform to traditional standards. This social stress is usually manifested in unhealthy ways to achieve the idealized appearance, and hence magnifies the prevalence of these disorders among young women relative to their male peers. Although general attitudes are that eating disorders occur in particular individuals, it is worth mentioning that such conditions also significantly affect men and boys and are likely to be plagued by their own pressures. Current studies show that men make up a quarter to a third of individuals with eating disorders, and they typically struggle with the muscular ideal, not the thin ideal that is predominantly present in women (Kiley, 2023). The unique expectations that are put on men can lead to body dysmorphia and an erroneous perception of self that can result in disordered eating behaviors. Besides, there is a strong need for more research into the male experience of eating disorders, specifically in society's pressure, towards the development of effective intervention programs aimed at helping this stigmatized group. Thus, it is essential to have the complete picture of eating disorders to develop effective and informed prevention.

Significance of Treating Eating Disorders

The treatment of eating disorders is crucial not only for the immediate health issues but also for fostering the eventual psychological and emotional well-being of the patients. The disorders may lead to severe complications in health, including cardiovascular disease, gastrointestinal disease, and malnutrition, which can, in extreme cases, lead to death.

The bodily consequences are due to both the sparse intake of essential nutrients and unhealthy dieting behaviors that disrupt the proper functioning of the body. It is imperative for health care systems to recognize the multi-dimensionality of these disorders and adopt an integral approach while planning treatment, especially in the context of combining psychological support with physical intervention. The necessity of an all-inclusive treatment plan is essential due to the interrelatedness between physical and mental well-being, indicating the need for these disorders to be treated promptly and efficiently to support a better quality of life for the patients. Psychological manifestations of eating disorders are no less pressing since they most often present alongside other mental disorders, leaving a tangled web of symptoms that can be challenging to separate. Empirical evidence indicates the necessity of employing transdiagnostic interventions that address the common psychopathological features of such conditions with a focus towards evoking psychological strength and recovery (Barlow et al., 2017). Being aware of the fact that patients can have any set of eating-related issues along with other mental illnesses, clinicians and psychologists can develop more efficient treatment plans that target different needs. These techniques enable the practitioner to focus not only on the eating disorder but also on other psychological disorders underlying it, thus enabling an integrated treatment framework. This integrative process can finally offer better recovery outcomes, demonstrating the importance of treating psychological conditions in eating disorder treatment. In addition, there is a need to establish a supportive environment that encourages recovery and challenges the prevailing societal norms that lead to the existence of eating disorders. It is common for many individuals affected by these disorders to be stigmatized, which triggers their sense of shame and isolation, thus discouraging them from seeking assistance. Effective advocacy and education are important in dismantling negative and unhealthy stereotypes about body image and health and therefore promoting greater understanding and sympathy in communities. By building awareness of the complexity of eating disorders, we can inspire individuals to understand the importance of early intervention as well as support networks. Such interventions may involve healthy food relationships, body positivity, and reducing society's pressures around appearance. Ultimately, treating the multifaceted nature of eating disorders is not just a medical necessity but a social obligation to ensure victims of these chronic conditions are healthy (Figure 11.2).

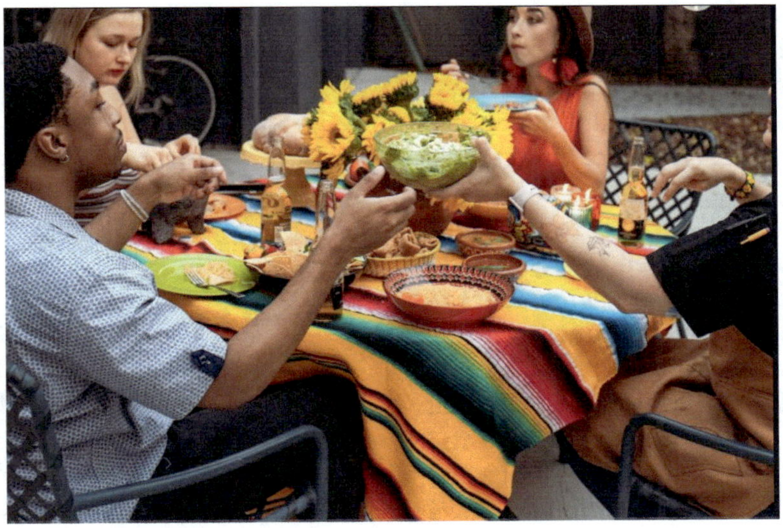

Figure 11.2. Group dining fostering connection and mindful eating.

Source: https://sanfordbehavioralhealth.com/wp-content/uploads/2023/01/group-dining-e1674215186688.jpg.

11.1. Types of Eating Disorders

Eating disorders encompass a spectrum of psychiatric conditions that are characterized by abnormal eating patterns and intense disturbance of body image. Of these conditions, anorexia nervosa represents an intense fear of fatness, leading to starvation and weight loss. Anorexic individuals typically have a distorted mental perception of their own body size, and they perceive themselves as fat even when they are severely underweight. The psychological and medical consequences of anorexia may be dangerous, sometimes leading to life-threatening situations , such as cardiac issues and thinning of bones. Other eating disorders, , such as bulimia nervosa, include repeated episodes of binge eating accompanied by attempts at compensation through vomiting or over-exercise. Both disorders highlight the urgent need to acquire knowledge regarding the underlying psychological issues and social stressors that are responsible for these illnesses, reiterating the need for early identification and multifaceted treatment approaches. Another significant type of eating disorder is binge eating disorder (BED), where repeated episodes of excessive eating occur regularly, typically triggered by emotional distress. Unlike bulimia, individuals with BED do not engage in compensation behavior, leading to such consequences as obesity and subsequent health outcomes. Diagnosis of BED illustrates that eating disorders manifest in varied forms, hence making it difficult to design effective treatment strategies. Emotional cues, including anxiety, stress, and depression, have been found to trigger episodes of binge eating, often initiating a vicious cycle of guilt, leading to more overeating. Approaching emotional health with a therapeutic approach, as well as creating a more wholesome relationship with food, is imperative in BED management. Recent studies demonstrate that combined treatment focusing on psychological health can be linked with improved recovery for individuals with this disorder, pointing towards a new area of research (Vos et al., 2017). Another less typical disorder is avoidant/restrictive food intake disorder (ARFID), wherein food is limited without the drive of concerns about weight or shape of the body. Individuals with ARFID may limit some food based on sensory problems or past trauma related to food. ARFID may lead to nutritional impairment and significant weight loss, impacting health. Since ARFID does not conform to the traditional criteria of other eating disorders, it usually remains undiagnosed and hence is treated belatedly. The intricacy of ARFID highlights the necessity of sensitivity among healthcare professionals and family members to enable people to seek the proper intervention. Treatment methods generally encompass a mix of cognitive-behavioral therapy and nutritional education with an aim to slowly increase the variety of foods in the diet and enhance the individual's comfort level with food. These interventions can have a strong positive impact on the quality of life of subjects with ARFID, demonstrating the demand for individualized treatment regimens in the treatment of eating disorders (Schiffman et al., 2014).

11.1.1. Anorexia Nervosa

Anorexia Nervosa, a highly acute eating disorder, is characterized by excessive caloric restriction secondary to a morbid fear of putting on weight. It usually appears in late adolescence or early adulthood with an extremely high prevalence among women. It is, however, increasingly being diagnosed in men too.

The psychological factors for anorexia involve several complex factors, including societal pressures, genetic tendencies, and individual characteristics , such as perfectionism and self-esteem. Treatment approaches generally target the physical consequences of starvation, yet these methods can also neglect the root psychological and emotional issues creating the condition. Thus, it is essential to understand the multifaceted nature of Anorexia Nervosa in designing treatment protocols that consider both the short-term medical complications as well as the psychological processes involved. The most common treatment regimen for Anorexia Nervosa is aimed at objective medical outcomes, i.e., weight gain, without adequate consideration of the psychological aspects of the disorder. A study evaluated the effectiveness of the common treatment programs and suggested an urgent need for a paradigm shift. Using theories , such as the Transtheoretical Model of Change and Social Networking Theory, it is possible to create a more holistic model that targets the root causes of anorexia and not merely medical symptoms. Here, recovery is viewed as both not merely physiological healing but change at the behavioral as well as the cognitive levels. An understanding of the inadequacies of traditional approaches necessitates a rethinking of treatment approaches to eating disorder treatments to guarantee that patients are offered comprehensive care that promotes recovery over the long term (Clites, 2012). Over the past few years, new treatment modalities have been introduced to improve accessibility and efficacy for patients with Anorexia Nervosa, especially adolescents. One of the encouraging options is the implementation of family-based treatment delivered via telemedicine, especially where families reside in rural or under-served areas. This method seeks to engage family members actively throughout the process of recovery, strengthening the social support groups that are critical to the treatment of eating disorders. Initial findings indicate that telemedicine can facilitate improved access to trained clinicians, cutting across geographical limitations to quality care (Anderson et al., 2015). By evaluating participants' treatment and experience feedback at the time of implementation, researchers attempt to find out how feasible this model is. Ultimately, such innovation can result in more availability of evidence-based practice, significantly improving the treatment of Anorexia Nervosa in various populations (Figure 11.3).

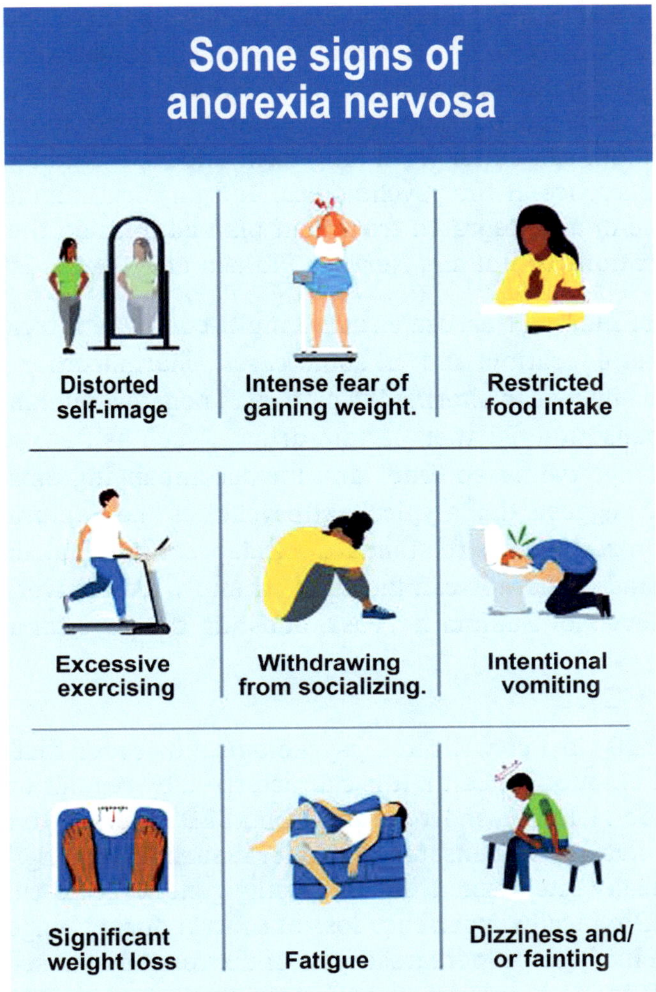
Some signs of anorexia nervosa
Distorted self-image
Intense fear of gaining weight.
Restricted food intake
Excessive exercising
Withdrawing from socializing.
Intentional vomiting
Significant weight loss
Fatigue
Dizziness and/ or fainting

Figure 11.3. Key warning signs of anorexia nervosa.

Source: https://my.clevelandclinic.org/-/scassets/images/org/health/articles/9794-anorexia-nervosa.jpg.

11.1.2. Bulimia Nervosa

Bulimia Nervosa, recurrent bouts of binge eating and compensatory behavior of self-induced vomiting, is a complex eating disorder with serious health implications. Individuals with this disorder commonly experience intense feelings of guilt, worry, and loss of control when they binge. The people afflicted with this disorder go through phases of restraint of diet and then subsequent bingeing, which results in the constant battle with weight and body image issues. The psychological factors of Bulimia Nervosa are very much intertwined with cultural and societal expectations, where pressures to conform to unrealistic body ideals reinforce the disorder. This condition is prevalent in adolescents, who are highly exposed to external pressures from media representation and peer groups, eventually influencing their body image and self-worth (Zhu, 2023). The physical consequences of Bulimia Nervosa can be challenging, as it produces a variety of medical complications that tend to undermine overall well-being. Repeated vomiting results in electrolyte imbalances, producing potentially fatal medical complications like cardiac arrhythmias. Moreover, frequent exposure to stomach acid results in dental erosion and damage to the esophagus, which can be medically repaired but may even require surgery. Apart from these short-term complications, the individual can suffer from long-term effects, including gastrointestinal disease and starvation. The concurrence of the psychological and physical manifestations of the disorder highlights the importance of an integrated treatment plan addressing the issues of mental illness and the medical complications of Bulimia Nervosa (Takaki and Okabe, 2015).

Effective treatment of Bulimia Nervosa entails a multi-component treatment plan that involves psychotherapy, nutritional education, and, in some cases, pharmacotherapy. Cognitive-behavioral therapy (CBT) has proved effective in altering the pattern of negative thinking and conduct associated with bingeing and compensation. Further, certain drugs, , such as fluoxetine, have been noted to be useful in inhibiting binge eating episodes and for accompanying anxiety or depression (Zhu, 2023). The literature also suggests that atypical antipsychotics like aripiprazole possess therapeutic value, particularly for non responders to standard antidepressants (Takaki and Okabe, 2015). The combination of these forms of therapy can facilitate an improved recovery process along with the healing of the complex levels of Bulimia Nervosa, boosting the physical and mental state.

11.1.3. Binge Eating Disorder

Binge Eating Disorder (BED) is a complicated psychological disorder that significantly impacts an individual's physical and emotional health. It is characterized by regular occurrences of consuming enormous quantities of food within a short duration, and BED differs from other eating disorders in that it does not typically involve compensatory behaviors , such as purging. The etiology behind BED is very complex and typically intertwined, encompassing genetic, socio-cultural, and psychological factors. Patients with BED typically experience loss of control during bingeing, followed by guilt or shame, which are in turn likely to perpetuate a cycle of distress and subsequent food consumption. Understanding these dynamics is critical to the identification of targeted interventions. Recent research focuses on the need for an integrated approach that takes into consideration both the physiological and psychological aspects of the disorder, noting its prevalence in different populations (Rao, 2025). BED's relationship with obesity is of interest since individuals who have BED are more likely to gain weight and have related health problems. Studies have shown that patterns of disordered eating and emotional eating can further compound obesity, resulting in a vicious cycle wherein increased body weight further deteriorates self-esteem and regulation of emotions (Burnatowska et al., 2023). Besides, the interconnection of obesity with diseases , such as polycystic ovary syndrome (PCOS) reveals how BED can initiate a series of health problems. Women with PCOS often face particular hormonal disturbances that are likely to complicate their treatment of BED and obesity. By revealing the interlinking of the disorders, clinicians can deal more effectively with the underlying causes of BED and reduce its adverse impact on overall health outcomes. Interventional approaches focused on determining food-evoked behaviors in the context of mental health are critical in the development of intervention approaches (Rao, 2025). Treatment of Binge Eating Disorder also requires a holistic strategy with an emphasis on psychological counseling along with nutrition education. Cognitive-behavioral therapy (CBT) has emerged as a method to alter the pathological thinking patterns that drive the binge-eating habit. CBT helps patients learn healthy coping mechanisms, establish a healthy body image, and bring about long-term behavior modification. In addition, pharmacotherapy, , such as the use of certain medications, can potentially reduce binge eating episodes, but it should be individualized according to the needs and circumstances of the patient. Engagement in a multidimensional treatment program not only proves useful in the management of BED but also can treat co-occurring psychiatric disorders like depression and anxiety, with which the disorder is commonly found. Lastly, interdisciplinary coordination among the caregivers to effectively assist those in their struggle with the Binge Eating Disorder (Burnatowska et al., 2023) (Figure 11.4).

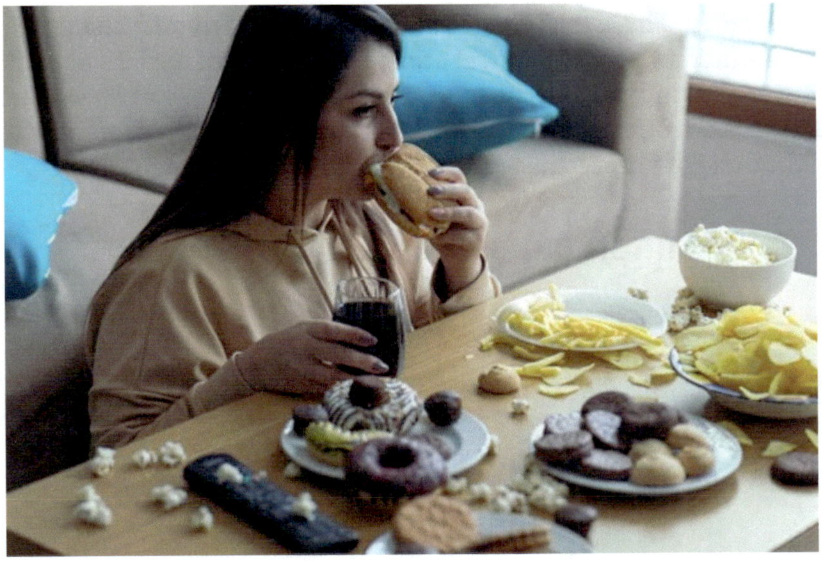

Figure 11.4. Binge eating episode with excessive intake of high-calorie foods.

Source: https://rainfordhall.com/wp-content/uploads/2025/02/Binge-eating-disorder.jpg.

11.2. Causes of Eating Disorders

The complex reciprocal interplay between eating disorders highlights the simultaneous presence of personal psychological determinants and broader sociocultural influences. Data demonstrates that eating disorder patients commonly view internal issues, , such as body dissatisfaction and psychological distress, as significant etiologic issues contributing to their illness. In a discussion among social media conversations of Chinese participants with self-reported eating disorders, over 90% of participants named individual reasons for their disorders, and among those, body image and eating were extremely prevalent (He et al., 2024). These are the type of individual factors that manifest as feelings of inadequacy or internalized perfectionism, where individuals attempt to achieve an unattainable ideal that in turn creates disordered eating behaviors. This shows how intrinsic psychological issues act as a central foundation for the formation of eating disorders. Sociocultural issues are also a significant reason for the occurrence and prevalence of eating disorders, especially in the areas of media exposure and societal pressures. Most people indicate that viewing idealized body ideals and the need to fit into culturally imposed expectations play a major role in their eating habits. In the above study, 35-51% of the participants reported experiencing the influence of sociocultural factors on their eating disorders, showing that environmental pressures may trigger personal vulnerabilities (He et al., 2024). The ongoing focus on certain body ideals in the media may lead to a skewed sense of self, fueling the process of self-doubt and pathological consumption. Understanding of such sociocultural forces informs an integrated understanding of how societal norms impact individual experience and lead to the development of eating disorders. In addition, the interconnectedness of eating disorders and health outcomes identifies the need for effective prevention and treatment strategies. A systematic review indicates a high correlation between eating disorders and mortality, emphasizing the severity of eating disorders. Most alarming is anorexia nervosa, which reveals a highly elevated standardized mortality ratio, illustrating the deadly risk of severe cases. This somber statistic presents a twofold challenge for intervention: countering the sociocultural and psychological etiology of eating disorders and enhancing screening and treatment policies. As individuals become enlightened, healthcare workers and society in general must create an environment that views mental well-being as valuable and minimizes the societal pressures that trigger these disorders (Figure 11.5).

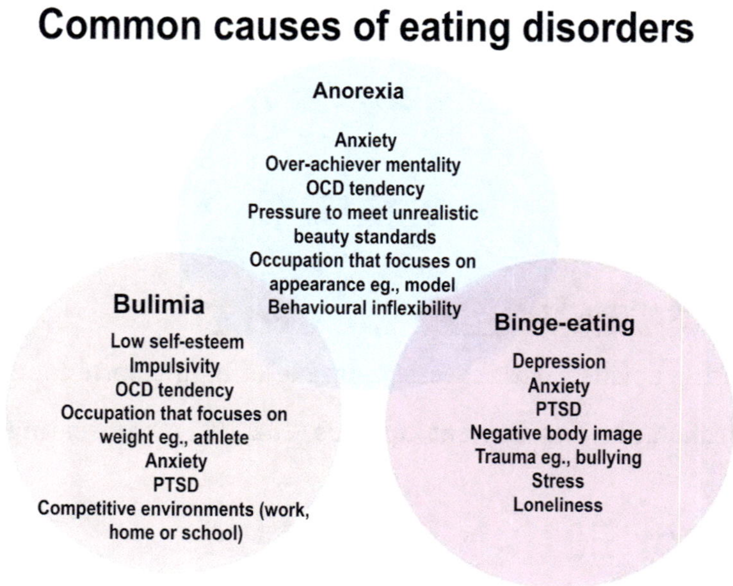

Figure 11.5. Venn diagram showing common psychological and environmental causes of anorexia, bulimia, and binge-eating disorders.

Source: https://cdn.ukat.co.uk/sites/ukat/wp-content/uploads/2022/07/eating-disorders-facts-2.jpg.

11.2.1. Genetic Factors

The complex relationship between eating disorders and genes has continued to be the subject of interest in modern studies in the etiology of multifactorial conditions. Genetic factors contribute significantly to influencing the susceptibility of individuals to eating disorders, , such as anorexia nervosa and bulimia nervosa. Evidence has established that eating disorder family history predisposes a person to the conditions, suggesting a hereditary factor that requires further study. Twin studies have also provided valuable insights, showing that genetics accounts for approximately half of eating disorder risk. This highlights the value of establishing genetic susceptibility as a significant component of eating disorder knowledge, ultimately facilitating treatment in a holistic way through integration of genetic evaluation with psychological and environmental factors. In addition to genetic determinants, some genetic markers are also associated with eating disorder behaviors and personality characteristics. Some genes responsible for the functioning of serotonin and dopamine receptors have been found to be associated with restrained eating, emotional control, and impulsivity. These tendencies are often typical of individuals with disordered eating. Secondly, the interplay between genetic risks and environmental factors, , such as media portrayal of body image, further illustrates the interconnectedness of these conditions. For instance, the influence of media presentation on body dissatisfaction is magnified in those who are genetically predisposed to disordered eating behaviors, as delineated in study where intense media exposure was linked with unhealthy conceptions and behaviors of the body (Maria et al., 2017). Thus, identification of these genetic factors is important for developing prevention programs and successful interventions. Furthermore, this knowledge about genetic factors in eating disorders also is not restricted to their interaction with environmental and psychological variables. For instance, responses to adverse life events, , such as trauma or loss, may be moderated by genetic risk, which can trigger or exacerbate disordered eating behavior. Research has confirmed that histories of nonconsensual sex during sexual initiation will forecast high levels of eating disorder attitudes and behaviors, linking both genetic risk factors and environmental variables (May 2019). The confluence at this site calls forth an inquiry into how genetics contributes to vulnerabilities while also being touched by their lived lives. As we continue to deconstruct the complexities in eating disorders and genetics, it is increasingly important that we adopt a multi-disciplinary approach that integrates biological, psychological, and sociocultural perspectives, paving the way for more holistic treatments.

11.2.2. Psychological Influences

The complex relationship between psychological variables and the etiology of eating disorders is a significant research domain that underscores the multifaceted nature of these disorders. Stress, among other psychological variables, has been demonstrated to play a significant role in the etiology and exacerbation of eating disorders. Research indicates that victims of such disorders have higher levels of stress than their counterparts. This added stress may be the result of internal psychological problems, , such as low self-esteem and body image distortion, or even outside pressures, , such as societal pressures and discouragement from other people. The interplay of these factors paints the complexity that comes with eating disorders, and the necessity of a comprehensive approach in both diagnosis and treatment measures, as emphasized in recent studies that determine the direct correlation between eating disorders and stress levels in psychology (Smutchak, 2024). Furthermore, the psychological component of eating disorders incorporates other factors, including genetic predisposition and cultural elements. The convergence of biological, psychological, and social elements offers an impoverished soil for the etiology of these disorders. For instance, cultural beauty ideals emphasizing thinness have a profound effect on one's body image, leading to maladaptive coping behavior that manifests as disordered eating behaviors. Psychological traits , such as perfectionism and social evaluation sensitivity have also been identified with an increased risk of developing eating disorders. It is crucial to understand the etiology from this multi-factorial context to plan effective treatment approaches. Researchers emphasize the importance of taking these complex interplaying factors into account to create personalized therapeutic interventions that address each individual's distinct collection of issues comprehensively (Tataryan et al., 2024).

The psychological impact of influence extends far beyond direct influence on eating behavior, with implications spanning into wider determinants of general health and well-being. Patients with eating disorders and elevated psychological stress have been found to complain of diminishing life satisfaction, increased depression, and a reduced sense of health. Conversely, patients who can effectively manage stress and start learning more effective coping mechanisms will experience increased well-being and life satisfaction. This correlation goes on to establish that psychological well-being needs to be addressed to address eating disorders. The instillation of psychological support systems , such as stress management abilities and cognitive behavioral therapy, is essential in promoting recovery and enhancing quality of life for the affected. Empathy for these psychological aspects, therefore, is essential not only in diagnosis and treatment but also in improving long-term outcomes for individuals who struggle with eating disorders (Smutchak, 2024) (Figure 11.6).

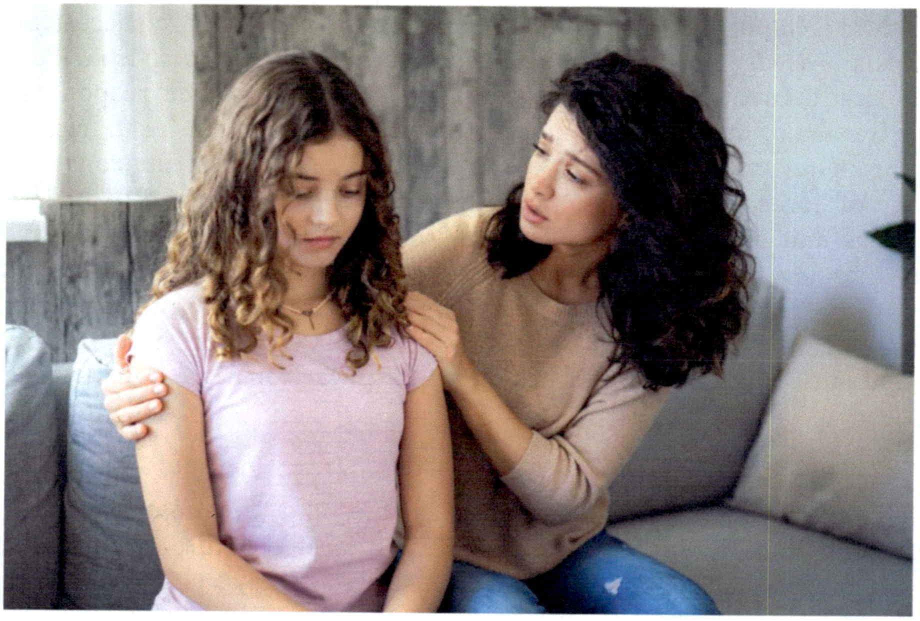

Figure 11.6. Mother comforting her daughter during an emotional moment.

Source: https://sierravistahospital.com/wp-content/uploads/2025/02/GettyImages-2150007714-1200x800.jpg.

11.2.3. Societal and Cultural Pressures

The wide-ranging influence of cultural and social pressures significantly shapes perceptions of body image, particularly for women. Such pressures predominantly manifest as media presentation reinforcing an extremely limited definition of beauty, typically encapsulated in the notion of never being fat. Endless pictures in periodicals, on screens, and through internet mediums continually flood women, reinforcing an unrealistic and psychologically damaging ideal. As highlighted in the research findings, frequent exposure to unnatural, unhealthy and unrealistic models communicates the subtle message that for a woman to be attractive, she has to achieve this extremely thin shape (Brien et al., 2012). These societal expectations promote poisonous comparisons that can cause a warped sense of self-perception, eventually driving people towards unhealthy habits to achieve an unattainable goal. Cultural narratives surrounding femininity also play a significant role in the causation of body dissatisfaction and eating disorders. Feminine identity is associated with beauty ideals, where conformity to these stereotypes is a measure of worth and acceptability. The social mandate that women are expected to be thin not only sustains negative body image but also impacts eating and exercise habits. Research reveals that several multiple regression analyses show that several female gender stereotypes have effects on body esteem, exercise and eating behavior (Sauerteig, 2017). This pressure to conform to such stereotypes can cause individuals to turn to disordered eating patterns and over-exercise, bringing forth the adverse relationship between societal expectations and individual health. Furthermore, the effects of these social pressures reach beyond individual behavior and impact wider social dynamics. The constant reinforcement of the ideal body figure contributes to a culture of criticism and comparison that fuels anxiety and low self-esteem in women. Because health becomes conflated with being thin, the prevalence of eating disorders is compounded by wanting approval and acceptance. The diet and physical appearance emphasis of culture can lead people to sacrifice their physical and mental well-being in pursuit of social acceptance. In order to combat such self-destructive norms, there needs to be a collective attempt at redefinition of what health and beauty are, and how they are more individualistic rather than conformist to self-destructive standards presented by mass culture (Figure 11.7).

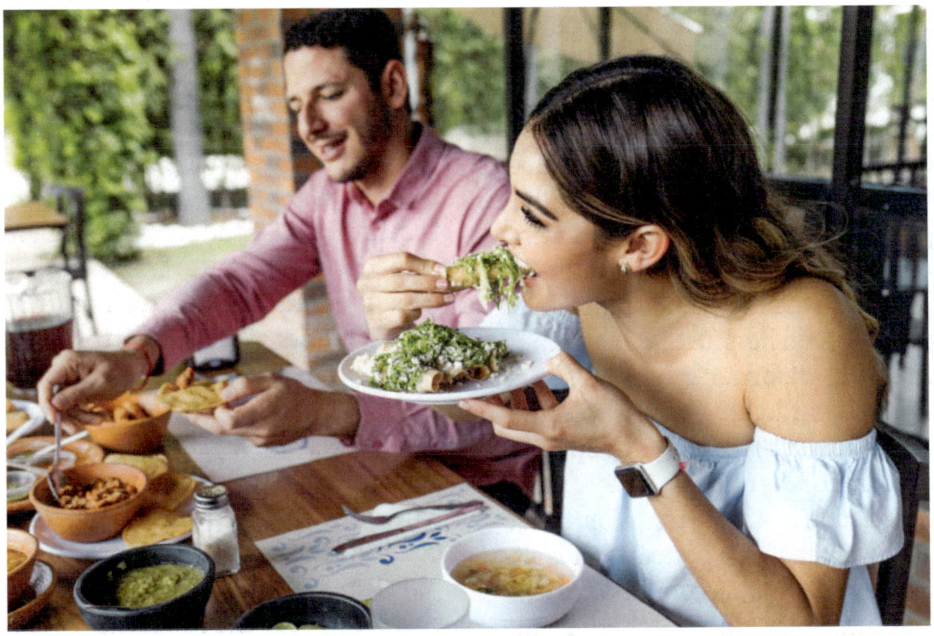

Figure 11.17. Sharing a joyful moment over a hearty meal.

Source: https://altoptions.com/wp-content/uploads/2023/02/iStock-1347161226-1-1024x683-1.jpg.

11.3. Symptoms and Diagnosis

Symptom identification in respect of eating disorders is necessary for proper diagnosis, followed by treatment. Certain subtypes , such as anorexia nervosa, bulimia nervosa, and binge eating disorder, all have their own symptomatology that needs to be recognized by practitioners. For example, individuals with anorexia have extreme weight loss, morbid fear of weight gain, and body distortion, whereas those with bulimia experience cycles of bingeing and purging. Symptoms become even more complex when the individual has other psychiatric disorders , such as depression or anxiety, which need close scrutiny in order to ascertain a complete comprehension of the individual's psychological state. Early and accurate diagnosis is important, as it allows for proper intervention measures related to the presenting symptoms of the patient, ultimately leading to improved treatment and outcomes for recovery. Knowledge of the process of diagnosis is also essential, as it encompasses various tools of evaluation that enable medical professionals to deliver accurate diagnoses of eating disorders. Among the most common approaches is through the application of standardized questionnaires, , such as the Eating Disorder Examination Questionnaire, which gauges eating behavior, food attitudes, and psychological distress surrounding eating behaviors. The assessment of early adaptive schemas, cognitive flexibility, and emotional regulation has also proved helpful in determining the severity of eating disorder symptoms. For instance, research has indicated that numerous predictors are more closely linked with specific subtypes and, hence, age and body mass index can be particularly important for binge eating disorder, whereas the concept of self-compassion can have a pivotal role in anorexia nervosa and bulimia nervosa (Mitchell et al., 2024). Hence, a more precise understanding of individual symptoms and the related diagnostic process is essential in treating eating disorders effectively. In addition to traditional diagnostic methods, growing technology adoption, , such as mobile applications, has started to transform eating disorder diagnosis. Recent research indicates that, through emotion, eating patterns, and body sensations monitoring that can be effective surrogates, these apps provide individuals with access to symptom monitoring and management resources (Guluzade and Sas, 2024). Furthermore, user-generated content, including reviews and comments on these apps, also captures the functional challenges and ethical concerns surrounding the utilization of digital technology to diagnose and treat. While beneficial as the tracking functions prove to be, the finesse required in developing such apps cannot be underestimated, considering the fact that they must convincingly address and track potentially self-harming behaviors without encouraging harmful habits. Thus, the combination of new technology with the diagnostic process can contribute to enhancing user participation and personal responsibility for self-managing symptoms, as well as to creating a more personalized treatment approach.

11.3.1. Physical Symptoms

Physical symptoms play a crucial role in the creation and identification of eating disorders, since they manifest as obvious indicators of hidden psychological pathology. Anorectic patients may experience weight loss, malnutrition, as well as various cognitive impairments, potentially resulting in impaired judgment and increased distorted perception of body image. The most common physical symptoms are bradycardia, hypotension, and electrolyte imbalances, which, if left untreated, can result in potentially life-threatening complications. These symptoms not only damage physical health but also reflect the emotional suffering of those with eating disorders. Because of this, familiarity with these physical symptoms is essential to early intervention, as early detection and intervention can greatly improve patient outcomes (van Doornik et al., 2024). Bulimia nervosa, in contrast, presents a different type of physical symptomatology that may be more subtle but no less problematic. Recurrent episodes of binge eating followed by compensatory behavior , such as self-induced vomiting and over-exercise may lead to severe dental erosion, gastrointestinal complications, and cardiac complications. They may also develop symptoms of dehydration and electrolyte imbalance, which are themselves responsible for additional health risks. The cycle of purging not only damages physical well-being but also creates a poisonous energy that reinforces the illness, and so it is crucial that medical practitioners can recognize such symptoms. Moreover, heightened awareness of the physical indicators makes for better education and understanding of the complexities in the cases of eating disorders and, therefore a holistic treatment strategy (Winer, 2014). Binge eating disorder (BED), the most prevalent of eating disorders, has a direct impact on a person's physical health profile. People afflicted with BED can acquire morbid obesity, hypertension, and type 2 diabetes due to chronic cycles of binge eating. Lack of compensatory behaviors, which differentiate this disorder from bulimia nervosa, has the potential to cause several metabolic complications as well as serious health consequences. Furthermore, BED patients experience psychological distress in the form of shame and loss of control. Such co-morbid physical and psychological disturbances create difficulties in treating the condition, necessitating an integrated treatment approach encompassing both medical and psychological care systems. With more research documenting the complex processes of eating disorders, identification of such specific physical symptoms remains fundamental in the formulation of effective interventions and improving patient prognosis (van Doornik et al., 2024) (Figure 11.8).

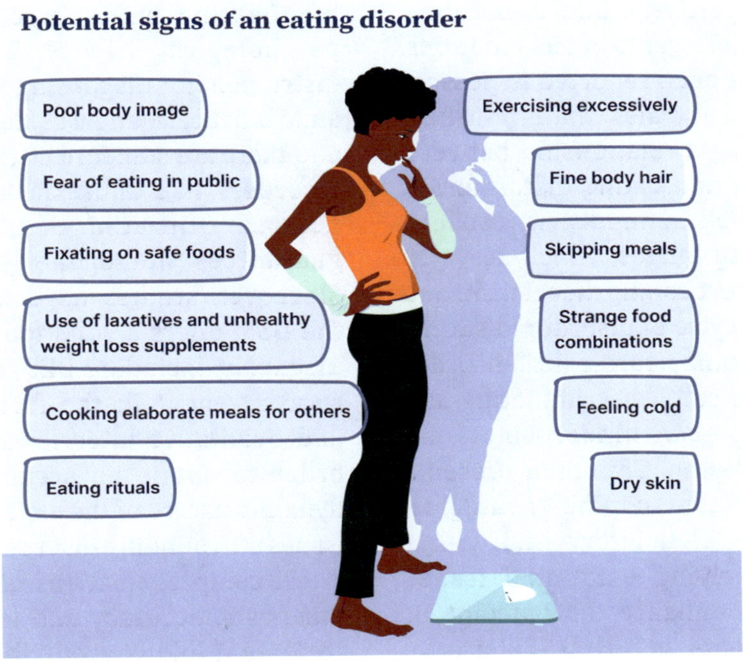

Figure 11.8. Signs of an eating disorder including behavioral and physical indicators.

Source: https://calmerry.com/wp-content/uploads/2021/03/Do-I-Have-an-Eating-Disorder.jpg.

11.3.2. Emotional and Behavioral Symptoms

Emotional and behavioral symptoms are prominent features of eating disorders, which have a significant contribution to their etiology and severity. Individuals with conditions , such as anorexia nervosa, bulimia nervosa, and binge eating disorder (BED) have predominantly been reported to experience more emotional dysregulation, which might, in turn, result in disordered eating. Research shows that individuals with emotional control issues in adolescence are at a higher risk of developing abnormal eating. Specifically, the parent's influence role, i.e., psychological control, increases emotional distress and thus raises vulnerability toward eating disorders. In a study of the association between paternal parenting and emotional symptoms in adolescents, it was found that emotional regulation issues were strongly correlated with psychological aspects of parenting, and this suggests that family functioning significantly adds to the emotional quality of adolescents who are at risk of these disorders (Flouri and McEwen, 2008). In the context of binge eating disorder specifically, behavioral and emotional symptoms appear as alexithymia and impulsivity, and it becomes harder for affected adolescents to feel emotions. BED adolescents have been reported to possess higher rates of these traits than non-BED adolescents, indicating a relationship between their emotional state and eating disturbances. The effects of high levels of impulsivity can lead to spontaneous eating binges, which serve as an emotional discomfort coping mechanism and further reinforce the cycle of disordered eating. Furthermore, alexithymia neurological disorder in which one has difficulty discriminating and describing emotions—can hinder emotional regulation and processing. This then presents a challenge to effective coping strategies, and hence, more targeted interventions that address these underlying emotional issues may be employed to enhance the outcome of treatment in adolescents with BED (Ballarotto, 2017). Importantly, the detection and treatment of emotional and behavioral symptoms of eating disorders in adolescents is critical in designing useful intervention programs. The interplay between emotion regulation, impulsive behavior, and maladaptive behavior indicates that treatment must be comprehensive in scope and go beyond the realm of eating behavior. Interventions that target emotion regulation and enhance emotional sensitivity can be very beneficial. Research indicates that targeting these skills may not only decrease emotional symptomatology but also decrease the risk of developing or maintaining disordered eating patterns. Although health professionals do consider these emotional factors in treatment plans, there is obviously a requirement to establish emotional resilience and adaptive coping mechanisms to enhance eating disorder and overall mental health management (Flouri and McEwen, 2008).

11.3.3. Diagnostic Criteria and Assessment

Measurement methods and the diagnostic test for eating disorders have evolved over time, highlighting shifts in clinical practice and psychological science. The most important instrument for diagnosing them is the Diagnostic and Statistical Manual of Mental Disorders (DSM), and there are standard criteria for various eating disorders like anorexia nervosa and bulimia nervosa. Utilization of DSM-5 in clinics also guarantees homogeneity in the diagnosis. Moreover, studies have indicated that while the DSM offers a solid foundation for disorder diagnosis, including BED, a methods approach to assessment in the form of questionnaires and qualitative interviews will be required in order to obtain an accurate portrayal of the dynamic nature of the experience and emotional issues surrounding disordered eating behaviors. These comprehensive assessments can enhance diagnostic accuracy and inform individualized treatment plans, contributing ultimately to enhanced outcomes for patients. Disordered eating behavior (DEB), which is often seen in adolescents and children, may render diagnosis challenging. A new Brazilian study of young people discovered that DEB were prevalent but in the majority of instances did not satisfy the strict DSM criteria for eating disorders. This highlights the importance of recognizing DEB as part of the broader eating disorder continuum.

The findings revealed that DEB was strongly associated with internalizing symptoms, particularly among girls, and that the behaviors may represent prodromes of more severe disorders , such as anorexia or bulimia. The developmental trajectory of DEB highlights the importance of having early assessment protocols that are able to identify at-risk youth in order to provide timely intervention before established eating disorders (Oliveira et al., 2024). In addition, research emphasizes the need for employing diverse assessment measures to quantify the incidence and impact of binge eating behaviors with precision. A systematic review of clinical trials indicated that while DSM-5 is an excellent tool in diagnosing BED, it is generally worthwhile including other standardized assessment tools. Measures like the Eating Disorder Examination and the Binge Eating Scale provide further dimensions of insight that could be useful in targeting qualitative and emotional determinants of eating. A multi-dimensional assessment not only enhances the validity of diagnoses but also facilitates the development of intervention strategies that more accurately target the needs of individual patients. Therefore, DSM criterion syncretism with corroborating assessment measures is required for enhancing the understanding and effective treatment of eating disorders (Escobar et al., 2021) (Figure 11.9).

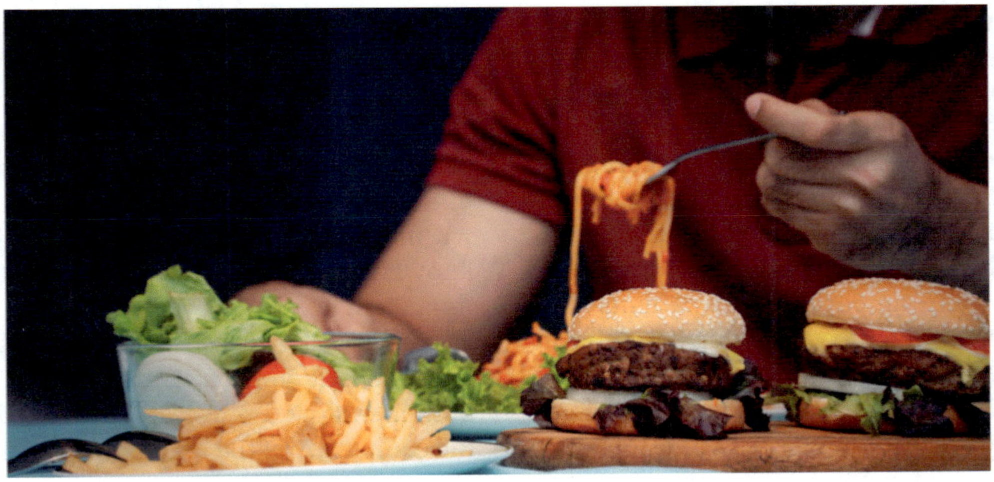

Figure 11.9. Binge eating behavior involves excessive consumption of high-calorie foods.

Source: https://cdn.rehabfiles.com/sites/ukrehab/wp-content/uploads/2024/01/uk-rehab-binge-eating.svg.

11.4. Consequences of Eating Disorders

The consequences of eating disorders extend past physical bodies; they also greatly affect psychological and social well-being. People with disorders , such as anorexia nervosa or bulimia nervosa can have serious mental health problems, ranging from anxiety disorders to depression. These issues are compounded, further promoting the eating disorder and thereby creating a cycle that is difficult to break. As can be seen in the literature, with the prominence in children and adolescents with autism, these comorbid conditions can have the consequence of an extremely limited diet, and a resultant impact upon physical health and emotional well-being (Bourne et al., 2022). Also, social consequences can be social isolation from peers, reduced self-esteem, and dysfunctional family dynamics. This multifaceted influence reflects the urgent need for comprehensive treatment approaches that address not only the eating disorder itself but also its psychological and social consequences. Furthermore, the recent global pandemic has brought about fairly dramatic alterations in the eating and physical exercise pattern, which has revealed the susceptibility of mental health in this regard. Research has indicated that individuals with pre-existing eating disorders had higher levels of restrictive, binge, and purging behaviors during the COVID-19 pandemic, which implied that the stressors of the pandemic exacerbated their conditions (Phillipou et al., 2020). Interestingly, the general population also changed, , such as increases in binge eating, suggesting an anxiety and uncertainty-driven trend towards disordered eating behavior. The pandemic has brought into prominence the inherent linkage between environmental stressors and the exacerbation of eating disorders, highlighting the need for intervention. It emphasizes how social issues tend to heighten underlying conditions, calling for extra caution and support for both patients with eating disorders and those experiencing shifts in eating patterns. Additionally, the consequences of eating disorders can have long-term health issues which are ongoing far into recovery from the disorder itself. Anorexia nervosa patients, for instance, will have complications like osteoporosis, cardiovascular issues, and gastrointestinal disturbances secondary to malnutrition and prolonged periods of starvation. The health effects in some cases are permanent, impacting life expectancy as well as quality of life. Besides, recent research has revealed that individuals suffering from eating disorders and, more so, those severely impacted can struggle with long-term psychological issues, thereby entering a cycle of health issues and deteriorated well-being (Bourne et al., 2022). Therefore, the aftereffects of eating disorders necessitate an integrated approach to overall health, incorporating medical, psychological, and dietetic treatment aimed at ameliorating both short-term effects and potential long-term consequences in a manner that allows patients to achieve and maintain overall health.

11.4.1. Physical Health Complications

The physical health issues that arise from EDs are profound and typically disastrous. Several forms of EDs, , such as anorexia nervosa, bulimia nervosa, and binge eating disorder, have different physiological effects that affect the overwhelming majority of body systems. Malnutrition, electrolyte imbalances, and severe weight fluctuations can afflict patients, causing cardiovascular complications, osteoporosis, and compromised immune status. Also, mortality risk is heightened, with anorexia nervosa being ranked as having the greatest mortality rates among all mental health disorders, as estimable evidence suggests that approximately 4% of patients die from associated complications within the disorder (Li et al., 2024). Therefore, knowledge of these physical consequences is important for both prevention and treatment strategies, and it serves to demonstrate the need for a holistic approach to care that considers both mental and physical welfare. Additionally, the complexity of the task in treating the physical symptoms of eating disorders is further fueled by an overall lack of knowledge among health professionals. A recent study found significant knowledge gaps among healthcare professionals with regard to the diagnostic, etiologic, and management aspects of EDs, particularly in the non-mental health specialties (Monteleone et al., 2024). While the majority of professionals are excellent at identifying physical complications, there is usually a lack of understanding of the psychological underpinnings that are associated with these disorders. Therefore, ED patients do not receive timely or adequate treatment, and their health is worsened. It underscores education and training of the health workforce that can make them competent to manage these sensitive physical and emotional bonds in an efficient manner. The need to address physical health conditions in the case of eating disorders is exacerbated by the most affected populations, namely adolescents and youth in the transitional age. This population has the highest prevalence of EDs, hence the need for early recognition and intervention all the more (Li et al., 2024). Adolescents are undergoing intense physiological change, and as such, they are particularly susceptible to the detrimental effects that eating disorders have on development and growth. Physical illness issues that this group of people face are not only temporary but may last well into adulthood, leading to long-term complications , such as gastrointestinal upsets and reproductive problems. A combined model that incorporates both physical health treatment and mental health care is therefore required to avert the long-term consequences of eating disorders (Figure 11.10).

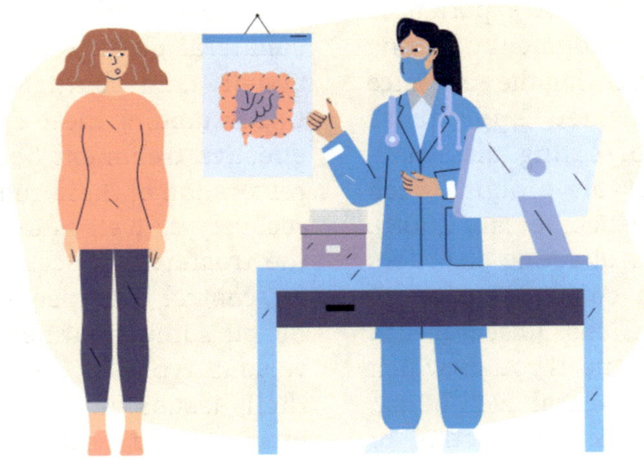

Figure 11.10. Doctor discussing digestive health symptoms with a patient during consultation.

Source: https://bulimia.com/wp-content/uploads/2022/08/symptoms-of-problem-1.svg.

11.4.2. Psychological Effects

The psychological consequences of eating disorders extend far beyond the physical health consequences at their root, often with the effect of making a very strong impact on the mental health of an individual. Anorexia nervosa, bulimia nervosa, and binge eating disorder are not merely eating impairments but complex psychological disorders that can have severe emotional distress as a result. These disorders usually make people fight with poor self-esteem, body dysmorphia, and excessive weight gain fear. Due to this, these disorders usually aggravate depression and loneliness, so it becomes more difficult for people suffering from them to approach people or engage in social activities. The internal struggle between the desire for acceptance and the impulse to have control over one's weight can perpetuate a cycle of anxiety and despair, justifying the psychological weight that becomes linked with these eating disorders. In addition, the relationship between trauma and eating disorders has attracted much research interest in the past few years. Sexual assault and harassment victims also experience traumatic effects that take the shape of eating disorders, which are psychological distress and maladaptive coping mechanisms. Disordered eating is found through research to be a way for individuals to regain control over their body to reverse the sensation of helplessness that tends to follow trauma. This identification underscores the importance of addressing the underlying psychological issues involved in both victimization and eating disorders because these conditions have the potential to create a feedback cycle that escalates emotional suffering. There is overwhelming evidence to affirm a relationship between the experiences of victimization and the development of eating disorder symptoms, underscoring the relevance of adopting trauma-informed approaches towards the treatment of eating disorders, particularly among vulnerable groups , such as students in colleges (Isaacs et al., 2008). The multifaceted character of eating disorders necessitates an in-depth comprehension of their psychological dimensions. Research has outlined various mechanisms through which such disorders influence mental well-being, most commonly through the intersection of cognitive distortions and unhealthily adaptive coping strategies. For example, individuals with eating disorders will often exhibit signs of anxiety disorder, depression, and even post-traumatic stress disorder, complicating their recovery process. As evident from recent studies, psychological concerns , such as internalization of cultural ideals of beauty and success, are also significant predictors of the emergence and continuance of eating disorders. These interacting psychological effects mean that successful treatments will have to target not only the eating disorder-related behaviors but also the associated cognitive processes and mental illness disorders underlying these diseases, providing a pathway for more extensive healing (Cavoli et al., 2011).

11.4.3. Social and Relational Impacts

The interpersonal and social consequences of eating disorders are broad and far-reaching, at times affecting more than the individual herself. People who have eating disorders can witness their relationships being gravely affected by their preoccupation with food, self-esteem, and body. By retreating from others through isolation or bypassing social meal situations, loved ones and friends become confused, annoyed, or helpless. This can lead to a breakdown of communication and support, further exacerbating loneliness and anxiety in the victim. The psychological morbidity of an eating disorder is in context; it impacts and alters social networks, and collateral damage is seen as reduced social activity and conflicted family relationships. Understanding these dynamics is important for effective treatment because it can result in a restoration of these connections that can foster recovery as well as overall health. In addition, the treatment process itself can be a catalyst for control over people's social relationships. By pursuing treatment, people will undergo various types of therapy that include facing their issues in a safe setting. Innovative interventions, , such as the proposed virtual reality (VR) café intervention, also illustrate the manner in which therapeutic environments can facilitate socialization and skill learning in a controlled setting. Through the provision of access to practice real-life social meal scenarios in a safe setting, the interventions can act as a template for gradual re-entry into social life. Of note in this regard is that both lived experience peers and their support networks expressed interest in such novel treatments, as they have the potential to facilitate not only personal recovery but also improve relational dynamics. Stakeholder engagement in the development of these treatment modalities places emphasis on the social nature of recovery, in which social support is a key element in addressing the larger relational impact of eating disorders (Shackshaft et al., 2024). Interpersonal psychotherapy (IPT) offers an evidence-based intervention to address the interpersonal nature of eating disorders and emphasizes the function of social support networks in recovery. IPT, with its focus on relational structure, asserts that psychological distress is a causal agent of influence over interpersonal functioning, which in turn can secondarily increase or decrease the impact of eating disorders. IPT encourages participants to address relationships as they learn communication skills to facilitate healthier relationships. As individuals get engaged with their social environment and get good at communicating their feelings and needs, they will feel less isolated due to their disorder. Moreover, IPT has also proved to be effective on diverse populations and in all age groups; thus, it is an effective treatment for responding to the complex social issues associated with eating disorders (Stuart et al., 2024). Lastly, relational healing is essential to successful long-term recovery, emphasizing the cooperative relationship between psychological well-being and social bonding (Figure 11.11).

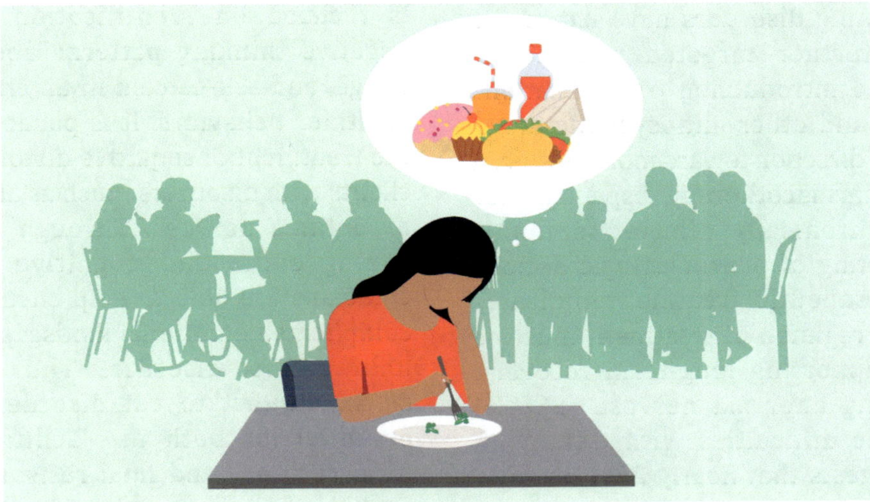

Figure 11.11. Craving high-calorie foods while restricting intake—an illustration of disordered eating behavior.

Source: https://assets.clevelandclinic.org/transform/9440ec8d-5b3b-4740-b554-f3bed4592b64/eating-disorders-1334045604.

11.5. Treatment Options

Effective therapy for eating disorders includes a multidisciplinary model that acknowledges the complex interplay between psychological, biological, and social variables. Cognitive Behavioral Therapy (CBT) is globally recommended as a sophisticated psychotherapy method, particularly in the treatment of disorders , such as Anorexia Nervosa and Bulimia Nervosa. CBT aims to modify adaptive thought processes and behaviors associated with disordered eating by establishing healthier cognitive processes. Research has also established its efficacy, particularly in tandem with nutritional counseling and medical treatment, regarding weight restoration as well as the overall mental state. The integration of such interventions into treatment plans ensures a holistic strategy that ultimately achieves optimal recovery rates among victims of eating disorders. Personalized treatment plans, formulated to treat the patient individually, are featured in recent literature, again calling for an approach to care with a holistic outlook in combating eating disorders. Another significant feature of the options in treatment is pharmacological treatment. Medications are not typically the first line of defense against eating disorders, yet they play an essential role as a complement to psychotherapeutic approaches for some patients. Antidepressants, particularly SSRIs, have been found useful to treat the symptoms of Bulimia Nervosa and binge eating disorders , such as anxiety and compulsive behavior. Additionally, advances in recent years regarding the neurobiological substrates of eating disorders have led to the possibility of further targeted treatments. For instance, the introduction of medications like dronabinol and other antipsychotic drugs represents a new direction toward more advanced treatment in pharmacotherapy, especially for severely and chronically affected patients. The complementing of pharmacologic options with psychotherapeutic treatment indicates that a complete regimen of treatment must be available for supporting long-term recovery. Chronic enduring anorexia nervosa (SE-AN) presents specific difficulties with treatment, as evidence suggests that nearly 20% of those diagnosed suffer from longstanding and long-term eating disorders. The patients will most frequently have more severe symptoms, higher hospitalization rates, and lower psychosocial functioning than individuals with short-duration illness (Marcolini et al., 2024). The treatment models for SE-AN today revolve around three general themes: psychotherapy, medication therapies, and brain stimulation therapies. Effective models of psychotherapy, , such as Specialist Supportive Clinical Management, have achieved variable levels of success, and the application of drugs, including certain antipsychotics, is useful for weight gain and symptom decrease, but has variable success. New brain stimulation treatments like Repetitive Transcranial Magnetic Stimulation have hopeful lines of research in psychiatric and emotional relief and serve as evidence of the urgent need for ongoing study into refining more targeted treatment methods and mitigating the long-term causes of this serious health issue (Marcolini et al., 2024).

11.5.1. Counseling and Therapy

Within the scope of eating disorders, therapy and counseling are important in facilitating healing and overall health. Numerous types of therapy have been created as effective interventions, including cognitive-behavioral therapy (CBT), which is one of the most widely used. CBT is focused on identification and changing negative thinking patterns about food, body image, and self-esteem in an effort to promote healthier behaviors. It is particularly useful in the treatment of cognitive distortions typical of clients with disorders , such as anorexia nervosa or bulimia nervosa. Through its teaching of coping skills and cognitive restructuring, clinicians are able to help clients navigate the complicated emotional landscape that typically follows these disorders. Thus, using therapy as an adjunct to eat disorder treatment is essential for both the facilitation of short-term recovery and final resistance to relapse. Family involvement is also another highly crucial aspect of therapy and counseling in treating eating disorders. Family-based therapy (FBT) has become a center modeled particularly on teens, where the family plays a key role in the recovery process. The process applied in such therapy aims at empowering families to take care of their loved ones and promote healthy eating, communication, and emotional support. By involving family, therapists can address sub-lying relational patterns that may be contributing to the maintenance of the disorder and ensure the support system is healthy and well-educated about the issues involved. Effective family engagement can help enhance outcomes, as it forms a team-based treatment method. In line with current research, the effectiveness of family-based treatments underscores the significance of a multidisciplinary team effort among patients, families, and clinicians during the process of recovery (Ram and Shelke, 2023).

Moreover, individualization of therapies is required to treat eating disorders successfully. Each individual's experience of an eating disorder is unique and influenced by a myriad of external and internal factors like previous trauma, culture, and personal history. From the experiences described by survivors, including Lorna Collins, it has been observed that mainstream treatment models do not tackle the complex aspects of these conditions, and hence, there is a call for tailored measures (Collins, 2024). Incorporating techniques like art therapy and mindfulness in the course of therapy can add depth to the healing experience, enabling patients to express themselves and their experiences artistically. These combined approaches not only facilitate symptom reduction but also enhance the quality of the patient's life with eating disorders. Therapy and counseling must, therefore, shift to encompass a broader variety of therapeutic approaches that resonate with the patient's recovery process (Figure 11.12).

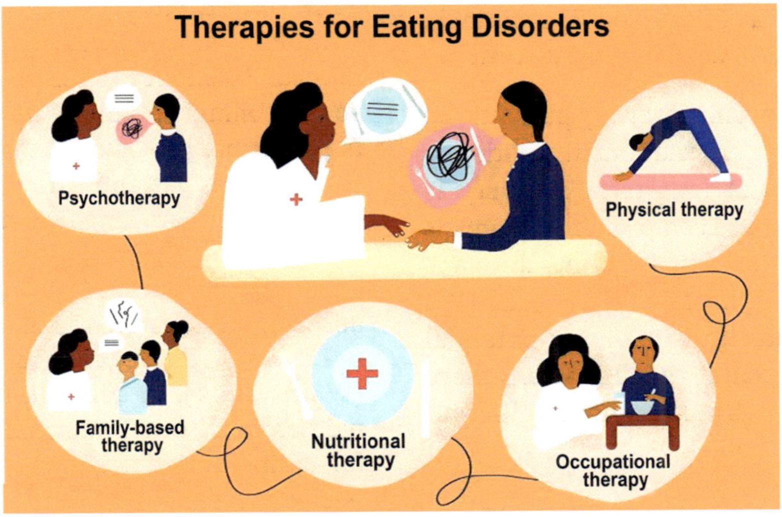
Therapies for Eating Disorders
Psychotherapy
Physical therapy
Family-based therapy
Nutritional therapy
Occupational therapy

Figure 11.12. Therapeutic approaches commonly used in the treatment of eating disorders.

Source: https://www.verywellhealth.com/thmb/BamUv1DsuI9mYBoopeqWlv0VDTQ=/1500x0/filters:no_upscale():max_bytes(150000):strip_icc()/Eating-disorders-treatment-5112475_final-7a652913ca284eaa9132401fd98f5942.jpg.

11.5.2. Nutritional Rehabilitation

Rehabilitation nutrition is an important part of treatment for eating disorders, particularly in the case of anorexia nervosa. It is a formal procedure directed towards nutritional status restoration and weight gain in severely malnourished individuals. As the body gradually acquires needs, clinicians monitor closely for such important signs, electrolytes, and overall health to neutralize dangers, including refeeding syndrome (RFS), during this risky time. Research has placed under the spotlight the potential incidence of RFS among nutritional rehabilitation patients; 33%, for example, of those participating in a study were found to have experienced some degree of RFS, highlighting the necessity for cautious prescriptions of energy and concern in this transition. Proper nutritional rehabilitation not only improves physical health but also lays the groundwork for psychological recovery, and it is thus an integral component of mass eating disorder treatment schemes (Brodie et al., 2024). The role of nutritional rehabilitation is greater than simple weight gain; rather, it is a multifaceted intervention that addresses both the physiological and psychological components of eating disorders. Effective nutritional treatment involves an individualized dietary plan that caters to individual patient requirements, i.e., caloric requirement and micronutrient requirements. This points towards the fact that nutritional inadequacy can prolong psychiatric symptomatology, again creating a cycle of recurrence of disordered eating behavior. In addition, integrating nutritional rehabilitation with psychotherapy may strengthen in the therapeutic impacts as cognitive and emotional problems are also crucial in eating disorders.

The focus is on empowering patients by establishing a healthier relationship with the body and food so that long-term recovery is facilitated. Integrated and comprehensive models become significant here in bridging the gaps usually found in existing treatment plans (Wu et al., 2024). Despite the significant potential benefits from nutritional rehabilitation, there remain issues in successful take-up in different clinical settings.

The majority of patients with eating disorders are resistant to treatment, often due to entrenched negative cognitive attitudes towards body image and food intake. This resistance can result in a delayed onset of treatment for nutritional care or poor compliance with dietary advice. The practitioners are required to operate under these challenges by leveraging trust and creating supportive settings that foster patient engagement towards their recovery journey. Research goes on progressing in the ways of best practice for nutritional rehabilitation as it attempts to optimize energy prescriptions in order to reconcile safety with adequate nutritional therapy. Through this, health practitioners can maximize treatment compliance and outcomes for individuals with eating disorders (Brodie et al., 2024).

11.5.3. Medication and Medical Intervention

Treatment of eating disorders most commonly necessitates the use of both medication and psychological therapy to achieve the optimal patient outcome. Of all such disorders, anorexia nervosa is particularly challenging due to its high morbidity and mortality, particularly in adolescents. The atypical antipsychotic olanzapine, though unlicensed for this specific application, has been noted to increase weight gain and diminish food and body image pathology anxiety. The National Institute for Clinical Excellence (NICE) has issued guidelines so that clinicians follow appropriate protocols in prescribing such medication in this condition to promote patient safety and effectiveness of treatment. An ongoing audit by the TEWV Trust revealed improvement in monitoring antipsychotic prescriptions and indications and calls for systematic assessment in clinical practice with regard to eating disorders (White, 2024). In addition to the psychotropic medications, other pharmacologic treatments for eating disorder co-morbid conditions have become established. Obesity, for instance, is now a pressing public health concern, and medical treatment efficacy for obesity is needed. Topiramate, primarily an anti-epileptic agent, is also frequently prescribed off-label for weight management in eating and mood disorders. The drug has garnered attention on the basis of its ability to induce weight loss through mechanisms that may be due to reduced calorie intake and effects on reward circuits for food. Clinical studies have provided robust support for its use, with documentation for beneficial weight loss in various patient groups, thereby putting the drug treatment in the limelight as an adjunct to nutritional and psychological treatment protocols (Wajid et al., 2023). Also, the complexity of eating disorders typically calls for multidisciplinary treatment consisting of both medical and psychological interventions. These patients require regular psychiatric assessment, particularly those with dual diagnosis or severe psychiatric comorbid conditions, where management of medication is also a crucial component. Treatment for eating disorders must be accompanied by a complete evaluation, including tracking of physical health, to prevent complicating both disorders and their pharmacologic treatment. Best communication between practitioners ensures that one will provide holistic care to individuals tailored to individualized needs. Through frequent monitoring of medication protocols and treatment adherence, healthcare systems are best positioned to address the complexity of eating disorder treatment while ensuring patient safety and quality of life (White, 2024) (Figure 11.13).

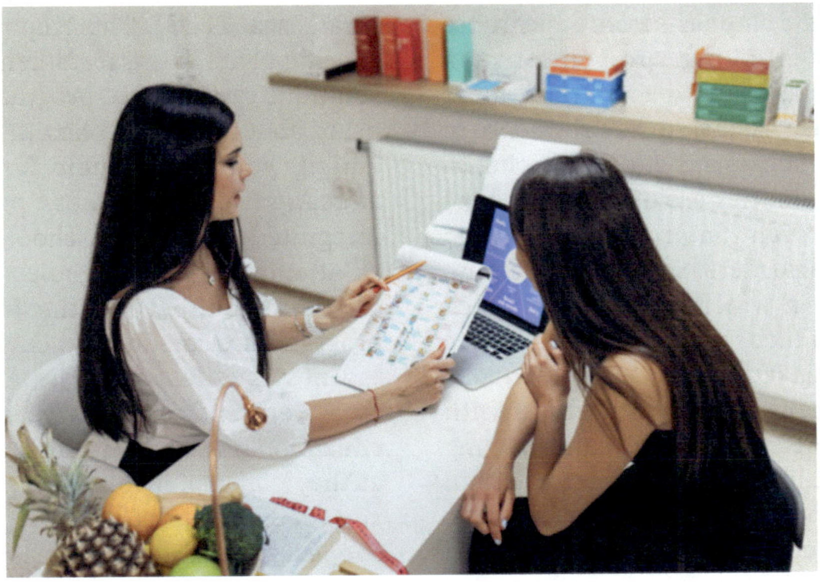

Figure 11.13. A dietitian offering personalized nutritional counseling during a client consultation.

Source: https://www.insidehighered.com/sites/default/files/styles/max_650x650/public/media/Screen%20Shot%202023-03-01%20at%2010.37.07%20AM.png?itok=pRnxAwW6.

11.6. Prevention Strategies

Successful prevention strategies for eating disorders are key to reversing the growing incidence of these severe psychiatric disorders. Identification of the appropriate levels of intervention is critical, as they can be classified as universal, selective, and indicated prevention programs. Universal prevention encompasses the general population with an attempt to strengthen positive body perception and nutrition information without identifying targeted individuals. Selective prevention targets groups at high risk, for example, those with a family history of eating disorders or body image concerns. Finally, indicated prevention offers specific interventions to individuals who exhibit early manifestations of disordered eating. All these strategies play a fundamental role in reducing risk factors and encouraging healthier food and body image attitudes, with a final aim of preventing eating disorders and their associated complications, as detailed in current evidence (Schlegl et al., 2025). The role of education and awareness in preventing eating disorders across different populations is continuously substantiated. Interventions that include media literacy education have proved particularly useful in countering societal body ideals and thinness. Social media has been noted as one of the leading causes of internalization of adverse body image ideals, it is thus important that prevention programs follow popular platforms and trends (Aylı et al., 2025). These educational interventions can contribute to fostering resilience in young people and adults to critically evaluate appearance messages in the media. By shifting the emphasis from appearance to health and well-being, prevention can empower individuals to build a healthier, more balanced body image, reducing the prevalence of disordered eating. Consensus efforts by schools, families, and communities are necessary for the effectiveness of prevention programs designed to combat eating disorders. Schools may offer a best environment in which to implement such programs through incorporating body positive and healthy eating classes in their curricula. Parents' involvement is also important, with education about healthy eating habits having the potential to facilitate open discussion within the home about body image and self-esteem. Programs at the community level that teach activity without weight as a priority can also establish a culture of appreciating health over appearance. These all-encompassing strategies need to be aligned with overall public health programs aimed at raising awareness of eating disorders. Lastly, effective prevention interventions must be well-versed in various underlying factors of eating disorders so that programs can be flexible and transferable across groups, as noted in ongoing research work (Schlegl et al., 2025).

11.6.1. Awareness and Education Campaigns

Effective education and awareness programs have an impact on the war against the rising rate of eating disorders among multicultural populations. The programs aim to introduce the public to healthy dietary habits as well as the psychological factors that predispose one to disordered eating behavior. The programs integrate specially designed material into educational curricula in order to reach students through interactive avenues that are culturally relevant to their composition. For instance, research emphasizes culturally sensitive nutrition education to report significant improvements in the attitudes and knowledge of students towards healthy eating following such interventions (Fransisca, 2025). The emphasis on culturally specific content is a testament to how regional solutions can enhance programs of education to bring about improved health habits awareness among youth and their families. Moreover, education and awareness programs must be integrated outside of school environments in an attempt to address the complexity of eating disorders. Supporting the functions of these programs are community activities that reinforce the messages delivered. The inclusion of parents, caregivers, and community leaders can increase educational interventions' access and influence as they play major roles in family environments and food consumption patterns. By promoting cooperation among schools and community groups, programs can foster consistency in the message across nutrition and mental health. There is evidence that supports parents' involvement in education programs, increasing the potential impact of such interventions towards healthier lifestyle choices for young people (Fransisca, 2025). A robust community structure lies behind the sustainability of such programs and fosters a healthy climate for open dialogue regarding body image and eating behavior. Furthermore, the cost-effectiveness of delivering all-around education and awareness programs should not be overlooked. There has been a recent evaluation of a school-based prevention intervention for high body mass index and eating disorders, which has indicated that such programs are apt to yield significant healthcare savings while maximizing health and well-being in adolescents. Research concludes that it takes long-term returns significantly more than the investment in targeted interventions, and hence, such an investment is advisable for public health. Such evidence-based prevention of eating disorders places education and awareness programs in a position to be powerful tools of primary prevention. Since research continues to indicate the benefits of such initiatives, policymakers and educators are encouraged to prioritize them and allocate funds towards them, not just so they can teach but also to provide a whole sense of health, thereby reducing the incidence of eating disorders among communities (Figure 11.14).

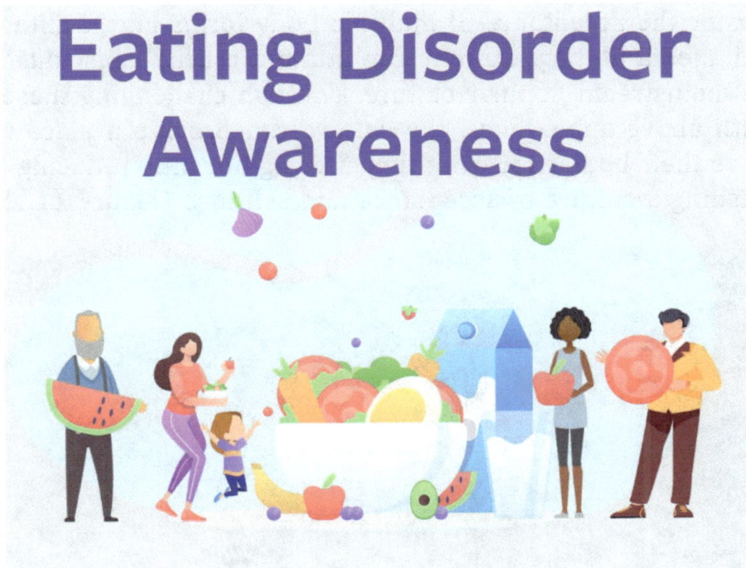

Figure 11.14. Eating Disorder Awareness: Promoting healthy eating habits for all ages.

Source: https://www.humangivens.com/wp-content/uploads/2021/02/eating-disorder-awareness_Card-01.jpg.

11.6.2. Promoting Healthy Body Image

Body satisfaction must be encouraged in the area of prevention of eating disorders, since the beauty ideal promoted by culture actually reinforces someone's dissatisfaction with his or her own body. It is important to understand the mechanisms of social comparison and how they can be explained on the basis of Social Comparison Theory. This hypothesis posits that individuals compare their body image with others, creating feelings of inadequacy against idealized images in media or social settings. Research in five major cities of Pakistan reveals that men engaging in upward social comparison are prone to increased body dissatisfaction and hence disordered eating habits. Thus, aiming at social comparison processes becomes a vital strategy in promoting healthy body image and preventing risk for eating disorder development in various groups, and evidence calls for intervention programs opposing these undesirable comparisons (Iqbal et al., 2024). Understanding and information regarding the factors of healthy body image become decisive in social environments, particularly among risk populations, , such as adolescents. For instance, body acceptance and body positivity educational interventions can lead to an appreciation of his or her personal body shape and size. Such intervention is crucial in consideration of the fact that poor body image is linked with higher eating disorder risk. The rise in body dissatisfaction that has been observed in studies, especially concerning some medical conditions like celiac disease, highlights the necessity for interventions focusing on psychological well-being as much as physical health. By educating patients in coping skills and positive body image affirmations, medical professionals can help to develop healthier lifestyle routines and increase mental health outcomes as a whole (Chodari et al., 2021). Encouraging a healthy body image also necessitates a collective effort to include families, educators, and the mass media. Involving parents in body image communication can significantly influence children's perceptions and attitudes towards their bodies, thereby averting the development of eating disorders. Second, schools must prioritize the creation of diverse-friendly environments that foster the acceptance of multiple body forms and facilitate open discourse of body positivity. Third, media literacy training can attain a crucial consciousness of the idealized ideals propagated by mainstream popular culture. Through challenging these norms and writing a tale that puts health above appearance, the culture can provide a place in which individuals feel empowered to love their bodies for what they are, significantly reducing the danger of eating disorders and establishing a culture of acceptance and self-love (Figure 11.15).

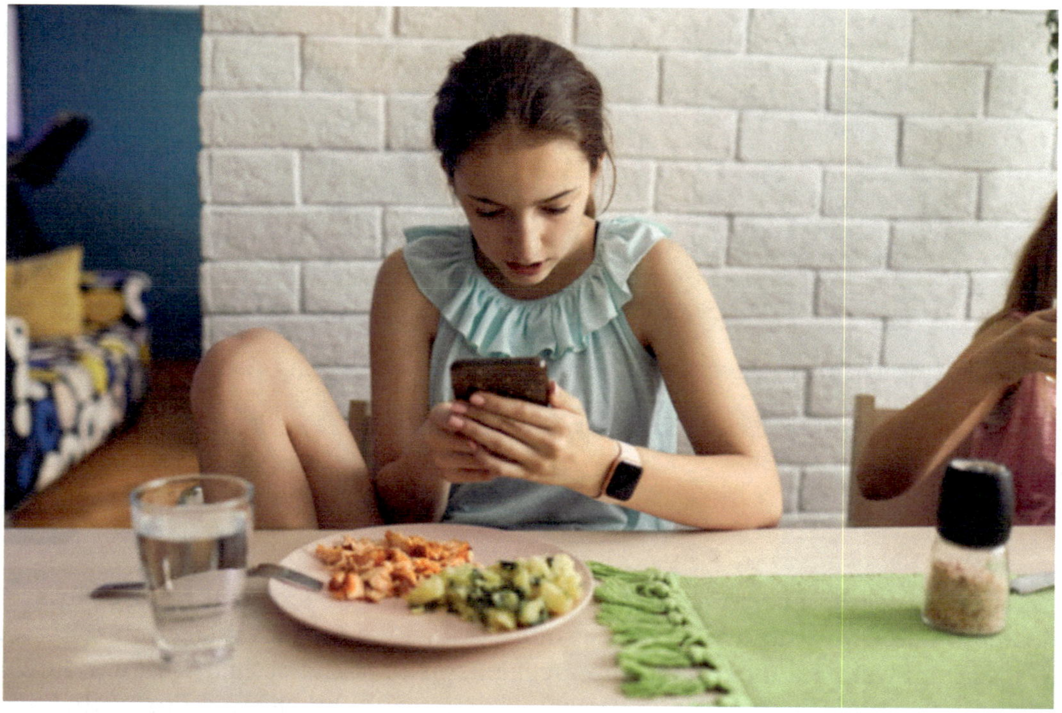

Figure 11.15. Distracted eating: A young girl focused on her phone during mealtimes.

Source: https://cfcenj.com/wp-content/uploads/2023/10/Screenshot-2023-10-12-171302.png.

11.6.3. Support Systems and Community Resources

Support systems and community resources play a critical role in the treatment and recovery of individuals who suffer from eating disorders. Eating disorders thrive in environments of isolation, secrecy, and stigma, so having strong support systems is imperative. Family members and friends can create a circle of understanding and support, providing emotional support that strongly aids the recovery process. Besides, structured community resources , such as support groups, create a judgment-free space for individuals to share their experiences and challenges and encourage a sense of belonging and legitimation. By connecting individuals experiencing the same warfare, support groups can combat the feeling of loneliness and despair that usually comes with eating disorders, validating the fact that recovery is not only possible but also achieved by strength in numbers (Herrera et al., 2021). Aside from peer and family aid, professional assistance is essential for full treatment. Mental health clinics and community centers offer referrals to therapists, nutritionists, and doctors who specialize in the dynamics of eating disorders. Professionals can then fashion treatment according to individual needs, opening the door to an interdisciplinary recovery. Apart from this, community outreach programs that encourage education on eating disorder symptoms and consequences can reduce stigma and encourage early treatment. By educating and providing timely intervention, these programs can provide a supportive environment for individuals to receive treatment and progress with their recovery (Volkow, 2020). The integration of technology has also maximized care services for those afflicted with eating disorders. Online discussions, virtual therapy sessions, and phone applications bring resources and support to an instant click for people. They can be especially helpful to those who are afraid of seeking face-to-face assistance due to stigma or fear of judgment. They enable users to converse with professionally trained people and people like them from the safety of their own homes, providing a sense of community and security. In addition, online sites are able to share learning materials, whereby people and their families are able to better understand the nature of eating disorders as well as the importance of treatment. Typically, technology combined with traditional systems can offer a more international and accessible recovery environment (Herrera et al., 2021).

CLOSER LOOK

BINGE EATING

Binge Eating is a serious eating disorder characterized by recurring episodes of consuming unusually large amounts of food in a short period, often accompanied by a loss of control and feelings of shame, guilt, or distress afterward. Unlike bulimia nervosa, binge eating is not followed by compensatory behaviors such as vomiting, excessive exercise, or fasting. This leads many individuals with binge eating disorder (BED) to struggle with overweight or obesity, although the disorder can occur at any body size.

During a binge, individuals may eat rapidly, continue eating even when not hungry, and eat until they feel uncomfortably full. Binges often occur in secret, and the person may feel powerless to stop the behavior. These episodes are not just occasional overeating—they are frequent, emotionally driven, and deeply distressing. The exact cause of binge eating is multifactorial, involving a combination of genetic, psychological, and environmental factors. Common contributing factors include emotional stress, depression, anxiety, low self-esteem, body dissatisfaction, and a history of restrictive dieting. In many cases, binge eating serves as a coping mechanism for dealing with negative emotions or traumatic experiences. Diagnosis is based on criteria outlined in the Diagnostic and Statistical Manual of Mental Disorders (DSM-5), which includes binge episodes at least once a week for three months, accompanied by significant distress.

Treatment involves a combination of approaches. Cognitive Behavioral Therapy (CBT) is considered the most effective, helping individuals understand and change patterns of thinking and behavior related to food and body image. Nutritional counseling, support groups, and sometimes medications such as antidepressants or appetite suppressants may also be helpful. The binge eating is a common but treatable eating disorder. Early intervention, emotional support, and a non-judgmental approach are essential for long-term recovery.

SUMMARY

The nature of eating disorders demands a system-wide comprehension of their implications on public health policies. The recent policies, such as the Calorie Labelling (Out of Home) Regulations in England, have attracted professionals' concern over their implications for people with eating disorders. Evidence that implies calorie labeling will exacerbate disordered behavior and thought requires considerate deliberation in policymaking. Surveys of participants affected by limiting eating disorders have determined that the availability of displayed calorie counts serves as a ubiquitous reminder that impedes recovery efforts. Hence, while public health policy continues to evolve, it is necessary to integrate the input of individuals with eating disorders when evaluating these policies so that they are not harmful and promote recovery-friendly environments (Duffy et al., 2023). In addition, the convergence of eating disorders and gender necessitates special intervention strategies in treatment practice. From observations in studies of gender-diverse populations, knowledge gaps remain regarding how gender identity influences the experiences of those who would prefer to be treated for eating disorders. The subjects of such studies reported feeling the impact of gender dysphoria on their eating and supported barriers while approaching standard treatment. This underscored the critical need for gender-affirming training in health practitioners, , such as dietitians. By bridging these gaps, the health system can ensure more equitable access to effective care for all, promoting recovery pathways responsive to patients' diversified needs (Joy et al., 2022). Ultimately, the complexities that accompany eating disorders require well-rounded, informed, and empathetic interventions on both the treatment and policy levels. Health practitioners and policymakers must collaborate to develop interventions that consider an individual's personal history, identity, and environmental conditions influencing their relationship with food. Furthermore, enhancing awareness and education on the unique issues in play for minority populations will allow for a more sensitive treatment strategy. These efforts not only reinforce the importance of person-focused care but also assist in reaching the ultimate objective of reducing the prevalence of eating disorders. Sustained commitment to review and revision of both health policy and treatment models is necessary to help those who struggle with eating disorders move toward recovery and positive relationships with food and body.

The increased prevalence of eating disorders (EDs) suggests a complex interplay of psychological, sociocultural, and biological factors that warrants thorough exploration. The evidence has accumulated to indicate that those with post-traumatic stress disorder (PTSD) are particularly vulnerable to the development of eating disorders. In the military population, a high positive correlation between ED and PTSD has been observed, with females being more likely to develop these comorbidities. Longitudinal studies underpin the suggestion that those with PTSD can be prone to later developing disordered eating patterns. The findings highlight the necessity for future exploration of this correlation, especially within cohorts other than U.S. military veterans, in an attempt to address how these factors would materialize in a broader model (Hughes, 2019). The cultural and gendered nature of eating disorders is also vital to awareness of their dynamics. Feminist and socio-cultural approaches position EDs as not merely individual health issues but as manifestations of broader societal constructs, most prominently gender identity. Female patient interviews who have endured anorexia and bulimia highlight the salience of gender in their individual histories and treatment interactions. Critically, they analyze how gender was or was not well managed in the treatment setting, believing that the dominant therapies are likely to neglect significant sociocultural contexts.

This neglect is likely to undermine effective treatment and recovery and therefore the significance of incorporating feminist rhetoric in clinical practice towards facilitating more diverse and effective models of treatment (Bartky et al., 2016). Finally, studies of eating disorders are improved by having a framework that is multidimensional and includes psychological, sociocultural, and gender-based factors. Integrating findings from various study contexts demonstrates the need for an appreciation of particular risk factors, including PTSD in military populations, as well as gender's cultural meaning in intervention. This more inclusive focus encourages reevaluation of treatment approaches to incorporate these vital variables, ultimately fostering optimism for greater efficacy for the individual with eating disorders. Further discussion around such issues, including careful critique of existing models, supports the necessity for integrative treatment practices that value the complicated intermixture of variables governing eating disorders in different populations (Bartky et al., 2016; Hughes, 2019).

References

1. Amiri, S., & Khan, M. A. (2024). Are eating disorders a risk agent for all-cause mortality: A meta-analysis. *Eating Disorders.* https://www.semanticscholar.org/paper/5d7df014cf74d358da61167bd17af44f74896c8a (accessed on 13th June 2025).
2. Anderson, K. E., Byrne, C., Goodyear, A., Le Grange, D., et al. (2015). Telemedicine of family-based treatment for adolescent anorexia nervosa: A protocol of treatment development study. https://core.ac.uk/download/287622307.pdf (accessed on 13th June 2025).
3. Apriady, H., Fitri, M., Paramitha, S., Sidik, T., et al. (2024). Psychology and sociology analysis of eating disorder factors among athletes: Age-based perspectives. https://core.ac.uk/download/640008693.pdf (accessed on 13th June 2025).
4. Aylı, B. I., & Bağcı Bosi, A. T. (2025). From risk to resilience: A comprehensive review of eating disorder prevention strategies. *International Journal of Research and Scientific Innovation.* https://www.semanticscholar.org/paper/b6c3109cc7548ce0dcdb8d246450093ed8891666 (accessed on 13th June 2025).
5. Ballarotto, G. (2017). Binge eating disorder in adolescence: The role of alexithymia and impulsivity. https://core.ac.uk/download/188828208.pdf (accessed on 13th June 2025).
6. Barlow, D. H., Boettcher, H. T., Bullis, J. R., Farchione, T. J., et al. (2017). Current definitions of "transdiagnostic" in treatment development: A search for consensus. https://open.bu.edu/bitstream/2144/40041/1/Current%20Definitions%20of%20Transdiagnostic%20-%206-10%20FINAL.pdf (accessed on 13th June 2025).
7. Bartky, S. L., Baumgardner, J., Bordo, S., Boskind-White, M., Boughtwood, D., Burns, M., M., et al. (2016). 'Blindness to the obvious'? Treatment experiences and feminist approaches to eating disorders. https://core.ac.uk/download/41993831.pdf (accessed on 13th June 2025).
8. Bourne, L., Mandy, W., & Bryant-Waugh, R. (2022). Avoid/restrictive food intake disorder and severe food selectivity in children and young people with autism: A scoping review. *Developmental Medicine & Child Neurology, 64*, 691–700. https://doi.org/10.1111/dmcn.15139 (accessed on 13th June 2025).
9. Brodie, E., van Veenendaal, N., Platz, E., Fleming, J., Gunn, H., Johnson, D., Griffin, H., et al. (2024). The incidence of refeeding syndrome and the nutrition management of severely malnourished inpatients with eating disorders: An observational study. *The International Journal of Eating Disorders.* https://www.semanticscholar.org/paper/d43af620aac7ccaba65edd00798cbabc1528483d (accessed on 13th June 2025).
10. Chodari, L., Bahrami, F., & Farshbaf, F. (2021). Eating disorders, body dissatisfaction, and health-promoting lifestyle: Comparing coeliac patients with healthy people. *Volume 12*, 25–37. https://www.semanticscholar.org/paper/99b93982d05f51ffd4104a29f5ec92c3419b7cef (accessed on 13th June 2025).
11. Cioch, M. J., Doman, K., Hermanowicz, K., Kaczmarska, K., et al. (2025). Comprehensive overview–Outcomes and challenges of bariatric surgery–Physical, psychological and nutritional considerations. https://core.ac.uk/download/646080057.pdf (accessed on 13th June 2025).

12. Clites, E. L. (2012). It is time to talk about it: Designing a health communication program for eating disorder recovery in an Appalachian university. https://core.ac.uk/download/232710271.pdf (accessed on 13th June 2025).
13. Collins, L. (2024). Applying Integrated Enhanced Cognitive Behavior Therapy (I-CBTE) to severe and longstanding eating disorders (SEED) Paper 1: I am no longer a SEED patient. *Journal of Eating Disorders, 12.* https://www.semanticscholar.org/paper/8d71bc9b3672cf8f7f396779592044eec760f6ea (accessed on 13th June 2025).
14. Escobar, M., Franzosi, O. S., Coelho, N., Halpern, S., Scherer, J., Ornell, F., Mendes Ceresér, K. M., et al. (2021). Instruments and diagnostic criteria for binge eating assessment in adults: A systematic review. *Volume 12*, 242–259. https://www.semanticscholar.org/paper/651d0bf0cff5650dba6443377c5974cb7d0347c0 (accessed on 13th June 2025).
15. Flouri, E., & McEwen, C. (2008). Fathers' parenting, adverse life events, and adolescents' emotional and eating disorder symptoms: The role of emotion regulation. https://core.ac.uk/download/pdf/82499.pdf (accessed on 13th June 2025).
16. Guluzade, L., & Sas, C. (2024). Functionality and user review analysis of mobile apps for mindfulness eating and eating disorders. *Proceedings of the 2024 ACM Designing Interactive Systems Conference.* https://www.semanticscholar.org/paper/7c37e1fb68419dcaaabec214ce2bdb8883301c85 (accessed on 13th June 2025).
17. Hughes, K. (2019). Disordered eating and the relationships with post-traumatic stress, self-criticism, and fear of compassion. https://core.ac.uk/download/228202636.pdf (accessed on 13th June 2025).
18. Iqbal, S., Sultana, S., & Malik, A. (2024). Examining the relationship between exposure to Avengers action figures and men's body dissatisfaction and eating disorders in Pakistan. *Pakistan Journal of Humanities and Social Sciences.* https://www.semanticscholar.org/paper/3823c9b411330bc4a4fb88cc853a2e2f269db677 (accessed on 13th June 2025).
19. Irish, L. A., Bottera, A., Manasse, S., Christensen Pacella, K. A., & Schaefer, L. M. (2024). The integration of sleep research into eating disorders research: Recommendations and best practices. *The International Journal of Eating Disorders.* https://www.semanticscholar.org/paper/94bac226b83f69da599f307d995e380feebd5fb5 (accessed on 13th June 2025).
20. Joy, P., White, M., & Jones, S. (2022). Exploring the influence of gender dysphoria in eating disorders among gender diverse individuals. *Nutrition & Dietetics: The Journal of the Dietitians Association of Australia.* https://www.semanticscholar.org/paper/108974e48ab1d9ef641e48fcfc04c513e2f481ef (accessed on 13th June 2025).
21. Kiley, M. (2023). A feminist perspective on social media's impact on body image and mental health in young people. https://core.ac.uk/download/568188763.pdf (accessed on 13th June 2025).
22. Li Cavoli, G., Mulè, G., & Rotolo, U. (2011). Renal involvement in psychological eating disorders. https://core.ac.uk/download/53273765.pdf (accessed on 13th June 2025).
23. Marcolini, F., Ravaglia, A., Tempia Valenta, S., Bosco, G., Marconi, G., De Ronchi, D., & Atti, A. (2024). Severe enduring anorexia nervosa (SE-AN) treatment options and their effectiveness: A review of literature. *Journal of Eating Disorders, 12.* https://www.semanticscholar.org/paper/249d4a95c1e2a67f704d2302089dd9279dca8dd2 (accessed on 13th June 2025).

24. May, C. (2019). The relationship between sexual debut and eating attitudes. https://core.ac.uk/download/227521295.pdf (accessed on 13th June 2025).

25. Novack, K., & Chadi, N. (2025). The hybrid space in eating disorder treatment: Towards a personalized approach to integrating telehealth and in-person care. *Journal of Eating Disorders, 13.* https://www.semanticscholar.org/paper/a0745a64c84f294864001c8894ad6fcc8f16cf4d (accessed on 13th June 2025).

26. Ram, J., & Shelke, S. (2023). Understanding eating disorders in children and adolescent population. *Journal of Indian Association for Child and Adolescent Mental Health, 19*, 60–69. https://www.semanticscholar.org/paper/f9baf444ea8c564bee3629723ec7b1877ac91e39 (accessed on 13th June 2025).

27. Rao, P. (2025). Investigating the psychological factors contributing to the eating disorder. *Innovative Research Thoughts.* https://www.semanticscholar.org/paper/3e3db836eced6a1ecf333a5e3ff496793df0037b (accessed on 13th June 2025).

28. Sauerteig, M. R. (2017). Conformity to gender stereotypes impacting body-esteem, eating, and exercise behaviors in female college students. https://core.ac.uk/download/212824322.pdf (accessed on 13th June 2025).

29. Shackshaft, L., Chapman, L., Biddle, L., Yardley, L., & Bould, H. (2024). Designing a virtual reality café to treat eating disorders: A thematic analysis of stakeholder viewpoints. *BJPsych Open, 10*, S80. https://www.semanticscholar.org/paper/d3de88cb296f1a6fb4b9098cb102d10579ff2f6e (accessed on 13th June 2025).

30. Smutchak, S. (2024). Analysis of psychological features of youth with eating disorders. *Bulletin of Postgraduate Education (Series Social and Behavioral Sciences; Management and Administration).* https://www.semanticscholar.org/paper/3f887a451b40e56b9968c66432f29198eb2b7379 (accessed on 13th June 2025).

31. Takaki, M., & Okabe, N. (2015). Aripiprazole may be effective as an add-on treatment in bulimic symptoms of eating disorders. *Journal of Clinical Psychopharmacology, 35*, 93–95. https://www.semanticscholar.org/paper/71596415fce7ccf373b262975127a21cb04307b4 (accessed on 13th June 2025).

32. Wajid, I., Vega, A., Thornhill, K., Jenkins, J. S., Merriman, C., Chandler, D., Shekoohi, S., et al. (2023). Topiramate (Topamax): Evolving role in weight reduction management: A narrative review. *Life, 13.* https://www.semanticscholar.org/paper/3c876f0af818148986c28f388357e4aedb364a00 (accessed on 13th June 2025).

33. Winer, M. H. (2014). Knowledge of and attitudes towards eating disorders of undergraduate nutrition majors at three Colorado universities. https://core.ac.uk/download/354443160.pdf (accessed on 13th June 2025).

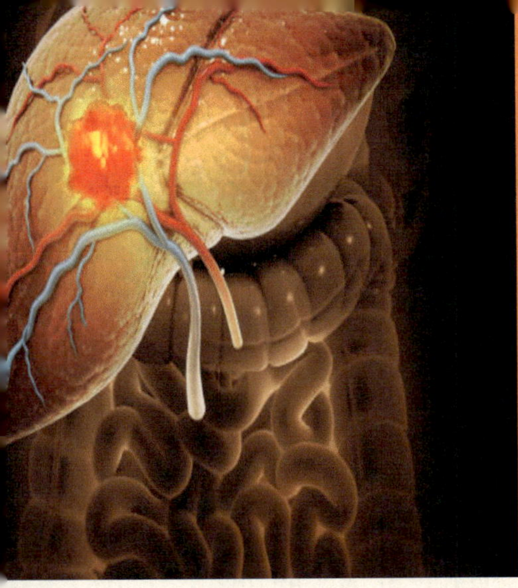

Chapter 12

GASTROINTESTINAL AND LIVER DISORDERS

Contents

Introduction....383
12.1. Anatomy and Physiology of the Gastrointestinal System....387
12.2. Common Gastrointestinal Disorders....391
12.3. Liver Disorders Overview....395
12.4. Diagnostic Strategies for Gastrointestinal and Hepatic Disorders....399
12.5. Treatment Options for Gastrointestinal Disorders....402
12.6. Pharmacological Treatments....406
Summary....411
References....413

Introduction

The gastrointestinal tract is crucial to the health of human beings, both as the pathway for nutrient uptake and as a critical component of immune and metabolic function. Gastrointestinal conditions range from minor to life-threatening and manifest with highly diverse symptoms that affect quality of life significantly. This diversity requires a good understanding of a number of conditions like inflammatory bowel diseases, gastroesophageal reflux, and peptic ulcers, all of which have unusual pathophysiological pathways. Moreover, the liver is heavily involved in the body's detoxifying process, metabolic regulation, and bile production, and thus liver disorders like hepatitis and cirrhosis are of equal importance to be treated. The interconnectedness of systems indicates the significance of the study of gastrointestinal and liver disease, as they contribute significantly to morbidity and mortality worldwide, which demands ongoing research and public health intervention. The prevalence of gastrointestinal and liver disease is a serious problem for healthcare systems worldwide. Diet transition, physical inactivity, and the emergence of antimicrobial resistance make managing and treating such diseases more difficult. Effective evaluation of these conditions often requires multispecialty care, such as gastroenterology, hepatology, nutrition, and surgery, which may be burdensome on health resources. Moreover, the economic burden of these diseases, driven by costly healthcare use and lost productivity, is a rationale for effective prevention efforts. Inadequate management of gastrointestinal diseases, according to recent studies, not only increases healthcare expenses but also exerts a profound impact on patients' quality of life, creating the necessity for improved clinical guidelines and patient education programs for early detection and management. Further research on gastrointestinal and liver diseases is continually untangling the biological, genetic, and lifestyle determinants of their development and progression. The influence of intestinal microbial flora, for instance, has been an emergent area of research, suggesting a causative link between dysbiosis and specific gastroenterological disorders. Moreover, growing evidence suggests the potential for pharmacogenomics to be the solution to personalized therapies, tailoring the result to the patient with specific genetic proclivities to liver disease. Thus, an interdisciplinary mechanism incorporating evidence-based research into clinical practice is essential to the development of treatment paradigms. Meeting the global burden posed by these diseases is not merely a question of awareness and knowledge but also one of creative solutions to improve patient care. It is this complex ballet of inquiry, clinical application, and healthcare policy that will inform future developments in the treatment of gastrointestinal and liver disease, as these studies continually redefine our understanding of digestive health.

Definition of Gastrointestinal Disorders

Gastrointestinal illnesses are a wide range of medical conditions that occur primarily in the digestive tract, including the esophagus, stomach, intestines, and accessory organs like the liver and pancreas. They occur as structural, functional, or inflammatory derangements that hamper the normal functioning of the gastrointestinal tract. Examples include irritable bowel syndrome (IBS), inflammatory bowel diseases (IBD) , such as Crohn's disease and ulcerative colitis, gastroesophageal reflux disease (GERD), and celiac disease. Their impact on patients can range from just discomfort to life-threatening complications, severely impacting quality of life and healthcare costs. Identification of the specific characteristics and pathogenetic processes of these diseases is significant in order to develop effective therapeutic regimens and public health measures, particularly for the control of the growing prevalence of these conditions all over the world. Clinical manifestations of gastrointestinal disorders can be quite disparate, often emerging with symptoms , such as abdominal discomfort, bloating, diarrhea, constipation, or altered bowel habits. These symptoms are not only expressive of internal gastrointestinal disturbances but also may express the presence of severe comorbidities that require urgent intervention. For instance, the gastrointestinal system not only impacts nutrition and absorptive processes but could further have implications that are systemic due to its relationship with the immune system. Recent studies have placed emphasis on the interconnections between gastrointestinal health and pathologies , such as obesity and metabolic syndrome, with gastrointestinal disease remaining pivotal within overarching contexts of health. Moreover, repeated gastrointestinal issues have been identified to increase psychiatric disorder risk, , such as depression and anxiety, and, as a result, there has been a focus on multifaceted treatment models targeting psychological as well as physiological factors. Therapies for gastroenterological disease are multidisciplinary in nature, typically consisting of lifestyle modification, drug treatment, and in some instances, surgery. Due to the intricacy of gastrointestinal disease, treating it is often interdisciplinary, with gastroenterologists, dietitians, and psychologists all playing their roles. Advances in medical science have also helped us understand the role of the gut microbiota in maintaining the health of the gastrointestinal system and managing disorders. As the understanding of these disorders evolves, it becomes increasingly important to implement guidelines that ensure patients receive evidence-based care tailored to their individual needs. For example, the recommendations by reputable health institutions highlight the need for early diagnosis, comprehensive management programs, and patient education to boost outcomes for patients with gastrointestinal disorders, indicative of the necessity for a systems approach to treatment and care (Visseren et al., 2021; Murray et al., 2022) (Figure 12.1).

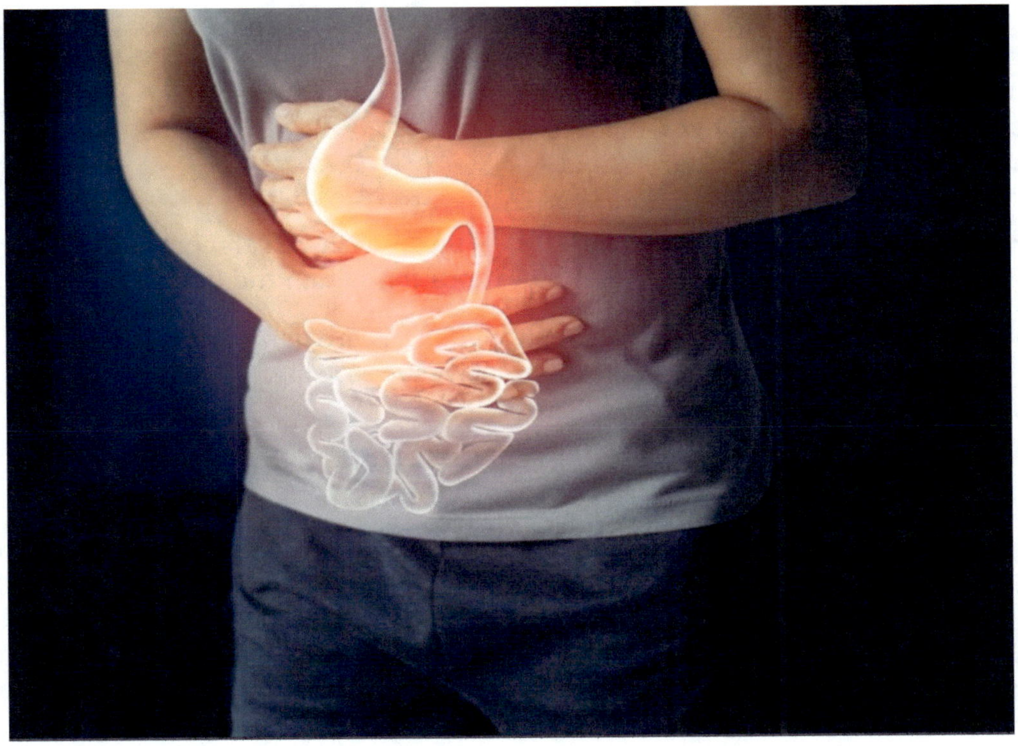

Figure 12.1. Visual representation of digestive discomfort in the stomach and intestines.

Source: https://d2jx2rerrg6sh3.cloudfront.net/images/Article_Images/ImageForArticle_22799_16572812576525563.jpg.

Overview of Liver Disorders

Liver disease encompasses a multifaceted group of diseases that can potentially have a significant impact on overall and gastrointestinal health. The most prevalent liver diseases are hepatitis, cirrhosis, and fatty liver disease, all with unique diagnostic and therapeutic difficulties. Hepatitis, often the consequence of viral infection, can bring about inflammation in the liver and acute and chronic disease. Chronic hepatitis can result in cirrhosis, which is severe scarring of liver tissue, causing compromised liver function and potentially fatal complications. Fatty liver disease, or non-alcoholic fatty liver disease (NAFLD), is increasingly being noted as a component of metabolic syndrome with severe health outcomes , such as liver failure and cardiovascular disease. The interaction between these disorders and their presentation in the gut necessitates a profound understanding to better approach paradigms of patient treatment and care. The interaction between gastrointestinal disease and liver disorders is also confounded by the potential for skin presentations that are predictive of underlying disease. Several autoimmune and neoplastic liver diseases have important dermatological presentations, , such as xanthomas and pruritus, which can precede gastrointestinal symptoms. The identification of liver disease can therefore be based on a general outlook, with these skin findings as possible indicators of the severity of liver disease. For instance, patients with Primary Biliary Cholangitis may have significant alterations in the skin that serve as sentinel markers for diagnosis, and intervention can be implemented at an earlier point. The discovery of these skin abnormalities underscores the necessity of a multidisciplinary treatment regimen for liver diseases and the interface of the liver with other systems, including the skin and gastrointestinal tract (Hajj et al., 2024). Additionally, knowledge growth in recent years regarding the gut-liver axis has generated new methods for treating liver diseases. Probiotics and immunonutrition have also been promising interventions to attain gut microbiota equilibrium, which is determinant in optimal liver function. The gut-liver axis is a crucial feature in the pathophysiology of liver disease, such that gut flora disruptions may exacerbate liver disease. While initial evidence is available to support the use of probiotics to enhance gastrointestinal functioning and reduce liver inflammation, clear evidence-based recommendations are absent. Meeting patients' nutritional requirements, particularly those suffering from liver disease, can make a real difference in outcomes. Thus, there's a pressing necessity to conduct more research to uncover the advantages of probiotics and immunonutrition in liver diseases and consolidate their position in treatment protocols (Figure 12.2).

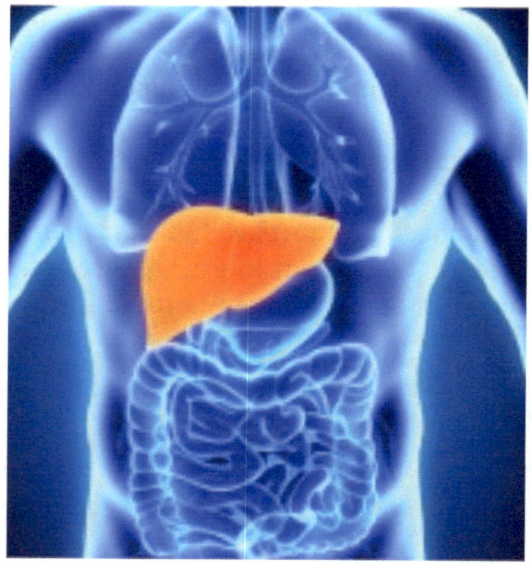

Figure 12.2. Visual representation of the liver's location within the human digestive system.

Source: https://medlineplus.gov/images/LiverDisease.jpg.

Importance of Understanding These Conditions

An in-depth understanding of liver and gastrointestinal diseases is important because they play an important role in determining the overall health and quality of life of individuals afflicted with them. By comprehending the complex relationship between the immune system and microbiome, researchers and medical professionals can better understand the processes through which imbalances evolve into many disorders.

As is described in recent research, microbiomes play a role in maintaining host homeostasis, and disruptions in this delicate balance can result in immune-mediated disease that tests the body's defense systems. Comprehending these interactions not only enables early detection but also forms the basis of developing specific therapeutic interventions to correct disequilibrium and promote health, thus highlighting the importance of further research and clinical awareness in this field (Zheng et al., 2020). Furthermore, gastrointestinal and liver disease comprehension is of great importance in maximizing health outcomes and guiding effective treatment strategies. Knowing the mechanisms of these conditions allows clinicians to develop individualized interventions according to patients' needs. Implementation of clinical guidelines, as provided by professional organizations, involves integration of current scientific evidence into practice. Guidelines facilitate patient-centered decision-making by practitioners, under which treatment procedures are best suited to current research, in addition to considering patient-specific factors and conditions. Such an informed reaction ultimately enhances the quality of care, reduces complications, and fosters a culture of teams among patients and practitioners, substantiating the argument that high-quality informed healthcare choices are a primary drive for effective treatment of gastrointestinal and liver diseases (Cosentino et al., 2019). Awareness and education about gastrointestinal and liver diseases also extend beyond clinical settings and touch public health. By elucidating the risk factors, symptoms, and prevention of these conditions, individuals can be empowered with the skill to make informed lifestyle choices that lower their risk. Increased awareness can also lead to earlier diagnosis, which is particularly important in furthering prognosis and outcomes. Furthermore, placing these conditions in social terms can result in public health campaigns aimed at reducing prevalence rates, thereby benefiting entire communities. As our understanding of the interactions between lifestyle, diet, and gut health grows, it becomes more and more clear that a vigilant and educated population is critical to fighting the increasing prevalence of these incapacitating illnesses (Zheng et al., 2020).

12.1. Anatomy and Physiology of the Gastrointestinal System

The GI tract, a system of organs that executes the processes of digestion and nutrient absorption, is made up of several organs with distinct functions. Starting from the oral cavity, mechanical breakdown of food occurs by mastication, and salivary enzymes initiate the chemical digestion of carbohydrates. The esophagus is a muscular tube that conveys food towards the stomach and gastric juices with hydrochloric acid and pepsin for protein breakdown. The entry into the small intestine that ensues is a pivotal site of digestion, where the combination of bile, pancreatic enzymes, and intestinal secretions optimizes the uptake of nutrients. This process is necessary, as disruptions can lead to disorders , such as gastroesophageal reflux disease (GERD) or peptic ulcer, and illustrate the need for maintaining GI homeostasis in preventing gastrointestinal disease. The six-meter-long small intestine absorbs nutrients, using its special construction to get the maximum amount of surface area. It is separated into three segments, duodenum, jejunum, and ileum, where the digestive system is different for every section. The duodenum is where stomach chyme is dumped and then mixed with pancreatic digestive juices and bile from the liver, ready to be sent on to the final digestion. Nutrient absorption occurs primarily in the jejunum by villi and microvilli, which extend into the lumen of the intestine to improve absorption. The ileum, which absorbs the remaining nutrients and bile salts, is connected to the large intestine, where water absorption and feces formation occur. Any dysfunction of a process will result in permanent health effects, , such as malabsorption syndrome or inflammatory bowel disease (Kansra et al., 2021). The liver, the GI system's crucial organ, is engaged multifunctionally in metabolic regulation, detoxification, and bile production. Bile, derived from hepatocytes, is vital for the emulsification of fats so that it is made accessible to enzymatic function. The liver also degrades absorbed nutrients from the small intestine, , such as glucose and amino acids, to make them accessible to the body. The hepatic portal system ensures maximal nutrient carriage from the GI tract to the liver, where the components can be metabolized or stored. Liver disease, , such as fatty liver disease or hepatitis, disrupts these functions and produces local as well as systemic effects that affect the overall condition and metabolism (Pyzik et al., 2019). It is critical to have knowledge of the anatomy and physiology of the liver when treating gastrointestinal and liver disease (Figure 12.3).

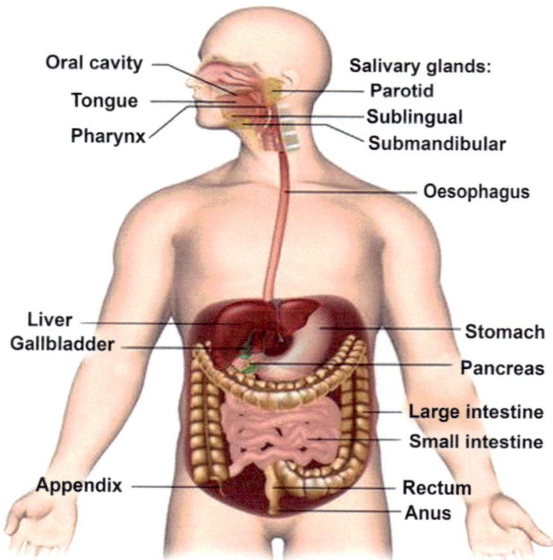

Figure 12.3. Digestive system diagram shows key organs from the oral cavity to the anus.

Source: https://www.magonlinelibrary.com/cms/10.12968/bjha.2018.12.3.110/asset/images/medium/bjha.2018.12.3.110_f01.jpg.

12.1.1. Structure of the Gastrointestinal Tract

The gastrointestinal system, which is a complex system, is the foundation of nutrient digestion and absorption. Every section, from the esophagus to the intestines, plays a particular role in digestion. The process begins in the mouth with mechanical disruption and enzymatic action that initiates the digestion process. Food thereafter passes into the esophagus, a muscular tube that employs peristalsis to propel the bolus into the stomach. The stomach further digests food using gastric enzymes and acids to create a semi-fluid material known as chyme. The tightly regulated mechanism is not only crucial for the absorption of nutrients but also for gut health, which is increasingly recognized to be linked with a wide variety of gastrointestinal and liver illnesses. Disruptions of this anatomy can lead to a variety of issues, emphasizing the significance of an awareness of the anatomy and function of the gut. After chyme emerges from the stomach, it moves into the small intestine, which is also subdivided into the duodenum, jejunum, and ileum. This is designed to enhance digestion and absorption greatly, with assistance from villi and microvilli that raise the surface area for nutrient uptake. This is where pancreatic enzymes and liver bile further digest food, allowing carbs, protein, and fat absorption into the bloodstream. The integrity of this section is crucial, as malabsorption or defects of permeability can generate states , such as celiac disease and inflammatory bowel diseases, emphasizing the relationship between clinical manifestations and structural dysfunction. Besides that, bile acids, which are necessary for fat digestion, are products of the liver's metabolism and are metabolized by gut microbiota, which modulates host immunity and potentially connects to gastrointestinal disorders through altered signaling pathways (Fiorucci et al., 2020). Following the small intestine, the remaining waste products advance to the large intestine, where water and electrolytes are absorbed, leaving solid waste. The architecture of the large intestine, which includes haustra and tenia coli, enables effective transit and storage of this waste before defecation. The large intestine is also a home for a dense microbiome, and it's where undigested carbohydrates are fermented with the production of significant vitamins. Disturbances in this microbiome may result in dysbiosis, leading to diseases , such as irritable bowel syndrome and colorectal cancer. The role of bile acids in enhancing communication between gut microbiota and the intestinal immune system is critical, with implications for unraveling inflammatory bowel diseases (Fiorucci et al., 2020). The structure of the gastrointestinal tract is hence closely tied to its function, as seen in the necessity to maintain its health against gastrointestinal and liver disease.

12.1.2. Functions of the Gastrointestinal System

The GI tract is central to the maintenance of overall health by its main functions: digestion, absorption, and defense against the barrier. Digestion starts in the mouth, where there is mechanical and enzymatic food breakdown, with activity thereafter in the stomach and small intestine. The stomach secretes gastric juices into proteins to digest them and mixes food with the juices into a liquid-like consistency known as chyme. When chyme reaches the small intestine, food particles are digested by pancreatic enzymes and bile to be absorbed for nutrient uptake. Nutrient absorption is crucial as it transforms the ingested food into accessible nutrients that are utilized for energy and cellular operations and thereby connects food intake to metabolic function and body operation. Additionally, the gastrointestinal tract is a formidable defense mechanism against toxins and pathogens, essentially safeguarding the internal environment of the body. The intestinal epithelium comprises specialized cells that create tight junctions to modulate permeability, ensuring selective passage of nutrients while keeping harmful entities out. Gut microbiota also reinforces this barrier by fermenting dietary fiber into short-chain fatty acids, which bolster the epithelial barrier as well as modulating the immune response. A healthy microbiome must exist because dysbiosis could interfere with barrier function and result in increased permeability and inflammatory disease, like inflammatory bowel disease. The complexity of this relationship emphasizes the gastrointestinal tract's function not only in digestion and absorption but even immunological health. The addition of these processes emphasizes the gastrointestinal system's integral part in the establishment of homeostasis. When gastrointestinal disease occurs, for example, gastroesophageal reflux disease or irritable bowel syndrome, it has the potential to destroy the harmony among digestion, absorption, and immune defense. Such a disease tends to cause malnutrition and systemic inflammation with huge impacts on general health. Additionally, hormonal and neuro-regulatory processes transmitting between the gut and the central nervous system highlight the gastrointestinal tract's impact on behavioral and physiological reactions. Close examination of such interactions recognizes how gastrointestinal malfunction can extend its impact beyond localized symptoms, presenting itself in widespread implications for both digestive and systemic health. This understanding also indicates the significance of appropriate approaches in the management of gastrointestinal and liver disease for the realization of complete well-being (Ghosh et al., 2021; Eom et al., 2022) (Figure 12.4).

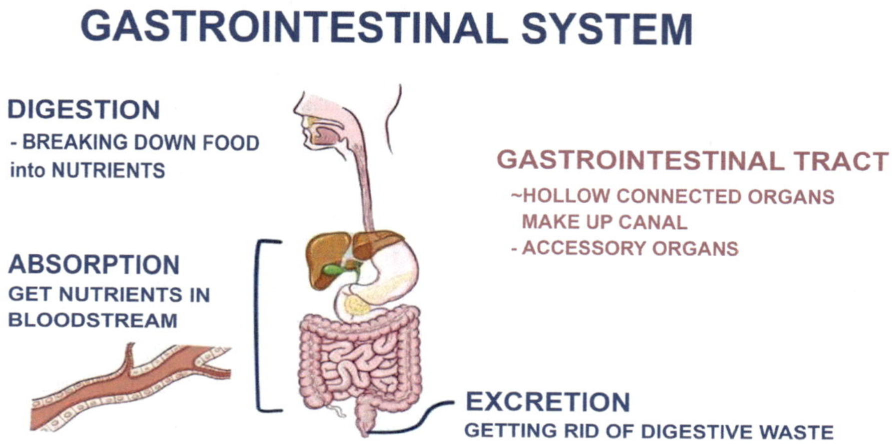

Figure 12.4. The gastrointestinal system shows digestion, absorption, and excretion functions.

Source: https://www.osmosis.org/_next/image?url=https%3A%2F%2Fd16qt3wv6xm098.cloudfront.net%2F3n-8nZVISVe1sAom6Myjr5xvSUebuU1X%2F_.jpg&w=3840&q=75.

12.1.3. Interaction Between the Gastrointestinal System and Liver

The intimate interaction between the liver and the gastrointestinal (GI) tract is a cornerstone in human physiology, characterized by a two-way communication network essential in maintaining metabolic homeostasis. The hepatic portal vein provides blood to the liver, which contains the ingested substances and signals absorbed through the intestines so that it may perform primary processes , such as detoxification and metabolism. This communication is important not only for nutrient processing but also for inflammatory control. The existing evidence suggests that the endocannabinoid system (ECS) plays a significant role in regulating GI function, including motility, secretion, and mucosal barrier integrity, and indirectly influences liver health and disease expression. Thus, the comprehension of the interaction between these systems is fundamental to the development of therapeutic interventions for disorders occurring as a result of dysregulation within either the GI tract or within the liver and highlights the interdependency of their functions in health and disease. Furthermore, the metabolic hub role of the liver highlights its involvement in many gastrointestinal disorders. Liver function changes can lead to alterations in bile composition and production, impacting the digestion process directly, particularly fat emulsification and absorption. GI disorders, however, can lead to hepatocellular inflammation and injury, hence conditions like non-alcoholic fatty liver disease (NAFLD). Aside from that, the ECS has also been implicated in conditions like IBS and IBD, where its dysregulation has been suggested to aggravate liver inflammation due to a compromised gut-liver axis. Furthermore, the identification of endocannabinoid-like compounds holds the promise of the creation of targeted therapies that would address both liver and GI pathologies. Thus, exploration of this gut-liver interaction becomes important for their efficient management of complex diseases. Another key aspect of the relationship between the gut microbiota and the liver is the effect that the gut microbiota has on the health of the liver. The gut microbiota plays a part in metabolite synthesis, which influences liver function, including short-chain fatty acids and bile acids. Besides, dysbiosis of the gut has been connected to numerous liver diseases, proving the role of gut health in the liver's pathobiology. In addition, parasites , such as helminths, offer an interesting perspective, as their immune-modulating function can decrease intestinal inflammation and therefore promote liver health. What is to be gleaned from such helminths may pave the way for new treatment methods that can decrease intestinal inflammation and promote liver function. As such, the dynamic interplays of the GI system and liver both highlight the complexity of human health as well as unveil the promise of integrative treatment modalities that treat both systems, which implies the necessity for holistic treatments of gastrointestinal and liver disease.

12.2. Common Gastrointestinal Disorders

Of the myriads of gastrointestinal diseases, irritable bowel syndrome (IBS) is among the most prevalent conditions that affect human beings globally. It is characterized by belly pain, bloating, and alteration in bowel habits leading to diarrhea, constipation, or both. In spite of the precise cause not being discovered yet, studies point towards multifactorial pathogenesis based on genetic, psychological, and environmental causes. The impact of IBS on lifestyle is severe, with a tendency to provoke serious morbidity due to distress and dietary restriction. While management of IBS is often attained through lifestyle modification, there is a significant contribution from gut-brain interactions to symptom worsening based on the current evidence. This directs towards the need for a complete understanding of the disorder, coupled with the management strategies directed towards both gastrointestinal and psychosocial aspects, to improve the quality of life in patients with the disorder. Another common gastrointestinal disorder is gastroesophageal reflux disease (GERD), defined by symptoms , such as chronic heartburn and regurgitation. The intrinsic cause of GERD is associated with the dysfunction of the lower esophageal sphincter, which leads to gastric content refluxing into the esophagus.

Exposures to stomach acid repeatedly might lead to mucosal injury as well as several complications like esophagitis or Barrett's esophagus. The incidence of GERD has increased markedly over the past few decades and is thought to be due to lifestyle, including dietary habits, obesity, and higher alcohol and caffeine consumption. Additionally, those with underlying diseases like diabetes or thyroid disease may have increased sensitivity to manifestations of GERD, making them more difficult to manage. Diet and lifestyle modification, as well as pharmacologic therapies, continue to be important in the management of GERD to avert esophageal complications in the long term. Inflammatory bowel disease (IBD), which comprises Crohn's disease and ulcerative colitis, is also a significant gastrointestinal health issue. IBD is chronic inflammation of the gastrointestinal tract with symptoms ranging from abdominal pain and diarrhea to emergent complications , such as bowel obstruction or systemic presentation. The pathophysiology of IBD is multigenetic, involving both genetic predisposition and immune system dysregulation, and is usually accompanied by prodigious flare-ups that call for vigorous management measures. Treatment generally involves a course of immunosuppressive medications and dietary adjustments for individual patients. In addition, evidence increasingly establishes the interconnection between IBD, nutrition status, and the population of gut microbiota. These results support the benefit of an interdisciplinary treatment approach to IBD, one that includes nutritional counseling and psychiatric consultation to enhance patient outcomes and quality of life (Figure 12.5).

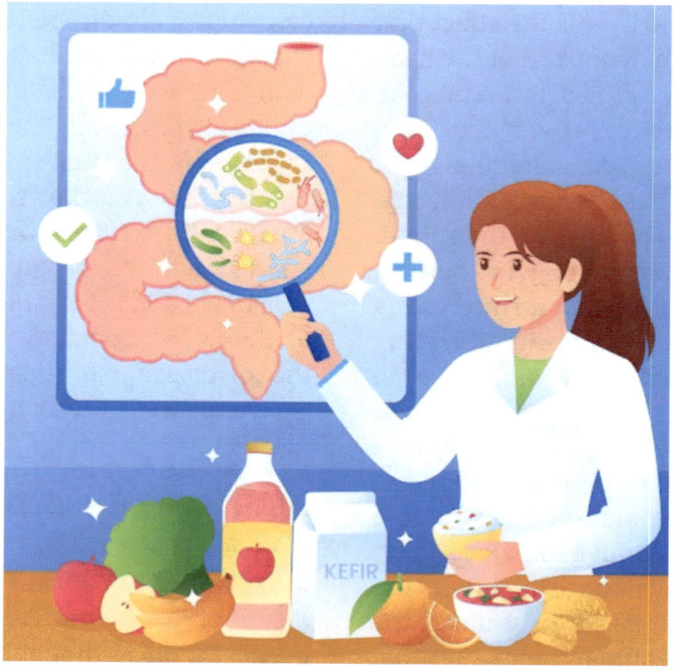

Figure 12.5. Healthy guts are supported by beneficial microbes and probiotic-rich foods.

Source: https://lh5.googleusercontent.com/proxy/RGnFsLbWVZGvidFCvq6247kS9-AiGp-k3ReUw0vzCK_A91Y8V1CNjtKOeY_B8KOc-0YbQsPvVyc3sabLm2JbgqcuUHjVWBYbCYJDmW3FMqU_qNmFav7JySECuOFZXrlZbB95ORZDfXHQ9xUDEDyZOWXowYVY-Z2Azk2LxHxRWezpi21TltWjBz9IOIZQdvuJyiqAQIN6IcfPmUSHlRdXiRlTmMZ7IscvEm-uAwMjAjskPjNoobBb9w.

12.2.1. Gastroesophageal Reflux Disease (GERD)

GERD is a common multifactorial gastrointestinal disorder in much of the Western world, as can be inferred from estimates, setting its prevalence at between 10% and 30% (Calabrese et al., 2024). The characteristic feature of GERD is the abnormal retrograde passage of gastric content into the esophagus, which yields a range of symptoms, both typical, e.g., heartburn, and cough and chest pain. The pathophysiologic mechanisms of GERD are many interrelated factors , such as hiatal hernia, esophageal motility disorders, and some food factors. The diagnosis is often supported by clinical evaluation and correlative tests like endoscopy, pH monitoring, and other functional tests that establish the severity and pattern of reflux, e.g., NERD and reflux hypersensitivity. The management of GERD is complicated, particularly given the variety of subtypes that need tailored therapeutic approaches. For instance, NERD has been defined by the presence of reflux symptoms without esophageal mucosal injury that can be demonstrated. Patients with reflux hypersensitivity may also have esophageal symptoms typical of reflux but lack well-documented structural or inflammatory etiologies, as listed in the Lyon Consensus 2.0 criteria (Calabrese et al., 2024). The presence of functional heartburn (FH), where heartburn is paired with normal test results, contributes to the therapeutic complexity. Therefore, successful treatment demands a personalized approach that encompasses pharmacotherapy, i.e., proton pump inhibitors, together with lifestyle modification and psychotherapy, in order to offer comprehensive care to patients. Furthermore, the role of lifestyle and diet cannot be overestimated when it comes to GERD therapy. Many patients undergo alternative therapies , such as herbal supplements, for the relief of symptoms, expecting greater tolerability than that of standard drugs. Indeed, a significant proportion of adults experience gastrointestinal disorders that drive them to seek out non-conventional therapies. Since gastrointestinal disorders are a generic term encompassing GERD, determination of dietary precipitants , such as fatty foods, caffeine, and alcohol, can help with better management. Furthermore, promoting healthy lifestyle behaviors, including exercise on a frequent basis and stress reduction, may minimize the symptoms of GERD and reduce medication requirements. Healthcare professionals will be able to enhance patient outcomes and overall quality of life by understanding the multifaceted nature of GERD and its control.

12.2.2. Inflammatory Bowel Disease (IBD)

IBD, encompassing Crohn's disease and ulcerative colitis, is perhaps the most critical of the entire spectrum of intestinal disorders. Characterized by chronic inflammation of the GI tract, IBD affects millions of individuals worldwide, causing an assortment of disabling signs and symptoms, including abdominal pain, diarrhea, and fatigue. The pathogenesis of IBD remains complex and multivariable, involving a combination of genetic predisposition, environmental insult, and abnormally regulated immune responses. Current research has shed light on progress made in the study of IBD's pathological mechanisms and has provided insights to open the gateway to innovative therapeutic approaches to improve patient care. Among numerous gastrointestinal diseases, IBD requires a multidisciplinary treatment plan with medical, nutritional, and psychological management to meet the different needs of patients suffering from this chronic condition. IBD patients typically experience comorbidities that complicate their overall health and quality of life, , such as psychiatric disorders like depression and anxiety and obesity. Studies indicate that chronic gastrointestinal disease are often affected by obesity due to overlapping pathophysiological mechanisms (Bischoff et al., 2022). Psych affective disturbances are also prevalent among IBD patients, and estimates have shown that 21% to 35% exhibit signs of anxiety or depression (Park and Jeen, 2016). This interaction can be bidirectional; increased psychological distress may increase physical symptoms and inflammation, creating a spiral that reduces patient well-being. Successful management of IBD thus demands an integrated treatment strategy incorporating nutritional counseling, psychotherapy, and adequate medical management to optimize patient care and enhance coping behavior. With the multifaceted play between physical and psychological well-being in IBD patients, tailored therapy methods are the solution to holistic care. Present advice is towards multidisciplinary treatment for obesity in chronic gastrointestinal disease patients, emphasizing collaboration among health workers like gastroenterologists, dietitians, and mental health workers (Bischoff et al., 2022). With appreciation of the prevalence of psychiatric illness, healthcare providers are urged to offer routine depression and anxiety screening to patients with IBD and to initiate personalized treatment plans that address not only the physical symptoms but the psychological impact of the disease as well (Park and Jeen, 2016). Through the provision of an environment of comprehensive care, clinicians are empowered to empower patients with IBD, optimizing disease control and quality of life as well as controlling the complex issues surrounding this disease (Figure 12.6).

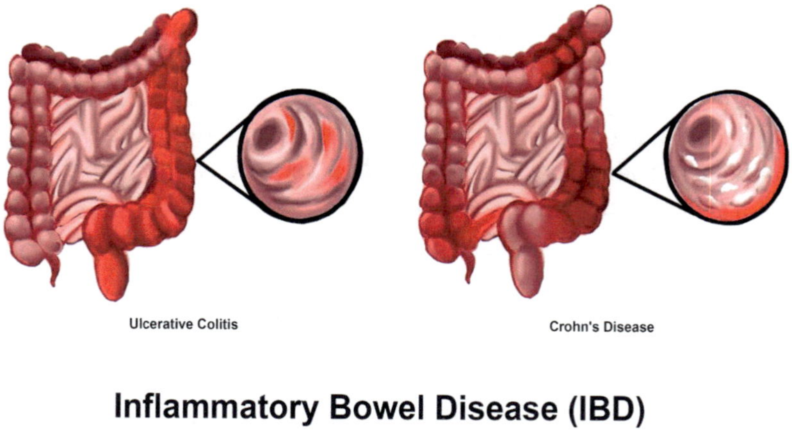

Figure 12.6. Ulcerative colitis and Crohn's disease are shown as types of inflammatory bowel disease (IBD).

Source: https://cdn.storymd.com/optimized/JdPvkNZFjA/original.jpg.

12.2.3. Irritable Bowel Syndrome (IBS)

IBS is a common functional gastrointestinal disorder that is defined by chronic abdominal discomfort, bloating, and changed bowel habits with diarrhea and constipation. Its etiology is multifactorial and includes genetic predisposition, environmental factors, and derangement of the gut microbiome. The evidence suggests that the composition of microbiota plays an important role in IBS pathogenesis, pointing to the significance of microbial well-being in determining gastrointestinal function. Microbiota dysbiosis, i.e., imbalance of the microbial community, has been implicated to result in aggravation of IBS symptoms, and therapeutic interventions targeting gut microbiota have promise in management and treatment (Hou et al., 2022). Furthermore, elucidation of mechanisms of gut-brain interactions illuminates why psychological stress and emotional issues tend to influence gastrointestinal health, further complicating the clinical presentation of IBS. The epidemiology of IBS reveals an alarming trend in its prevalence and the health cost associated with it, as shown by an incidence rate of 106.54/10,000 population reported in a Taiwanese study (Lai et al., 2021). Prevalent comorbidities identified among IBS patients included anxiety, dyslipidemia, and gastroesophageal reflux disease (GERD). This suggests that IBS is often associated with other gastrointestinal conditions that complicate diagnosis and treatment. Besides, the study notes a downward trend in incidence and prevalence between 2012 and 2018, dispelling the assumptions that IBS is increasing in prevalence globally. The newly emerging data calls for a cautious interpretation of the status of IBS, suggesting the need for both therapeutic interventions tailored to the gastrointestinal symptoms and dealing with the concomitant psychological and physiological comorbidities. While therapeutic strategies for IBS are plenty, dietary modifications, drug treatments, and behavioral therapies to manage the disorder's multidimensional nature are among them. Among the therapeutic means, the most common prescribed medication is antispasmodics, followed by laxatives and antidiarrheals (Lai et al., 2021). Interestingly, despite the treatment of over two-thirds of diagnosed patients, rates of follow-up after diagnosis are low, suggesting a missing link in ongoing management and compliance of patients with therapies. The evolving perspective of IBS management must aim at patient education regarding the chronicity of the disease and the requirement of ongoing treatment to effectively manage symptoms. While scientific findings continue to unravel the interrelational phenomena of IBS with, e.g., gut microbiota, interdisciplinary management combining diet, pharmacology, and behavioral medicine is paramount to optimizing patient outcomes in this pervasive gastrointestinal disorder (Figure 12.7).

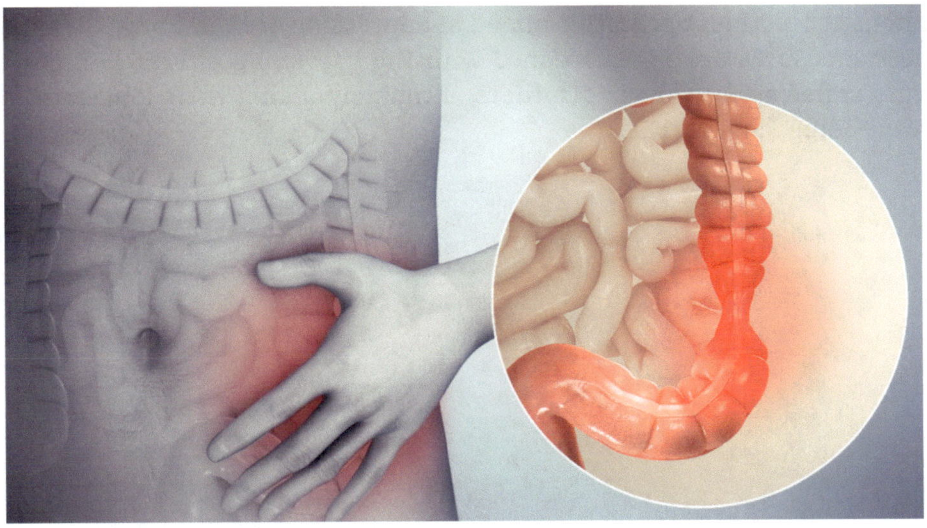

Figure 12.7. Irritable bowel syndrome (IBS) showing abdominal pain and colon inflammation.

Source: https://upload.wikimedia.org/wikipedia/commons/1/1a/Irritable_bowel_syndrome.jpg.

12.3. Liver Disorders Overview

Liver disease encompasses a wide range of diseases that affect the structure and function of the liver, with numerous potential etiologies, from viral infections, alcohol consumption, to metabolic disorders. Hepatitis resulting from viral infections , such as hepatitis A, B, and C, is a major global health problem due to the risk of progression to chronic liver disease or cirrhosis. Non-alcoholic fatty liver disease (NAFLD) has become a top contributor to liver diseases, largely correlated with obesity and metabolic syndrome. The increasing rates of liver disease are also due to lifestyle choices, making it a priority to raise public awareness and education regarding risk factors and preventive measures. Knowledge of liver disease pathophysiology is essential in designing successful therapy and maximizing outcomes in an increasingly health-aware population with liver-related illness. Liver disease can lead to a continuum of complications like hepatic encephalopathy, coagulopathy, and ascites that make management and recovery progressively more challenging. All the crucial functions of the liver, including detoxification, protein synthesis, and metabolic regulation, are impaired in chronic liver disease. Furthermore, patients with concurrent liver disease are often at risk of gastrointestinal bleeding and, in the worst scenario, multi-organ failure. Effective management is thus paramount not only to reduce the severity of liver dysfunction but to prevent the onset of end-stage liver disease requiring transplantation. Early identification of liver disease is paramount, necessitating routine screening and monitoring for symptomatically involved patients to enable immediate intervention. New studies continue to enlighten us on the various aspects of liver diseases. Recent studies have established that lifestyle intervention through dietary modification and physical exercise can significantly contribute to improving liver function and arresting disease progression. It is important that clinicians adopt a multidisciplinary model, unifying both medical and lifestyle management of liver disease. Second, mental health's contribution to liver disease cannot be discounted, as patients become more anxious and depressed as a result of their chronic condition. Such a relationship between body and mind reinforces the importance of holistic treatment protocols aimed at addressing both in a way that enhances overall well-being. These measures are in accordance with the prevailing efforts to improve the quality of life of patients suffering from liver disorders, ultimately aiding their long-term prognosis and their general well-being (Figure 12.8).

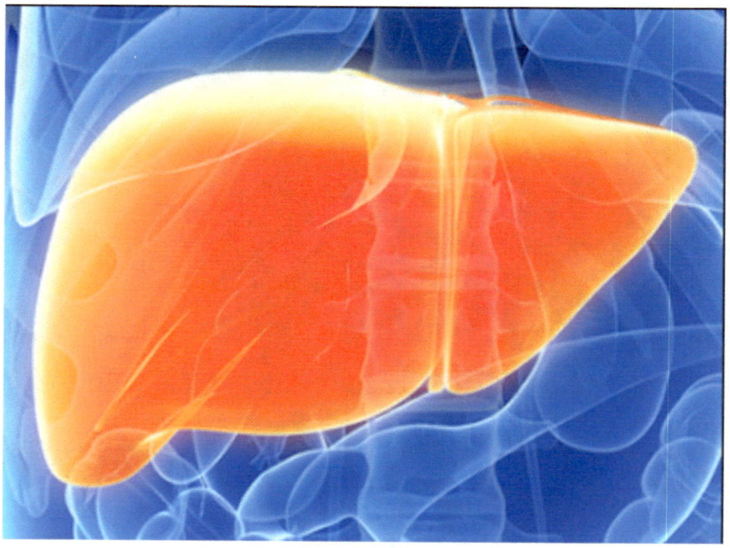

Figure 12.8. The human liver is shown in anatomical position within the abdominal cavity.

Source: https://www.niddk.nih.gov/-/media/Images/Health-Information/Diabetes/landing/liver.png.

12.3.1. Types of Liver Disorders

Liver diseases are an unlimited group of conditions that can profoundly impair the liver's crucial functions. Hepatitis is one of the important liver diseases, an inflammatory disorder that may develop as a result of viral infections, autoimmune reactions, or chemical damage from substances like alcohol and drugs. Viral hepatitis is the most challenging, with hepatitis A, B, C, D, and E all having unique patterns of transmission and epidemiologic characteristics. Chronic hepatitis is liable to result in serious complications like fibrosis, cirrhosis, and even hepatocellular carcinoma and therefore early diagnosis as well as effective management are of prime importance. The clinical importance of untreated hepatitis underlines the requirement for public health interventions through vaccination, safe conduct, and education against these infections. Fatty liver diseases are another essential group of liver diseases that are characterized by fat deposits within liver cells. Non-alcoholic fatty liver disease (NAFLD) is of growing concern due to its association with metabolic syndrome, which is characterized by obesity, insulin resistance, and type 2 diabetes. Strong evidence has shown that vitamin D deficiency plays a role in the progression and worsening of NAFLD, which further adds to its prevalence among populations receiving limited sun exposure or poor diet (Cai et al., 2016). The spectrum of NAFLD ranges from simple steatosis to non-alcoholic steatohepatitis (NASH), a more severe form with inflammation and liver damage. With its rising global prevalence, recognition and control of the risk factors for fatty liver conditions are crucial in preventing late hepatic complications. Liver conditions can also be a consequence of autoimmune conditions, where the body's immune response mistakenly attacks liver cells. Autoimmune hepatitis is a very severe condition that may lead to extensive inflammation and cumulative liver damage if left untreated. Autoimmune disease pathogenesis is complex and typically includes both genetic susceptibility in combination with environmental triggers. Dysbiosis of gut microbiota has received some recognition in the recent past, suggesting gut changes may affect liver diseases like metabolic syndrome and non-alcoholic fatty liver disease (Cai et al., 2016). Effective management of autoimmune hepatitis often includes the use of immunosuppressive therapies, reinforcing the need for ongoing research into the relationship between the immune system, gut, and liver. Generally, the heterogeneity of liver disorders necessitates a polymeric strategy for diagnosis, treatment, and prevention in the clinic.

12.3.2. Causes of Liver Disorders

Liver diseases are caused by an enormous number of causative agents that disrupt the liver's essential functions. Prominent among these is viral hepatitis, namely hepatitis B and C, which have chronic infections that can snowball into inflammation, fibrosis, and eventually cirrhosis. Blood-borne and body fluid-borne viral etiologies are the most prevalent agents and contribute largely to the overwhelming public health burden worldwide. Other than viral diseases, conditions , such as autoimmune hepatitis may also produce inflammation and damage to the liver, where the immune system of the body targets liver cells erroneously. The resulting tissue injury is compounded by this immune assault, and scarring can have adverse effects on liver function in the long run. The disseminated and heterogeneous presentation of viral and autoimmune etiologies demonstrates the complexity of liver disease, for which specific diagnostics and interventions are required to effectively manage the conditions and prevent long-term sequelae. A final key etiology of liver disease is the consumption of harmful substances and alcohol and certain toxins. Chronic alcohol consumption is a leading global cause of liver disease, affecting millions of individuals and leading to alcoholic liver disease, which encompasses fatty liver, alcoholic hepatitis, and cirrhosis. The liver metabolizes alcohol, yet excessive use exceeds the detoxifying capacity of the organ, leading to cellular damage and inflammation. Furthermore, exposure to environmental toxins, , such as deoxynivalenol (DON), have been found to induce oxidative stress and inflammation, which are detrimental to liver health. Research has proved that DON may lead to increased alkaline phosphatase levels and fibrosis of liver tissues, which reflect tissue injury. An understanding of alcohol and toxin action is necessary to develop preventive measures and therapeutic models and consequently eradicate liver disorders caused by these chemicals. Last but not least, metabolic conditions like non-alcoholic fatty liver disease (NAFLD) have become extremely significant causes of liver disorders in recent years. NAFLD is a spectrum of liver disease with fat accumulation in the absence of excessive alcohol intake and is most commonly associated with obesity, diabetes, and dyslipidemia. With lifestyles trending towards increased sedentary and high-calorie diets, NAFLD has become increasingly common, which poses a risk for liver inflammation and fibrosis. Comorbidities , such as those that arise from low socioeconomic status and reduced access to medical care, can heighten these risks. In addition, lifestyle food intake, including the consumption of extrinsic food, has been linked to high rates of hepatic injuries and metabolic disturbances. Management of these lifestyle and metabolic factors is paramount to the prevention of the advancement of liver disease and overall gastrointestinal and hepatic health (Figure 12.9).

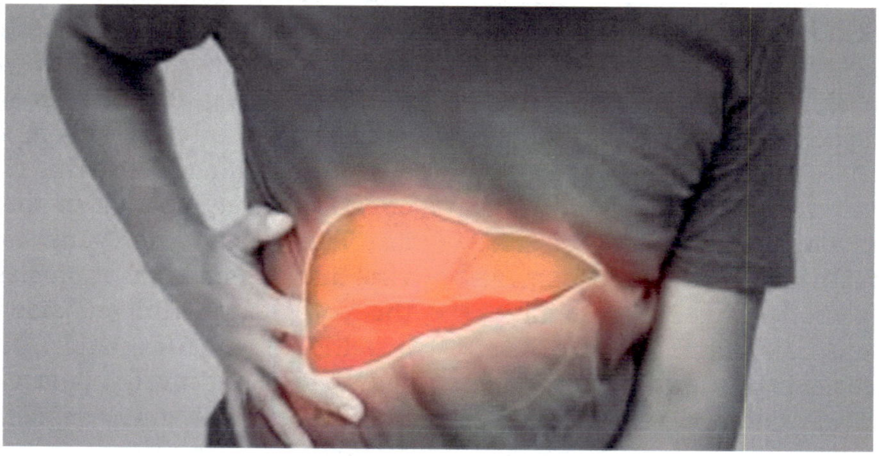

Figure 12.9. Liver pain indicating potential inflammation or liver-related disorder.

Source: https://encrypted-tbn0.gstatic.com/images?q=tbn:ANd9GcSyYGqtTXVPvi2GzQ3wEltZW7U5iNceP3pLBA&s.

12.3.3. Symptoms Associated with Liver Disorders

The liver, which is a vital component of the body's metabolic processes, is tasked with detoxification as well as storage. Symptoms of liver diseases vary significantly with the disorder of the liver, but are primarily jaundice, tiredness, and pain in the stomach. Jaundice, or yellowish pigmentation of the skin and eyes, is caused by the result of a deposit of bilirubin in the bloodstream as a result of dysfunctional liver cells. Fatigue is a common complaint, most often because of the liver's decreased ability to process nutrients into energy or as a result of the metabolic derangement secondary to liver disease. Abdominal pain or discomfort, most commonly in the right upper quadrant, may be secondary to liver enlargement or inflammation due to such underlying conditions as cirrhosis or hepatitis. It is crucial to recognize these symptoms because they can lead to premature diagnosis and treatment of liver disease, ultimately leading to improved patient outcomes. In addition to the classic symptoms, other presentations may be seen in individuals with liver disease. For instance, alcoholic liver disease might lead to withdrawal symptoms on cessation of alcohol intake, e.g., insomnia, anxiety, and mood alterations. These symptoms are capable of producing worse deterioration in the quality of life of the individual and, most time, are misdiagnosed as other mental illness disorders. Also, complications from deranged liver function can result in gastrointestinal symptoms like vomiting, nausea, and even gastrointestinal hemorrhage. For instance, with further development of liver insufficiency, varices or dilated veins develop in the esophagus as a result of portal hypertension, with severe health implications. This complex interaction of liver function and gastrointestinal condition emphasizes the necessity for an overarching diagnosis and treatment response covering both liver-specific indicators and associated gastrointestinal complications (Acharjee, 2025). The impacts of liver disease extend to the gastrointestinal system in profound and fundamental ways, especially in the framework of contemporary healthcare crises , such as the COVID-19 pandemic. Evidence indicates that patients with compromised liver function can experience heightened gastrointestinal symptoms as a result of viral infections, including those caused by SARS-CoV-2. The heightened abdominal pain, as well as liver enzyme abnormalities, not only complicate the progression of the viral infection but also increase liver health management difficulties. Moreover, impaired liver function may lead to systemic inflammation, severely weakening gut microbiota and intestinal barrier integrity. These changes are involved in a vicious cycle of metabolic derangement in which the failure of the liver to regulate toxins and nutrients will tend to worsen the gastrointestinal signs and advance liver disease. Therefore, therapeutic interventions aiming at correcting gastrointestinal imbalance and liver function are mandated in holistic treatment protocols (Grinevich and Kravchuk, 2021).

12.4. Diagnostic Strategies for Gastrointestinal and Hepatic Disorders

The clinical setting for the diagnosis of gastrointestinal and liver disease has been transformed and now includes a range of techniques to facilitate the sensitivity and rapidity of the detection of disease. Traditional techniques , such as endoscopy and imaging studies, including ultrasound, CT scanning, and MRI, play a significant role in monitoring structural deficits and evidence of lesions. Emerging endoscopic modalities, , such as endoscopic ultrasound (EUS), enhance diagnostic yield for both conditions of the gastrointestinal tract and the liver by facilitating real-time acquisition of tissue and accurate tumor staging. In addition, the use of biomarker testing, including serum liver enzymes and new markers, has become more significant in clinical care, helping to distinguish benign from malignant processes in the liver, thus informing the treatment and tracking the progression of the disease (N/A, 2022). Non-invasive examinations have become an adjunct to traditional techniques in gastroenterology, following the demand for minimizing patient discomfort and complications from invasive procedures. Assessments of fecal biomarkers, including calprotectin and fecal immunochemical tests (FIT), present an encouraging route towards the identification of inflammatory bowel disease (IBD) and colorectal cancer. These methods not only contribute to early diagnosis but also facilitate monitoring of treatment responses, hence being very useful in chronic disease care. Furthermore, the development of breath tests, particularly for the detection of Helicobacter pylori and malabsorption syndrome testing, is an enormous leap in diagnostic techniques. These non-invasive tests demonstrate the shift towards patient-centered care as well as enhance gastrointestinal diagnostics precision (Hertlein et al., 2012). With every advancement in our understanding of the pathophysiology of gastrointestinal and liver illnesses, the development of new diagnostic technology continues to be a cornerstone in improving patient outcomes. The latest research highlights the potential benefit of merging multi-omics technologies that analyze genomic, proteomic, and metabolomic data for identifying prospective biomarkers for early detection and risk stratification of various disorders. For instance, exploration of new biomarkers, , such as those from bile or provoked as a result of liver dysfunction, might uncover mechanisms of the disease process and allow for population screening on an expanded level. These technologies not only hold promises for enhancing diagnostic accuracy but also for individualizing personalized treatment regimens in patients with liver and gastrointestinal diseases, thus leading to more effective and comprehensive treatment (Hertlein et al., 2012) (Figure 12.10).

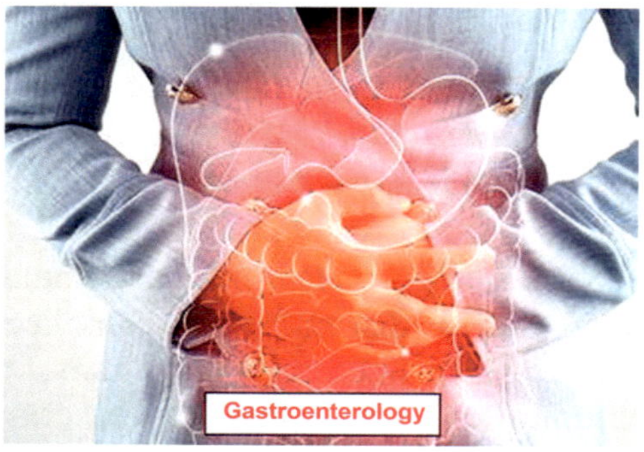

Figure 12.10. Gastroenterology concept image showing abdominal discomfort and the digestive tract.

Source: https://www.edhacare.com/storage/departments/1683901670gastroenterology.jpg.

12.4.1. Imaging Techniques (e.g., Ultrasound, CT scan)

Imaging techniques play a key role in the diagnosis and treatment of liver and gastrointestinal illness, significantly enhancing the doctor's capability to visualize inside the body. Among available methods, ultrasound stands out as non-invasive and offers real-time imagery. European Federation of Societies for Ultrasound in Medicine and Biology emphasizes the broad function of gastrointestinal ultrasound (GIUS) in diagnosis and the creation in October 2014 of a task force to promote its use in the clinic. The activity of this group has led to the publication of guidelines that allow clinicians to interpret correctly anatomical and physiological features of an organ or system through various ultrasound modalities, emphasizing the diagnostic function of GIUS in the evaluation of biliary obstruction, liver cirrhosis, and inflammatory bowel diseases (Calabrese et al., 2016). Apart from ultrasound, computed tomography (CT) scans provide highly accurate cross-sectional images and are hence valuable in the diagnosis of complex gastrointestinal conditions. CT scans are particularly valuable in diagnosing conditions like pancreatitis, gastrointestinal malignancies, and liver metastases, where accuracy and visibility are of utmost importance. The modality's ability to image from many different angles allows extensive studies of the abdominal and pelvic cavities. Furthermore, advanced CT technologies , such as CT angiography, provide evaluation of vascular involvement in liver disease and gastrointestinal hemorrhage. Such broad-ranging imaging capability makes CT scans valuable tools for clinicians to design accurate treatment plans based on the unique needs of individual patients, managing the wide scope of gastrointestinal disorders. Despite continuing advances in imaging technology, the incorporation of these technologies into clinical applications remains crucial in delivering comprehensive patient care. Ongoing research to optimize imaging protocols and improve resolution will continue to increase diagnostic precision. For instance, newer ultrasound has improved visualization of minor abnormalities and facilitated dynamic assessment of organ function. Standardized protocols and guidelines, as put out by the GIUS task force, ensure the utilization and interpretation of imaging data consistently across clinical settings (Hertlein et al., 2012). Therefore, clinicians become increasingly capable of detecting, diagnosing, and monitoring gastrointestinal and liver disorders, finally optimizing patient outcomes through prompt and effective intervention.

12.4.2. Endoscopic Procedures

Endoscopy has emerged as an integral diagnostic and therapeutic modality in liver and gastrointestinal diseases. Through minimally invasive techniques, doctors are able to visualize, diagnose, and manage a number of disorders of the digestive system. Two of the most sought-after endoscopic methods are esophagogastroduodenoscopy (EGD) and colonoscopy, which enable adequate examination of the upper and lower gastrointestinal tracts, respectively. Technology has evolved significantly, with improved precision of diagnosis as well as quick recovery times for patients. Endoscopic intervention can also provide procedures , such as biopsies and resections of polyps, which play a crucial role in the prevention of possible malignancies. This diagnostic and therapeutic capability synergy highlights endoscopy's pivotal position in contemporary gastroenterological practice, enhancing both patient management and results. Video capsule endoscopy (VCE) has expanded the diagnostic arsenal for the study of the small intestine, which is challenging because of its topographical intricacy. Based on recent publications, VCE possesses particular indications in obscure gastrointestinal bleeding or suspected inflammatory bowel disease. Personnel with training, , such as nurses, can significantly assist in the preliminary assessment of VCE images in regard to detecting abnormalities, hence streamlining the process for gastroenterologists. For example, the agreement identified among trained nurses and gastroenterologists in lesion detection has proven that a team-based approach could improve efficiency and diagnostic yield in clinical practice (Guarini et al., 2018). In addition, using trained personnel for initial assessments can significantly cut the time that experts spend reviewing recordings, thus making it easier to allocate medical resources effectively. In addition to traditional endoscopic techniques, recent imaging technologies are enhancing our ability to assess esophagogastric and gastrointestinal tract pathology. Multidetector computed tomography (MDCT), often used for determining hiatal surface area (HSA), offers a quantifiable measure that is useful for preoperative planning for hiatus defects (Boru et al., 2017). The technique used in studies allows precise measurements inaccessible through preoperative endoscopy. The combination of endoscopy with emerging imaging modalities has the potential to detect complex disorders, facilitate specific treatments, and ultimately contribute to improved patient outcomes. As the progress in gastroenterology continues to be fueled by technology, the integration of such procedures will form the backbone of effective care for gastrointestinal and liver diseases (Figure 12.11).

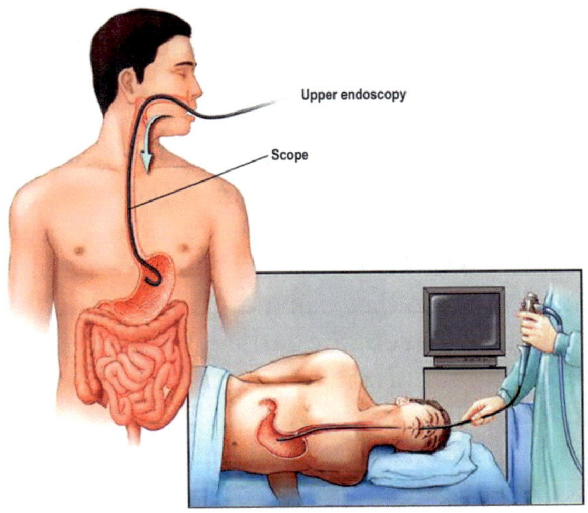

Figure 12.11. Upper endoscopy showing the scope inserted to examine the upper digestive tract.

Source: https://www.mayoclinic.org/-/media/kcms/gbs/patient-consumer/images/2016/05/02/14/44/mcdc7_endoscopy-8col.jpg.

12.4.3. Laboratory Tests (e.g., Liver Function Tests)

Laboratory investigation plays a critical role in the diagnosis and management of gastrointestinal and liver illness. Among the several tests that come under this umbrella, liver function tests (LFTs) serve a particular purpose because they reflect the functioning of the liver's metabolic activity. Most LFTs search for the concentrations of enzymes, proteins, and chemicals produced by the liver and consist of alanine aminotransferase (ALT), aspartate aminotransferase (AST), alkaline phosphatase (ALP), and bilirubin. Greater quantities of these enzymes typically suggest inflammation or injury to the liver, and this can be an indicator for many disorders, for instance, hepatitis or cirrhosis. Moreover, LFTs have the ability to track disease advancement in the liver as well as therapeutic efficacy and therefore guide clinical intervention. Apart from LFTs, other laboratory tests are utilized in the assessment of the severity of and complications of liver disease. For instance, coagulation factor test measurements are important in the evaluation of liver hemostatic function, especially for cirrhotic patients. The liver synthesizes glycoproteins required for blood clotting and impaired synthesis can lead to bleeding complications. These, in turn, can have extensive management as they can induce such conditions as hepatic encephalopathy, which causes a great deal of damage to patient morbidity and mortality (Bacalbașa et al., 2019). The interconnection between coagulopathy and liver disease indicates the importance of systematic laboratory examination in optimizing the results in patients with liver disease. In addition to the routine LFTs and coagulation profiles, more specific investigations are warranted based on clinical suspicion. For example, when autoimmune liver disease is suspected, autoantibody screening can characterize the pathology. Similarly, monitoring serum ammonia is crucial in the case of hepatic encephalopathy due to the fact that variations in ammonia levels may indicate declining liver function and necessitate immediate intervention. Last but not least, laboratory testing is an invaluable diagnostic modality that not only helps to direct diagnosis and treatment but also enhances our understanding of the complex interface between the gastrointestinal and hepatic systems. With the inclusion of regular and specialist laboratory testing, practitioners are better able to adopt a more evidence-based and holistic management of liver disease (Balasubramanian et al., 2016).

12.5. Treatment Options for Gastrointestinal Disorders

The treatment of gastrointestinal disease is commonly a multidisciplinary approach, unique to the patient's condition and needs. Medication is the foundation of treatment and may be antacids, proton pump inhibitors, and antibiotics for conditions , such as gastroesophageal reflux disease (GERD) or bacterial illnesses , such as Helicobacter pylori. Medication that influences motility, , such as prokinetics, is also useful for patients with gastroparesis or functional dyspepsia. Determination of root causes is important in appropriate treatment; thus, advanced diagnostic equipment like endoscopy will elucidate issues ranging from peptic ulcers to IBD. The advent of biologic treatments, particularly in IBD, is another fine example of advancement in treatment options, with targeted therapies that improve patient care in chronic inflammatory diseases (Northup et al., 2020). Apart from pharmacotherapies, lifestyle changes also form an integral part of the treatment of gastrointestinal diseases. Dietary changes, for example, fiber supplementation, fat limitation, and exclusion of specific trigger foods, form a significant component of treatment in cases of irritable bowel syndrome (IBS). Exercise has also been found to aid in gut health and symptom improvement for conditions , such as constipation. In addition, the psychological aspect of stress management and cognitive-behavioral treatment are becoming more widely acknowledged, particularly in cases where there is involvement of the brain-gut axis. The holistic approach highlights the necessity of addressing both physiological and psychological aspects of gastrointestinal management, especially in view of the bidirectional influence between mental and gastrointestinal well-being (Alexander et al., 2020).

Procedure-based interventions might be occasionally necessary for more long-standing gastrointestinal issues. Endoscopic interventions , such as balloon dilatation for strictures or polypectomy to remove growth, are increasingly the norm in sophisticated management techniques. Severe IBD or malignant disease might have resections or ostomy creation as surgical procedures, bringing into play the coordination of specialists. Additionally, studies on new therapies , such as gene therapy and microbiome-related therapy, also remain promising for gastrointestinal treatment in the future. Effective management often includes a multidisciplinary approach by gastroenterologists, surgeons, dietitians, and mental health professionals in creating an integrated care plan specific to the multifactorial pathogenesis of gastrointestinal disease (Northup et al., 2020) (Figure 12.12).

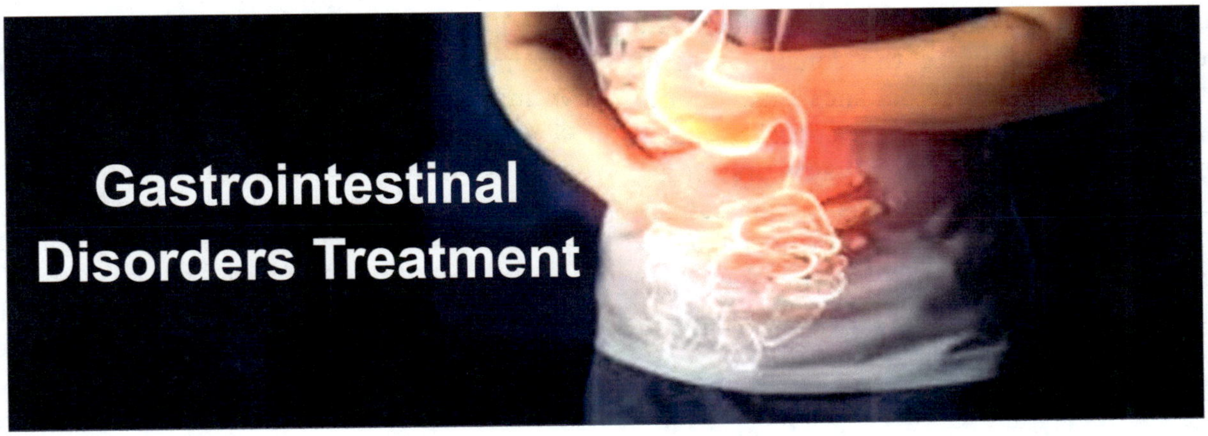

Figure 12.12. Gastrointestinal disorders treatment targeting digestive tract issues.

Source: https://encrypted-tbn0.gstatic.com/images?q=tbn:ANd9GcQWvtb6xkp4RfQcRRNyJw8ZGHqC7BepaAbqIA&s.

12.5.1. Dietary Modifications

Nutritional adaptation is a critical component in the treatment of gastrointestinal and liver illnesses since adequate nutrition can reverse person deficiency and complications due to the illness. For instance, individuals with gastrointestinal disease become malabsorptive, hence unable to absorb sufficient nutrients. Such conditions call for nutritional strategies for enhanced nutrient availability and consideration of the functional capacity of the aged gastrointestinal tract. The drop in mechanical, sensory, and chemical digestion processes in the elderly is impressive; these processes can complicate digestion and nutrient intake. Nutritionists advocate the intake of diets with high macronutrient and micronutrient contents that are easily digested and micronutrient supplements that complement the particular needs of the elderly population's physiological problems, thus averting malnutrition and associated complications (Rémond et al., 2015). In addition to management of malabsorption, dietary modification also needs to consider the specific needs according to liver disease. Diets for liver function tend to concentrate on reducing consumption of saturated fat and sugar and increasing intake of antioxidant foods. Dietary modification tends to reduce the burden of liver metabolism and improve liver function. Dietary intake of foods high in omega-3 fatty acids, including flaxseeds and fatty fish, may contribute to aiding anti-inflammatory processes that maximize the recovery of the liver. Furthermore, the incorporation of complex carbohydrates and fiber can optimize digestive function and normality and subsequently reduce the risks of gastrointestinal disturbance often associated with liver disease.

Through supplementation of these food groups, individuals can better manage their liver diseases, optimize the consumption of nutrients, and therefore enhance their quality of life. Lastly, the addition of specific dietary components can also go a long way in preventing recurrent forms of urolithiasis, particularly calcium oxalate (CaOx) stones, which involve both gastrointestinal and liver function. Recognition of the role of dietary oxalates in urolithiasis is important so that specific preventive strategies can be devised. Evidence suggests that the provision of commercially available CaOx stone-preventative diets may be inadequate to prevent recurrence due to their borderline efficacy (Baal et al., 2011). Hence, it is important to continue investigating dietary risk factors and also incorporate knowledge about the metabolic pathways involved. Appreciation for the metabolism of oxalate and its implications in the detoxification and metabolism of dietary intake by the liver could lead to more effective dietary modifications capable of successfully preventing the incidence and recurrence of uroliths, proving the complex correlation between dietary practices and treatment of gastrointestinal and liver disorders using technological knowledge, integration of these processes will likely become the solution for proper management of gastrointestinal and liver disorders.

12.5.2. Laboratory Tests (e.g., Liver Function Tests)

Laboratory tests play a major role in the treatment and diagnosis of liver and gastrointestinal diseases. Among the laboratory tests, liver function tests (LFTs) are specifically required because they indicate the functional capacity of the liver to perform its metabolic functions. The tests are most frequently applied to assess enzymes, proteins, and liver products, , such as alanine aminotransferase (ALT), aspartate aminotransferase (AST), alkaline phosphatase (ALP), and bilirubin. Elevated levels of these enzymes typically reflect liver inflammation or injury, and such can result from a range of conditions including hepatitis or cirrhosis. LFTs can also be utilized to monitor the progression of liver disease and the effectiveness of treatment interventions, finally guiding clinical management. Apart from LFTs, various laboratory tests help to measure the severity and complications of liver disease. For instance, coagulation factor assays are important in determining the hemostatic function of the liver, which is especially significant in the case of patients with cirrhosis. The liver synthesizes glycoproteins used in blood coagulation, and their reduced synthesis might be a consequence of bleeding complications. These typically need extensive therapy since they can lead to conditions like hepatic encephalopathy, which significantly aggravates morbidity and mortality in patients (Bacalbașa et al., 2019). The interaction between coagulopathy and liver function highlights the significance of systematic laboratory tests in optimizing the outcome for liver disorder patients. Besides standard LFTs and coagulation tests, more specific tests may also be indicated depending on clinical suspicion. For instance, when autoimmune liver disease is suspected, autoantibody testing can be done to clarify the underlying pathology.

Similarly, monitoring serum ammonia levels is critical for hepatic encephalopathy, as elevated ammonia indicates waning liver function and needs prompt treatment. Laboratory testing, ultimately, is a precious tool that not only assists diagnosis and treatment but also the comprehension of the complex interplay between the liver and gut. By using both standard and specialty laboratory tests, physicians are able to make a more informed and comprehensive treatment decision for liver disease (Balasubramanian et al., 2016) (Figure 12.13).

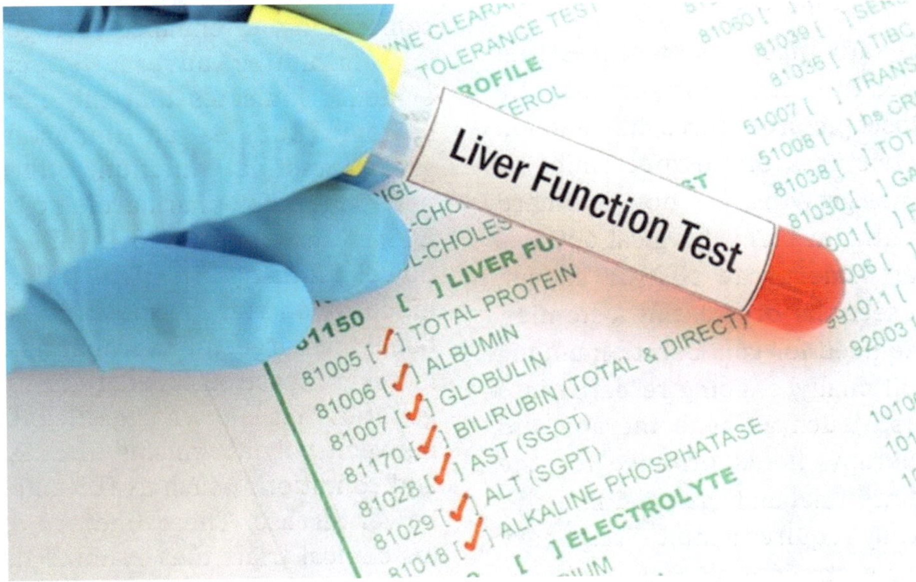

Figure 12.13. Liver function test sample used to evaluate liver health markers.

Source: https://www.labtestpk.com/wp-content/uploads/2022/03/Liver-Function-Test.jpg.

12.5.3. Treatment Options for Gastrointestinal Disorders

Therapy for gastrointestinal illnesses usually involves a tailored approach that considers both the specific condition and the individual patient. Medications are a key part of the treatment and can include antacids, proton pump inhibitors, and antibiotics for issues like gastroesophageal reflux disease (GERD) or Helicobacter pylori infections. Additionally, medications that affect motility, , such as prokinetics, can be helpful for patients dealing with gastroparesis or functional dyspepsia. Identifying the root cause is crucial for effective treatment, which is why modern diagnostic methods like endoscopy are valuable for clarifying conditions ranging from peptic ulcers to inflammatory bowel disease (IBD). The rise of biologic therapy, especially in IBD, shows the advancement of treatment options, offering targeted therapies that enhance patient outcomes in chronic inflammatory diseases (Northup et al., 2020).

Alongside medication, lifestyle changes are also important in managing gastrointestinal disorders. Adjusting one's diet, such as,, such as increasing fiber intake, reducing fat consumption, or avoiding specific trigger foods, can be beneficial for conditions like irritable bowel syndrome (IBS). Regular exercise contributes to intestinal health and can alleviate symptoms of constipation. Moreover, addressing psychological factors, including stress management and cognitive-behavioral therapy, is becoming increasingly recognized, especially when the brain-gut connection is involved. This comprehensive approach highlights the importance of treating both physiological and psychological aspects of gastrointestinal health, as mental well-being is closely linked to digestive health (Alexander et al., 2020).

For more advanced gastrointestinal diseases, procedural interventions may be necessary. Endoscopic procedures, like balloon dilatation of strictures or polypectomies to remove abnormal growths, are now standard in advanced treatment plans. Surgical options, particularly for widespread IBD or cancer, may involve resections or creating ostomies, emphasizing the need for collaboration among specialists. Additionally, ongoing research into new treatments, , such as gene therapy and microbiome therapy, holds promise for the future of gastrointestinal management. Effective treatment typically requires a multidisciplinary team of surgeons, gastroenterologists, dietitians, and mental health professionals to develop a comprehensive plan that addresses the complex nature of gastrointestinal disorders (Northup et al., 2020).

12.6. Pharmacological Treatments

Pharmacologic treatments of gastrointestinal and liver disease are key to symptom relief and quality-of-life enhancement for patients. Medications are frequently employed to treat chosen pathways within the pathophysiology of these conditions. For instance, prokinetic medications induce motility of the gastrointestinal tract and thus reduce gastroparesis and functional dyspepsia. Antispasmodics, however, are employed to alleviate abdominal pain with irritable bowel syndrome (IBS) and another gastrointestinal dysfunction. Importantly, the effectiveness of these treatments not only resides in the individual pharmacologic agents themselves but also in understanding the pathophysiologic mechanisms of gastrointestinal disorders. The development of pharmacotherapy should consider individualized factors of the patient, including genetic predisposition and comorbidity, to enhance therapeutic response and minimize adverse effects. Emerging evidence indicates that the endocannabinoid system (ECS) is an important player in gastrointestinal function, offering potential new targets for pharmacologic treatment. The ECS is also implicated in the modulation of bowel motility, intestinal inflammation, and mucosal barrier permeability and has thus been the target of therapeutic interventions in several gastrointestinal diseases. Molecular genetics has shown significant associations between polymorphisms of ECS-related genes and conditions , such as IBS and inflammatory bowel disease. These findings open the door for clinical trials that examine the therapeutic potential of endocannabinoid agonists and antagonists for symptom control. But the current lack of robust randomized controlled trials (RCTs) warrants prudence. Ethical, political, and economic concerns regarding cannabis-based medications complicate their use in the clinic, yet they have tremendous promise to ease gastrointestinal symptoms (Alessandra et al., 2018). In addition to modulating specific pathways, pharmacologic treatments must consider multimodal approaches pairing chemical treatments with behavioral treatments. For instance, advances in imaging techniques enable a better understanding of the brain-gut interactions that are characteristic of gastrointestinal illness. Studies conducted with these techniques have demonstrated the part dysregulated visceral signals contribute to symptomology while simultaneously highlighting the brain's complex role in interpreting these signals (Aziz et al., 2019). A multidisciplinary approach based on pharmacotherapy, diet counseling, psychological therapy, and physical therapies provides the most optimal outcomes. The synergy of these modalities promises to provide hope for the successful treatment of the multifaceted nature of gastrointestinal and liver diseases. Ongoing research should aim to validate these multimodal strategies by rigorous clinical trials, thereby ushering the way for following innovations in treatment protocols that optimize patient care (Figure 12.14).

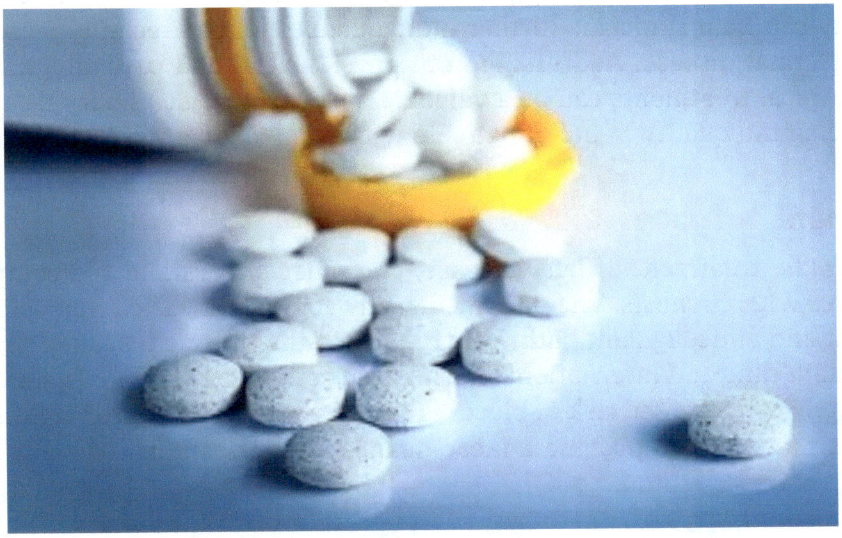

Figure 12.14. Medications used for treating injuries or medical conditions.

Source: https://assets.yourpractice.online/2259/3d-images/pharmacological-interventions-for-knee-injuries.jpg.

12.6.1. Surgical Interventions

Gastrointestinal and liver disease surgery has become a necessity in the management of various pathologies, especially where conservative treatment is not adequate. A good example is the treatment of severe obesity, which is connected with very dangerous health complications like type 2 diabetes and cardiovascular conditions. As highlighted in research, medical interventions , such as nutrition and behavior therapy generally experience low success rates among severe obesity populations, hence the viability of bariatric surgery. Bariatric surgery, including gastric bypass and sleeve gastrectomy, not only results in marked weight loss but also optimizes co-morbidities of obesity. Surgical intervention has a high degree of efficacy in practice, underlining the importance of surgical treatment of illnesses not manageable with traditional approaches. Secondly, this is the role of surgical intervention in treating gastrointestinal diseases , such as colorectal cancer, inflammatory bowel disease, and hernias. Operations , such as laparoscopic resections and colostomies provide techniques that are minimally invasive yet suit the demands of modern patient care. The development of surgical techniques and technologies facilitates earlier diagnosis and customized treatment strategies that have the potential to significantly improve patient outcomes. Moreover, patients experience shorter recovery times and fewer risks for postoperative complications, which is important in the care of chronic conditions often associated with gastrointestinal disease. Individualizing the surgical procedure to the specific pathology and patient condition is important because these procedures not only produce symptomatic relief but are a possible cure for many debilitating illnesses. The complex interaction between surgery and the psychological aspects of gastrointestinal illness must also be considered. Conditions , such as irritable bowel syndrome (IBS) are stress-related, hence pointing towards the need for a comprehensive treatment system that combines surgical and psychological management. Evidence attests that stress plays a dominant role in causing gastrointestinal symptoms and outcomes of treatment. Understanding of the brain-gut axis and the mechanisms by which stress influences visceral sensitivity can help clinicians further individualize surgical techniques and postoperative care for gastrointestinal disease. Addressing both physiological and psychological components of these diseases, surgical treatments can be a valuable part of interdisciplinary treatment programs, ultimately enhancing the quality of life of patients with complex liver and gastrointestinal disease.

12.6.2. Treatment for Liver Disorders

When considering the treatment of liver disease, one must understand the complex interplay of hemostatic changes with cirrhosis. The patients usually come with varied hemostatic profiles with both procoagulant and anticoagulant pathways, rendering the routine means of procedural control tedious. Prothrombin time and international normalized ratio, the routine coagulation tests, cannot be used to accurately estimate the risk of bleeding from liver disease. Newer techniques, like global trials of hemostasis, attempt to provide a more nuanced understanding of hemostatic balance.

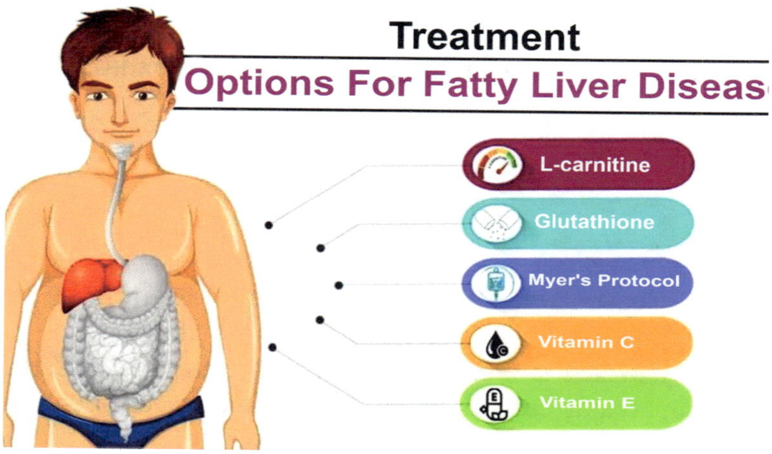

Figure 12.15. Treatment options for fatty liver include L-carnitine, glutathione, vitamins C and E, and Myer's protocol.

Source: https://www.carewellmedicalcentre.com/wp-content/uploads/2025/03/treatment-options-for-fatty-liver-1200x675-1-1024x576.jpg.

These innovations potentially allow the clinician to more accurately evaluate risk for bleeding and choose ideal therapies for procedures that are low risk superficially but that genuinely threaten the patient with compromised liver function, thus enhancing overall management of liver disease (Northup et al., 2020). In pharmacologic management, newer agents are promising in controlling liver disease with thrombocytopenia. Avatrombopag and lusutrombopag, thrombopoietin receptor agonists, have been effective at increasing platelet counts before procedures. Precaution is taken because clinical evidence shows that simply increasing the platelet count is not inversely proportional to a reduction in the incidence of bleeding complications. This highlights the need for a personalized approach based on patient profiles and the nature of the procedure. The role of liver function, nature of procedure, and systemic components is still crucial in developing treatment plans for the successful management of patients with chronic liver disease (Alexander et al., 2020). Non-pharmacological measures are also vital in the management of liver conditions. For instance, dietary and lifestyle modifications play an important role in the modulation of liver disease and health. Patients are typically advised to have a properly balanced diet with high fruit, vegetables, and lean protein and low saturated fats and alcohol consumption through processed food. The control and monitoring of co-morbid conditions , such as obesity and diabetes, also come with liver disorder treatments. Moreover, increasing evidence suggests that lifestyle modifications along with mindfulness skills can calm patients and enhance their well-being, which ultimately culminates in enhanced outcomes in the treatment of liver disease. Integrative approaches target not just the physiology of liver disease but also the psychological and social aspects during recovery (Northup et al., 2020) (Figure 12.15).

12.6.3. Lifestyle Changes and Dietary Recommendations

To minimize the risk of gastrointestinal and liver disease, the inclusion of lifestyle changes in conjunction with diet is essential. A vital part of the facilitation of the gastrointestinal tract is the application of a well-balanced diet that includes high levels of dietary fiber, fruits, and vegetables. These elements aid in regulating bowel movements and ensuring the proper functioning of the digestive system. Notably, long-term improper nutrition can lead to a whole range of health issues, including obesity and gastrointestinal system disorders, due to a deficiency in the consumption of dietary fiber (Krotova et al., 2024). Insertion of fiber-rich food into the diet and reduction of consumption of processed food containing carcinogenic additives would greatly lower the possibility of such disorders' development. Encouraging whole food intake benefits not just better digestion but also facilitate enhanced lifestyle practices that foster general wellness. In addition to diet, lifestyle modifications are essential in managing gastrointestinal disease. Stress-reducing therapies , such as meditation, yoga, or exercise, are useful strategies for individuals with symptomatology from functional gastrointestinal disorders. Syndromes like irritable bowel syndrome (IBS), which include symptoms of bloating and abdominal pain, typically have stress as a major trigger (Akyüz et al., 2024). Therefore, creating a stronger mind-body relationship is essential in symptom control. Also, creating a pattern of regular eating rather than irregular eating may maintain the normality of the gut. Emphasizing the importance of hydration is also crucial, with appropriate water intake aiding digestion and nutrient uptake, thus avoiding gastrointestinal distress complications. Finally, individual dietary recommendations should also be considered in terms of the individual patients' particular symptoms and underlying conditions. In diagnosed patients with IBS, a personalized approach with diet and lifestyle changes can create dramatic relief in symptoms. For instance, the implementation of a low-FODMAP diet can significantly alleviate symptoms as well as enhance the quality of life in the patient (Akyüz et al., 2024). Furthermore, follow-up consultations and visits with medical professionals can provide sufficient support to refine such dietary interventions in the long term. It is necessary to realize that lifestyle and dietary changes are not short-term measures but fundamental pillars that facilitate long-term wellness. Ultimately, an integrative approach that includes nutrition, stress management, and medical advice is critical for the effective treatment of gastrointestinal and liver disease.

CLOSER LOOK

INFLAMMATORY

Inflammation is the body's natural defense response to injury, infection, or harmful stimuli. It is an essential part of the immune system, designed to protect and heal the body. There are two main types of inflammation: acute and chronic. Acute inflammation is short-term and occurs immediately after tissue damage—for example, swelling and redness after a cut or infection. It involves the release of immune cells, cytokines, and increased blood flow to the affected area, which helps eliminate pathogens and start the healing process. However, when inflammation becomes chronic, it can lead to long-term tissue damage and contribute to a range of diseases. Chronic inflammatory conditions include rheumatoid arthritis, inflammatory bowel disease (IBD), psoriasis, asthma, and even chronic diseases such as heart disease, diabetes, obesity, and cancer. In these cases, the immune system mistakenly attacks healthy tissues, or the inflammatory response remains active longer than necessary, causing harm instead of healing.

Several factors contribute to chronic inflammation, including poor diet, physical inactivity, chronic stress, smoking, pollution, and infections that don't completely resolve. Pro-inflammatory foods such as refined sugars, trans fats, and processed meats can worsen inflammation, while anti-inflammatory foods like fruits, vegetables, fatty fish, nuts, and whole grains can help reduce it. Symptoms of chronic inflammation can be subtle, such as fatigue, joint pain, digestive problems, and general malaise, making it harder to detect early. Treatment focuses on identifying and managing the underlying cause, using anti-inflammatory medications, lifestyle changes, and dietary interventions. The while inflammation is a protective response, chronic inflammation can be harmful and is linked to many serious health conditions. Understanding and managing inflammation through a healthy lifestyle is key to long-term wellness and disease prevention.

SUMMARY

The complex interplay between liver and gastrointestinal illnesses necessitates a detailed understanding of pathophysiology and treatment. The complexity of these diseases, particularly those involving bile acid homeostasis and gut microbiota, signifies deep therapeutic challenges. Studies , such as the evaluation of maralixibat for pruritus of primary biliary cholangitis (PBC) show the inadequacy of existing therapies and underscore the necessity of new strategies. While maralixibat was promising, the fact that there was no significant difference in pruritus reduction in the treatment and placebo groups implies the need for ongoing research into effective interventions. This attests to the dynamic nature of gastrointestinal and liver diseases that call for ongoing research to explore new therapies and modify current treatment regimens to suit patients better (Apostol et al., 2019). Furthermore, the gut microbiota has emerged as a central element in gastrointestinal disease etiology. Current research emphasizes that dysbiosis can be the source of mucosal alterations with far-reaching implications for gastrointestinal motility and health. Because microbiota could influence inflammatory responses and neuromuscular control, therapeutic potential of microbiome manipulation by probiotics and other interventions must not be overlooked. Such findings suggest that subsequent studies for microbiota-gastrointestinal disease interactions can open doors to novel therapeutic strategies that target the gut-brain axis and neuromuscular systems. Studying these interactions expands our understanding regarding how lifestyle factors, diet, and microbiotic community contribute to the pathogenesis of various conditions (Cicala et al., 2016). Lastly, management of gastrointestinal and hepatic illnesses primarily calls for multi-disciplinary collaboration in the form of medical research, clinical practice, and patient education. Increased awareness of symptomatic overlap between these conditions can lead to proper diagnosis and tailored treatment regimens. The intersection of novel pharmacological treatments with microbiome-directed therapies presents a window of opportunity for resilience against these often-disabling illnesses. In addition, public health initiatives aimed at the improvement of gastrointestinal well-being can be an addition to preventive interventions, reducing the prevalence of such disorders among the population. Thus, the creation of cooperation among researchers, clinicians, and patients will be essential in bringing about greater knowledge of gastrointestinal and liver disorders as well as the provision of effective treatments to the sufferers.

In elaborating on the context of gastrointestinal and liver diseases, it is required to describe the complex nature of the health threats involved. Among the most prominent issues in this line of inquiry is the escalating incidence of antimicrobial resistance (AMR) as a compelling problem for treatment effectiveness among various infections. The repercussions extend far, considering that AMR has been linked to nearly 4.95 million deaths due to bacterial infections globally in 2019, a sign that the intervention measures need to be substantial. Also, increased resistant infections , such as *Escherichia coli* and *Staphylococcus aureus,* underscore the clinical significance of AMR in gastrointestinal and liver disease, especially because these infections easily superimpose on pre-existing conditions and cause higher morbidity in the affected populations (Murray et al., 2022). Another critical area is in the pathophysiological pathways to such disorders. Recent studies have identified ferroptosis as a form of iron-dependent oxidative cellular death that plays a central role in numerous diseases of gastrointestinal and liver dysfunction. From the studies, ferroptosis is not an isolated process but is intimately associated with multiple diseases like ischemia-reperfusion injury and autoimmune disease. The accumulation of reactive oxygen species in ferroptosis induces massive cellular damage and raises the risk of gastrointestinal and liver disease burden. Understanding such mechanisms can provide valuable insights into potential targets for intervention (Li et al., 2020). Lastly, the roles of public health programs and policy responses cannot be overemphasized when addressing gastrointestinal and liver disease complexities. To combat AMR and the associated mortality rates, a multi-faceted approach comprising enhanced infection prevention practices and robust surveillance systems is necessary. Closing data gaps, particularly in low-resource settings, is paramount to successful policy implementation. With enhanced microbiology laboratory capabilities and study into new treatments, the healthcare community can better understand and combat the risks of AMR. Further study of ferroptosis in gastrointestinal disease also offers promising avenues forward for novel treatments, thereby reinforcing public health interventions and improving patient outcomes (Li et al., 2020; Murray et al., 2022).

References

1. Acharjee, D. (2025). Ayurvedic management of alcohol withdrawal: A case study. *International Journal of Ayurvedic Medicine*. https://www.semanticscholar.org/paper/01c3d0fc38d0c7fd02968e9e987a172a3c3f42bf (accessed on 13th June 2025).
2. Akyüz, F., Çelebi, A., Doğan, İ., Erzin, Y., Kav, T., Soytürk, M., Oğuz, D., et al. (2024). Functional bowel disorder management in routine practice with tips for hot topics: Expert opinion review. *The Turkish Journal of Gastroenterology, 35*, 423–439. https://www.semanticscholar.org/paper/488a4007e66922beeb834ba0f23e439d9deb07e1 (accessed on 13th June 2025).
3. Alvina, R., Kansra, S., Lakkunarajah, S., & Jay, M. S. (2021). Childhood and adolescent obesity: A review. *Frontiers in Pediatrics, 8*. https://doi.org/10.3389/fped.2020.581461 (accessed on 13th June 2025).
4. Hertlein, L., Stieber, P., Kirschenhofer, A., Krocker, K., Nagel, D., Lenhard, M., & Burges, A. (2012). Human epididymis protein 4 (HE4) in benign and malignant diseases. *Clinical chemistry and laboratory medicine, 50*(12), 2181–2188. https://doi.org/10.1515/cclm-2012-0097(accessed on 13th June 2025).
5. Guarini, A., De Marinis, F., Hassan, C., Manta, R., De Francesco, V., Annibale, B., & Zullo, A. (2018). High concordance between trained nurses and gastroenterologists in evaluating recordings of small bowel video capsule endoscopy (VCE). *Journal of gastrointestinal and liver diseases: JGLD, 27*(2), 271. https://doi.org/10.15403/jgld.2014.1121.272.bch (accessed on 13th June 2025).
6. Apostol, G., Bacon, B., Bowlus, C. L., Dorenbaum, A., et al. (2019). A randomized, controlled, phase 2 study of maralixibat in the treatment of itching associated with primary biliary cholangitis. https://core.ac.uk/download/323068939.pdf (accessed on 13th June 2025).
7. Aziz, Q., Borsook, D., Elsenbruch, S., Kilpatrick, L., et al. (2019). Role of brain imaging in disorders of brain-gut interaction: A Rome Working Team report. https://core.ac.uk/download/323078713.pdf (accessed on 13th June 2025).
8. Baal, J., van Dijcker, J. C., Hendriks, W. H., et al. (2011). Influence of nutrition on feline calcium oxalate urolithiasis with emphasis on endogenous oxalate synthesis. https://core.ac.uk/download/pdf/29235447.pdf (accessed on 13th June 2025).
9. Bacalbașa, N., Banu, P., Bălălău, C., Ghinghină, I., et al. (2019). The risk of bleeding and encephalopathy in surgical patients with liver cirrhosis. https://core.ac.uk/download/216811033.pdf (accessed on 13th June 2025).
10. Bax, B. E. (2020). Mitochondrial neurogastrointestinal encephalomyopathy: Approaches to diagnosis and treatment. https://core.ac.uk/download/287649788.pdf (accessed on 13th June 2025).
11. Bilzer, M., Ehrentraut, S., Gerbes, A. L., Kapfhammer, H. P., et al. (2002). Psychiatric and psychosocial outcome of orthotopic liver transplantation. https://core.ac.uk/download/16432271.pdf (accessed on 13th June 2025).
12. Rémond, D., Shahar, D. R., Gille, D., Pinto, P., Kachal, J., Peyron, M. A., Dos Santos, C. N., Walther, B., Bordoni, A., Dupont, D., Tomás-Cobos, L., & Vergères, G. (2015). Understanding the gastrointestinal tract of the elderly to develop dietary solutions that prevent malnutrition. *Oncotarget, 6*(16), 13858–13898. https://doi.org/10.18632/oncotarget.4030(accessed on 13th June 2025).

13. Boru, E. C., Guida, A., Iossa, A., Rengo, M., et al. (2017). 25th International Congress of the European Association for Endoscopic Surgery (EAES) Frankfurt, Germany, 14–17 June 2017: Oral presentations. https://core.ac.uk/download/141696623.pdf (accessed on 13th June 2025).

14. Cai, L., Chen, Z., Duan, Z., Han, X., et al. (2016). Vitamin D signaling through induction of Paneth cell defensins maintains gut microbiota and improves metabolic disorders and hepatic steatosis in animal models. https://core.ac.uk/download/323071972.pdf (accessed on 13th June 2025).

15. Calabrese, F., Marabotto, E., Mari, A., Pasta, L., et al. (2024). The clinical spectrum of gastroesophageal reflux disease: Facts and fictions. https://core.ac.uk/download/643641496.pdf (accessed on 13th June 2025).

16. Cicala, M., Guarino, M. P., Putignani, L., Severi, C., et al. (2016). Gastrointestinal neuromuscular apparatus: An underestimated target of gut microbiota. https://core.ac.uk/download/98336463.pdf (accessed on 13th June 2025).

17. D'Alessandro, A., Esposito, G., Gigli, S., et al. (2018). Endocannabinoid-related compounds in gastrointestinal diseases. https://core.ac.uk/download/127586499.pdf (accessed on 13th June 2025).

18. Eom, Y. S., Wilson, J. R., & Bernet, V. (2022). Links between thyroid disorders and glucose homeostasis. *Diabetes & Metabolism Journal, 46*, 239–256. https://doi.org/10.4093/dmj.2022.0013 (accessed on 13th June 2025).

19. Fleming, J. O., Maizels, R., & Varyani, F. (2017). Helminths in the gastrointestinal tract as modulators of immunity and pathology. https://core.ac.uk/download/80697189.pdf (accessed on 13th June 2025).

20. Ghosh, S., Whitley, C. S., Haribabu, B., & Jala, V. R. (2021). Regulation of intestinal barrier function by microbial metabolites. *Cellular and Molecular Gastroenterology and Hepatology, 11*, 1463–1482. https://doi.org/10.1016/j.jcmgh.2021.02.007 (accessed on 13th June 2025).

21. Grinevich, V., & Kravchuk, Y. (2021). Diseases of the digestive organs and COVID-19. *Russian Military Medical Academy Reports*. https://www.semanticscholar.org/paper/d01280a7715c1bc7675bb788a5b89810670c7c88 (accessed on 13th June 2025).

22. Hou, K., Wu, Z. X., Chen, X. Y., Wang, J. Q., Zhang, D., Xiao, C., Zhu, D., et al. (2022). Microbiota in health and diseases. *Signal Transduction and Targeted Therapy, 7*. https://doi.org/10.1038/s41392-022-00974-4 (accessed on 13th June 2025).

23. Krotova, O., Efimov, D., Detochenko, L., Orobinskaya, V., Kholodova, E., & Eroshenko, A. (2024). Problems and prospects of functional nutrition in Russia: Industry and social aspect. *BIO Web of Conferences*. https://www.semanticscholar.org/paper/bab2a43b04433951fc051e69fd6da79befb8f0a7 (accessed on 13th June 2025).

24. Larauche, M., Mulak, A., & Taché, Y. (2011). Stress-related alterations of visceral sensation: Animal models for irritable bowel syndrome study. https://core.ac.uk/download/323080393.pdf (accessed on 13th June 2025).

25. Leissner, P., Olsson, E. M. G., Rondung, E., Sundelin, R., Spaak, J., Ulvenstam, A., Nordenskjöld, A. M., et al. (2025). Mental health status and quality-of-life after an acute myocardial

infarction with non-obstructive coronary arteries or takotsubo syndrome: A systematic review. *European Journal of Preventive Cardiology*. https://www.semanticscholar.org/paper/fcdd6bb5bfc66ca1778a324c1e8226576c3a3b7f (accessed on 13th June 2025).

26. Li, J., Cao, F., Yin, H., Huang, Z., Lin, Z., Mao, N., Sun, B., et al. (2020). Ferroptosis: Past, present and future. *Cell Death and Disease, 11*. https://doi.org/10.1038/s41419-020-2298-2 (accessed on 13th June 2025).

27. Magrin, L., Contiero, B., Cozzi, G., & Gottardo, F. (2022). Data on gastrointestinal and claw disorders as possible predictive factors in beef cattle and veal calves' health and welfare. *Data, 7*, 43. https://www.semanticscholar.org/paper/0dca5bdf4e2a7820f85efeb2393f0cf5d87713d5 (accessed on 13th June 2025).

28. Northup, P. G., García-Pagán, J. C., García–Tsao, G., Intagliata, N. M., Superina, R., Roberts, L. N., Lisman, T., et al. (2020). Vascular liver disorders, portal vein thrombosis, and procedural bleeding in patients with liver disease: 2020 practice guidance by the American Association for the Study of Liver Diseases. *Hepatology, 73*, 366–413. https://doi.org/10.1002/hep.31646 (accessed on 13th June 2025).

29. Park, S. C., & Jeen, Y. (2016). The mental health state of quiescent inflammatory bowel disease patients. *Gut and Liver, 10*, 330–331. https://www.semanticscholar.org/paper/4534fff46b83ec8458ee3fa2b23eb73a762bb53a (accessed on 13th June 2025).

30. Pyzik, M., Sand, K. M. K., Hubbard, J. J., Andersen, J. T., Sandlie, I., & Blumberg, R. S. (2019). The neonatal Fc receptor (FcRn): A misnomer? *Frontiers in Immunology, 10*. https://doi.org/10.3389/fimmu.2019.01540 (accessed on 13th June 2025).

31. Visseren, F. L. J., Mach, F., Smulders, Y. M., Carballo, D., Koskinas, K. C., Bäck, M., Bénétos, A., et al. (2021). 2021 ESC guidelines on cardiovascular disease prevention in clinical practice. *European Heart Journal, 42*, 3227–3337. https://doi.org/10.1093/eurheartj/ehab484 (accessed on 13th June 2025).

32. Zheng, D., Liwinski, T., & Elinav, E. (2020). Interaction between microbiota and immunity in health and disease. *Cell Research, 30*, 492–506. https://doi.org/10.1038/s41422-020-0332-7 (accessed on 13th June 2025).

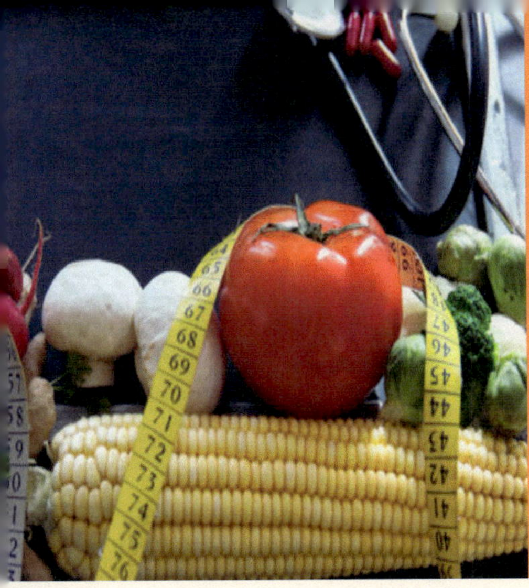

Chapter 13
NUTRITIONAL DISORDERS IN SPECIAL POPULATIONS

Contents

Introduction....417
13.1. Nutritional Disorders in Children....420
13.2. Nutritional Disorders in the Elderly....424
13.3. Nutritional Disorders in Pregnant Women....428
13.4. Nutrition Disorders Among Athletes....432
13.5. Nutritional Disorders Among Persons with Disabilities....436
13.6. Cultural Influences on Nutritional Disorders....440
Summary....445
References....447

Introduction

Understanding the complexities of nutritional disorders requires careful study of special populations that include vulnerable segments , such as ethnic minorities, students, and the elderly. These populations are inclined to have unusual dietary needs and are also subject to peculiar challenges that increase their exposure to nutritional disorders. Reality proves that eating disorders (EDs), usually associated with stereotypes of certain groups, in fact cross racial and ethnic boundaries. Even as recognition of eating disorder behavior in diverse populations has grown, discrepancies in diagnosis and treatment persist, which suggests systemic deficits in proportionately impacting minority ethnic populations to appropriate care (Tuomainen et al., 2024). This points to a critical need for more representative research and intervention strategies that are tailored to meet these disparities. Further, the dietary and health status of students remains a particularly relevant concern in this regard. When students are dealing with academic stress and pressures, their eating habits suffer, resulting in a host of complications to their health. A study at Felix Houphouët University illustrates how students are subject to a number of gastrointestinal disorders due to poor diet and environmental factors (Anon et al., 2024). With 5.29% of the students being underweight and others suffering from obesity or being overweight, the health implications are enormous.

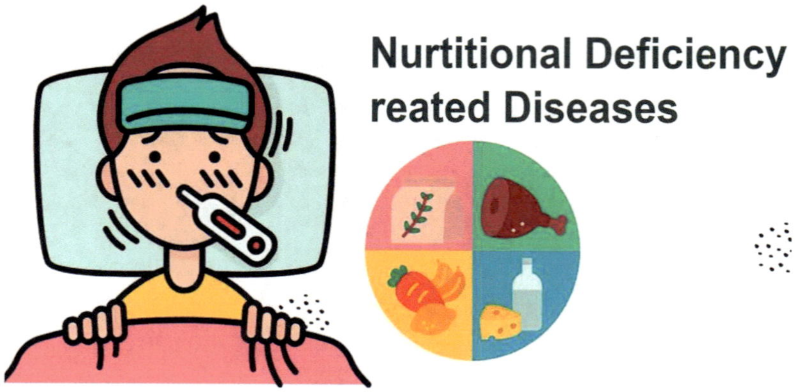

Figure 13.1. Nutritional deficiencies can lead to diet-related diseases and poor health.

Source: https://anthroholic.com/wp-content/uploads/2024/03/Nutritional-Deficiency-Related-Diseases-in-Anthropology.webp.

In addition to the stress of university life, these findings underscore the necessity of addressing nutrition education and awareness on university campuses to minimize the risks of nutritional disorders in this group. With these findings, it is clear that nutritional disorders among special populations are worthy of attention and intervention. The solution to the challenges, therefore, needs to be multi-dimensional, addressing the socio-cultural, economic, and psychological determinants of disordered eating and inadequate diet. Existing literature on the topic indicates a pressing need for specialized research that goes beyond prevalence to examine access to care and treatment. Through focusing attention on collective efforts between researchers, clinicians, and policymakers, policies can be created that would enhance access to healthy food and healthier dietary habits among these individuals. Ultimately, such steps are necessary in ushering into a healthier future and reducing nutritional disorder prevalence among high-risk populations (Figure 13.1).

Definition of Nutritional Disorders

In the complex setting of health and wellbeing, nutritional disorders provide a fascinating instance of the intersection of physiology, diet, and health. Nutritional disorders are characterized by a dealignment of nutritional supply and consequential adverse health consequences, which can occur in the form of deficiencies, overloads, or malabsorption of important nutrients. Nutritional disorders have varying effects on different groups, particularly those susceptible due to social, economic, or medical factors. For instance, developmentally disabled children may have unique problems that complicate their nutritional needs and require them to their growth and overall health. The complications point to the need for a precise definition of nutritional disorders that not only consider the physical manifestations of the inadequate or excessive consumption of nutrition but also the psychosocial factors affecting dietary habits and food intake. Nutritional disorders have extended to appreciate the multidimensional nature of the conditions, particularly in special populations. PFDs, for example, have emerged to symbolize a distinct class of nutritional disorders that underscore the subtlety of addressing low intake that is most frequently interwoven with medical and psychosocial dysfunction. According to new paradigms, PFDs are characterized as feeding difficulties that involve inappropriate oral intake and multiple related functional limitations, therefore requiring an interdisciplinary team approach for efficacious treatment and management. This change in definition emphasizes needing to consider more than simply social functioning and incorporates other such variables as feeding skills and the psychosocial context within which feeding choices are made, ultimately resulting in practitioners prescribing more holistic and targeted interventions for those affected (Browne et al., 2019). Also, the overlap of nutritional and mental health disorders has important implications for treatment and definition, particularly when discussed within special populations like children and adolescents. Mental illness can disrupt adherence to necessary diet regimens and therefore, exacerbate nutritional disorders. The recognition of the importance of mental health in enabling nutritional adherence means that effective interventions must address not only the physical realm of nutrition but also the psychological basis of diet behavior. Special groups , such as street children and repatriated child soldiers, are the best examples of this challenge because they hardly enjoy the stable contexts required for healthy development and eating patterns. The comprehension of subtleties in these interactions allows for a wider framework for detection and intervention of nutritional disorders, ultimately supplementing physical and mental health outcomes in such high-risk populations (Belfer, 2005).

Importance of Studying Special Populations

The study of special populations is crucial in understanding the complicated nutrition disorders that exist among these populations. Special populations like children, the elderly, pregnant individuals, and chronically diseased individuals have different dietary needs that differ from those of the normal population. Iron deficiency, for instance, is prevalent in risk groups like young children and pregnant women and hence needs special nutritional interventions to ensure adequate iron status and prevent anemia. An understanding of the risk factors and nutritional requirements of such groups enables health professionals to provide proper dietary recommendations and advice. As noted from existing research, continuous monitoring of the status of iron and appropriate supplementation can significantly enhance the health status of patients with increased risk of deficiency, demonstrating the necessity for targeted research and clinical interventions in special populations (Mć-Ćirić et al., 2023). Moreover, the implications of special population taste disorders indicate the necessity for comprehensive studies. These conditions can seriously compromise individuals' quality of life through the diminution of their ability to enjoy food and lead to malnutrition. Accurate diagnosis and the best possible treatment of taste disorders are central to enhancing dietary behavior in affected individuals, , such as the elderly or patients undergoing medical treatments that inhibit the perception of taste. The lack of current clinical expertise and effective treatments for taste disorders reflects the acute need for research establishing effective therapeutic modalities. Prioritizing research into taste disorders would allow clinicians to more effectively design treatment regimens that operate in harmony to address the physical and psychological effects of these disorders, ultimately improving overall nutritional intake and health in special populations (Hsieh et al., 2022). Incorporating interventions that respond to the unique nutritional requirements of special populations has a critical influence on public health initiatives. Targeting individualized diet advice from the distinct features of such populations can allow for early identification and treatment of nutritional disorders. Early intervention is required in reversing common issues , such as obesity, malnutrition, and chronic diseases that disproportionately affect members of special populations. By giving prominence to the importance of research on special populations, health practitioners can formulate evidence-based and culturally tailored nutrition plans. Not only do these programs facilitate healthier diet habits, but they also inform individuals about the tools and information vital for effective management of nutritional health. The importance of studying special populations, thus, extends beyond pedagogy to include actionable plans that have immediate impacts on health outcomes (Figure 13.2).

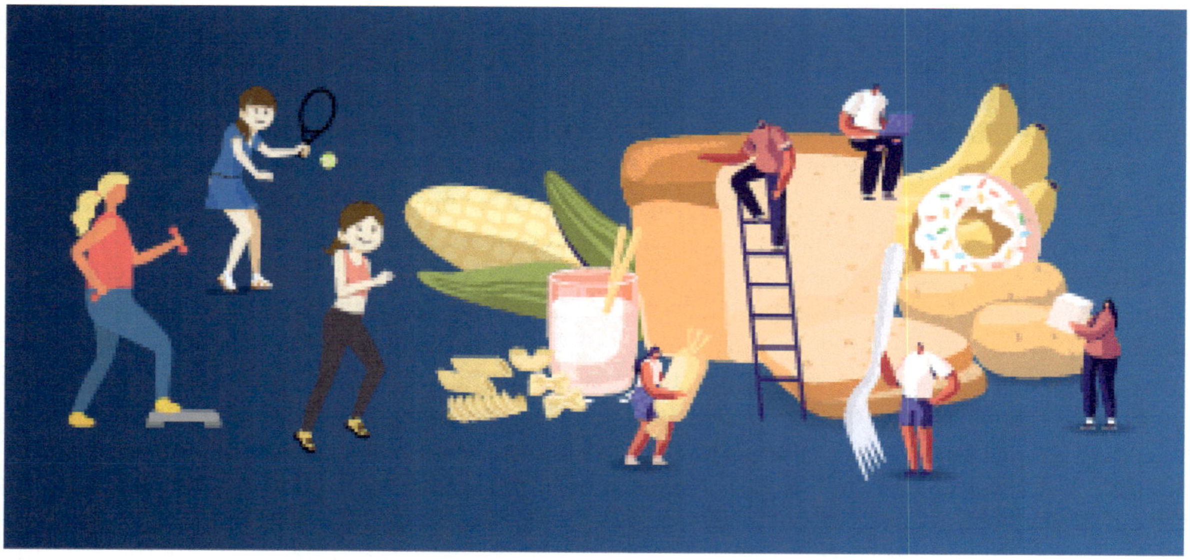

Figure 13.2. Balanced nutrition and physical activity tailored to special populations for optimal health.

Source: https://dosily.com/wp-content/uploads/2020/10/General-Medicine_Nutrition-For-Special-Population.png.

13.1. Nutritional Disorders in Children

The incidence of nutritional disorders in children reflects the critical need to appreciate comprehensively the complex factors underlying these conditions. Among the many manifestations of nutritional disorders, the malabsorption syndromes are particularly remarkable for their complexity and the significant developmental impact they have in pediatric populations. Malabsorption may be caused by a wide variety of congenital as well as acquired disorders, such as cystic fibrosis and coeliac disease. Early detection of such disorders is crucial as they can lead to malnutrition and, as a result, growth issues. Nutritional care plays a central role in the management of malabsorption, and it usually consists of individualized dietary therapy and supplementation according to the specific requirements of each child, thus emphasizing interprofessional care between pediatric experts as well as primary healthcare practitioners (Lenti et al., 2025). Treating such disorders, in addition to guaranteeing physical health, also benefits overall psychological and intellectual development in children. The nutritional needs of children with autism spectrum disorder (ASD) are another field that needs successful research under the subject of nutritional disorders. Children with ASD are selective eaters and show aversions to certain textures or tastes, which result in an inappropriate intake of nutrition. It has been found that most children with ASD are at a high risk for developing deficiencies of critical vitamins and minerals, , such as calcium, vitamin D, and iron. Recent evidence indicates that the occurrence of specific dietary patterns in such children, , such as low carbs or high sugar, may worsen behavior-related issues and inhibit social interactions (Kim et al., 2025). Thus, nutrition interventions that are targeted towards children's food preferences and sensory sensitivities can be fundamental to guaranteeing their growth and development and minimizing behavioral issues. One must collaborate with dietitians and nutritionists when coming up with appealing diet plans that will encourage sound eating behavior. Generally speaking, the overlap among nutritional disorders and the unique needs of special groups , such as children, requires an all-embracing response to assessment and management. Preventive interventions are vital in an attempt to identify high-risk children, particularly those with longstanding medical conditions or neurodevelopmental disorders, who are at potential risk for deficiency. Regular nutritional screening and assessment can facilitate early intervention, modifying dietary advice to promote optimal growth and health outcomes. Family and education are also important because caregivers must be taught to make smart nutritional choices in the presence of their children's varying needs and wants. By creating an interdisciplinary system that incorporates medical, educational, and psychological perspectives, health professionals can make a significant contribution to the children's quality of life with nutritional disorders (Lenti et al., 2025; Kim et al., 2025) (Figure 13.3).

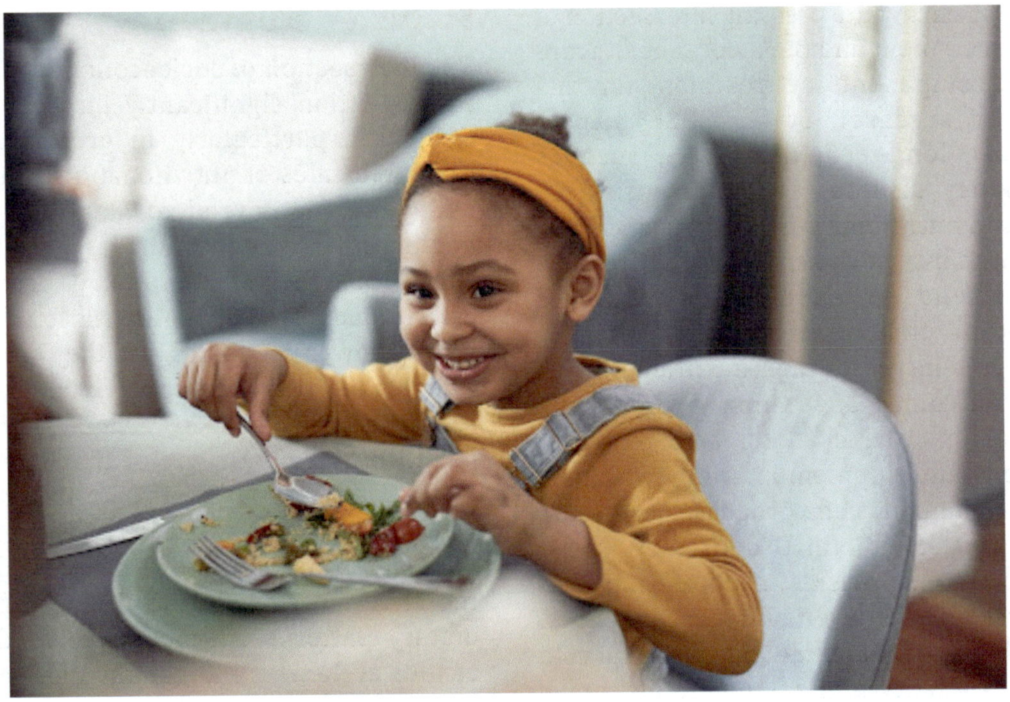

Figure 13.3. A child enjoying a nutritious meal, promoting healthy eating habits from a young age.

Source: https://wakeforestpediatrics.com/wp-content/uploads/2023/09/unnamed.jpg.

13.1.1. Common Disorders Affecting Children

Childhood nutritional disorders can be compounded by the common developmental and behavioral disorders that exert a significant impact on their food intake and overall health. Autism Spectrum Disorder (ASD), a neurodevelopmental disorder affecting social interaction and communication, is likely to result in dietary deficiencies due to sensory sensitivities and selective food consumption characteristic of affected children. Evidence shows that most children with ASD have unbalanced diets, leading to less than adequate consumption of such nutrients as vitamins D, B1, iron, and calcium, which are important for their development and growth. These nutritional imbalances can have widespread implications, causing physical sickness in concert with the psychic symptoms of autism, thereby emphasizing the pressing intersection of nutrition assessment and behavioral healthcare as integral components of treatment for this population (Jørgensen et al., 2025). Apart from autism, long-term illnesses, , such as chronic kidney disease (CKD), are also very susceptible to nutritional deficiency, particularly in major vitamins , such as vitamin D. Children with CKD tend to experience metabolic dysregulation that inhibits their dietary absorption and increases their nutritional need. The poor outcomes of vitamin D deficiency in CKD highlight the need for stringent diet management and supplementation regimens. Current recommendations propose monitoring and treatment of vitamin D deficiency in the children to diminish risks , such as impaired bone health and its attendant consequences. Nutritional interventions can play a pivotal role in improving quality of life and care outcomes among children with chronic diseases in the face of adversity from the diseases (Jørgensen et al., 2025). Additionally, gastrointestinal issues are more likely to occur with various developmental disorders, increasing the complexity of nutrition. Gastrointestinal symptoms in most children with ASD include diarrhea and constipation, which impede their ability to consume a balanced diet. These gastrointestinal issues can result in malabsorption of nutrients, with a resultant large deficiency that compromises growth and development. Interventions , such as parent nutrition education programs, are critical to addressing the challenges since they can help families establish well-formulated diets suited to the special nutritional needs of children. Collaboration between healthcare practitioners, nutritionists, and families can assist in ensuring the delivery of adequate nutrition to children despite developmental and gastrointestinal disorders, which subsequently will result in enhanced long-term health effects (Alp et al., 2025).

13.1.2. Impact of Socioeconomic Status on Nutrition

The intersection of socioeconomic status (SES) and nutrition significantly impacts outcomes of health, particularly in groups at risk of increased rates of nutritional disorders. Lower SES populations tend to have less access to healthy sources of food and, as such, their diets consist of higher consumption of processed and caloric foods. The economic restrictions curb the buying power of families, and they have to resort to using more affordable food, which is usually less healthy and leans towards obesity and other health problems. On top of that, the residents of food deserts also have limited options to visit grocery stores that carry fresh fruits and vegetables and other healthy food, making the situation even worse. These variations in dietary patterns and access to food create a vicious cycle where unhealthy diet perpetuates health inequality, illustrating the important link between SES and nutritional status in vulnerable populations. Moreover, the impacts of SES on nutrition extend beyond individual food choice behaviors to include broader, more systematic factors, including education and health literacy.

Individuals from lower SES backgrounds often have less access to nutritional education, which hinders their ability to make informed dietary choices. This lack of knowledge regarding healthy eating practices can lead to misconceptions about nutrition, thus perpetuating unhealthy eating patterns. For instance, individuals may prioritize calorie-dense foods that offer short-term satiation, neglecting essential nutrients needed for long-term health. In addition, cultural and community factors also influence food patterns and hence contribute to a complex set of determinants to regulate nutrition in low-SES populations. Bridging these educational gaps is crucial in implementing effective public health interventions that can improve nutritional outcomes as well as reduce health disparities in marginalized groups.

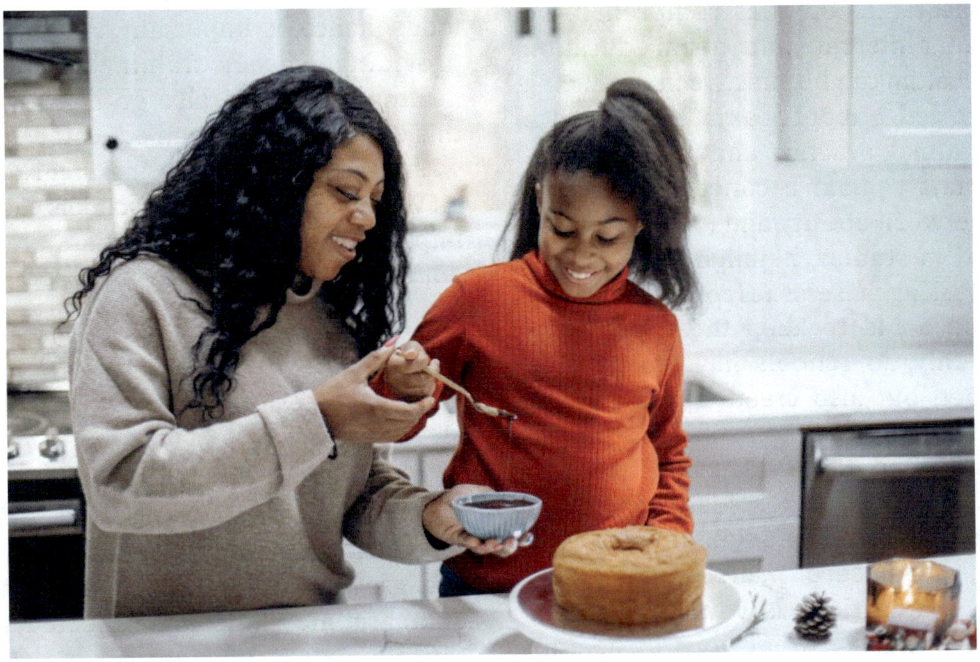

Figure 13.4. Mother and daughter cook together, promoting healthy eating and bonding.

Source: https://culinahealth.com/wp-content/uploads/2024/04/mother-daughter-cooking-scaled.jpg.

Lastly, socioeconomic status affects nutritional outcomes by playing a role in access to, as well as utilization of, healthcare. Low SES patients are frequently confronted with several barriers to healthcare, and this serves to restrict them from receiving appropriate nutritional counseling as well as prevention services. This lack of access plays its role in the higher incidences of nutrition-disease, including diabetes, hypertension, and obesity, particularly among special populations. Furthermore, during health crisis periods, , such as the COVID-19 pandemic, these problems are exacerbated, as evidenced by the necessity for targeted interventions in individuals with substance use disorders (Volkow, 2020). Furthermore, food insecurity can also affect vulnerable populations, which becomes more relevant within the present economic situation. Substantial policies that narrow these disparities and promote equitable access to nutritional and health care resources will be essential to altering the impact of socioeconomic status on health and well-being among these groups (Figure 13.4).

13.1.3. Role of Schools in Promoting Healthy Eating

Schools play an important part in enhancing the diet and health condition of children, especially among those at high risk of nutritional problems. Schools are in a good position to influence the attitudes of students towards food through organized programs and activities aimed at promoting healthy eating. In studies, it has been established that comprehensive approaches that integrate nutritional education into the curriculum can be effective in enhancing students' knowledge about healthy eating habits. However, minimal practice and evaluation of these programs remain a concern. The very strong link between obesity and food insecurity, as delineated in studies, highlights the urgent need for addressing these issues comprehensively in schools. In a bid to keep these problems at bay, not only do schools have to provide nutritious food but also create a culture that prioritizes health literacy to facilitate students in making informed dietary decisions (Laitsch et al., 2009). To add on, stakeholder cooperation cannot be emphasized enough. Involvement of families, healthcare professionals, and community organizations is vital in terms of recruiting an inclusive framework of healthy eating. The partnership can be through workshops or public gatherings in which not only are individuals enlightened, but families are also involved in the children's nutrition process. The academic pressure closes the gap for healthy nutrition among students, hence propagating existing health disparities. Schools are assisted in preventing obesity complications and their accompanying health indicators when they emphasize and promote healthy eating. Such inter-disciplinary collaboration would be of great value to health outcomes across varying groups of people, ranging from economically disadvantaged individuals, who are similarly disadvantaged in terms of access to healthy food Edwards et al, 2022). Finally, ongoing support and firm funding are essential for the sustenance of school eating healthy programs. Schools lack the requisite resources necessary to implement comprehensive programs due to insufficient finances. As concluded in several studies, one of the key challenges to effective nutritional education is the shortage of funding allocated for such programs, which may hinder schools from offering wholesome food regularly. Raising awareness for fostering policies that provide sustained funding and access to healthy foods, hence, is important. Programs aimed at providing teacher training in nutrition and healthy eating can also go hand in hand with this effort and create an educated support base within schools. By creating a culture centered on well-being and health, schools can reduce the impact of nutritional disorders among special populations considerably and create a healthier future for all students (Edwards et al, 2022).

13.2. Nutritional Disorders in the Elderly

Malnutrition among older adults is a primary and growing concern in population health, as demographic shifts are expected to increase the population of older adults. Older adults are susceptible to many chronic conditions, including musculoskeletal disease and cognitive impairment, which adversely affect their nutritional status. As stated by older individuals tend to have a combination of conditions and thus are extremely prone to nutrient deficiencies. Poor nutritional attention not only causes physical worsening but also intensifies further cognitive deterioration, bringing about a cycle that perpetuates overall worsening in health. Thus, addressing nutritional issues among this population must be a well-rounded approach that considers individual nutritional needs, socioeconomics, and underlying medical issues, which can be barriers to eating healthy foods. One of the root causes of nutritional disorders among the elderly is the prevalence of age-related physiological changes that impact appetite, in addition to nutritional assimilation. For instance, senescence tends to cause changes in the perception of taste and smell, leading to the decreased desire to eat and consequently to less caloric intake. In addition, older individuals may suffer from chewing or swallowing impairment due to dental disease or other disorders, thereby contributing to their nutrition-related impairments. Edwards et al. (2022) posit that health care systems should develop targeted programs designed to reverse these unique barriers to the aged. Efficacious strategies may involve increasing the education of healthcare professionals and carers to detect and treat these conditions promptly, encouraging better diet and nutrition, and increasing quality of life. The social functions related to eating and nutrition also cannot be overlooked when talking about nutritional disorders among the elderly. Most of the older people are socially isolated and hence their motivational levels to prepare nutritious food diminish, and convenience foods become a prerequisite, which are mostly devoid of essential nutrients. Social interaction plays a vital role in encouraging healthy eating habits, and therefore, interventions by communities can help this segment immensely by not just boosting nutrition but also by giving them companionship and a feeling of psychological well-being. Collaborating with multidisciplinary groups, as outlined by Edwards et al. (2022), including geriatricians, dietitians, and social workers, can yield a comprehensive approach to meeting the nutritional needs of the elderly. The holistic care model is striving to enhance physical and psychosocial results, producing improved health outcomes for this vulnerable population (Figure 13.5).

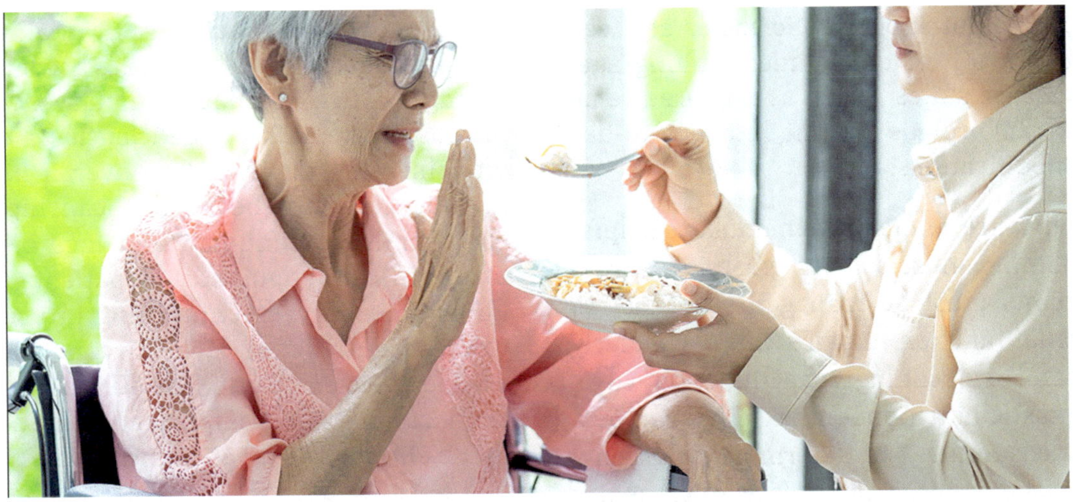

Figure 13.5. Elderly woman refusing food, highlighting nutritional challenges in aging populations.

Source: https://www.samvednacare.com/blog/wp-content/uploads/2020/01/5-Ways-to-Improve-Nutrition-in-the-Elderly.jpg.

13.2.1. Age-Related Changes Affecting Nutrition

With increasing age, certain changes occur in the body that impact nutritional requirements and dietary habits. One of the common alterations is a drop in metabolic rate with corresponding reduction in energy needs, which in turn tends to result in involuntary weight gain unless dietary adjustments are appropriately made. Taste and smell perception also decline with increasing age, which will impact appetite and food intake with resulting in poor nutrient consumption. These changes require a refined understanding of the specific nutritional needs of older individuals, emphasizing the importance of tailored dietary strategies to achieve adequate nutrient quality with respect to personal tastes and pathological conditions. These strategic planning actions can be successful in counterbalancing the risks of malnutrition, the most prevalent nutritional disorder among elderly people. Precision nutrition becomes increasingly relevant in addressing aging-related changes in nutrition. Individualized dietary guidance to fit the life cycles and consequent nutritional requirements of an individual may enhance nutrient intake and health. In the elderly, this means giving higher priority to essential vitamins and minerals that are often in short supply due to compromised absorption and dietary restrictions. Yoon et al. (2024) emphasize that tailored guidance, supported by country-level survey data, ensures these specific nutritional deficiencies are well managed. On top of that, understanding age-related disease states, , such as impaired renal function, can provide insight into day-to-day dietary modifications.

For instance, while protein intake is helpful in maintaining muscle mass, protein sources and amounts must be managed so as not to add to renal function impairment, particularly in the case of declining renal function. Also, the prognostic nutritional index (PNI) can be a helpful measurement to determine nutritional status in the elderly and relate it to health outcomes , such as renal function. Poor nutritional status, as indicated by lower PNI scores, has been seen to correlate with greater progression of renal impairment over time (Park et al., 2024). This relationship emphasizes the importance of surveillance of nutritional markers in the elderly to prevent compromise of vital health markers. The implementation of dietary interventions that retain or increase the PNI can therefore serve as a preventive strategy against nutritional abnormalities. Therefore, enhancement of nutritional awareness and implementation of age-related interventions can allow older people to sustain their health and nutrition and enjoy a healthier life in their older ages.

13.2.2. Common Deficiencies in Elderly Populations

Since the population of older persons are growing, it is becoming increasingly vital to detect and treat prevalent nutritional deficiencies. Malnutrition is one of the key issues present in about 12.9% according to Body Mass Index (BMI) assessment, as well as in 19.6% according to the Mini Nutritional Assessment (MNA) criteria. Malnutrition in the elderly can be precipitated by various factors like drugs, socioeconomic condition, and loss of appetite, which tend to lead to inadequate caloric and nutrient intake. This is complemented by comorbidities accompanying old age, which complicate dietary needs and increase vulnerability to deficiencies in essential vitamins and minerals. The overall impact of malnutrition can be severe, causing frailty, compromised immunity, and loss of quality of life in this population of patients and the importance of screening and interventions towards nutritional care. Sarcopenia, or the gradual weakening and loss of muscle strength and mass, is another important deficit prevalent in the elderly. The diagnosis rates of sarcopenia tell us how serious it is, and a staggering prevalence rate of 49.1% as per the Ishii criteria has been shown by studies. Malnutrition, or chronic energy deficit and physical inactivity, is statistically correlated with sarcopenia and carries repercussions beyond muscle loss. Muscle mass loss can significantly impair mobility and increase the risk of hospitalization, falls, and fractures. Thus, sarcopenia treatment is not only required to maintain physical function but also for the elderly's health and independence as well. Food interventions, generally including supplementation with high-quality protein sources and exercise, become crucial steps in reversing this alarming trend among aging populations. Moreover, micronutrient deficiencies also remain a significant issue among older people, more precisely trace elements and vitamins. These deficiencies are typically unsuspected but can have potentially severe health effects, including cognitive decline, impaired immunity, and osteoporosis. Leafy chenopods, which are rich in essential micronutrients, could hold the solution to combating these widespread deficiencies. Their high nutrient content of iron, zinc, calcium, and vitamins A, C, and E make them plants with major potential to enhance nutrition among older adults. Their ability to thrive under poor conditions makes them ideally adapted to cultivation in various environments, hence providing a sustainable food supply that addresses the twin problems of malnutrition and climate resilience. As such, efforts at advocating for the consumption of nutrient-dense foods like leafy chenopods can potentially be key in improving the nutritional status of the elderly and halting common deficits among the vulnerable age group (Figure 13.6).

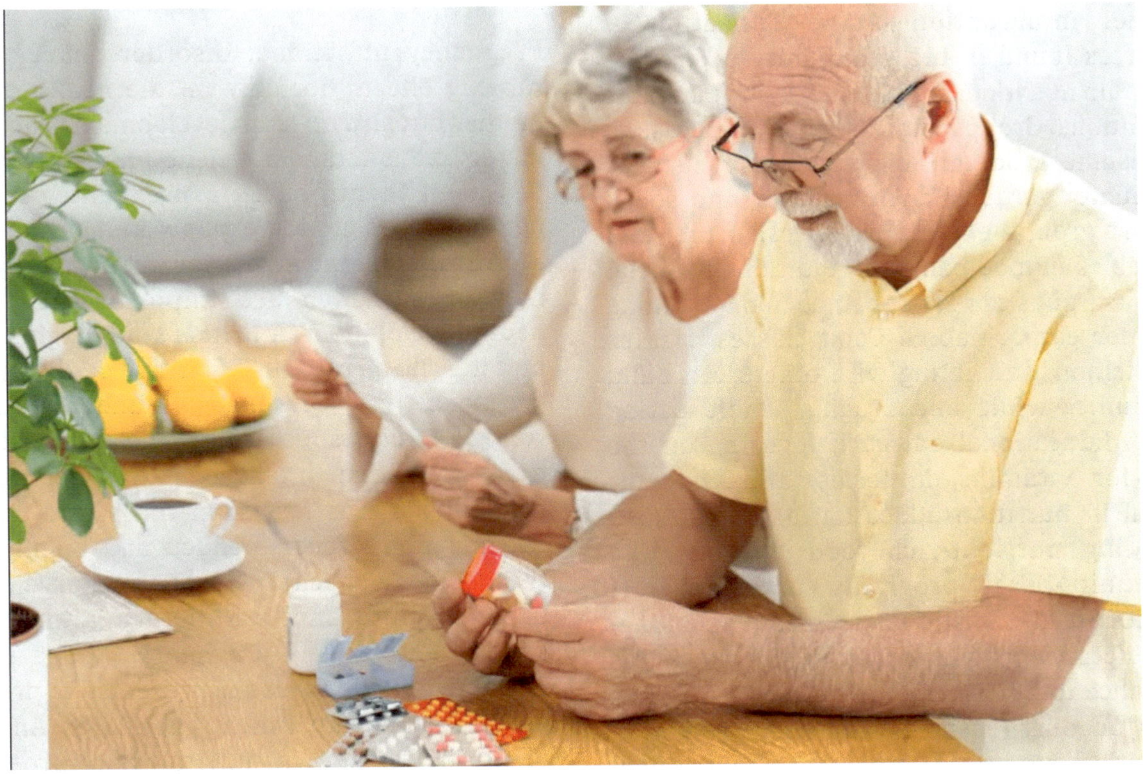

Figure 13.6. Older adults managing medications for common age-related health issues.

Source: https://colonialassistedliving.com/wp-content/uploads/2023/05/10-Most-Common-Health-Problems-The-Elderly-Face.jpg.

13.2.3. Strategies for Improving Nutritional Intake

In the management of nutritional disorders in special populations, enhancing nutritional intake needs to be tackled using a multi-faceted approach. Specialized dietetic interventions are of paramount significance in enhancing the nutritional value of foods consumed by specific groups like the elderly, developmentally disabled children, or patients with chronic diseases. Having collaborations with health professionals, , such as dietitians, can ensure that dietary regimens are not only adapted to personal needs but also adhere to established dietary guidelines. Educating the public about the importance of nutritional intake can translate into healthier eating habits and increased surveillance regarding dietary deficiencies, particularly in needy populations. Furthermore, pragmatic interventions like meal planning and preparation can enable patients to control their diets, finally translating into better eating practices that minimize the risk of nutritional disorders (Vilstrup et al., 2014). Another intervention is the utilization of resources found in the community to provide support in nutritional requirements in vulnerable populations. Groups may also provide access to wholesome food through activities , such as community gardens, farm markets, and social support groups emphasizing fresh fruits and vegetables in food pantries. Additionally, social support groups can assist people in maintaining healthier eating habits. Cook classes, classes on nutrition, and eating with others can build community while encouraging whole eating habits. Educational outreach focusing on the need for vitamins, minerals, and water is critical in nutrition education of populations regarding nutrient-rich food options. The community-based programs target not just the short-term nutritional needs but also long-term dietary lifestyle change, which promotes resistance to nutritional diseases (Ekor, 2014). Lastly, ongoing research and policy promotion are critical factors for maximizing nutritional intake initiatives. The regulators should strive to implement regulations that make food safe and fortify the staple foods in areas where malnutrition occurrences are high. Research testing the effectiveness of various interventions provides empirical bases for the implementation of best practices in nutritional education and food distribution. Funding programs among the vulnerable also can be optimized through public-private partnerships, offering long-term strategies in countering nutritional deficiencies. Prioritizing these measures, thus, can help us to create an environment that promotes healthier eating in an interactive way and satisfies the sophisticated nutritional needs of special groups, hence reducing the occurrence of nutritional disorders (Vilstrup et al., 2014).

13.3. Nutritional Disorders in Pregnant Women

Pregnancy nutritional disorders have wide-ranging effects not only on the health of the mother but also on fetal development. The most major one is iodine deficiency, a disorder that has been identified as a pregnant woman's health hazard in some populations. Iodine is a critical element in the formation of thyroid hormones, which are important for fetal neurodevelopment. A British study highlighted that despite an overall knowledge of diet during pregnancy, very few mothers understood the role of iodine specifically. The study stated that the median intake of iodine among the participants was less than the World Health Organization's recommended and highlighted the need for specific education interventions on the importance of dietary iodine and supplements during pregnancy (Bouga et al., 2015). This deficit must be prevented to prevent developmental impairments in children. Another of the better-known nutritional disorders is alcohol intake, which poses an enormous risk to fetal development. The effects of prenatal alcohol exposure can lead to a variety of disorders collectively known as Fetal Alcohol Spectrum Disorders (FASD). Alcohol's teratogenic impact is capable of causing physical abnormalities, retarded growth, and severe cognitive impairments, which manifest in most domains , such as memory and executive function. FASD sufferers often have difficulties throughout life, so intervention and treatment need to occur early. Because no minimum safe amount of alcohol consumption during pregnancy has been established, absolute abstinence is strongly recommended. Alcohol drinking among pregnant women should be detected and strong methods must be utilized to create awareness and prevent alcohol-related damage to future generations (Carito et al., 2016).

Finally, social conditions must be realized in the context of nutrition and health habits among pregnant women. Socioeconomic status heterogeneity, health beliefs, and healthcare resources influence food composition and overall nutritional contribution. Poor women are prone to food insecurity, limited access to nutrient-dense foods, and inadequate prenatal care, all of which can potentially cause nutritional disorders. Moreover, culturally associated eating practices can either compromise or enhance nutrition during pregnancy based on the nutrients emphasized. Therefore, public health interventions need to be sensitive to culture and aimed at addressing the needs of different groups. Interventions that promote learning on healthy nutrition, enhance social networks, and augment access to healthy foods are essential to avoid risks of nutritional disorders during pregnancy, ultimately leading to a better mother and child health status (Figure 13.7).

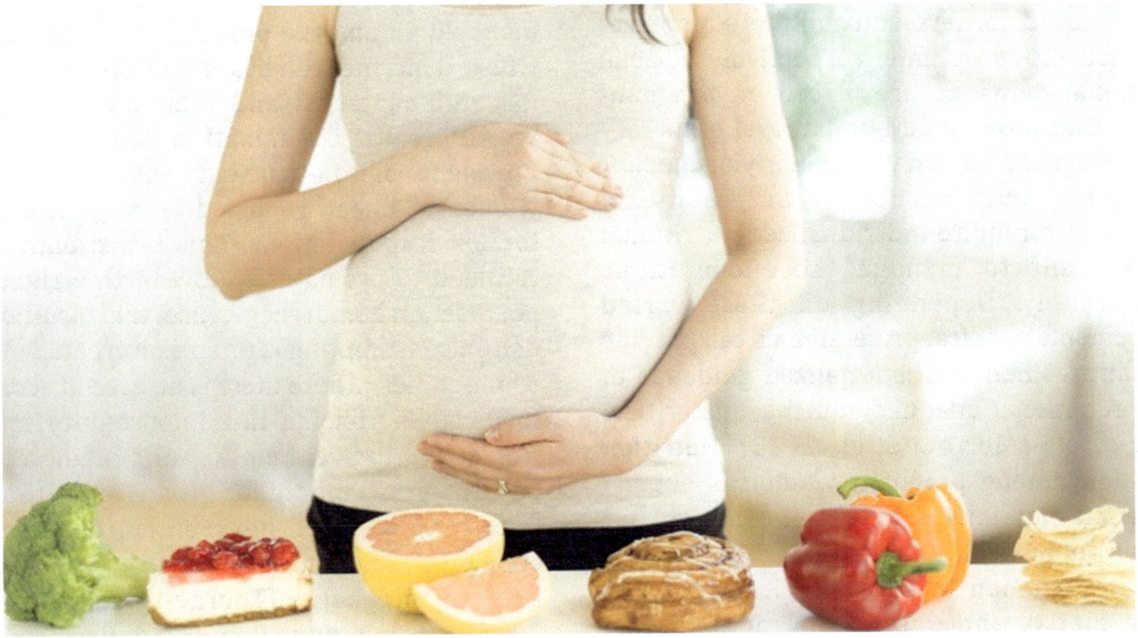

Figure 13.7. Pregnancy nutrition choices affect fetal growth and maternal health.

Source: https://cdn.prod.website-files.com/5ee7039040ea6efb80d7521c/5feafd71cbbb62541388f47a_Impact-of-nutritional-deficiencies-in-pregnancy-%E2%80%93-On-the-foetus.jpg.

13.3.1. Importance of Nutrition During Pregnancy

Correct nutrition during pregnancy guarantees the health of the mother and the developing fetus. The nutritional requirements are greatly enhanced during pregnancy due to the higher metabolic demands and need for fetal growth and development. It should be particularly pointed out that malnutrition in key nutrients results in severe issues, including low birth weight and developmental abnormalities. For instance, iodine is crucial in thyroid hormone synthesis, which is vital in fetal brain development. In the UK, where the population is mildly iodine-deficient, awareness of the role of iodine during pregnancy is extremely low. It was reassuring to find that in a study, 96% of pregnant women were aware of general nutrition recommendations, yet only 12% were aware of the significance of iodine, highlighting a large gap to be bridged to ensure healthier maternal and fetal outcomes (Bouga et al., 2015). Moreover, a well-planned diet rich in macronutrients and micronutrients is the ticket to preventing pregnancy complications. The benefits are not merely in short-term health but also in long-term well-being of the child. For example, some nutrients like folic acid, iron, and calcium are needed for the prevention of neural tube disorders and for the support of increased blood volume, respectively. Special nutritional demands are placed on pregnant women that pose an additional level of dietary needs. Pregnant women with underlying medical conditions , such as obesity or gestational diabetes, can require individualized nutritional management to manage these conditions appropriately. Depending on these varied requirements, medical professionals can provide pregnant women with specialized guidance to meet nutritional adequacy during this critical phase of life (Morrow et al., 2012). Nutrition education among pregnant women is equally important not only for personal health but also for public health policy. Greater awareness can allow women to eat more healthfully in a way that is appropriate for their specific needs. This is particularly relevant in the management of conditions like gestational diabetes and nutritional deficiencies, which affect some groups more than others. Failure to offer adequate diet instruction can result in long-term consequences, not only for maternal health but also for the development of the child. Hence, health professionals ought to emphasize the importance of nutrition through providing accessible and appropriate cultural resources and support. By creating an environment of knowledge that is supportive of the proper nutrition during pregnancy, we are able to contribute towards reducing the prevalence of nutritional disorders in special groups, thereby allowing healthier generations in the future (Morrow et al., 2012; Bouga et al., 2015).

13.3.2. Common Nutritional Deficiencies Among Pregnant Women

The physiological requirements of pregnancy elevate a woman's dietary requirement significantly, rendering her susceptible to many dietary deficiencies. One among these deficiencies that arise during this critical phase is that of iron, which is vital in the production of hemoglobin and the prevention of anemia, and whose deficiency can bear harmful consequences for both maternal and fetal well-being. The World Health Organization reports that the prevalence of iron-deficiency anemia in pregnant women has been reported to range from 20% to 70% in populations. This is a situation that can lead to prematurity, low birth weight, and postpartum hemorrhage. Also, this insufficiency of iron consumption is often exacerbated in poor communities, where there is no ease in accessing food high in iron. It is thus important to improve iron status to avoid mother and infant adverse outcomes in vulnerable groups, and the goal is to have targeted intervention and nutrient supplementation protocols in order to encourage a healthy pregnancy (Thorne-Lyman and Webb, 2025). Calcium and vitamin D deficiencies also present difficult problems for pregnant women, particularly in groups where the diet is not rich in sources of these nutrients. Calcium is critical to fetal bone health, and deficiency will lead to unfavorable growth effects on the mother and child's bone health. Vitamin D deficiency can also interfere with calcium absorption and further complicate the situation. Pregnant women, particularly those who are from low socioeconomic backgrounds, might not have the diet and sun exposure, putting them at risk for deficiencies. According to research, up to 80%

of pregnant women in some regions have been found to be lacking in vitamin D, and this may lead to pregnancy complications like preeclampsia and gestational diabetes. Thus, public health interventions should aim at educating pregnant women on calcium and vitamin D consumption, fortification of food, and sun exposure recommendations (Balgir, 2011). Folate deficiency is also another prevalent condition, significant in fetal neural tube formation, particularly during early pregnancy. This B-vitamin is essential for DNA synthesis and cell division, and adequate intake of folate needs to be ensured to prevent neural tube defects. Despite a high level of awareness, it has been shown that a high percentage of pregnant women ingest less than the recommended dietary amount of folate, especially in at-risk communities where access to fortified foods is poor. The implications of such a deficiency are severe, having long-term effects on the intellectual development and general health of the child. Public health interventions must address increased intake of folate-containing foods like green vegetables, legumes, and fortified breakfast cereals, along with additional counseling for prenatal vitamins. By addressing folate deficiency with education and the distribution of resources, both mothers and their offspring can have their health risks reduced, leading to healthier populations in general (Thorne-Lyman and Webb, 2025) (Figure 13.8).

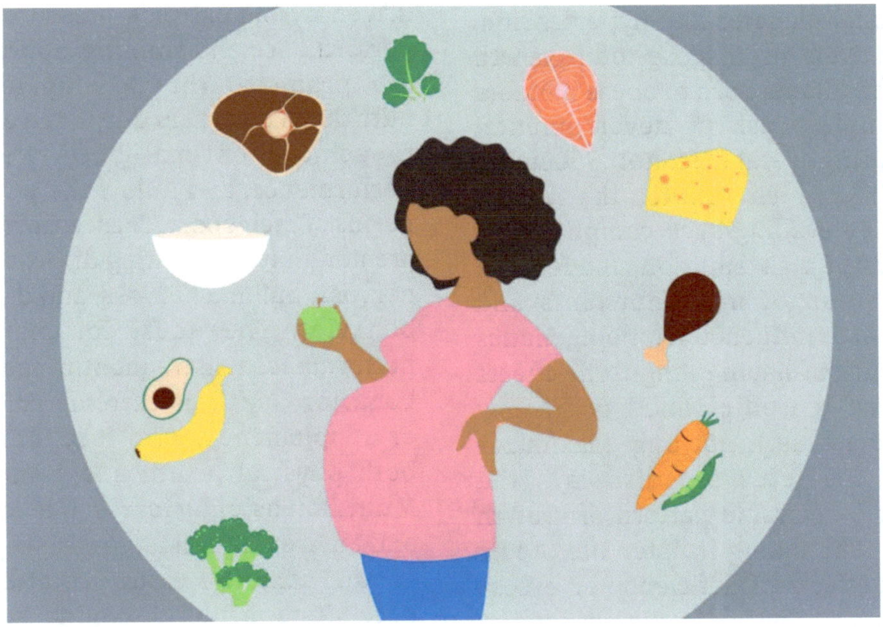

Figure 13.8. Balanced nutrition during pregnancy supports the mother and baby's health.

Source: https://assets.clevelandclinic.org/transform/29b77398-af06-4231-a4da-446e35e1f8b8/pregnant-Healthy-Eating-1344587580_770x533_jpg.

13.3.3. Effects of Maternal Nutrition on Fetal Development

Maternal nutrition is an important factor affecting fetal development, with consequences that persist beyond gestation into the lifetime health of the offspring. The nutritional status of the mother during pregnancy directly impacts the supply of essential nutrients required for fetal growth and organ formation. Insufficient intake of basic nutrients , such as folic acid, iron, and omega-3 fatty acids, has adverse effects, , such as low birth weight, neural tube defects, and impaired brain functioning in the offspring. Furthermore, studies have found that maternal malnutrition can also interact with genetic risk factors to exacerbate developmental disorders. The need to understand is that the consequences of maternal nutrition are not only on the physical well-being of the child but also on their neurocognitive development, thus establishing a huge link between the dietary habits of the mothers and the subsequent overall health of the children, highlighting the need for interventions specifically during pregnancy (Morrow et al., 2012). The nutritional quality of mothers is important for the development of metabolic processes and fetal metabolic programming. Maternal obesity and excessive nutrient intake have been shown to increase the risk for gestational diabetes and hypertension, which can negatively predispose fetal growth and development. Infants born to obese mothers may be at a higher risk of developmental disorder, including Fetal Alcohol Spectrum Disorders (FASD), which denotes the role of a balanced diet in evading such complications (Carito et al., 2016). In addition, inadequate or overconsumption of macronutrients and micronutrients may influence fetal epigenetics and the possibility of having long-term effects on health. Hence, a well-planned pregnancy diet is most crucial, as it not only maximizes the growth of the fetus but also lays the groundwork for a favorable pattern of growth and behavioral functioning in later life. Apart from the direct effects of deficiency or excess of nutrients, maternal nutrition also possesses psycho-social dimensions that shape fetal growth. The majority of mothers have limited access to nutritious foods, depending on limited availability and economic constraints, and limited nutrition knowledge. All these socio-economic determinants can lead to a cycle of poor nutrition for the mothers and poor fetal outcomes. Public health programs should include awareness and education on maternal nutrition to avoid nutritional disorders among vulnerable groups. Moreover, inter-disciplinary approaches involving health professionals, nutritionists, and community interventions are key to addressing the complex issues of maternal nutrition. By promoting improved nutritional access and food practices, fetal development results can be enhanced for healthier generations in the long term (Morrow et al., 2012).

13.4. Nutrition Disorders Among Athletes

The sporting world typically presents unique challenges in terms of nutritional disorders, driven by the extreme pressure of competitive performance and training. Sporting individuals are prone to the development of various nutritional disorders due to the extreme stresses to achieve optimal body weight, enhance performance, and follow the physical aesthetic norms of their sport. These disorders include, but are not limited to, eating disorders like anorexia nervosa, bulimia nervosa, and disordered eating behavior. The quest for maximal physical performance will frequently lead to undesirable behavior, , such as extreme caloric restriction or supplement abuse, that ultimately negates both physical health and competitive ability. Multidimensional forces like cultural, social, and environmental forces are key determinants of an athlete's food relationship, which necessitates a multidisciplinary approach to the deconstruction and correction of these issues in the best possible manner. The consequences of nutritional disorders on athletes are not merely physical but also mental, and this is crucial to accomplish peak performance. The prevalence of eating disorders among athletes has grown compared to non-athletes since the 1980s, as proven by a host of studies. With the heightened competition and often idealized physical body image of an athlete, athletes are at heightened risks, which serve to underscore a compelling need for specific healthcare interventions.

Proper management and treatment guidelines attempt to educate athletes to recognize symptoms and adopt healthier lifestyles; however, guidelines from the likes of NICE and UK Sport exhibit telltale inadequacies, particularly in accomplishing effective screening measures and proper interventions for specific sports. Coaches, sporting leaders, and doctors must collaborate to create settings in which mental well-being is prioritized along with performance to reduce help-seeking stigma. Education and awareness are major factors in avoiding and managing sports nutritional disorders. By creating an enabling culture within sporting programs, stakeholders are able to substantially influence the body image and nutritional attitudes of athletes. This is cultural change that entails initiating open discussion around the aspects of nutrition and mental health and creating a balanced system for diet and training. Proper training programs that address the importance of nutrition and performance can make it possible for athletes to make the appropriate choices and seek help when needed. Including psychological support in sporting training programs can also reduce the risk factors for nutritional disorders. Effective strategies should embrace preventive measures and responsive care and management specifically tailored to the unique needs of the athletes, as per current guidelines, hence leading to a healthier sporting community dedicated to well-being and performance excellence (Aerenhouts et al., 2019; Hilling et al., 2023) (Figure 13.9).

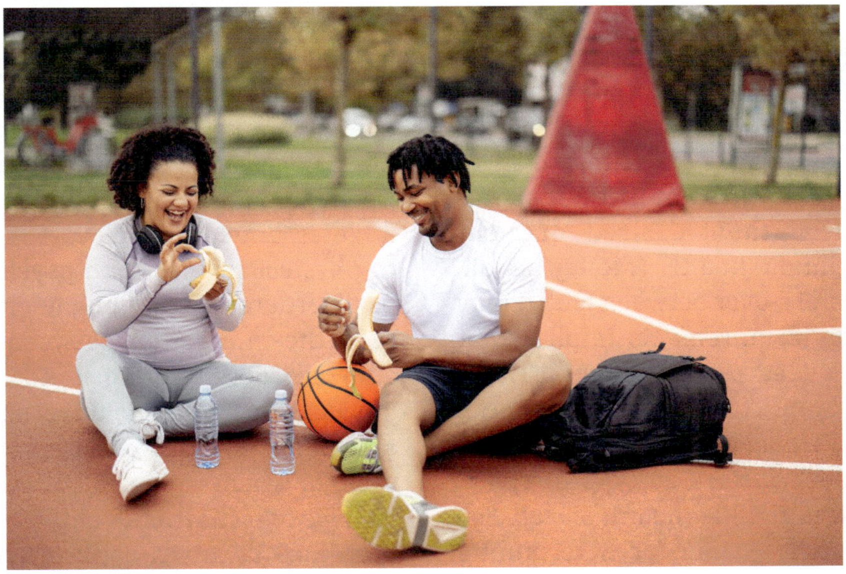

Figure 13.9. A couple refueling with bananas and water after playing basketball.

Source: https://cdn.sanity.io/images/ibmh0om4/production/2bcc46d71230ea5821635eebe8d54064d67fb3ac-3864x2576.jpg?w=3840&q=75&fit=clip&auto=format.

13.4.1. Unique Nutritional Needs of Athletes

Athletes require specific nutritional requirements that are of primary importance for optimal performance and recuperation. The demands of training and competition establish a specific balance of macronutrients—carbohydrates, proteins, and fats—to provide the energy requirements of the body and assist in muscle repair and building. Carbohydrates are the primary fuel source for high-intensity exercise, and their appropriate consumption is critical. Meanwhile, protein intake is essential not only for muscle development but for the recovery from intense exercise as well. Interestingly, the responsibility for providing enough nutrition falls on a collective burden on the coaches, sports leaders, and the athletes themselves, as the importance of a supportive environment in any sport is deemed as the central idea (Aerenhouts et al., 2019). Moreover, micronutrients , such as vitamins and minerals, also play a significant role in optimizing athletic performance. Since their fast turnover during training requires the athletes to make it a priority to take them to prevent deficiency that can impair performance, specific mention should be made of the role of iron in oxygen delivery and energy production as well as that of calcium and vitamin D in maintaining bone health, particularly among female athletes who are more prone to osteoporosis. Many athletes, especially women, struggle to meet the needs for energy intake, thereby leading to an insufficient replenishment of nutrients. Therefore, while a food-first approach is the best, supplementation may be entertained in certain conditions to guarantee that sports performers achieve their desired nutrient uptake and maximum health (McKay et al., 2023). Lastly, the cross-over between food habits and overall energy requirements implies that sports performers need personalized nutrition approaches. Individual evaluations are essential in establishing individual nutrient requirements with respect to such factors as type of sport, training level, and individual health status. For instance, an effective system for determining nutritional requirements should not only account for the athletes' eating patterns but also their biological and clinical characteristics. Moreover, factors , such as gender can play a crucial role in affecting the needs for nutrients and the effectiveness of supplementation. Hence, personalized dieting regimens must be created, paying special heed to proper timing and co-administration with other nutrients for greater absorption and effectiveness. Overall, a deep understanding of these advanced dietary needs is the greatest priority in working within the greater context of nutritional pathologies among special populations, specifically sports individuals (McKay et al., 2023).

13.4.2. Risks of Disordered Eating in Sports

Incidence of eating disorder in sport is a significant concern, especially among those sports athletes who are engaged in weight-sensitive or aesthetic sports. These athletes face a huge burden of pressure in order to satisfy societal and cultural demands of thinness, which might lead to adverse energy balance as well as intentional and unintentional calorie restrictions. According to Miller et al. (2013), low caloric intake in athletes makes them at risk for severe and long-term consequences, , such as menstrual disturbance in female athletes. These complications do not only hinder an athlete from performing but can have lasting impacts on an athlete's health, which hampers vital physiological functioning to recover and endure. By neglecting their nutritional needs, these athletes, unwittingly, elevate their susceptibility to physical sickness and psychological distress of disordered eating behaviors. In addition to that, the interaction between energy balance and disordered eating is not only short-term physical but also includes psychological and emotional effects. Athletes then fall into a cycle in which rigid control over diet produces feelings of insufficiency and fear of performance, therefore reinforcing disordered eating. The psychological load is great, and athletes tend to have increased stress levels accompanied by potential withdrawal from social and competition settings. The humiliation of having problems , such as their weight and eating, in addition to the stigma that typically accompanies discussing these issues within sporting settings, hindering athletes from seeking assistance. This alienation will complicate matters, as it maintains confidentiality over their struggles while further cultivating unhealthy dietary behaviors (Currie et al., 2016). To address these pressing issues, it is critical that sports organizations implement conducive systems that enable open discussion of nutrition and mental health for athletes. Educational programs for coaches, trainers, and athletes themselves could also provide some insight into the risks of disordered eating while promoting good eating and emotional well-being. There should be regular screening of energy balance and nutritional status adopted as regular protocol such that those at risk can be identified early (Miller et al., 2013). In addition, building a culture that values the importance of mental health can encourage players to talk openly without being afraid of being stigmatized. By emphasizing physical and psychological resilience, the sports community can go a long way in steering clear of the risks of disordered eating and making room where all players can thrive (Figure 13.10).

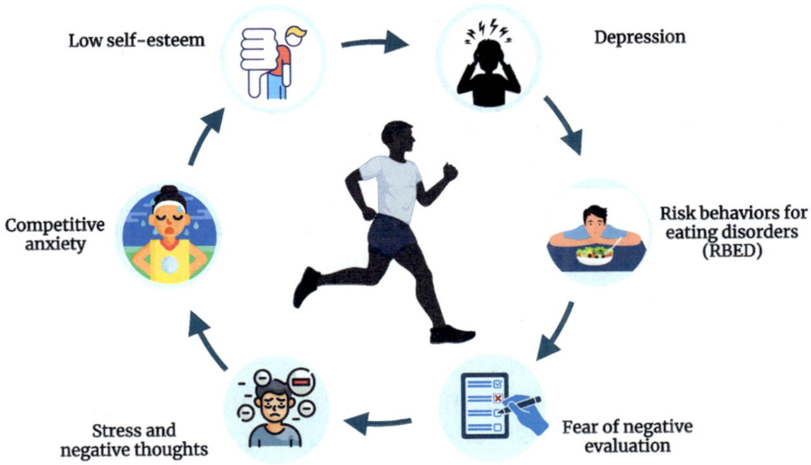

Figure 13.10. Cycle showing how low self-esteem and stress contribute to eating disorders in athletes.

Source: https://www.nutritional-psychology.org/wp-content/uploads/2023/10/unnamed-1-1.png.

13.4.3. Importance of Hydration and Recovery Nutrition

Recovery nutrition and hydration are prominent factors in the maximization of sporting performance, particularly in special populations, , such as youth athletes or those with specific health conditions. Adequate hydration is crucial, as it plays a significant role in temperature regulation, maintenance of cardiovascular function, and facilitation of nutrient transport. In the absence of optimal hydration, athletes can experience declines in performance and an increased risk of injury or heat illness. Competitors must familiarize themselves with their individual hydration needs, which can vary based on intensity levels and activity time. A recent study emphasizes that hydration is an exercise performance-limiting factor, citing its connection to the intake of essential nutrients, , such as carbohydrates and proteins, as a reason for proper nutrition education targeted at special groups (Heikkilä, 2020). Recovery nutrition also directly contributes to general well-being and sporting performance when the training and competition load causes additional stress to the body. Proper recovery nutrition entails prompt carbohydrate, protein, and electrolyte consumption after exercise to assist in muscle repair, glycogen repletion, and hydration. For some individuals, , such as endurance athletes or chronically ill patients, personalized recovery strategies are necessary. It has been revealed through studies that nutrition information among athletes is generally inadequate, leading to inappropriate eating habits that hinder recovery and performance (Heikkilä, 2020). Having systematic nutrition programs specifically for recovery introduced can not only enhance athletic performance but also provide long-term health benefits. It should also be considered that hydration and recovery nutrition extend beyond individual nutritional choices and involve sociocultural and economic factors. Most young athletes do not have access to the correct educational resources on hydration and nutrition, which can foster myths that influence their decisions. Additionally, the exponential growth of the commercial food market with its inaccurate products creates an obstacle course for athletes, especially special populations, as they make diet decisions amidst conflicting information. By establishing comprehensive hydration and recovery nutrition education programs, sporting organizations can potentially allow athletes to make informed dietary choices, ultimately improving their overall well-being and performance outcomes. Such targeted interventions can potentially build resilience and flexibility in athletes with particular nutritional requirements, which highlights the importance of official assistance in sporting teams (Gil-Izquierdo et al., 2015).

13.5. Nutritional Disorders Among Persons with Disabilities

Nutritional disorders in individuals with disabilities frequently arise from complex interactions between physical, mental, and environmental factors. These are manifest in a range of expressions from undernutrition through to obesity and micronutrient deficiencies, varying with the type and relative severity of the disability. For example, individuals with mobility impairments can have challenges with physical activity, leading to weight gain and obesity, while individuals with cognitive disabilities can have challenges with food preparation and planning, leaving them susceptible to improper nutrient consumption. Therapy of nutritional disorders thus requires careful assessment and individualized treatment that not only considers the individual's specific needs but also the creation of supportive settings to facilitate the development of good eating habits. Educating caregivers in nutrition is also a central area of concern in averting these disorders as well as improving the general health status of disabled individuals. Furthermore, the prevalence of nutritional disorders in the disabled is worsened by socio-economic factors, thus making healthy foods accessible an integral barrier. The majority of individuals with disabilities possess limited incomes that might limit their access to healthy foods, thus supporting malnutrition and nutritional imbalances. This factor is particularly applicable in low-income communities where fresh fruit and healthy foods are not readily available. Interventions to combat such inequalities include advocating for policy reform towards improved food security and the institution of community-driven programs improving access to nutritional resources. By addressing the affordability and accessibility of healthy foods, stakeholders are in a position to design environments that enable healthier food choices, leading to the decline of the prevalence of nutritional disorders among such vulnerable populations. Education and outreach programs, specifically designed to address the special challenges of people with disabilities, can further promote awareness and encourage change. Finally, healthcare professionals have a key role to play in the early detection and treatment of nutritional disorders in people with disabilities. Nutritional screening should be made an integral part of regular health care for such populations so that timely interventions can be initiated once deficiencies or imbalances are identified. Multidisciplinary intervention by dietitians, physical therapists, and social workers can offer integrated care, not just for nutritional aspects but also for physical training, psychosocial guidance, and access to resources. Furthermore, further research is needed to establish the most effective methodologies and practices suited to disabled individuals' multiple needs. By facilitating collaboration between health systems and community organizations, and through an emphasis on the primacy of nutrition to overall health, the fight against nutritional disorders in individuals with disabilities can make tremendous strides towards better health outcomes (Figure 13.11).

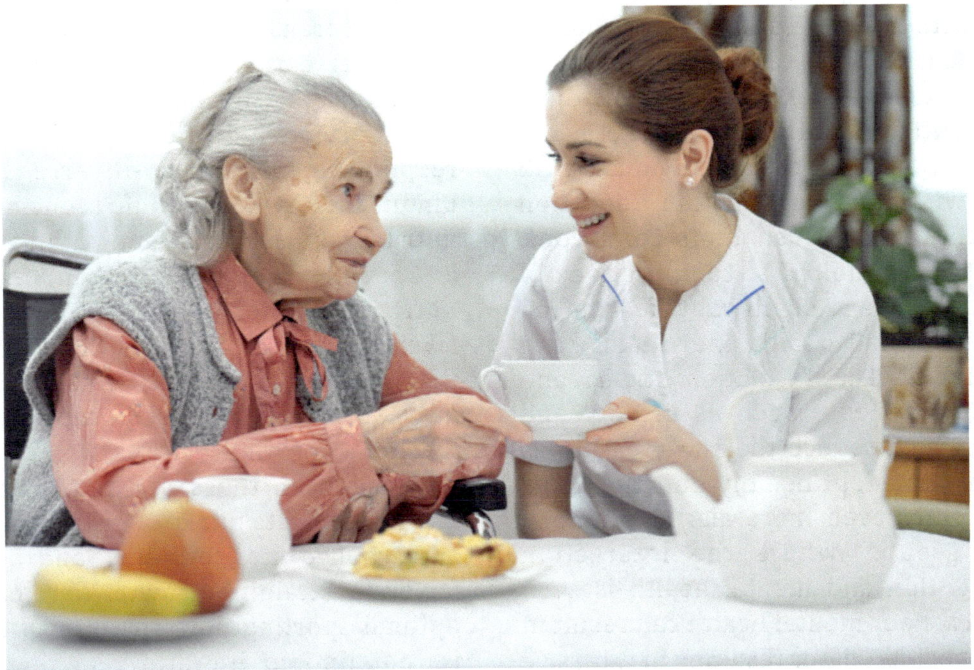

Figure 13.11. Caregiver assisting elderly woman at mealtime, encouraging nutrition and care.

Source: https://images.squarespace-cdn.com/content/v1/5e573566bb687c386d29f4b9/1614636525277-MT5S1VN98QL2RVUF0AIA/AdobeStock_51210281.jpeg.

13.5.1. Challenges Faced by Individuals with Disabilities

The problems faced by disabled individuals are sophisticated and reach various aspects of life, for example, access to significant services. One of the most prevalent challenges is the unavailability of healthy food, which is a cornerstone in managing medical issues and preventing nutritional diseases. The majority of the disabled will encounter obstacles , such as physical inaccessibility to retail outlets, limited transport, and insufficient assistance in food preparation that will exacerbate dietary deprivation and lead to general ill health. Besides, people who belong to lower socioeconomic statuses experience greater food insecurity, and hence, acquiring a balanced diet becomes even harder (Herrera et al., 2021). This overlap between disability and socioeconomic status highlights the need for more inclusive food systems that can cater to the special requirements of such groups and therefore ensure equal access to nutrition. Apart from issues of accessibility, individuals with disabilities also have healthcare service-based barriers that complicate their nutritional status. The majority of healthcare systems lack provisions required by disabled individuals, , such as equipment appropriate to their needs and skilled staff who understand their specific needs. This lack of provision limits preventive treatment and dietary counselling, essential components in the management of nutritional disorders common in this population (Herrera et al., 2021). In addition, nutritional health-focused public health programs tend to overlook the specific needs of individuals with disabilities, and hence, there is a lack of special services. Creating an enhanced healthcare system to make it more accessible involves sensitizing healthcare workers and implementing policies to equip individuals with disabilities with tailored nutrition education and intervention based on their conditions. Ultimately, the psychological complications of disability also have a significant bearing on nutrition and overall health. Individuals with disabilities are at risk of isolation, stigma, and mental health issues, , such as anxiety and depression, which reduce their interest in, as well as ability to adopt healthy nutrition. This concern becomes even more alarming among vulnerable groups, where the interaction between nutrition and mental health is even more complex. Poor mental health can result in erratic eating habits, either resulting in excessive consumption of unhealthy foods or starvation due to loss of appetite (Masonbrink et al., 2020). For that reason, it is important to pay attention to the mental health aspect of nutritional disorders in individuals with disabilities when designing comprehensive treatment regimens. These programs should consider psychological treatment as well as nutrition education to establish a more comprehensive approach to treat special populations.

13.5.2. Specific Nutritional Needs and Considerations

In the deliberation of the unique nutritional needs of special populations, one must also be mindful of the diverse experiences and health issues that influence dietary needs. Gender-diverse populations, for instance, typically have nutrition- and eating-related difficulties that are distinct from gender-conforming populations. Research shows that such groups may use food restriction not only for health but as a means of suppressing secondary sex characteristics or fulfilling societal expectations (Mittertreiner et al., 2024). This will lead to disordered eating patterns, particularly in healthcare settings that lack trans-affirmative care. Recognition of such diverse experiences encourages healthcare providers to design inclusive environments that prioritize nutrition literacy and a safe space, responding to gender-diverse individuals' unique dietary needs while reducing the risk of nutritional disorders. Young athletes represent a special population requiring modified nutritional interventions due to their high level of physical demands. Research indicates that the dietary requirements of children and adolescents, particularly those engaged in frequent sporting activities, are significantly different from those of adults (Amawi et al., 2024). Adequate intake of macronutrients , such as carbohydrates, proteins, and fats is a key factor in attaining growth, development, and optimal sporting performance. Of significance is that limited literature on the population translates into a requirement for adequate knowledge of their nutritional status and food habits. Because adolescent athletes are also at risk of succumbing to pressures that encourage poor eating habits, addressing these conditions with counseling and education can lower the risk for diet disorder development and finally secure their long-term health and athletic potential. In addition, creating effective dietary interventions in special populations needs to be an interdisciplinary process that brings together nutrition science, psychology, and health activism. Professionals need to develop further insight into the emotional and psychological resistances that discourage maximum nutrition in diverse populations. Considering the experience of gender-diverse people, as described in the literature, is a central part of maximizing therapeutic relationships and client gains (Mittertreiner et al., 2024). Likewise, in the case of child athletes, comprehensive diet plans, instead of merely tackling body performance, must also provide for healthy nutritional habits with a focus on mental well-being. Adopting evidence-based practice and promoting collaboration between healthcare professionals, dietitians can better meet the multifaceted nutritional needs of such populations, thereby reducing the incidence of nutritional disorders and improving overall well-being (Figure 13.12).

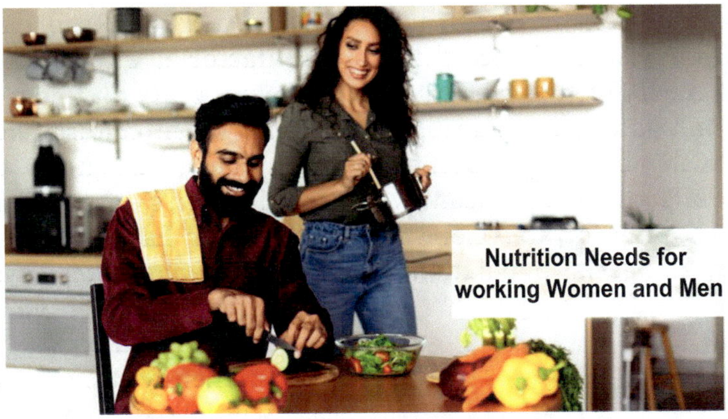

Figure 13.12. Healthy meal prep highlighting nutrition needs of working men and women.

Source: https://continentalhospitals.com/images/blogs/4bbf5a36ca7ad0569c300f30973096f5.webp.

13.5.3. Role of Caregivers in Managing Nutrition

Caregivers are the focal persons in managing nutrition among individuals with nutritional disorders, particularly in special populations , such as disabled, chronic diseases, or cognitive impairment. These caregivers, typically family members or paid caregivers, not only prepare meals but also tailor diet programs based on individual nutritional needs. For example, in the case of Alzheimer's disease patients, caregivers must be observant to note that the food provided not only stays healthy but is also appetizing, as changes in taste and preference make mealtime challenging. They serve as watchdogs over the nutritional health of their clients, having to ensure complex diet restrictions that may be triggered by related medical conditions. The caregivers' enormous responsibility goes beyond cooking food; they also oversee eating habits and hydration status, which are pivotal in the prevention of malnutrition and dehydration, the most prevalent problems in such groups (Liu et al., 2020). Furthermore, the emotional and psychological dimensions of caregiving have a huge influence on nutrition management. Caregivers become stressed and emotionally drained, often compromising their own health and well-being. This stress can lead to trouble with daily meal planning and preparation. Furthermore, emotional support provided by caregivers can make the eating process more enjoyable for individuals, rendering eating less stressful, particularly for those with decreased appetites or cognitive impairment. Care recipient nutritional status and caregiver health being interactive implies that effective support systems need to be established for caregivers, too. They require resources, education, and rest to help eliminate their charges and to enhance their ability to provide good nutrition care (Liu et al., 2020). Education and training of caregivers are essential components in optimizing nutritional management. Training programs focused on nutritional information enable caregivers to prepare well-balanced food that is compliant with the dietary needs suitable for their loved ones or patients. Equally vital is learning how to recognize nutritional deficiencies because these can be such serious complications if not caught. Also, caregivers' understanding of the importance of socialization during eating will help make mealtimes a better experience, one that is so crucial to the overall health of the individual with eating challenges due to sickness or old age. Through the establishment of nurturing environments and the provision of necessary education, caregivers can influence healthier nutrition habits and mitigate the conditions of malnutrition. Eventually, caregivers' ability to perform nutrition effectively significantly contributes to the shaping of the health conditions of members in special populations (Liu et al., 2020).

13.6. Cultural Influences on Nutritional Disorders

Cultural factors significantly play a role in the development of dietary habits that have direct implications for nutritional disorders within special groups. Every culture has certain food habits, belief patterns, and practices that not only decide what and how much is consumed but also how it is prepared and consumed during group meals. Cultural origin can thus influence the prevalence of several nutritional disorders like obesity, undernutrition, and eating disorders. For example, some cultures may focus on particular food groups to the extent of creating an imbalance between nutrients consumed. In addition, these culturally learned eating patterns can be at odds with clinical dietary advice, thereby complicating nutrition disorder management. Through appreciation of the cultural context surrounding food preferences, healthcare professionals can develop more efficient, culturally sensitive interventions that are aware of and respect such beliefs while catering to dietary requirements. In children, cultural issues strongly impact pediatric feeding disorders (PFDs), making it imperative to have an in-depth knowledge of related nutritional issues. The absence of a universally accepted definition for PFDs reflects the complexity of diagnosing and managing these disorders in various populations. The earlier paradigms might have been shortsighted regarding the multifactorial etiology of feeding disorders, focusing only on medical or psychosocial factors. When cultural elements are added to the model of diagnosis, as the World Health Organization's International Classification of Functioning has been proposed, it is possible to better define feeding dysfunctions. Accepting that PFDs can result from cultural forces in food consumption and cooking routines encourages a comprehensive treatment approach. Improved care will follow from an understanding of the complex interplay between cultural influences and nutritional deficiencies, particularly in children at a susceptible phase of growth and development. Finally, socioeconomic status combined with cultural influences confers a further layer of complexity to the prevention and management of nutritional disorders, particularly in vulnerable groups. Cultural practices can amplify or dampen the effects of food insecurity, often reflecting a community's historical relationship with food availability. The entitlement theory describes that disparities in the accessibility of essential micronutrients in case of emergencies can contribute to the vulnerability of populations to nutritional disorders, especially in vulnerable groups (Thorne-Lyman and Webb, 2025). It requires not only an understanding of eating habits but also socioeconomic determinants of food access and utilization analysis. Interventions should then be planned to fit the economic conditions as well as the cultural values of those targeted populations. Finally, the creation of economically feasible and culturally appropriate nutrition programs can do much to reduce the effects of nutritional disorders in heterogeneous special populations (Figure 13.13).

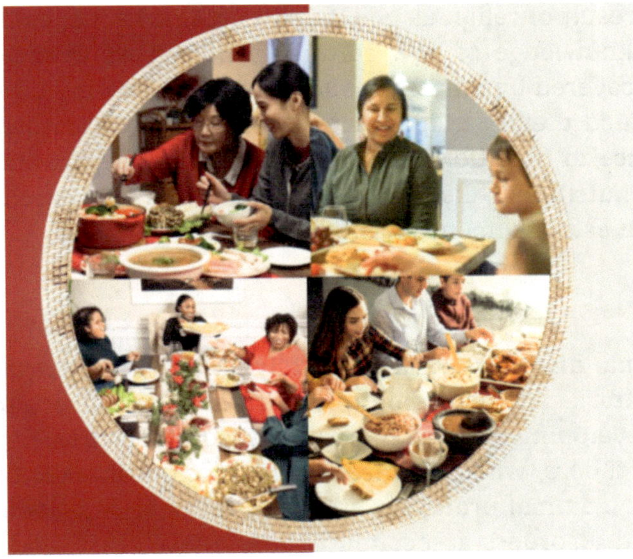

Figure 13.13. Families enjoy traditional meals, highlighting the culture's role in healthy eating.

Source: https://www.nhlbi.nih.gov/sites/default/files/styles/16x9_crop/public/2023-08/Culture-Centered%20Dietary%20Interventions%20NHLBI%20Public%20Site-%202160x1080px.png?h=bb1a4d8b&itok=bK-Wtuj8.

13.6.1. Impact of Cultural Beliefs on Dietary Practices

Cultural beliefs have a powerful influence on diet, not only dictating food consumption but also concepts of health and well-being. In most populations, foods consumed traditionally embody values and beliefs central to their existence, and these may include special nutritional attributes. In indigenous populations, for instance, they tend to use as their foundation foods that are locally grown and keep them healthy and well based on millennia of farming knowledge. Conversely, when dietary needs confront food availability, individuals may develop nutritional disorders and, as a result, have general health effects. It is hence important to be aware of the relationship between food culture and eating habits in addressing nutritional disorders among special populations, particularly those undergoing extreme lifestyle changes resulting from globalization and urbanization. Moreover, cultural ideology infuses social ritual and group practice around food, affecting the manner of eating meals and the frequency of their consumption. In most cultures, the consumption of a meal is a shared ritual that enhances bonding among household members and consolidates social unity. However, as fast foods and convenience meals gain popularity, often for their perceived efficiency and novelty, these crucial social forms can be undermined, leading to unhealthier patterns of consumption. Evidence suggests that as individuals prioritize convenience above traditional foodways, they will tend to experience an increase in risk of obesity and related morbidities. Displacement of traditional foodways is generally symptomatic of larger social alterations and demands culturally relevant interventions to offset the adverse effects of dietary change, leading to nutritional disorders in affected groups. Also, cultural beliefs influence the perception of health and, therefore, dictate strategies towards dietary consumption and maintenance of health. For example, in some cultures, the understanding of food as a healing factor promotes the utilization of particular ingredients in light of traditional medicinal practices. Nevertheless, misconceptions about specific foods or dietary restrictions, as a result of religious beliefs, restrict nutritional consumption and contribute to deficiency. Moreover, knowledge of how cultural beliefs cross over health matters in today's world, , such as those uncovered by illnesses , such as PASC following COVID-19, is necessary. The need for culturally informed dietary guidance that respects and tolerates cultural environments can increase the adherence to nutrition interventions and enable healthier status among special populations affected by nutritional disorders, directing future research and community health interventions towards the establishment of tolerant dietary practices.

13.6.2. Nutritional Disorders Prevalent in Specific Cultures

The incidence of nutritional disorders varies radically among different cultural settings, typically set by traditional food patterns and accessibility of various food sources. Malnourishment remains a vital concern in most developing regions. In certain African societies, for example, the core foods are primarily grains and tubers, which can lead to insufficient intakes of essential vitamins and minerals, particularly when animal protein is limited. Conversely, city populations can suffer from an increase in obesity and disorders associated with increased fast-food intake, reporting a shift in cultural patterns.

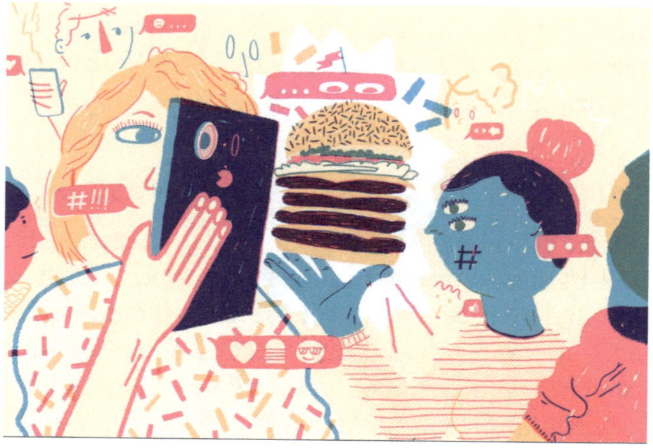

Figure 13.14. Social media influence on food choices and eating behaviors.

Source: https://global-studies.shorthandstories.com/from-disordered-eating-to-eating-disorders/assets/naMe2iICnz/burger-1200x800.jpeg.

This double burden signifies that cultural eating habits can contribute to both undernutrition and overnutrition at the same time, posing the need for specific public health interventions that take cognizance of these unique cultural factors affecting nutrition. In addition to malnutrition and obesity, certain cultures also have certain nutritional diseases related to lifestyle and genetics. For instance, Mediterranean individuals who rely heavily on olive oil and fish typically have lower rates of heart disease. Nevertheless, the traditional Mediterranean diet is fast becoming history with increasing consumption of processed foods and, as a result, increased cases of diabetes and high blood pressure. Similarly, lactose intolerance is common in Asian populations, where long-standing low intake of dairy foods can result in gastrointestinal disease upon the introduction of dairy products into the diet. Such distinct nutritional disorders are best understood through an understanding of cultural practices that both influence food choice and dictate the status of health status of specific groups. In addition, management of nutritional disorders within cultural groups may be complex. For example, the diagnosis of polycystic ovary syndrome (PCOS) is based on cultural understandings of women's health and diet. Obesity stigma, in all but a few cultures, can thwart one's desire to seek assistance, reinforcing inadequate dietary patterns and exacerbating symptoms (Teede et al., 2018). Therefore, culturally sensitive interventions that consider typical food choices and beliefs locally are integral to effective management. Where cultural foods play a significant role in communities, integrating these into health promotion can enhance adherence to dietary advice and overall health outcomes. Accordingly, there is a need to design health programs to not only promote nutrition disorders but also to acknowledge and respect cultural values, thereby making interventions relevant and sustainable (Figure 13.14).

13.6.3. Strategies for Culturally Sensitive Nutrition Education

Successful culturally responsive nutrition education methods are a central element in addressing nutritional disorders within special populations. A pivotal starting point is to find out about the distinctive cultural aspects of said groups, not only food preferences and aversions, but also exact foods and food preparation patterns. By integrating contextually suitable materials into nutrition education courses, practitioners can create an atmosphere of respect and recognition among group members. This approach not only enhances participation but also enhances the likelihood of behavior change, as individuals are more likely to be responsive to information that resonates with their norms and cultural values. As noted in the literature, the effectiveness of nutrition interventions is significantly improved when education is tailored to the particular characteristics of the population, hence enhancing greater acceptability and utilization of better food options (Birnbaum et al., 2011). From the culturally targeted programs as the foundation, combining family-centered and community-based interventions has become a key strategy in nutrition education. Involving families in interventions allow families to have a support system that reinforces healthy behavior, and hence they become more effective. With the support of the community, whether through workshops or through community organizations, the families are again supported because the nutrition message is rendered relevant and community tailored. Evidence indicates that involving families and leveraging community resources can lead to a greater effect on weight loss and nutritional improvement, particularly for Latino populations. Adding social support during educational sessions not only increases participants' knowledge but also promotes feelings of belonging and obligation, hence laying the groundwork for successful life change (Burgos and Rivera, 2012). In addition, ongoing assessment and revision of nutrition education strategies are the key to long-term effectiveness in culturally competent initiatives. Regular feedback from participants will help nutrition educators modify their approaches to ensure ongoing responsiveness to the evolving needs of the community. Through the use of tools like surveys or focus groups, practitioners can identify areas of knowledge gaps and areas requiring further focus. Secondly, a responsive program structure enables instructors to incorporate emerging cultural patterns and tendencies into their programs. According to the literature, an open and dynamic approach involving community involvement optimizes the efficacy and relevance of nutrition education programs, thereby contributing to the reduction of nutritional morbidity among diverse populations (Birnbaum et al., 2011; Burgos and Rivera, 2012).

CLOSER LOOK

EATING DISORDERS

Eating disorders are serious mental health conditions that involve persistent disturbances in eating behaviors, thoughts, and emotions related to food, body weight, and shape. These disorders can significantly affect a person's physical health, psychological well-being, and social functioning. The most common types include anorexia nervosa, bulimia nervosa, and binge eating disorder (BED). Other recognized eating disorders include Avoidant/Restrictive Food Intake Disorder (ARFID), pica, and rumination disorder.

Anorexia nervosa is characterized by extreme food restriction, an intense fear of gaining weight, and a distorted body image. People with anorexia often become dangerously underweight and may suffer from malnutrition, organ damage, and even death if untreated. Bulimia nervosa involves cycles of binge eating followed by compensatory behaviors such as vomiting, excessive exercise, or laxative use. Binge eating disorder, the most common of all, involves repeated episodes of eating large quantities of food without purging, often leading to obesity and emotional distress.

The causes of eating disorders are complex and multifactorial. They often stem from a combination of genetic, psychological, environmental, and sociocultural factors. Risk factors include low self-esteem, perfectionism, trauma, peer pressure, and exposure to unrealistic body ideals in the media. Early recognition and intervention are crucial. Treatment typically involves a multidisciplinary approach, including psychotherapy (especially Cognitive Behavioral Therapy), nutritional counseling, medical monitoring, and sometimes medication. Family involvement is also essential, especially in children and adolescents. Eating disorders can affect anyone, regardless of age, gender, or background. Without treatment, they can lead to severe health complications or become life-threatening. However, with proper care and support, recovery is possible.

SUMMARY

The exploration of nutritional disorders within special populations highlights key challenges that must be addressed to effectively mitigate their prevalence and impact. Results from studies indicate a concerning upward trend in conditions , such as hypertension, particularly among older adults, who comprise a significant portion of the affected demographic. Specifically, the Korea Hypertension Fact Sheet reports that 28.0% of Korean adults were influenced by hypertension in 2021, with under-treatment and awareness rates which have been hindering effective control (Kim et al., 2024). The above highlights the importance of targeted interventions based on nutritional training and enhanced access to healthier foods, as dietary inadequacies immediately correlate with the prevalence of these conditions. Implementing strategies targeting the unique needs of each age group, particularly the elderly, is essential to improving health outcomes and preventing the exacerbation of nutrition-related diseases. Additionally, conditions like amyotrophic lateral sclerosis (ALS) emphasize the complex role of nutrition in the development of the disease in vulnerable populations. The outstanding weight reduction and muscle mass loss in the rapidly evolving ALS patients reflect an urgent need for more vigorous nutritional support measures. Despite the crucial interconnection between nutritional status and quality of life, timely measures are still absent for the majority of patients, as evidenced by low gastrostomy tube insertion and special therapeutic nutrition rates (Ermilov et al., 2024). Filling these gaps by means of extensive monitoring and intervention programs can enhance the outcomes for the patients. The culmination of this process lies in creating an understanding of nutritional requirements among physicians, who have to provide support for early nutritional screening as these illnesses progress to avoid declining in the patients' health further. In summary, solving nutritional disorders in vulnerable populations requires an interdisciplinary approach that incorporates healthcare, education, and policy change. The data illustrate that while some improvement has been made in the areas of awareness and treatment guidelines, the majority of patients are still poorly cared for, particularly where chronic degenerative conditions like ALS and elderly hypertension are involved. Future plans must tackle the issue of individualized care, considering the diverse needs of these populations, so that effective nutritional interventions can be applied regularly. Policymakers and health care professionals must collaborate to develop comprehensive programs that offer constant nutrition observation and intervention to ultimately enhance the quality of life for individuals suffering from such nutritional challenges in the world today. The research is conclusive in its call to action because ignoring these issues can have the potential to widen health disparities and elevate morbidity rates among already vulnerable populations.

Understanding of the broad range of special population nutritional disorders involves a detailed assessment of both demographic and health variables. More recent studies indicate that new eligible Medicaid members may have varying health profiles from current members, suggesting that differential interventions may be necessary. The age and health status variables will determine not only access to nutritional services but also the overall cost of care provision. These conclusions emphasize the necessity of examining participation levels among such groups to be able to effectively address the issues they pose, since changes in health demographics severely burden health care systems and economic sustainability (Kenney et al., 2010). In addition to issues of access to health care, age-related changes in physiological processes significantly impact nutritional intake among the elderly. More and more studies recognize that the aging gastrointestinal tract undergoes noteworthy alterations, which can affect digestion and absorption of essential nutrients. Knowledge of the alterations is crucial as they contribute to raising the prevalence of malnutrition among elderly individuals, which predisposes them to numerous illnesses. The confluence of the functional decline in the gastrointestinal tract with subsequent malnutrition highlights the necessity of wide-ranging dietary advice and interventions tailored to the unique needs of this group (Rémond et al., 2015). Moreover, the impact of malnutrition is not merely individual but extends into community health infrastructure and well-being. Because malnutrition leads to increased vulnerability to numerous pathological conditions, including those affecting the nervous, musculoskeletal, cardiovascular, immune, and integumentary systems, not only can the overall burden on health care facilities be large, but interventions for the prevention of malnutrition must consider not only the biochemistry of nutrient intake and availability, but the psychological, economic, and societal factors influencing food selection. Finally, developing an integrative approach that allows for these considerations is key to enhancing the nutritional status of special populations and their overall health outcomes.

References

1. Aerenhouts, D., Aerenhouts, C., Aerenhouts, R., Aerenhouts, S., Aragon-Vargas, L., Aragon-Vargas, F., Artal, R., et al. (2019). Nutrition for special populations: Young, female, and masters' athletes. https://core.ac.uk/download/334951624.pdf (accessed on 13th June 2025).
2. Balgir, R. S. (2011). Genetic disease burden, nutrition and determinants of tribal health care in Chhattisgarh State of Central-East India: A status paper. https://core.ac.uk/download/pdf/332892.pdf (accessed on 13th June 2025).
3. Belfer, M. L. (2005). Child and adolescent mental health around the world: Challenges for progress. https://core.ac.uk/download/pdf/86268.pdf (accessed on 13th June 2025).
4. https://core.ac.uk/download/286575279.pdf Rémond, D., Shahar, D. R., Gille, D., Pinto, P., Kachal, J., Peyron, M. A., Dos Santos, C. N., Walther, B., Bordoni, A., Dupont, D., Tomás-Cobos, L., & Vergères, G. (2015). Understanding the gastrointestinal tract of the elderly to develop dietary solutions that prevent malnutrition. *Oncotarget*, *6*(16), 13858–13898. https://doi.org/10.18632/oncotarget.4030 (accessed on 13th June 2025).
5. Burgos, G., & Rivera, F. I. (2012). Review of body mass index reduction interventions among Mexican origin Latinos and Latinas. https://core.ac.uk/download/267865529.pdf (accessed on 13th June 2025).
6. Currie, A., Plateau, C., & Arcelus, J. (2016). Eating disorders. https://core.ac.uk/download/288371375.pdf (accessed on 13th June 2025).
7. Edwards, K. J., Maslin, K., Andrade, J., Jones, R. B., & Shawe, J. (2022). Mobile health as a primary mode of intervention for women at risk of or diagnosed with gestational diabetes mellitus: a scoping review. *JBI evidence synthesis*, *20*(9), 2195–2243. https://doi.org/10.11124/JBIES-21-00294
8. Ekor, M. (2014). The growing use of herbal medicines: Issues relating to adverse reactions and challenges in monitoring safety. *Frontiers in Pharmacology, 4*. https://doi.org/10.3389/fphar.2013.00177 (accessed on 13th June 2025).
9. Heikkilä, M. (2020). Nutrition knowledge and skills among young endurance athletes. https://core.ac.uk/download/286389712.pdf (accessed on 13th June 2025).
10. Hilling, J. J., Robertson, C. E., & Hilling, J. J., et al. (2023). A review of the nutritional guidance for athletes to prevent eating disorders. https://core.ac.uk/download/586147205.pdf (accessed on 13th June 2025).
11. Kenney, G. M., Pelletier, J. E., & Holahan, J. (2010). The health status of new Medicaid enrollees under health reform. https://core.ac.uk/download/71347859.pdf (accessed on 13th June 2025).
12. Liu, Q., Luo, D., Haase, J. E., Guo, Q., Wang, X. Q., Liu, S., Xia, L., et al. (2020). The experiences of health-care providers during the COVID-19 crisis in China: A qualitative study. *The Lancet Global Health, 8*, e790–e798. https://doi.org/10.1016/s2214-109x(20)30204-7 (accessed on 13th June 2025).
13. McKay, A. K. A., Peeling, P., & Sim, M. (2023). Considerations for the consumption of vitamin and mineral supplements in athlete populations. https://core.ac.uk/download/587262144.pdf (accessed on 13th June 2025).

14. Park, I. H., Ko, N., Jin, M., & Lee, Y. J. (2024). Lower prognostic nutritional index is associated with a greater decline in long-term kidney function in general population. *Nutrition Journal, 23*. https://www.semanticscholar.org/paper/6421f0be579d7568c43449ffb3869401c42f061e (accessed on 13th June 2025).

15. Prajapati, N. K., Pasawan, S., Ram, M., & Kumar, S. (2024). Leafy chenopods: A nutritional powerhouse. *Journal of Agriculture and Ecology*. https://www.semanticscholar.org/paper/a07d1d19ab0cf2cb8ae05a1ba55ebfa867e69f0b (accessed on 13th June 2025).

16. Teede, H., Misso, M., Costello, M., Dokras, A., Laven, J. S. E., Moran, L., Piltonen, T., et al. (2018). Recommendations from the international evidence-based guideline for the assessment and management of polycystic ovary syndrome. *Clinical Endocrinology, 89*, 251–268. https://doi.org/10.1111/cen.13795 (accessed on 13th June 2025).

17. Thorne-Lyman, A., & Webb, P. (2025). Entitlement failure from a food quality perspective: The life and death role of vitamins and minerals in humanitarian crises. https://core.ac.uk/download/pdf/6380030.pdf (accessed on 13th June 2025).

18. Vilstrup, H., Amodio, P., Bajaj, J. S., Córdoba, J., Ferenci, P., Mullen, K. D., Weißenborn, K., et al. (2014). Hepatic encephalopathy in chronic liver disease: 2014 practice guideline by the American Association for the Study of Liver Diseases and the European Association for the Study of the Liver. *Hepatology, 60*, 715–735. https://doi.org/10.1002/hep.27210 (accessed on 13th June 2025).

19. Volkow, N. D. (2020). Collision of the COVID-19 and addiction epidemics. *Annals of Internal Medicine, 173*, 61–62. https://doi.org/10.7326/m20-1212 (accessed on 13th June 2025).

20. Yoon, Y. S., Lee, H. I., & Oh, S. W. (2024). A life-stage approach to precision nutrition: A narrative review. *Cureus, 16*. https://www.semanticscholar.org/paper/a2a2c43079a2c8d2eae2f63f5508760f693ff409 (accessed on 13th June 2025).

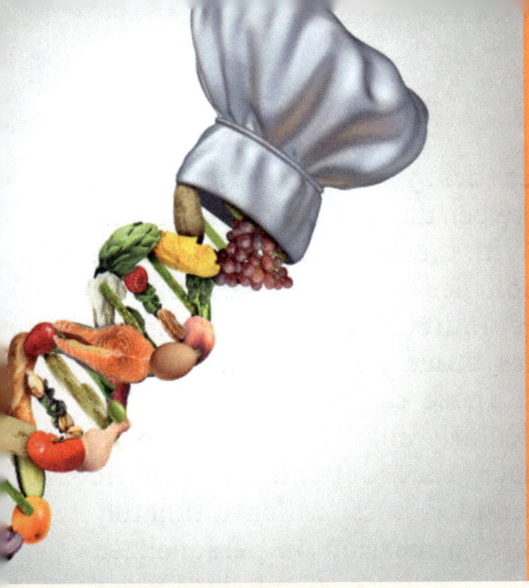

Chapter 14

NUTRIGENOMICS AND PERSONALIZED NUTRITION

Contents

Introduction....449
14.1. The Science of Nutrigenomics....452
14.2. Historical Context....457
14.3. Applications for Nutrigenomics....460
14.4. Benefits of Personalized Nutrition....464
14.5. Challenges and Limitations....468
14.6. Future Directions in Nutrigenomics....472
Summary....478
References....480

Introduction

The intersection of genetics and diet, or nutrigenomics as it is also referred to, is an area of study of utmost interest to scientists. Essentially, it involves studying how an individual's genetic makeup influences his or her nutritional requirements and metabolic responses. It is not a task for experts only; it has far-reaching implications for public health, food selection, and disease risk reduction. The establishment of genomic technology has caused researchers to begin revealing single genetic variants, , such as single-nucleotide polymorphisms (SNPs), that control nutrient metabolism and health outcomes. This information holds the potential for tailoring food recommendations based on people's genetic background, a significant improvement over traditional, one-size-fits-all dietary advice, and providing avenues for personalized nutrition (Zhang et al., 2024). With advances in nutritional science, the importance of personalized dietary advice continues to become clearer. Nutrigenomics is central to resolving the question of why some people react differently to eating plans, helping to reveal the genetic basis for such differences. For instance, individual SNPs involved in mineral homeostasis have been associated with varying risks of deficiency or toxicity, demonstrating how hereditary elements influence nutritional requirements. Nutrigenomics research has begun focusing on the key role genetic differences play in optimizing the intake of nutrients and overall health. Notably, Chickpea research as a functional food brings into focus how knowledge of genetics can be transferred to agriculture and nutrition programs. With new evidence on the health benefits of legumes, like chickpeas, a greater understanding of their genetic correlations can contribute significantly to dietary strategies for reducing poor health globally (Zhang et al., 2024). Public health policy integrating nutrigenomics is a groundbreaking strategy for more effective and holistic nutritional strategies. Through the acceptance of genetic diversity in populations, public health programs are able to come up with customized dietary recommendations with the purpose of lessening prevalent health conditions resulting from poor nutrition. However, it is important to embrace the limitations and ethical concerns associated with customization nutrition. For instance, research that has largely been done on Caucasian populations will be prone to exclude genetic diversity in favor of other populations and therefore distort the range of findings (Bösch et al., 2024). To address these problems, future research must ensure enhanced demographic representation in its genetic research. This way, nutrigenomics will not only enhance the well-being of human beings but also promote fair well-being results that represent the diverse genetic population of mankind.

Definition of Nutrigenomics

Nutrigenomics can be defined as the science of studying the effect of nutrients on gene function and how individual genetic variations influence reactions to nutritional factors. The new branch of study seeks to bridge the gap between nutrition and genetics by focusing on the complex relationship between dietary intake and genetic susceptibility. With the use of highly developed genomic technologies, nutrigenomics renders nutrition more individualized to maximize health outcomes based on one's own unique genetic factors. These can provide significant benefits, particularly for the prevention of chronic diseases that depend on genetic and environmental factors, which ultimately leads to a general discussion on personalized nutrition. As the database of nutrigenomics increases, its implications are more than mere dietary recommendations. Nutrigenomics can potentially allow for the design of functional foods that not only are healthy but are designed to combat a particular genetic type. It is worth mentioning that the role of nutraceuticals overlaps with this innovation; compounds found in various foods have been discovered to have profound effects on health at a molecular level. Nutraceuticals, as they are also characterized as required food constituents with nutritional as well as therapeutic or medicinal value, may be concerned with this.

Their bioactive molecules can modulate gene expression, thereby witnessing the molecular mechanisms of the benefits of nutrigenomics as we research its implementations in personalized nutrition (Al Ali et al., 2021). Despite the promising future of nutrigenomics, several challenges still exist, particularly regarding standardization and regulation. A universal definition of functional foods, including nutrigenomic principles, is still awaited, preventing concerted research and development. The lack of an integrated strategy reduces the chances of creating well-designed personalized nutrition programs that are both scientifically sound and compliant with the law. Various stakeholders, including scientists, regulatory agencies, and marketers, have a tendency to operate within siloed organizations where it becomes challenging to build a shared definition of functional foods and their implications. Addressing these challenges from a systems point of view is crucial to propel the nutrigenomics discipline forward and make it capable of meeting consumer needs based on stringent scientific standards (Alongi and Anese, 2021) (Figure 14.1).

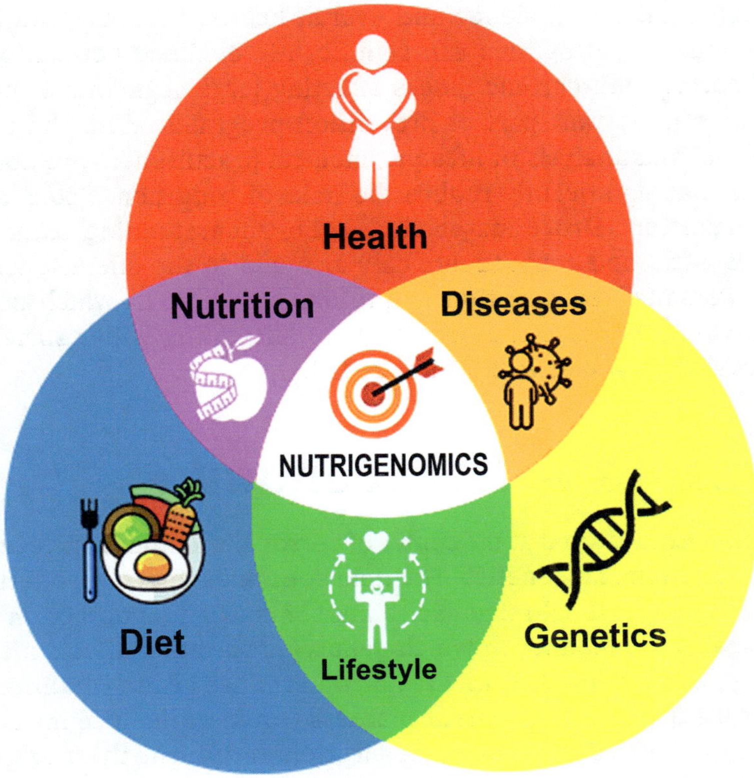

Figure 14.1. Nutrigenomics links diet, lifestyle, genetics, and health.

Source: https://welocitygenetics.com/website/html/assets/img/nutrigenomics-2.png.

Importance of Personalized Nutrition

The significance of personalized nutrition is that it can revolutionize nutrition guidance based on individual genetic, metabolic, and lifestyle traits. While traditional models of nutrition depend on standardized guidelines, personalized nutrition utilizes the principles of nutrigenomics in a bid to tailor dietary programs based on the unique genetic expression and health status of an individual. Using this specific method, one attempts to attain greater health benefits and address chronic conditions more effectively. The possibility of personalized nutrition emerges with regard to the prevalence of lifestyle diseases , such as obesity and cardiovascular diseases. By examining people's genetic risk factors, nutritionists can recommend food interventions that not only accommodate the individual's needs but also trigger acceptability and continuance of healthy eating behaviors. Furthermore, with rising evidence of the connections between diet and genetics, it is more and more evident that an across-the-board solution is not sufficient. The complex dance between genomic differences and dietary reactions serves to emphasize the need for accuracy in nutritional advice. Research suggests that people metabolize macronutrients differently and have different results in weight control and disease prevention. For instance, those genetically predisposed to gain weight can be assisted with a personalized regimen that involves higher protein and lower carbohydrate intake, focusing on their individual metabolic profiles. Not only is the aim to provide recommendations based on population means but to create more understanding of how individual differences may influence dining efficiency and overall health. Secondly, the use of personalized nutrition to inform population programs can significantly enhance population health outcomes. With rising levels of obesity and chronic illness affecting large segments of populations, tailored dietary advice can be an important part of prevention programs. With the use of instruments , such as genetic screening and analysis of lifestyle, medical practitioners are able to design focused intervention programs that significantly reduce the risks of conditions , such as dyslipidemia and obesity-induced hypertension (Dro Dżdż et al., 2021). Understanding oxidative stress profiles and their relationships with food constituents may also add to the effectiveness of individualized programs. Therefore, personalized nutrition is a future paradigm in which not just the personal health needs are addressed, but also the possibility of alleviating wider societal impacts of diet-related diseases is present (Senoner and Dichtl, 2019).

14.1. The Science of Nutrigenomics

The science of nutrigenomics is located at the center of personalized nutrition, focusing on the complex relationship between nutrition and genetics. The field continues to evolve, offering groundbreaking insights into the tailoring of personal response to nutrients as a function of one's genetic makeup. Nutrigenomics investigates the manner in which genotypic variation affects metabolic, absorptive, and utilization pathways of nutrients and, as a result, determines health conditions and vulnerability to chronic disease. For instance, certain genetic markers would be likely to make people susceptible to insulin resistance or enhanced cholesterol absorption and might thereby guide individualized dietary counseling for at-risk patients. This is not only descriptive of interventions for clinician audiences but also toward a more encompassing public health approach that includes genetic literacy in populations. By adopting the foundations of nutrigenomics, it is possible to shift from one-size-fits-all dietary advice to more personalized nutrition that can positively impact individual health and reduce disease risk. In addition to its implications for individual health, the impact of nutrigenomics also goes beyond that to food production and sustainability considerations. The use of nutrigenomics in agricultural engineering facilitates the alleviation of crop production that is specially made to fulfill specific nutritional needs, balancing farming operations with personalized nutrition concepts. For example, crops enriched with essential vitamins and minerals can be developed using processes grounded in nutrigenomic science. This intersection not only addresses personal health disparities but also contributes to global food security by providing nutrient-rich sources of food that have the potential to combat malnutrition. The activities of food sciences are also important, as scientists can create functional foods that cater to certain health needs by exploiting the results under nutrigenomics. This combined system develops a sustainable food production system that facilitates the reinforcement of health and environmental management to provide nutrient-rich foods to the general public. Nutrigenomics is also crucial in managing today's public health issues, typified by the pandemic of obesity. With increased rates of obesity levels being linked with increased cardiometabolic disorders risks, personalized dietary interventions guided by nutrigenomic data can be crucial in preventing these risks. Through the identification of the genetic risks of an individual developing obesity and obesity-related disorders, targeted nutritional interventions can be developed. For instance, research shows how certain genetic factors influence appetite, metabolism, and the body's response to different macronutrients. Based on these genetic factors, individualized eating regimens can be developed by healthcare professionals that maintain long-term weight control and reduce diet-associated chronic conditions , such as type 2 diabetes and high blood pressure. As a result, incorporating nutrigenomics into public health programs can motivate people to make informed food choices, with ultimate long-term positive effects on their health and improvement of the well-being of the overall population, which is essential in solving the increasing problems related to obesity and its long-term effects on health, as mentioned in Dro Dżdż et al. (2021) (Figure 14.2).

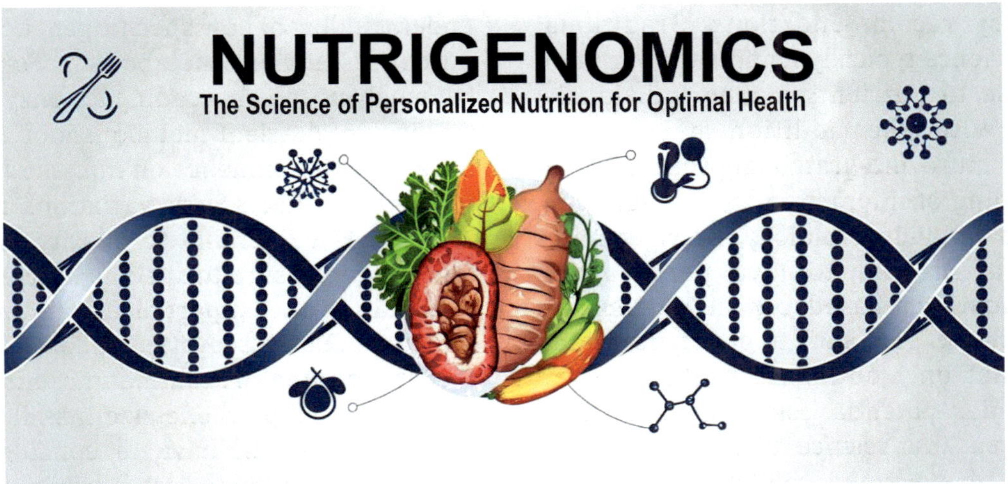

Figure 14.2. Nutrigenomics connects nutrition and genes for personalized health.

Source: https://mapmygenome.in/cdn/shop/articles/Nutrigenomics_-_The_Science_of_Personalized_Nutrition_for_Optimal_Health.jpg?v=1736400461.

14.1.1 Genetic Variations and Their Impact on Nutrition

Understanding the complex interplay between genetic variation and diet is the cornerstone of the complex emerging science of nutrigenomics. Genetic variation, in the form of single-nucleotide polymorphisms (SNPs), profoundly affects the way people metabolize nutrients and hence their health outcomes. Research has shown that these polymorphisms can significantly influence vitamin metabolism, with associations between them and critical vitamins like B vitamins, Vitamin D, and Vitamin E. Genetic factors related to the GC gene, for instance, have been linked with lower 25(OH)D concentrations, which means that those who have particular SNPs may require different amounts of vitamin D to maintain health. These findings point to the necessity of personalized nutrition advice based on genetic susceptibilities to facilitate more effective disease prevention and maintenance of health, as encapsulated in the systematic review of the literature (Bösch et al., 2025). The significance of ancestry should not be overstated regarding genetic variation and dietary adaptation. People with various ancestral origins can have diverse nutrient metabolism due to evolutionary adaptations that are in harmony with their former diets. Ancestral effects on SNP associations imply that one-size-fits-all nutrition might not be sufficient. Instead, individually adapted nutritional guidelines can enable us to identify people who are at risk for obesity, type 2 diabetes, and cardiovascular diseases. By identifying such variations, healthcare professionals can create personalized interventions that are tailored to certain genetic profiles and enhance overall wellness and health (Elsayed et al., 2024). Such a practice facilitates better insight into personalized nutrition's function in meeting various needs in different populations globally. The ongoing advancements in nutrigenomics are destined to change the future of diet and dietary recommendations. Traditional nutrition science typically ignores the variation in response to nutrients among individuals; however, with the addition of genetics, there is a more integrated approach. By an understanding of interaction among nutrition, genes, and individual biology, nutrigenomics allows practitioners to give personalized recommendations based on an individual's genetic makeup. This shift to genotype-guided nutrition not only optimizes healthy results but also holds potential for lowering chronic disease threats. As science advances, it will be important to overcome challenges , such as translating genetic information into effective dietary recommendations and scaling up these interventions to be effective and accessible in diverse populations, hence realizing the full potential of personalized nutrition (Elsayed et al., 2024).

14.1.2. Mechanisms of Gene-Nutrient Interactions

Clarifying the mechanistic basis of gene-nutrient interactions is crucial to drive nutrigenomics and personalized nutrition. At the molecular level, they could be understood via an array of mechanisms that modulate gene expression upon consumption of food constituents. For example, certain dietary bioactive compounds can act as signaling molecules, influencing transcription factors governing gene expression. This complex interplay results in convergent physiological responses based on a person's unique genetic makeup. Therefore, individuals metabolize nutrients differently, affecting disease susceptibility and overall health outcomes. With researchers unraveling these processes, there is the promise of targeted dietary recommendations, paving the way for innovative approaches to disease prevention and management, and ultimately optimizing individual health via nutrition. New breakthroughs in genomics sequencing and metabolomics have accelerated our understanding of how specific genetic variations influence nutrient metabolism. For instance, gene polymorphisms coding for enzymes in the pathway of nutrient metabolism or absorption have a crucial influence on individual response to dietary intake. Such variations may make individuals vulnerable to obesity or diabetes following exposure to specific nutrients, hence revalidating the importance of individualized nutrition. Such discoveries enhance the notion that nutritional recommendations will not be able to adopt a one-size-fits-all approach. Instead, they will have to consider genetic predispositions and the complexities of nutrient-gene interactions, with potential advantages for more tailored dietary interventions according to individual health needs. The implications of this personalized approach extend to public as well as personal health, foretelling a revolution in the concept of nutrition in the context of modern healthcare strategies for healthier populations. Although with highly promising progress toward characterizing the mechanism of gene-nutrient interactions, implementation of nutrigenomics is plagued with problems. While some of the correlations between specific genotypes and reactions to nutrients have been well established, many are inconsistent or unexplored, identifying a significant area of knowledge deficit in the discipline. The limitation renders the application of nutritional techniques to clinical practice difficult, where all the stakeholders may be uncertain of the reliability of genetic tests and their recommendations for diets. Furthermore, sociocultural factors like consumer acceptance and understanding of genetic concepts influence the use of nutrigenomic approaches. These challenges can be overcome through concerted effort on the part of scientists, clinicians, and educators to translate advances in the field into actual gains in health. To that end, additional research and debate are needed to navigate the complexities of this new science and to realize the full potential of personalized nutrition strategies to improve health outcomes (Castle et al., 2007; Beckett et al., 2017) (Figure 14.3).

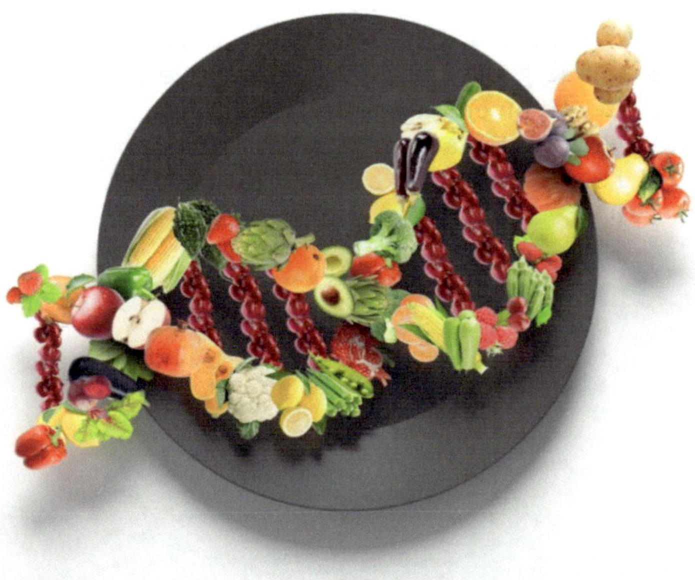

Figure 14.3. Fruits and vegetables forming a DNA strand to represent the nutrition–gene connection.

Source: https://thepoultrypunch.com/wp-content/uploads/2023/10/fjdhgs-1024x683.jpg.

14.1.3. Role of Epigenetics in Dietary Responses

The complex interplay of epigenetics and diet-induced responses is better elucidated in the fields of nutrigenomics and personalized nutrition. DNA methylation and histone modification are examples of epigenetic modifications that regulate gene expression without affecting the inherent genetic code. These modifications are, in turn, most often triggered by dietary components, i.e., macronutrients and bioactive foods. For example, certain polyphenols in vegetables and fruits have been shown to change epigenetic marks, which can lead to epigenetic changes in gene expression patterns that affect metabolism and disease susceptibility. Since individuals are unique genetically and epigenetically, they might also react uniquely to dietary treatments. The identification of these differences is essential to designing individualized dietary plans in line with an individual's epigenetic makeup in order to optimize health and effective disease prevention, particularly chronic disease associated with obesity (Allayee et al., 2017). Additionally, the role of the gut microbiota adds another layer of complexity to dietary inputs on epigenetics. The pertinent interplay between the human host and gut microbiome is complicated, mediating the effects of what we consume. The metabolism stage by bacteria in the gut can create both short-chain fatty acids and other metabolites that can modulate host gene expression via epigenetic modification. This interaction highlights the need for a more comprehensive nutrigenomics approach that considers not only human genomics but also the food genome and gut microbial genome (Martin et al., 2011). Personalized nutrition interventions must take these interactions into account in order to ensure that dietary guidance is not only based on genetic predispositions but also considers the impact of the microbiome on epigenetic consequences. Finally, the implications of these findings for public health and clinical nutrition are important. As our understanding of epigenetic mechanisms deepens, it becomes apparent that dietary interventions can serve as powerful tools for modifying epigenetic status and, subsequently, health outcomes. This is particularly important for populations at high risk for chronic diseases, where lifestyle and nutritional changes could lead to significant epigenetic alterations that mitigate these risks. For instance, individually optimized dietary interventions based on the individual's unique genetic and epigenetic patterns can optimize health pathways throughout life. Thus, the integration of epigenetic data into nutrition science not only introduces the prospect of new dietary interventions but also facilitates a more comprehensive understanding of health maintenance and disease prevention by supporting the connection between diet and gene expression (Martin et al., 2011; Allayee et al., 2017) (Figure 14.4).

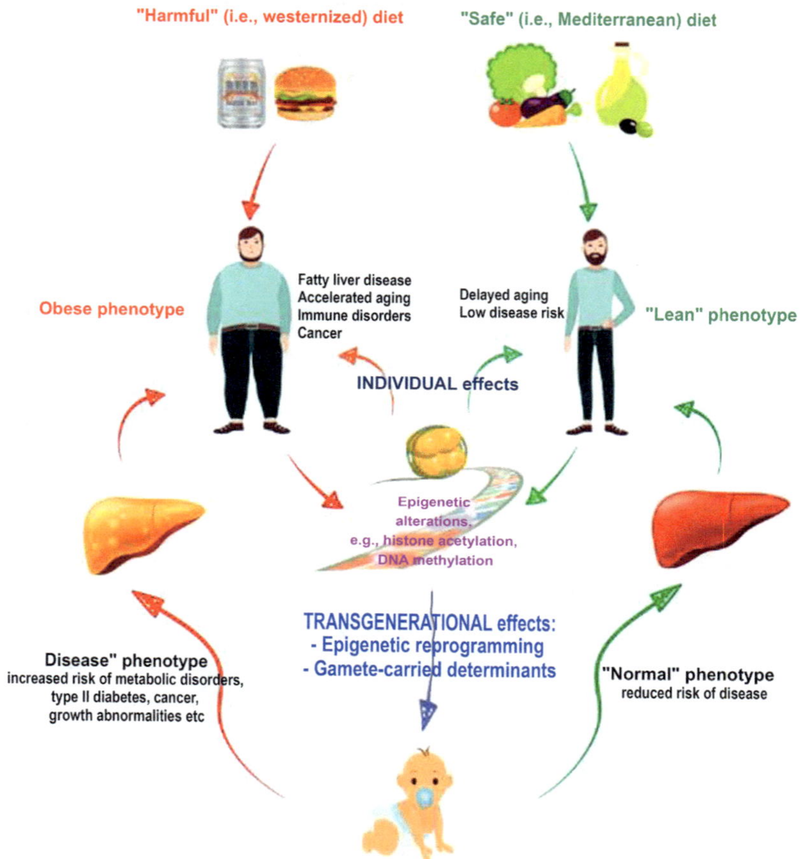

Figure 14.4. Diet influences health and disease risk through epigenetic and transgenerational effects.

Source: Tiffon C. The Impact of Nutrition and Environmental Epigenetics on Human Health and Disease. *International Journal of Molecular Sciences*. 2018; 19(11):3425. https://doi.org/10.3390/ijms19113425

14.2. Historical Context

The search for diet-gen interaction has made remarkable strides in recent decades, heralding the onset of nutrigenomics as a scientific field in biomedical research. Initially, the concept of individualized nutrition was mainly stimulated by food consumption and dietary advice emanating from large population surveys. However, the advent of high-throughput genomic technologies has triggered a paradigm shift, enabling researchers to investigate how genetic variations regulate nutritional responses at a more personalized level. Looking back in history, one could trace some of the advancement in this area to early 20th-century research that linked vitamins and minerals with allied deficiencies, providing the platform for contemporary investigation into the extent to which an individual's genetic makeup can provide personalized dietary recommendations (Castle et al., 2007). As discoveries in genomics and molecular biology expanded, the translation of such findings to the nutrition space became apparent, and nutrigenomics was born. Nutrigenomics integrates the analysis of genetics with what an individual consumes to account for how nutrients are involved in gene-expression modification. The transition to individualized nutrition follows parallel currents in healthcare as a whole, where more focus is given to personalization rather than the employment of one-size-fits-all treatments. This is particularly pertinent in the management of complex, multifactorial illnesses subject to both environmental factors and genetic predispositions. The convergence of nutrition and genetic data can, therefore, inform more effective diet methodologies for disease control and prevention, representing a fundamental historic shift in nutrition policy (Argano et al., 2019). While commenting on the history of nutrigenomics, one must commend various scientific advancements and societal changes that have affected its development. The completion of the Human Genome Project in 2003 was a landmark achievement, providing detailed data on human genetic variation and driving advances in related fields. As scientists began to identify genetic markers for various health ailments, they began to understand that diet could potentially have a pivotal role in modifying the impact of health based on these markers. Moreover, the increasing prevalence of lifestyle diseases again confirmed the necessity for customized nutritional interventions, culminating in an even stronger interest in how individual genetic profile might shape nutritional needs and tolerance. This historical background is crucial in the understanding of the evolving landscape of nutrigenomics and its potential to revolutionize strategies for individualized nutrition that address individualized health profiles (Castle et al., 2007).

14.2.1. Evolution of Nutritional Science

Nutrition science has progressed significantly since its humble origins, growing from basic diet observations to an extremely sophisticated comprehension of the biochemical complexities of food and disease. Early nutrition science was first interested in avoiding deficiency diseases, and vitamins and minerals became central components of human well-being. With the creation of the first dietary guidelines, nutrition was revolutionized, as there was now a system for well-balanced nutrition. As technology improved, the identification of biochemical processes facilitated scientists in investigating more intensely the metabolism of nutrients and interactions within the human body. This breakthrough led to more personalized dietary counseling, opening the path for future discovery of nutrigenomics as a science that investigates how genetic difference affects nutritional requirements and response. The history of nutritional science is thus central to appreciating the focus on personalized nutrition today. Genomic research has been funded, which has brought great implications for the field of nutrition, particularly in nutrigenomics. With the mapping of the human genome through the Human Genome Project, researchers obtained unparalleled access to genetic variations that can affect health and dietary needs. This early work reinforced the fact that genetic predisposition could modulate the impact of diet on the health of an individual, and this has prompted reevaluation of the one-size-fits-all dietary recommendations. The understanding that food components interact with gene expression has ushered in an era of customized nutrition. By providing diet advice that is genetically determined for the individual, nutrigenomics holds the potential to not only to enable overall well-being but also treat and prevent chronic disease more effectively. This turns in nutritional science heralds a significant change from traditional approaches and emphasizes the use of genetics in dietary treatment.

In addition, the clinical application of nutritional medicine is a major advance in the field of nutrition research and also in individualized health care. Advances in genomic nutrition are helping to enhance the understanding of how certain foods can affect gene expression, eventually leading to personalized nutritional strategies for an individual. For instance, certain eating habits have been linked to reduced inflammation or improved metabolic health, depending on genetic variation that controls how one reacts to specific nutrients. The results of this study are groundbreaking in that they enable health professionals to devise personalized nutrition plans that closely align with an individual's own DNA. As such, nutrigenomics not only broadens the purview of nutritional science but also promises more optimal prevention and intervention strategies for various diseases. The evolution of nutritional science thus takes on a paradigm where individualization with respect to genetic data is paramount to the achievement of optimal health outcomes (Castle et al., 2007; Butorac et al., 2011).

14.2.2. Key Milestones in Nutrigenomics Research

Nutrigenomics discipline has evolved dramatically since its conception, identifying critical milestones in the history of the interaction between genetics and nutrition. One of the earliest breakthroughs was the discovery of certain gene-diet interactions that affect metabolic processes. This work provided a foundation for appreciating how genetic differences among individuals can result in varying responses to nutritional elements. Therefore, the emergence of genome-wide association studies (GWAS) was a milestone for nutrigenomics, and with this advancement, scientists have been able to link genetic variation with many diet-dependent health endpoints. These links underscore the application of a personalized nutrition strategy, in which dietary guidance can be based on an individual's genetic profile. With nutrigenomics' continued growth, new technologies have played a significant role in pushing the research frontier further. The development of high-throughput sequencing technologies has revolutionized research into genetic information so that very extensive gene expression analyses of the reaction to specific nutrients are possible. Technology has enabled the identification of how food components, , such as fats and carbohydrates, can control the activity of genes and what the underlying processes are that couple diet and health. Additionally, the advancement of metabolomics has revealed how nutrients from diet affect biomarkers and metabolic pathways, with consequent more tailored dietary interventions and recommendations. Continued advancements in these technologies are pivotal for finding new potential disease risk biomarkers and to response to diet, further facilitating individualized nutrition interventions. Recognizing that health conditions have a complex etiology has led to a greater focus on the inclusion of behavioral, environmental, and genetic variables in nutrigenomics studies. Recent focus has been on the holistic approach to understanding lifestyle components in interaction with genetic factors influencing health outcomes, particularly in the case of non-communicable diseases. This complexity makes it essential to realize that the diet is only one piece of a complex jigsaw puzzle of genetic, environmental, and lifestyle factors. The design of personalized nutrition advice must thus consider all of these interconnected factors to optimally maintain health and prevent disease. The ongoing debate in the scientific community regarding how to incorporate these factors will guide future research and clinical practice in nutrigenomics towards ultimately enhancing the efficiency of personalized nutrition interventions (Chrousos et al., 2014; Baixauli, 2022) (Figure 14.5).

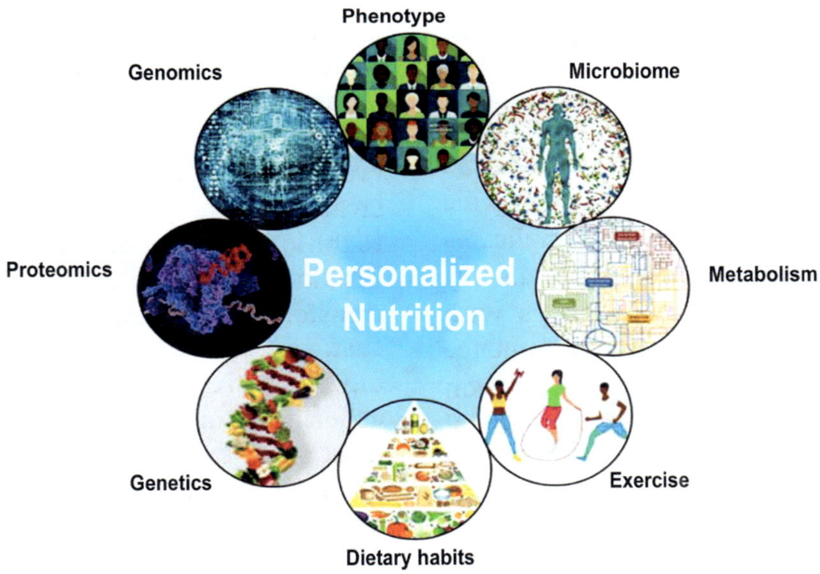

Figure 14.5. Personalized nutrition shaped by genetics, lifestyle, and metabolic factors.

Source: https://media.springernature.com/lw1200/springer-static/image/art%3A10.1186%2Fs40246-023-00561-w/MediaObjects/40246_2023_561_Fig1_HTML.png.

14.2.3. Development of Personalized Nutrition Concepts

Conceptualization of personalized nutrition is based on the realization that nutritional requirements are greatly different among individuals. Personalized nutrition considers the impact of genetics on metabolism and the possibility to craft meal plans that appeal to the unique genetic identity of an individual. In contrast to conventional dietary recommendations, which tend to follow a one-fits-all policy, personalized nutrition stresses customized dietary advice to enhance healthy outcomes depending on genetic susceptibility. This paradigm shift is exemplified by advances in nutrigenomics, which is the study of complex food and gene interactions. Such research describes the way diet components influence individual health, forming the basis of more successful and personalized nutritional treatment that promotes well-being (Ganesh et al., 2024). As the premise of personalized nutrition evolves further, it is based largely on valuable lessons gained through the investigation of nutrigenetics. Genetic profiling makes people aware of how their body processes a variety of nutrients and makes food choices based on their biology. It helps them to prevent potential health risks associated with individual genetic vulnerabilities, , such as obesity or metabolic syndrome. In addition, omics technologies like metabolomics and microbiomics have facilitated the attainment of deep new insights into the interaction of diet with gene expression. By integrating genetic information with intensive phenotyping, personalized nutrition recommendations can be derived to address the complex interaction of biology and environment responsible for dietary responses (Lagoumintzis and Patrinos, 2023).

While there is huge potential in personalized nutrition, its widespread acceptance is threatened by a number of factors. The polygenic etiology of most nutrition disorders complicates the challenge of developing worldwide dietary recommendations, as numerous genes with minimal individual effects collectively influence health outcomes. In addition, the interaction of these genetic elements with environmental elements complicates things further. To overcome these challenges, ongoing research must refine methods for successful genotyping, as well as simultaneously integrate findings from microbiome studies. These advancements will not merely enhance the precision of personally optimized dietary recommendations but also further establish avenues for understanding the interaction between genes, diet, and health (Lagoumintzis and Patrinos, 2023; Ganesh et al., 2024). With the advancement of the personalized nutrition field, so will its role in creating healthier lifestyles with unique demands.

14.3. Applications for Nutrigenomics

The emerging science of nutrigenomics has significant implications for personalized nutrition, revolutionizing the way dietary recommendations are tailored to suit an individual's genetic makeup. Through the study of genetic differences and how they interact with specific nutrients, nutrigenomics provides information on how individuals metabolize food, respond to dietary changes, and manage diet-related diseases. This information is critical in developing personalized diet regimens that can prevent or manage diet-related diseases, , such as obesity and diabetes. With precision nutrition advancing, the integration of advanced tools like bioinformatics and machine learning helps uncover complex interactions between genetic markers and food nutrients to lay the groundwork for more effective public health strategies and personal health management techniques (Ramos-López et al., 2024). Ultimately, nutrigenomics is the backbone in transforming conventional dietary advice into customized solutions that consider the individual differences in genetic and metabolic responses, ushering in improved health results. One of the most significant applications of nutrigenomics is in preventing obesity and associated metabolic disorders. As obesity is becoming more prevalent across the globe, integrating nutrigenomics into food science is introducing novel solutions with a focus on stimulating better diets and avoiding obesity. Through designing functional foods that act on specific metabolic pathways, nutrigenomics enables one to add nutrients to diets that have the potential to alter gene expression and augment physiological responses. Moreover, customization of diet plans for individuals based on their genetic makeup allows for simpler management of weight and protection against chronic diseases. Utilizing dietary interventions based on genetic data streamlines the fight against obesity and thus offers healthier benefits that are more long-lasting as well as healthier individuals who are engaged in decision-making for foods (Lynrah et al., 2024). Besides, nutrigenomics holds the promise to enhance the sustainability and equity of food systems. The greater the research that is conducted to open up the connections between nutrition, genes, and the environment, the more effective interventions can be designed that address not only the special needs of individuals but also consider broader social issues , such as food insecurity and access to nutritious food. Evidence-based nutrition interventions informed by nutritional technology can lead to more effective public health interventions that ensure equitable access to healthy foods across various populations. Here, application of nutrigenomic principles not only improves individual well-being but also facilitates the shift towards healthy and sustainable food systems for the globe. By producing an integrated understanding of food cultures, nutrigenomics will be in a position to advise policy interventions that address both personal wellbeing and the public good of the community, in the end improving general quality of life (Lynrah et al., 2024; Ramos-López et al., 2024) (Figure 14.6).

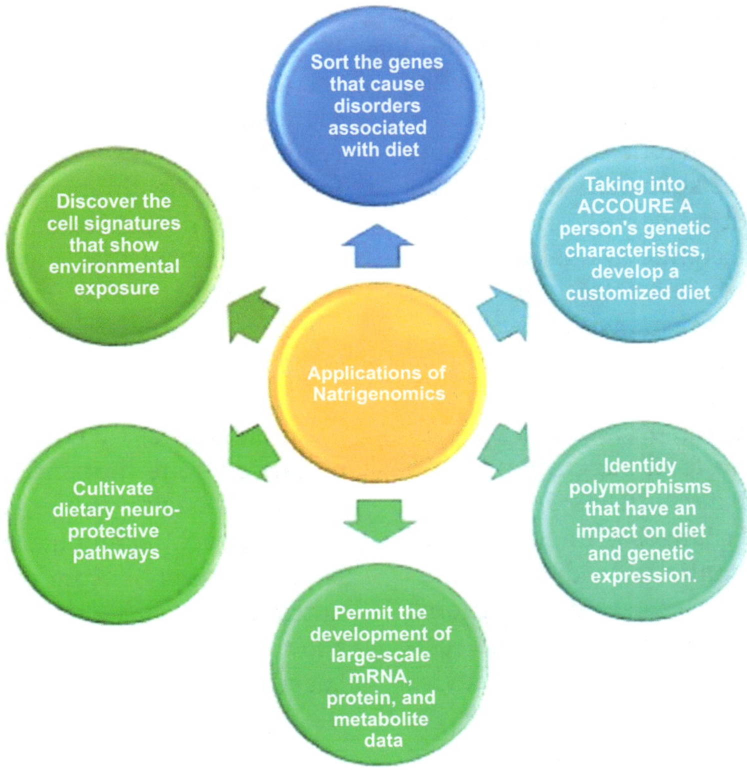
Sort the genes that cause disorders associated with diet
Taking into ACCOURE A person's genetic characteristics, develop a customized diet
Identidy polymorphisms that have an impact on diet and genetic expression.
Permit the development of large-scale mRNA, protein, and metabolite data
Cultivate dietary neuro-protective pathways
Discover the cell signatures that show environmental exposure
Applications of Natrigenomics

Figure 14.6. Applications of nutrigenomics in personalized diet and gene interaction.

Source: https://www.researchgate.net/publication/378244052/figure/fig2/AS:11431281224174279@1708086666462/Representation-of-nutrigenomics-applications-including-polymorphism-detection-diet.ppm.

14.3.1. Tailored Dietary Recommendations

The concept of personalized nutrition guidance is on the forefront of the new science of nutrigenomics, where scientists examine the relationship between an individual's genotype and their responses to food. Since genetic variation affects the effectiveness of metabolism and nutrient absorption, medical professionals can design nutrition programs for each individual to maximize health outcomes. For example, genes involved in lipid metabolism may influence dietary decisions about fat consumption , such as enabling individuals with particular genetic profiles to modify risks for disorders like cardiovascular disease. Personalized nutrition counseling not only increases adherence to nutrition counseling but also overall effectiveness by offering solutions to the unique needs and wants of every individual, fostering a more sustainable approach to nutrition and health care (Singar et al., 2024). Integration of artificial intelligence (AI) and machine learning (ML) into developing personalized dietary counseling is a significant advancement in personalized nutrition. Traditional dietetic strategies were prone to neglecting the specificity of individual response to food, but newer AI solutions are revolutionizing the discipline by analyzing large data sets with gene-based data, food intake patterns, and metabolic responses. Deep neural networks (DNNs) enable these newer systems to identify complex relationships between food inputs and personal health profiles and increase prediction accuracy in food suggestions. Such a solution based on data makes suggestions dynamic, adapting as changes in an individual's lifestyle and health continue to develop, thus enabling a better holistic view of nutritional needs (Vegesna, 2024). Furthermore, the real-world applicability of personalized diet advice through nutrigenomics also includes challenges along with opportunities. As scientists explore the complex relationships between genes and diet, there is an increasing call for full educational courses to equip healthcare professionals with the knowledge necessary to implement it properly. The ethical issue of genetic data confidentiality and potential misuse of information also needs to be addressed with care in order not to create public distrust and noncompliance. In that regard, the encouragement of interdisciplinary collaboration between data scientists, geneticists, and nutritionists will be paramount in the development of personalized nutrition. As science deepens, not only will the opportunity for large-scale application of personalized dietary advice have the potential to offer superior health outcomes for individuals but also create a healthier population at large (Singar et al., 2024).

14.3.2. Nutrigenomic Assessment and Testing

Nutrigenomic analysis and testing are an important driver of personalized nutrition based on the association of individual genetic profiles with dietary needs. Through a study of the influence of genetic variation on nutrient metabolism, the topic allows for tailored dietary recommendations aimed at optimizing health outcomes. The combination of various genetic information facilitates easier detection of polymorphisms that may influence a person's response to specific nutrients and thereby give way towards nutritional strategies that optimize health. One such instance is the employment of bioinformatics and compilation of data from databases like the GWAS catalog that enhances gene-diet interaction and possible effects on health. While research continues to enhance such techniques, nutrigenomic testing is progressively becoming a go-to resource for nutritionists and healthcare practitioners, which allows them to provide customized diet regimens based on the personalized genetic profiles of their patients (De, 2023). The accessibility of nutrigenomic testing has completely transformed the mentality of individuals regarding their dietary intake. These tests give an insight into how one's genetic predispositions can affect the absorption, metabolism, and utilization of numerous nutrients. Therefore, individuals can make realistic diet choices depending on their genes to prevent chronic conditions and improve overall health. Moreover, the application of systems biology in nutritional components make possible the examination of the complex interaction between genes, environmental exposures, and nutritional components. This holistic approach highlights the worth of an integrative approach to nutrition, one that not only considers individuals' genetic background but also their lifestyle and surroundings, advocating for personalized nutrition as a dynamic, multifaceted science (Özdemir, 2015). To the extent that the significance of nutrigenomic analysis grows louder, numerous issues and ethical concerns ensue, above all concerning access and confidentiality. The cost of genetic testing may restrict access to some groups, thereby maintaining health disparities. Additionally, individuals must be educated on how their genetic data will be stored, used, and protected, and this leads to consent and misuse concerning intimate information. These concerns will have to be addressed as nutrigenomics becomes more deeply rooted and is more integrated into routine care. Ensuring that nutrigenomic testing is equitable and ethically safe will be important in establishing public trust and encouraging the application of personalized nutrition methods that benefit different groups of people (De, 2023) (Figure 14.7).

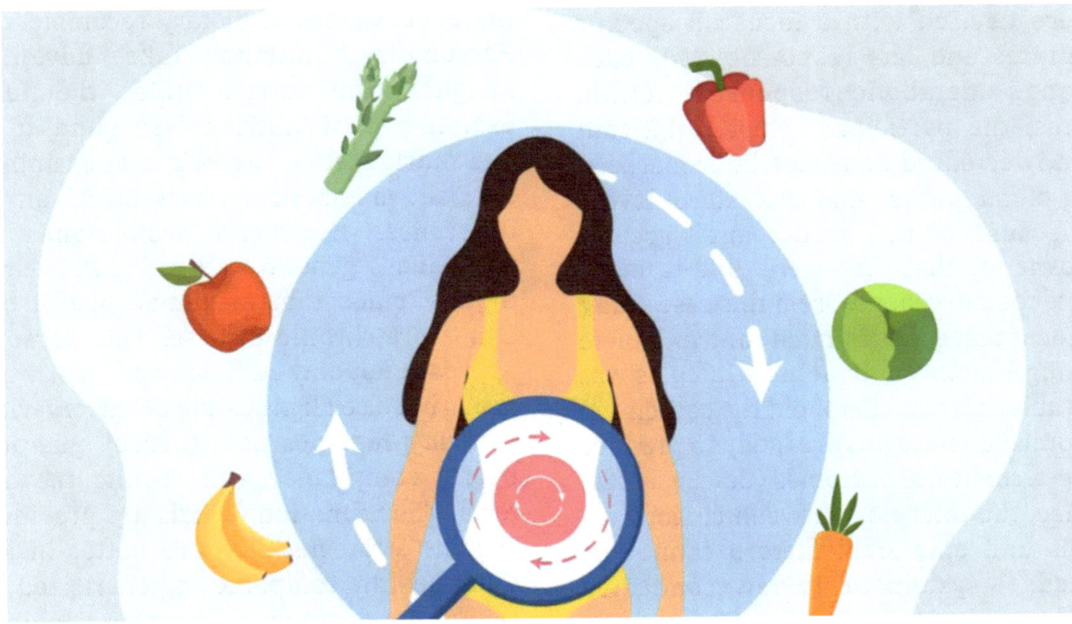

Figure 14.7. Nutrition influences gene expression and overall health.

Source: https://assets.clevelandclinic.org/transform/LargeFeatureImage/ce257e33-8d7c-436c-a1c8-113c152da07a/Nutrigenomics-1289259444-770x533-1_jpg.

14.3.3. Case Studies of Successful Personalized Nutrition Plans

Customized nutritional regimens are now a key component of nutritional components and have great potential to enhance health outcomes across different populations. An excellent case was a patient cohort with chronic kidney disease (CKD), where personalized diet interventions were at the core of treatment. The patients were treated with individualized low-protein diets (LPDs) supplemented with ketoanalogues. This approach was employed to reduce the kidney strain on their organs and still ensure adequate nutritional supplementation. The results indicated a remarkable decrease in CKD progression in the group that adhered to the tailored regimen. The long-term adherence difficulties, however, revealed the intricacy of maintaining dietary restrictions in chronic disease. These findings point out the significance of developing strategies that enhance patient retention within individualized nutrition plans, and point out that even though LPDs are beneficial, whether or not they succeed relies on individual circumstances and long-term commitment (Alobaidi, 2025). Another compelling case study illustrates the efficacy of individualized nutrition to sustain weight and metabolic well-being. The patients included in this study, who were primarily overweight patients, underwent genetic screening to ascertain their unique responses to macronutrient profiles. According to these genetic results, individualized meal plans were devised with a focus on specific carbohydrates and fats responsible for each participant's metabolic responses. Within 12 months, the participants lost significant weight and decreased their metabolic markers, including blood glucose and cholesterol levels. It was because of the participants' greater body knowledge that they were able to make reasonable food decisions. From this case study, it was evident that genetics' main contribution to determining effective nutritional strategies was indispensable and helped uphold the contention that customized strategies are likely to produce more long-term health outcomes (Gonzaga et al., 2025). Also, the interplay between customized diet plans and emotional factors cannot be overlooked. A systematic review conducted with students preparing for the Civil Service Examination showed that the incorporation of mental readiness and emotional health in tailored dietary programs had a strong impact on levels of achievement. The subjects possessed better focus and reduced stress when their diet was synchronized with their study calendars. Moreover, the integration of online materials and nicely structured meal programs offered another reinforcement and engagement dimension. This case study sheds light on the complex nature of individualized nutrition, wherein nutritional approaches intersect with mental and emotional health. Such types of findings encourage researchers and practitioners to consider well-rounded strategies that not only address the biological aspects of nutrition but also the cognitive and emotional aspects, so that interventions by individualized nutrition become more impactful (Gonzaga et al., 2025).

14.4. Benefits of Personalized Nutrition

The advantages of personalized nutrition lie in its capacity to take individual genetic profiles into account, which can significantly increase the effectiveness of dietary recommendations. Personalized nutrition takes advantage of insights from nutrigenomics, the field that examines how nutrients respond to genes, and nutrigenetics, the field that examines how nutrient metabolism varies based on genetic differences. Healthcare professionals use an individual's genetic data to create customized dietary plans that maximize health benefits and avert chronic disease. This personalized approach not only addresses particular nutrient needs but also aligns eating behaviors with one's genetic predisposition, thereby guaranteeing better compliance and results in the long term. Therefore, individuals are provided with specific strategies that are better in keeping them healthy compared to generalized dietary recommendations, suggesting significant improvements in personalized health management and disease prevention (Wang et al., 2025). The incorporation of technology into personalized nutrition has been found to multiply with its effect. Online platforms , such as mobile applications and wearable technology, allow for continuous tracking of dietary patterns, physical activity, and other health metrics. They can include real-time feedback and personalized recommendations based on individuals' genetic information, which can significantly improve health. For instance, research has indicated that such AI-powered programs can obtain a mean weight loss of 4.6 kg, as well as major glycemic and cardiovascular improvements (Wang et al., 2025). The dynamic nature of these interventions increases user engagement and improves motivation, yielding a stronger environment for habit formation and health gain. Furthermore, the adaptability of the instruments is capable of facilitating ongoing alterations to diet regimens to ensure that they remain effective based on changing individual progress. Another crucial advantage of personalized nutrition is its capability of promoting public health program improvements through challenging the intricacies of global obesity and trends of chronic diseases. Personalized nutrition interventions are particularly beneficial in at-risk group identification and in framing prevention strategies based on their specific needs. With the implementation of knowledge obtained through genetic testing, healthcare professionals are able to develop more effective outreach programs that provide individualized nutrition counseling. Not only are these programs able to empower patients to make well-educated food decisions, but they also increase health literacy among communities. Lastly, tapping into the power of individualized nutrition from genetics and technology can deliver more sustainable gains in health and a radical reduction in healthcare spending on diet-related disease (Kibibi, 2024) (Figure 14.8).

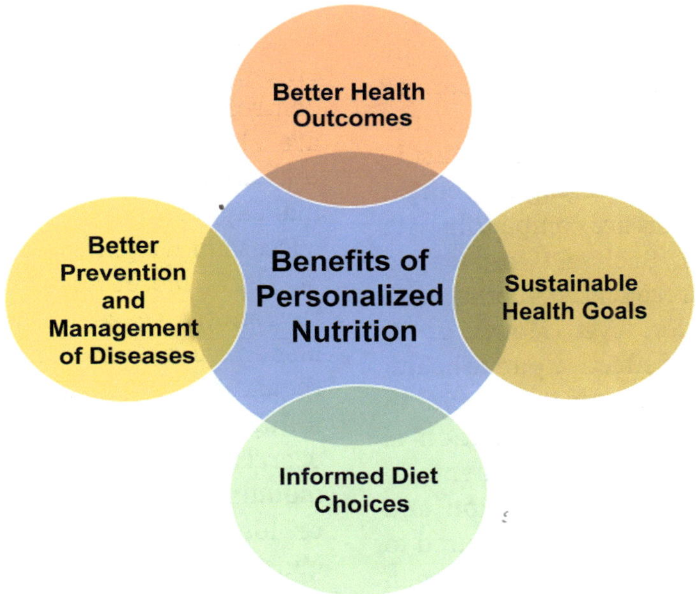

Figure 14.8. Benefits of personalized nutrition for health, diet, and disease prevention.

Source: https://www.techsciresearch.com/blog/personalized-nutrition-enhanced-living-through-science/169.html.

14.4.1. Improved Health Outcomes

The relationship of nutrigenomics to improved health outcomes becomes increasingly evident through research emphasizing the importance of personalized nutrition based on genetic makeup. Personalized nutrition based on the genetic makeup of an individual has the potential to determine dietary food choices that help in lowering the risk of chronic diseases. For instance, the need for specific micronutrients may vary significantly among individuals due to genetic variation affecting the metabolism and absorption of nutrients. These tailored needs can be an important preventative strategy against obesity, diabetes, and cardiovascular diseases. By targeting dietary interventions based on genetic propensities, nutrigenomics enables the creation of personal nutrition recommendations for the highest health impact, ultimately optimizing the efficiency of dietary interventions in the control of chronic disease (Pandarinathan et al., 2024). The role of ultra-processed foods (UPFs) also cannot be precluded in addressing health outcomes. The rise in consumption of UPFs is attributed to the expanding epidemic of obesity and various chronic diseases globally. They are characterized by high sugars, unwholesome oils, and additives with low levels of essential nutrients. The harmful health effects of UPFs emphasize the importance of promoting eating habits that are friendly to whole, minimally processed food. By promoting such dietary changes, nutrigenomics can be integrated into public health programs aimed at reducing UPF consumption and encouraging movement towards healthier diets that are compatible with genetic characteristics. Such a two-pronged strategy can lead to unprecedented public health benefits at the population level (Monda et al., 2024). Implementation of effective public health interventions that capitalize on the results of nutrigenomics and personalized nutrition is the key to achieving lasting improvements in health outcomes. Both public education and practitioner education programs are required to enhance awareness of the connection between food and genetics. Policy reforms that increase access to whole food and limit access to UPFs are also needed. By creating a setting conducive to healthier food selection, communities can better address the complicated issue of chronic diseases. Current research studies need to focus on examining the longitudinal effects of tailored nutritional intervention and determining how genetic tailoring of the diet approach influences long-term health outcomes in diverse populations. This combined strategy reflects the vast potential of nutrigenomics to transform models of public health and improve global health trends.

14.4.2. Enhanced Weight Management Measures

In the context of augmented weight management strategies, nutrigenomics is a central integration into personalized nutrition interventions. As an emerging field, it considers the manner in which genetic differences dictate an individual's response to specific nutrients and provides a foundation for personalized nutritional advice. For instance, individuals metabolize carbohydrates differently following genetic sensitivities, which affect weight gain and retention. Treatment of these unique metabolic pathways with individualized nutrition regimens, as well as maximizing compliance, also optimizes efficacy in achieving objectives for weight control. Using genetic information, physicians are able to establish the ideal form of diet that aligns with each person's unique genetic makeup, enhancing the likelihood of intended success in weight control programs (Allayee et al., 2017). Moreover, precision nutrition extends to genetic susceptibility; epigenetic factors also have an important function in weight regulation. The mounting evidence points to the influence of lifestyle, for example, dietary and exercise habits, in modifying gene expression, modulating an individual's propensity to gain or lose weight. Such insight facilitates the generation of personalized strategies that consider not only the genetic composition but also environmental and lifestyle elements. For example, specific diet components, e.g., omega-3 fatty acids and polyphenols, have been found to exert a beneficial influence on the expression of genes involved in body weight regulation. Integration of such information into tailored nutrition interventions enables the leverage of nutrient power against obesity as well as overall health improvement (Arsenault et al., 2017). Additionally, multicomponent weight control necessitates behavioral modification as well as dietary modification. Methods , such as deep phenotyping enable health professionals to analyze individuals' diet, activity, and psychology. Such a comprehensive assessment leaves the way open for the creation of tailored interventions that account for the unique needs and problems of each patient. In embracing the fact that one diet does not fit all, incorporating behaviorally informed methods into a nutrigenomic strategy has the potential for more effective and long-term weight control strategies. By bridging the gap between scientific evidence and actual practice, enhanced methodologies for weight control have the potential to enable individuals to achieve and maintain healthy weights more efficiently (Allayee et al., 2017) (Figure 14.9).

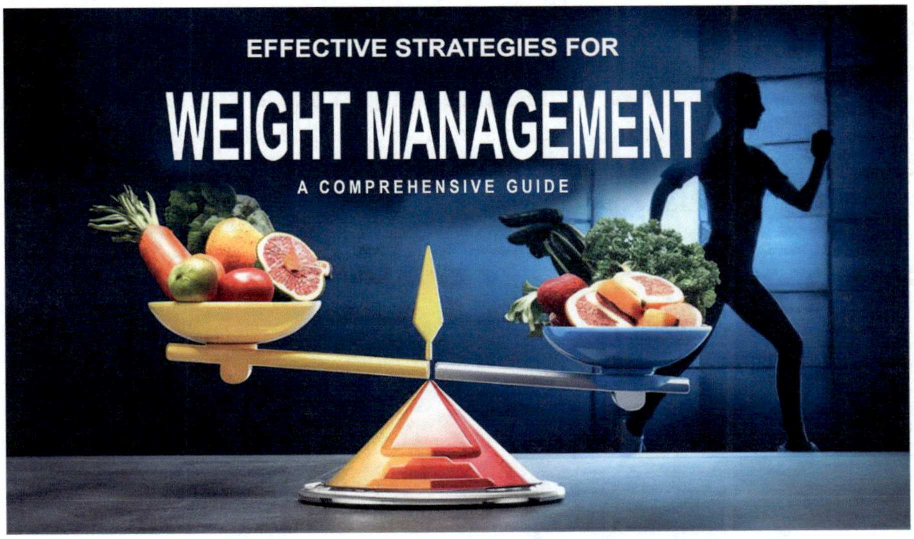

Figure 14.9. A balanced diet and exercise support effective weight management.

Source: https://mapmygenome.in/cdn/shop/articles/Effective_Strategies_for_Weight_Management.webp?v=1720248101.

14.4.3. Prevention of Diet-Related Diseases

The rising rates of diet diseases, , such as obesity, diabetes, and cardiovascular disease, have put the imperative for preventive interventions based on personalized nutrition into sharp focus. Nutrigenomics, or the study of how foods interact with genes, has emerged as a key strategy for addressing these diseases. By understanding how genetic variation influences the way individuals react to what they consume, health practitioners can offer individualized dietary recommendations that not only prevent but also control chronic diseases. The individual approach is more than what usual dietary recommendations can offer, flexible to the individual's own biochemical and genetic make-up, hence making preventive interventions more efficient. Greater understanding of these interactions can allow individuals to make informed food choices that promote long-term health and well-being, potentially cutting the incidence of diet-related illness spectacularly. As scientists delve more comprehensively into the gene-diet interface, ever greater need for a multi-disciplinary strategy for personalized nutrition becomes evident. Integrating knowledge from genomics, biochemistry, and epidemiology can unlock the potential for the design of holistic dietary models applicable to broad populations. For instance, different genetic predispositions may determine how individuals metabolize macronutrients, thus the need for individualized diet plans to maximize health results. In addition, advancing technologies in nutritional genomics provide real-time dietary individualization according to the genetic profile of an individual, permitting targeted interventions. These developments are poised to enhance not only individuals' health but also the efficiency of public health interventions for preventing diet-related disorders, ensuring that all demographic groups will be in a position to take advantage of the new developments in nutrition approaches. The fate of nutrigenomics is not only going to hinge on scientific progress but also on addressing ethical issues related to genetic screening and data protection. As with personalized nutrition in the limelight, stakeholders must deal with issues over the meaning of genetic information, particularly with respect to personal control and discrimination. Availability of access to personalized dietary strategies not create social disparities is critical so that nutrigenomic benefits are available to all. Public health policies thus play a vital role in creating an environment in which tailored nutrition can thrive while addressing potential challenges of access and ethical use. Through the focus on inclusivity as well as ethical practice, the promise of nutrigenomics can be realized, leading to a healthier population and effectively reducing the incidence of diet-related disease among a range of populations. (Singar et al., 2024; Tamboli et al., 2024) (Figure 14.10).

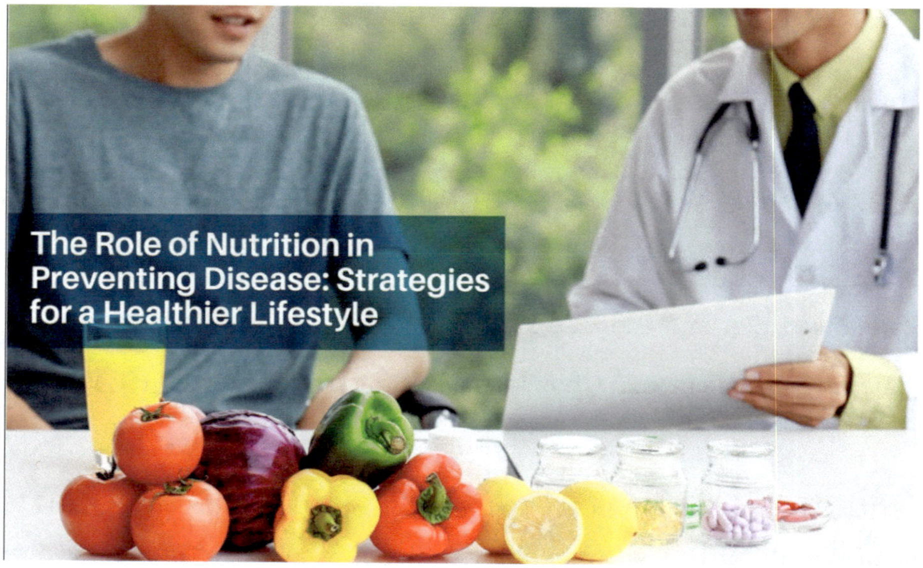
The Role of Nutrition in Preventing Disease: Strategies for a Healthier Lifestyle

Figure 14.10. Nutrition guidance supports disease prevention and healthy living.

Source: https://www.saraswatihospitals.com/wp-content/uploads/2024/04/Blog-Banners_1140-x-696-px_English_Saraswati-03.jpg.

14.5. Challenges and Limitations

The landscape of nutrigenomics and personalization is full of significant hurdles and deficits, particularly in practice translation to heterogeneous populations. Primarily among the hindrances is the inherent complex nature of human biology, which makes it difficult to predict response to specific dietary interventions based on genetic or epigenetic traits. For instance, while nutrigenomics can answer questions about bioactive compounds from the diet affecting gene expression, personalized counsel traditionally requires comprehensive, nuanced information about many external variables that affect the health of an individual. Additionally, as mentioned in recent literature, the integration of dietetic interventions into clinical frameworks necessitates the collaboration of practitioners across a number of professions, i.e., nutrition and gastroenterology, and thus makes it even more challenging to develop tailored dietary therapies (Dhaliwal et al., 2025). Furthermore, there is another significant limitation of personalized nutrition that arises from variation in the strength of evidence supporting individual dietary interventions. While scientific advancement holds the promise of yielding good outcomes, present literature is typically marred by methodological flaws, variations in study designs, and scarcity of large-scale randomized controlled trials. The majority of studies are conducted on animal models that are very much removed from entirely reflecting the complexity of human metabolism and nutrition, which becomes an issue about the applicability of the findings to human health (Dhaliwal et al., 2025). Apart from that, technical difficulties, including the intricacy of obtaining and analyzing precise genomic and food data, restrict the establishing of such universally effective guidelines for personalized nutrition. While researchers try to trace the influence of particular foods on gene expression, the problem of guaranteeing constant data acquisition and correct analysis is most essential in confirming personalized dietary advice. Consumer uptake is also a major barrier to the realization of nutrigenomics in conventional nutrition. The potential of innovations , such as in vitro cultured meat to revolutionize diets, faces skepticism from consumers, owing to fear regarding safety and ethical production methods. As noted in the literature, concerns regarding genetically modified organisms and the long-term health consequences of new sources of food raise very serious issues regarding consumer trust and acceptance of these alternatives. Furthermore, the ability to navigate the intricacies of dietary advice with existing eating habits needs good communication strategies from health practitioners so that they are able to help people understand and accept. To overcome these challenges, it is essential to engage public perception through education and transparent research, ensuring that evolving nutritional paradigms align with consumer needs and preferences while addressing potential health risks.

14.5.1. Ethical Considerations of Nutrigenomics

The ethical dimensions of nutrigenomics are complex and multifaceted, in essence revolving around genetic privacy, informed consent, and access to tailored nutrition therapies. As the incidence of genetic testing increases in analyses of food systems, abuse of genetic data may be problematic. Genetic discrimination is likely to take place, particularly within healthcare insurance and workplace environments. Second, there must be informed consent; the patients must be well informed about the implications of genetic testing and what is to be done with their data. Ethical guidelines must be created that protect individual rights but also facilitate personalized nutrition advancement. Third, there must be equal access to nutrigenomic services; unequal access to medical care could prevent disadvantaged groups from being in a position to benefit from these advances, increasing present health disparities even more. Moreover, the intersection of nutrigenomics and public health policy brings new ethical issues, particularly in regulating genetic testing and nutritional interventions. The rate of advancement in genetic science is unprecedented and outpaces current regulation mechanisms for the purpose of safeguarding public health. This could lead to non-regulated genetic tests that are providing false or misleading dietary advice on a large scale and could cause consumers' harm. To bridge this gap, ethical guidelines must be created for the regulation of nutrigenomic services so that therapeutic claims are supported by evidence from science. Regular debate with bioethicists, healthcare professionals, and policymakers is required to create a balanced strategy that supports innovation without undermining public interest. Monitoring and evaluation mechanisms must also be established in order to ensure social responsibility in deriving the benefits from nutrigenomics. Finally, the ethical considerations of nutrigenomic research lie in broader societal spheres, namely the global impact on diet and identity. Tailored nutrition commercialization can commoditize traditional diets and lead to a homogenization of diets as individuals resort to genetically directed, science-based counsel. It can diminish the cultural significance of the traditional diet, provoking ethical questions about dietary sovereignty. Furthermore, with nutrigenomics promoting individualized nutrition, the ethical issue of maintaining individual agency takes center stage; citizens must remain capable of controlling decision-making that is in harmony with their cultural heritage rather than being forced into acquiescence with scientifically determined diets. To address these issues, there needs to be interdisciplinary efforts that involve nutritionists, ethicists, and cultural anthropologists to have a discourse that addresses the implications of nutrigenomics in depth and breadth. The objective should be to strike a balance that honors personal preference but brings nutrigenomic science developments to global food habits (Figure 14.11).

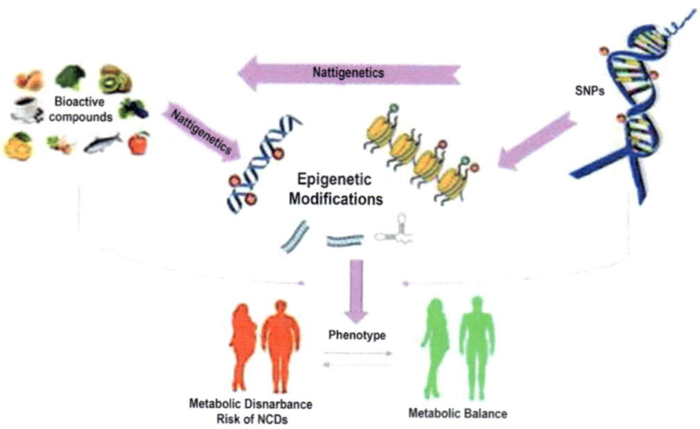

Figure 14.11. Nutrigenetics and nutrigenomics influence metabolism and disease risk through gene–diet interactions.

Source: Franzago M, Santurbano D, Vitacolonna E, Stuppia L. Genes and Diet in the Prevention of Chronic Diseases in Future Generations. *International Journal of Molecular Sciences*. 2020; 21(7):2633. https://doi.org/10.3390/ijms21072633

14.5.2. Accessibility and Affordability of Testing

The relationship of affordability and accessibility for nutrigenomics screening is a critical component in the real-world adoption of personalized nutrition. While technology has the potential to expand access to genetic testing, there remain significant barriers. Economic disparities and the overall cost of these tests can prevent individuals from accessing tailored dietary advice. One's primary concern is that even while nutrigenomics science improves, the affordability of such interventions could prevent the lower-income segments of society from accessing personalized nutrition interventions. That raises ethical questions regarding the fairness of genomic-based health interventions, given that more economically poorer individuals could be deprived of cost-effective dietary changes that could enhance their health status. The promise of nutrigenomics should therefore be examined critically through the costing prism to ensure overall public health gains are fostered while preventing inequalities in accessibility and affordability (Godard et al., 2013). Second, test applicability is another critical factor employed to determine accessibility. Not only must people be in a position to go for genetic testing but also put into practice what these results mean daily. There is often a discrepancy between the advanced data generated by genetic tests and interpreting the meaning of that information in making daily food choices. Such intricacy may deter engagement with personalized nutrition, particularly from consumers who are overawed by technical jargon or imprecise advice. Studies show that customers value convenience and simplicity, which means that dietary advice needs to be developed in harmony with daily habits and preferences (Bouwman et al., 2009).

Therefore, efforts to make nutrigenomic testing more prevalent need to focus on streamlining the return of results so that the information is useful and applicable to different populations. Finally, there is a call for an expedited participatory approach for the development of nutrigenomic testing methods based on accessibility and affordability. Engaging a wide range of stakeholders, like consumers, healthcare professionals, and policymakers, can make the discussion of the implications of personalized nutrition more inclusive. This multi-stakeholder process can establish a knowledge exchange that is public demand-driven and confidence-building for the new innovations.

By addressing affordability and access concerns within an inclusive framework, the nutrigenomics science can better integrate social demands and expectations. Such a process would have to involve consumers as active co-designers of the various applications of nutrigenomic information so that social and ethical values are built into test design and subsequent nutritional interventions to enhance health equity upon implementation of personalized nutrition strategies (Bouwman et al., 2009).

14.5.3. Variability in Individual Response to Diets

The response heterogeneity to diets is a fundamental issue in the field of nutrigenomics and individualized nutrition. Heterogeneity comes from an immensely large number of variables, including genetic predisposition, metabolic rate, and even psychological responses to food. Experiments have revealed that individuals do not respond to diet interventions the same way and hence the need to embrace personalized dietary recommendations. Recent research into personalized nutrition suggests that having the ability to comprehend these differences will make them more effective in weight-loss and disease-prevention management. Picking one's way through the complexity of individual variability, the hope of nutrition researchers is to refine dietary advice that is relevant to specific genetic and phenotypic patterns with the ultimate intention of maximizing health impact across different populations (Arsenault et al., 2017). Beyond genetic factors, environmental forces also significantly determine dietary responses. Individual lifestyle practices, , such as physical activity level, socioeconomic standing, and access to healthy food, interact with genetic predispositions to produce varying effects on health. This interaction complicates the formulation of universally acceptable dietary advice. Current studies underscore the role of deep phenotyping and metabolomics in elucidating the complex mechanisms of dietary response. Through the use of sophisticated analytical tools, researchers are able to develop a better understanding of a person's individual physiological and metabolic traits, which can be used in guiding tailored dietary measures. Such approaches are particularly critical in addressing the rising prevalence of obesity and related metabolic diseases, through the identification and acceptance of interindividual variation in the development of interventions (Arsenault et al., 2017). Profiling the microbiome of one's diet is a field with great potential to advance personalized nutrition. The human microbiome is made up of trillions of microorganisms that reside in the gut and play a crucial role in nutrient metabolism and health. Diversity of microbiomes can also produce varying dietary responses in individuals, thereby emphasizing the need for individualized nutritional strategies. State-of-the-art investigations now probe interactions between diet, microbiota, and individual health outcomes, further proving that the same dietary recommendations work for all is no longer effective. The more scientists understand interactions between genetics, environment, and microbiome, the more promising the prospect of even more precise and effective nutritional counseling becomes. This changing knowledge is essential to addressing public health problems, , such as metabolic syndrome, by targeted, evidence-based dietary interventions (Figure 14.12).

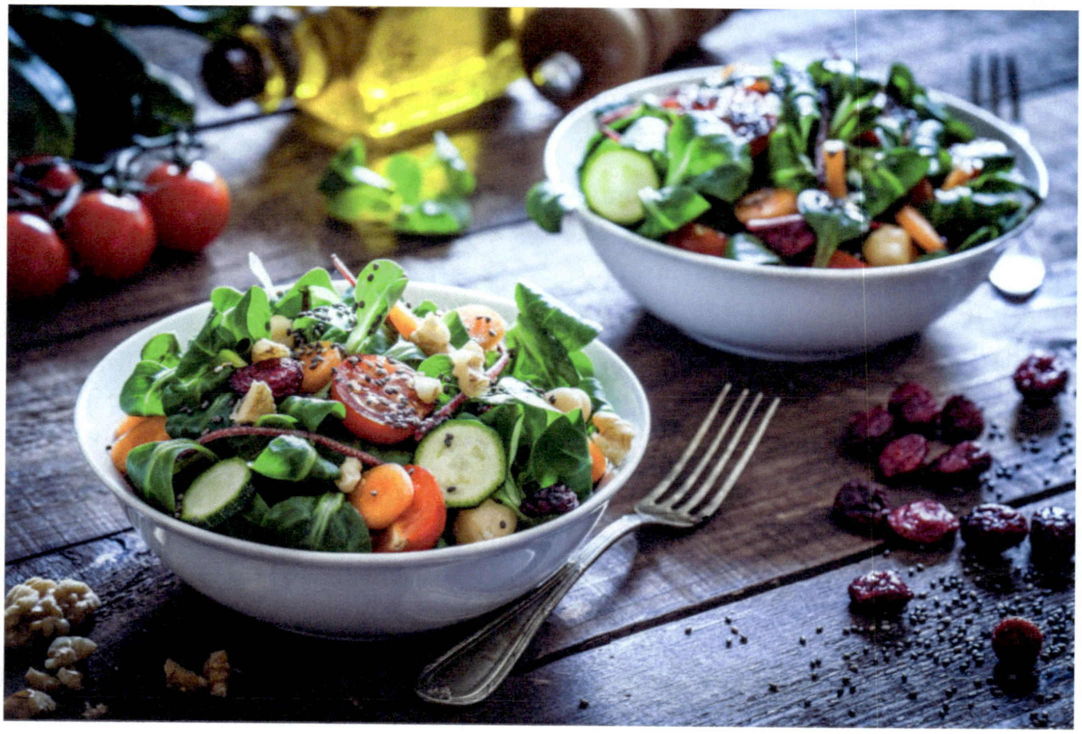

Figure 14.12. Fresh vegetable salads rich in nutrients, promoting a healthy and balanced diet.

Source: https://static01.nyt.com/images/2019/06/10/multimedia/10nutrition/447bc37a1bcb42caa95d2785123ef972-superJumbo.jpg.

14.6. Future Directions in Nutrigenomics

The future of nutrigenomics stands at the intersection of genetic study and personal nutrition, promising to revolutionize diet solutions based on specific genetic makeup. With new research uncovering complex relationships between genes and how one responds to food, greater emphasis is being put on using this knowledge to develop personal dietary advice. These tailored nutrition strategies offer the potential to optimize health gain and manage chronic disease more effectively, particularly as we begin to discover significant gene-diet interactions that influence diseases , such as obesity and diabetes. The inclusion of advanced genetic testing will also take these activities further by providing patients with clear, actionable data regarding how their metabolism responds to various nutrients, thereby allowing targeted dietary intervention closely correlated to their unique genetic profile (Singar et al., 2024). Coupled with genetic data, technological advancements are transforming the practice of nutrigenomics and personalized nutrition. The merging of genomic data analysis programs with bioinformatics is vital to compact vast amounts of genetic information and translate them into actionable dietary recommendations. New platforms , such as mobile programs and personal meal-planning programs, are being developed to permit real-time diet revision using individual genetic information. These technologies, in addition to enhancing access to personalized nutrition, also facilitate active health management to allow consumers to make informed dietary decisions. As multidisciplinary science continues to grow, stakeholders must find ways to address data privacy and ethical considerations to allow proper use of genetic testing in nutrition applications (Singar et al., 2024). In the coming years, nutrigenomics as a science is likely to expand immensely in health and wellness businesses, marking the beginning of personalized medicine. The therapeutic value of personalized nutrition, particularly in the management of chronic conditions, could be enhanced with the convergence of new therapeutic strategies, , such as innovative antidiabetic drugs that have added-value effects besides glycemic regulation. For instance, the use of glucagon-like peptide-1 receptor agonists and sodium-glucose co-transporters shows how breakthroughs in the field of drugs can be supplemented with dietary changes to exert a synergistic effect on cardiovascular and metabolic health. With the promotion of collaboration between nutritionists, geneticists, and doctors, patient-focused models of personalized care will become increasingly prevalent, ultimately leading to more targeted approaches to managing disease conditions like type 2 diabetes.

14.6.1. Advances in Genomic Technologies

Genomic integration has radically redefined our understanding of nutrigenomics and personalized nutrition, opening up novel opportunities for diet interventions upon individual genetic backgrounds. Advances in high-throughput sequencing technologies allow researchers to analyze complex genetic information at a level never before seen, revealing complex interconnections among dietary lifestyles and genetic compositions. This capacity makes it possible to find genetic markers for specific responses to foods, resulting in ultimate personalized dietary recommendations. For instance, various capacities to break down food from one individual to another based on genetic make-up, , such as the manner people respond to caffeine or lactose, make it possible for nutritionists to make tailored meal plans that optimize wellness and health outcomes. As genetic information widens, so does the scope for precision nutrition, which is about matching food with genetic types to promote health and prevent diet-related disorders. Additionally, the application of nutrigenomics is not only in individualized dietary counseling but in the agriculture sector as well, particularly in maximizing feed efficiency. With the application of genomic tools in cattle breeding and nutrition, farmers can identify genetic elements maximizing nutrient utilization. This nutrigenomics function allows for the creation of precision feeding schemes, which adjust diets based on the genetic profile of individual animals. These steps not only optimize productivity and profitability for cattle farmers but also align farm activities with the increasing demand for green and environmentally friendly food production. With the discovery of genetic markers and integration into breeding schemes, the livestock sector can combat both financial and environmental issues head-on, hence validating the contribution of genomic advancement towards enhanced food security and sustainability (Olorunkoya et al., 2024). Despite the promising advancement of genetics, there are obstacles surrounding the ethical appreciation and practical integration of genetic data into everyday dietary practices. Genetic information interpretation necessitates careful monitoring to ensure that dietary advice is scientifically valid and comprehensible by the public. Issues of privacy and genetic information misuse also necessitate ethics regulations that protect individuals while optimizing person-specific nutrition. Resolving these matters is important in providing assurances of public trust in nutrigenomics. The future of customized nutrition will rely on the formulation of strong regulatory guidelines and the development of evidence-based guidelines that consider both the complexities of individual genomics and the broader social impacts of genomics technologies (Ghazanfar, 2024). As research continues, the overlap between genetics and nutrition will increasingly become more complex, holding out the potential for a finer appreciation of how individual eating habits may be tailored for optimum health and prevention of disease (Figure 14.13).

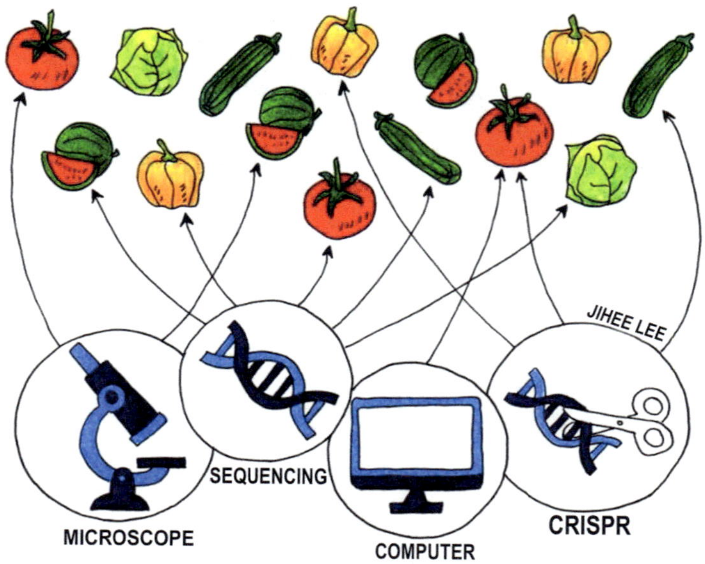

Figure 14.13. Tools like CRISPR and sequencing enhance fruit and vegetable genetics.

Source: https://specialtycropgrower.com/wp-content/uploads/2019/01/TGLee_VSC_Nov2018_Figure-1024x772.jpg.

14.6.2. Integration of Nutrigenomics into Healthcare

The integration of nutrigenomics into health care represents an important step towards personalized nutrition, where genetic information guides dietary recommendations. This new approach has the promise to enhance patient care through making nutritional therapies tailored to patient-specific genetic differences that affect nutrient metabolism and clinical outcomes. The effective integration of nutrigenomics into regular practice is fraught with numerous challenges. According to the Indian dietetic expert study, one of the major deterrents for its incorporation is that genetic testing is extremely costly, and access for both providers and patients is limited by this (Rosario et al., 2025). There is also a significant lack of standardized test protocols and clinical trials demonstrating efficacy, due to which there are professional doubts about its usefulness in real-world, clinical practice (Rosario et al., 2025). Transcending these challenges is necessary for developing an environment in which nutritional technology can thrive and result in improved health outcomes. For nutrigenomics, interprofessional collaboration emerges as an important plan for dismantling existing barriers to integration. Because the field is so new, interprofessional alliances among dietitians, geneticists, and healthcare professionals can facilitate knowledge exchange and evidence-based practice construction. An Indian study emphasizes the need for higher education among dietetic practitioners towards raising awareness and understanding of genetic testing's potential; this education can be crucial in promoting its application in clinical practice. Secondly, public awareness campaigns are needed to demystify genetic testing, therefore raising patients' acceptance (Rosario et al., 2025). In combined efforts, all this can yield robust frameworks that support the integration of nutrigenomics so that personal nutrition strategies can be rendered effective and feasible. Moreover, investigations of genetic diversity and dietary reactions provide a basis for arguments for embracing nutrigenomics as an element in healthcare systems. One study highlighted the significance of having individual genetic profiles in guiding the use of dietary supplements, illustrating variability in response based on genetic status. The study indicates genetically directed personalized nutrition to enhance the effectiveness of nutraceuticals and improve patient safety through minimizing side effects. This information is valuable for health care providers striving to develop personalized recommendations for nutrition that are based on individualized genetic profiles. Therefore, the integration of nutrigenomics not only helps in individualized dietary counseling but also optimizes the overall effectiveness of nutrition interventions, eventually leading to improved health and wellbeing outcomes in diverse populations. This highlights the need for health systems to evolve and incorporate nutrigenomics as part of the very fabric of personalized health care provision (Figure 14.14).

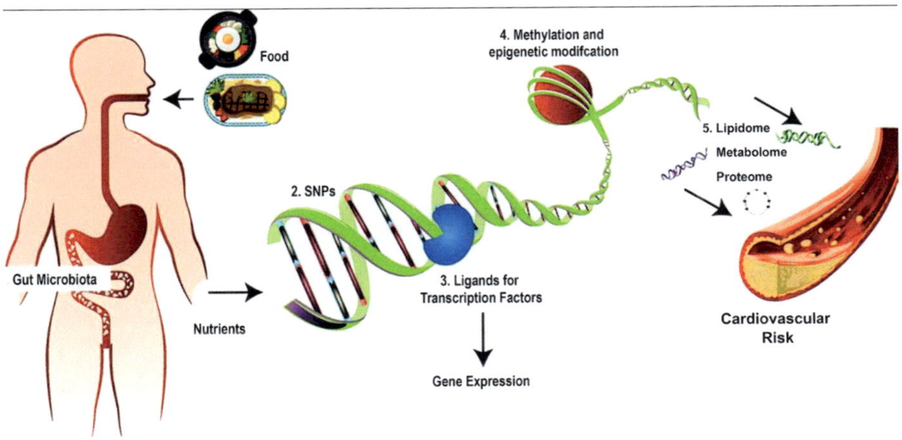

Figure 14.14. Gut microbiota and nutrients affect gene expression and cardiovascular risk.

Source: https://www.ahajournals.org/cms/10.1161/HCG.0000000000000030/asset/8497d53e-bd2f-48db-9897-fcc726a980a6/assets/graphic/291fig01.jpeg.

14.6.3. Potential for Public Health Initiatives

There are enormous public health opportunities in the field of nutritional nutrition and personalized nutrition, particularly with awareness of genetic influences on nutritional needs on the increase. Understanding how an individual's genetic makeup determines nutritional needs and responses, public health initiatives can be more effectively planned to address the far-reaching needs of the population. Nutrigenomically founded programs could lead to individualized dietary advice that consider genetic diversity for optimal intake of nutrients for better health. Such individualized strategies can be particularly beneficial in the management of chronic disease, where nutritional therapy has the potential to have significant influences on health status and reduce healthcare costs. Emerging technologies, including 3D food printing, could have extensive implications for public health initiatives aimed at promoting personalized nutrition. Emerging technology allows for precise personalization of meals to meet the diverse nutritional requirements and taste, allowing for the addressing of issues related to food accessibility and food compliance. Through the addition of targeted macronutrients and micronutrients to foods, 3D printing could help provide healthier diets. But to make these interventions worthwhile, there is a need for monumental efforts in consumer education and the removal of concerns regarding the affordability and acceptability of printed foods. With increased public engagement, so will public acceptance of such technologies will expand our potential impact on public health through personalized nutrition interventions. In addition, integration of genetic research into public health initiatives can maximize the effectiveness of nutritional guidance. Evidence for genetic variation in mineral metabolism, as outlined in recent reviews, underscores the potential for personalized nutrition recommendations. For example, the identification of SNPs influencing iron absorption can guide practice, , such as supplementation in at-risk groups. Such findings not only create potential for better health outcomes at an individual level but can be projected to community-based interventions aimed at preventing nutrient deficiency diseases. Collective shifting towards personalized nutrition facilitated by progress in nutrigenomics brings dramatic opportunities for the public health interventions aimed at promoting well-being and reducing health inequities within populations (Bösch et al., 2024; Do Rosario et al., 2025).

CLOSER LOOK

NUTRIGENOMICS

Nutrigenomics is an emerging field at the intersection of nutrition, genetics, and molecular biology that explores how individual genetic variations influence responses to specific nutrients and dietary patterns. It is grounded in the idea that food is not only a source of energy but also a powerful environmental factor that can interact with the genome to affect health outcomes. By understanding how genes and nutrients interact, nutrigenomics aims to enable more personalized dietary recommendations, moving away from one-size-fits-all approaches to nutrition. For example, a person with a genetic variant affecting lipid metabolism might benefit from a diet lower in saturated fats compared to someone without that variant. This field also investigates how nutrients can affect gene expression — a concept known as "nutritional epigenetics" — which has implications for disease prevention, especially chronic conditions like obesity, diabetes, and cardiovascular disease. One of the most promising aspects of nutrigenomics is its potential role in preventative healthcare. By identifying genetic predispositions to certain diseases early in life, individuals can adopt tailored diets that may reduce their risk of developing those conditions. This is particularly relevant in the context of the growing global burden of non-communicable diseases, many of which are diet-related. However, nutrigenomics is not without challenges. The science is complex, and the translation of genetic data into actionable nutritional advice requires robust, evidence-based research. There are also ethical concerns regarding genetic privacy, accessibility, and the potential for misuse of genetic information by insurers or employers. Moreover, the effectiveness of personalized nutrition depends not only on accurate genetic testing but also on individuals' willingness and ability to make sustainable dietary changes. Despite these hurdles, nutrigenomics holds significant promise for revolutionizing the future of nutrition and healthcare. Advances in DNA sequencing technology and bioinformatics are accelerating discoveries in this field, making personalized nutrition increasingly feasible and affordable. As research progresses, we can expect a more precise understanding of how diet influences health at a molecular level, leading to interventions that are both more effective and more aligned with an individual's unique biological makeup.

SUMMARY

The union of nutrigenomics and personal nutrition is a promising field for diet science, one that promises to transform public health trends and individual well-being. While researchers examine the genetic drivers of nutrient metabolism, a growing awareness is emerging regarding how tailored dietary information can be designed in an effort to optimize health. This scientific development provides a culture in which food selection is more responsive to the genetic individual, potentially leading to enhanced metabolic efficacy and protection against disease. The knowledge that is achieved through study in this discipline positions nutrigenomics not only as a theoretical paradigm but as a literal vehicle by which to promote population health and personalized nutrition planning. Thus, the implementation of this new science could bring a new dawn when nutritional treatment is as tailored as the individual for whom it is designed. But the potential of nutrigenomics has to be weighed against caution in relation to the ethical problems that arise from its application. The risk of abusing or misinterpreting genetic information can have the potential to generate socioethical problems like those of privacy, consent, and autonomy of dietary choice. Scholars in the research field have been optimistic about the potential of nutrigenomics to offer personalized nutrition recommendations without fundamentally altering concepts of food consumption. But one must consider the broader implications of using such personalized interventions in light of rights at the individual level and social norms. As has come into focus with recent studies, the issue of stigmatizing individuals who don't eat according to nutritional advice or creating a preconceived assumption that health can be sold on the basis of genes necessitates a close examination of the socioethical context within which nutrigenomics operates (Godard et al., 2013). In the long term, the successful integration of nutrigenomics into personalized nutrition depends on collaboration between scientists, physicians, ethicists, and policymakers. Assuring that the fruits of nutrigenomic research are translated into practice in an effective manner entails a full strategy that, while being mindful of scientific advances, also accommodates the necessary ethical frameworks. As discipline progresses further, visionary debate about the implications of such genetic findings for population health policy and individual dietary behavior will be essential in fostering confidence and acceptance among the population. Continuous grappling with such ethical concerns will strive to guide the ethical use of nutrigenomics, eventually guiding a future in which personalized nutrition not only leads to the health of the individual but also strives to deliver equal health outcomes from various populations (Castle et al., 2007).

The rapidly evolving science of nutrigenomics is leading the way in personalizing nutrition by deciphering how the unique genetic makeup of an individual influences food responses and health status in general. Central to this strategy is the integration of genetic data into dietary counseling so that people can make wise food choices based on their personal biological profile. This approach not only enhances the efficacy of diet therapy but also can prevent nutritional disorders. In addition, the idea of genomic nutritional profiling offers new mechanisms for achieving the maximum nutrient absorption that allows it to offer a more tailored form of health care that is in touch with the advancements in molecular biology and genetics in the field of nutrition (Castle et al., 2007). Consumer acceptance of nutrigenomics and personalized nutrition is also critical to its successful utilization. Research estimates total interest in personalized nutrition; however, acceptability varies significantly across different populations. One piece of research on Dutch consumers highlighted that acceptability is higher when individuals feel they are in control of their genetic data and that obtaining named and tangible advantages of personalized diet interventions. Learning from seasoned stakeholders is also essential in creating trust and enthusiasm regarding such innovation. This means that an effective educational strategy, through the emphasis on the advantages of nutrigenomics while addressing potential challenges as well, is the key to attaining acceptance and enhancing public engagement in individualized nutrition programs (Ronteltap et al., 2009). Briefly, the convergence between nutrigenomics and tailored nutrition is a new direction in learning about the impact of diet on health. The application of tailored dietary strategies not only reflects advances in scientific research but also needs to be accompanied by strategic communication to best motivate and inform the consumer. As technology continues to come into being, we need to consider consumer beliefs and the psychological drivers of adoption. Lastly, by supporting efficient communication and ensuring functional advantages, nutrigenomics can transform dietary patterns, propagating an active lifestyle towards health and wellness, appealing to the customer on an individual level (Ronteltap et al., 2009).

References

1. Akordor, V. L., Devi, C., Choudhuri, S., Vidhya, C. S., Niharika, M., Singh, R., Pandey, S. K., et al. (2024). The role of food science in combating obesity and related metabolic disorders. *European Journal of Nutrition & Food Safety*. https://www.semanticscholar.org/paper/7d2c481af79334db77a349b7028b94baad916e26 (accessed on 13th June 2025).
2. Allayee, H., Chmurzynska, A., Choi, M. S., Curi, R., et al. (2017). Guide for current nutrigenetic, nutrigenomic, and Nutri epigenetic approaches for precision nutrition involving the prevention and management of chronic diseases associated with obesity. https://core.ac.uk/download/304664691.pdf (accessed on 13th June 2025).
3. Alobaidi, S. (2025). Protein consumption and personalized nutrition in CKD: A comprehensive review. *Nutrition Research Reviews*. https://www.semanticscholar.org/paper/75ba148d025061590405aebf46fb04642549f175 (accessed on 13th June 2025).
4. Alongi, M., & Anese, M. (2021). Re-thinking functional food development through a holistic approach. *Journal of Functional Foods, 81*, 104466–104466. https://doi.org/10.1016/j.jff.2021.104466 (accessed on 13th June 2025).
5. Argano, V., Balistreri, C. R., Giarratana, R. M., Lio, D., et al. (2019). On the road to accurate biomarkers for cardiometabolic diseases by integrating precision and gender medicine approaches. https://core.ac.uk/download/268910274.pdf (accessed on 13th June 2025).
6. Arsenault, B., Després, J. P., de Toro Martin, J., Vohl, M. C., et al. (2017). Precision nutrition: A review of personalized nutritional approaches for the prevention and management of metabolic syndrome. https://core.ac.uk/download/442626140.pdf (accessed on 13th June 2025).
7. Baixauli, J. H. (2022). Multi-omics biomarkers of metabolic homeostasis of risk factors associated to non-communicable diseases. https://core.ac.uk/download/532364671.pdf (accessed on 13th June 2025).
8. Beckett, E., Jones, P., Lucock, M., Veysey, M., et al. (2017). Nutrigenetics—Personalized nutrition in the genetic age. https://core.ac.uk/download/225617935.pdf (accessed on 13th June 2025).
9. Chatzianagnostou, K., Gaggini, M., Florentin, A. S., Simonini, L., & Vassalle, C. (2024). New molecules in type 2 diabetes: Advancements, challenges and future directions. *International Journal of Molecular Sciences, 25*. https://www.semanticscholar.org/paper/a324411af6ff54aae428b5276a9466c10ae60cc2 (accessed on 13th June 2025).
10. Chrousos, G., Dafermos, C., Featherstone, K., Haliassos, A., et al. (2014). National strategic framework for research & innovation. 2014–2020. https://www.econstor.eu/dspace/bitstream/10419/102713/1/798025204.pdf (accessed on 13th June 2025).
11. De, G. M. (2023). Computational strategies in nutrigenetics: Constructing a reference dataset of nutrition-associated genetic polymorphisms. https://www.semanticscholar.org/paper/4c48449be5d7f4bde9d5cda478cc97512fcc32cf (accessed on 13th June 2025).
12. Dias Do Rosario, N. A., Gokhale, D., & Gore, M. (2025). Exploring the future of nutrigenomics: Dietitians' perceptions on integration in Indian practice. *Genes & Nutrition, 20*. https://www.semanticscholar.org/paper/2cef26dbb713c82bb548baa1338f23a0be6e834e (accessed on 13th June 2025).

13. Drożdż, D., Álvarez-Pitti, J., Wójcik, M., Borghi, C., Gabbianelli, R., Mazur, A., Herceg-Čavrak, V., et al. (2021). Obesity and cardiometabolic risk factors: From childhood to adulthood. *Nutrients, 13,* 4176–4176. https://doi.org/10.3390/nu13114176 (accessed on 13th June 2025).

14. Ferguson, L. R., Mathers, J. C., Ordovas, J. M., Tai, E. S., et al. (2018). Personalized nutrition and health. https://core.ac.uk/download/226307558.pdf (accessed on 13th June 2025).

15. Ghazanfar, S. (2024). The diet equation: Linking food, genetics, and wellness. *DIET FACTOR (Journal of Nutritional and Food Sciences).* https://www.semanticscholar.org/paper/77079c92588df31f085b1bd3052c427c80d89c77 (accessed on 13th June 2025).

16. Godard, B., Graham, J. E., Hurlimann, T., Menuz, V., et al. (2013). Risks of nutrigenomics and nutrigenetics? What the scientists say. https://core.ac.uk/download/442618824.pdf (accessed on 13th June 2025).

17. Kussmann, M., & van Bladeren, P. (2011). The extended nutrigenomics–Understanding the interplay between the genomes of food, gut microbes, and human host. https://core.ac.uk/download/pdf/8676207.pdf (accessed on 13th June 2025).

18. Lagoumintzis, G., & Patrinos, G. (2023). Triangulating nutrigenomics, metabolomics and microbiomics toward personalized nutrition and healthy living. *Human Genomics, 17.* https://www.semanticscholar.org/paper/165cd51a16cdf96c4801969dc6411146a48b068a (accessed on 13th June 2025).

19. Monda, A., de Stefano, M. I., Villano, I., Allocca, S., Casillo, M., Messina, A., Monda, V., et al. (2024). Ultra-processed food intake and increased risk of obesity: A narrative review. *Foods, 13.* https://www.semanticscholar.org/paper/08a29d0ff38c583a25c982e1a26c5485d44b80c3 (accessed on 13th June 2025).

20. Olorunkoya, S. O., Fijabi, O., Alagbe, O. V., & Olatinwo, M. (2024). Harnessing the role of nutrigenomics for feed efficiency utilization in cattle: Opportunities and challenges. *Engineering Science & Technology Journal.* https://www.semanticscholar.org/paper/eaeb19ec35bec21a5faa4edec9535d9de0fb6b1c (accessed on 13th June 2025).

21. Pandarinathan, S., Khatri, A., Niharika, M., Karthikeyan, K., Jagadeesan, R., Mohapatra, R., & Jena, J. P. (2024). Role of micronutrients in preventing chronic diseases: A review. *European Journal of Nutrition & Food Safety.* https://www.semanticscholar.org/paper/762da0690d29a78c39707c8f2558cdf52f181180 (accessed on 13th June 2025).

22. Pawar, T. G., Mehta, S. P., Auti, S. S., & Gage, P. K. (2024). Personalized nutrition plan based on DNA. *International Journal of Advanced Research in Science, Communication and Technology.* https://www.semanticscholar.org/paper/f01c34dd6c613139080c7168e41076d381668871 (accessed on 13th June 2025).

23. Ronteltap, A., van Trijp, J. C., & Renes, R. J. (2009). Consumer acceptance of nutrigenomics-based personalised nutrition. *The British journal of nutrition, 101*(1), 132–144. https://doi.org/10.1017/S0007114508992552(accessed on 13th June 2025).

24. Senoner, T., & Dichtl, W. (2019). Oxidative stress in cardiovascular diseases: Still a therapeutic target? *Nutrients, 11,* 2090–2090. https://doi.org/10.3390/nu11092090 (accessed on 13th June 2025).

25. Tamboli, F. A., Salunkhe, A. A., Zade, M. S., Kore, M. D., & Mhakle, R. A. (2024). Nutrigenomics: A new approach to the diagnosis and prevention of diseases. *IP Journal of Nutrition, Metabolism and Health Science*. https://www.semanticscholar.org/paper/ecf8b1db448496dcee0336ec7cad0975e6cd4455 (accessed on 13th June 2025).

26. Zhang, J., Wang, J., Zhu, C., Singh, R. P., & Chen, W. (2024). Chickpea: Its origin, distribution, nutrition, benefits, breeding, and symbiotic relationship with *Mesorhizobium* species. *Plants, 13*. https://www.semanticscholar.org/paper/1540661f694dce7dc36308d2d0fbbefef38ca461 (accessed on 13th June 2025).

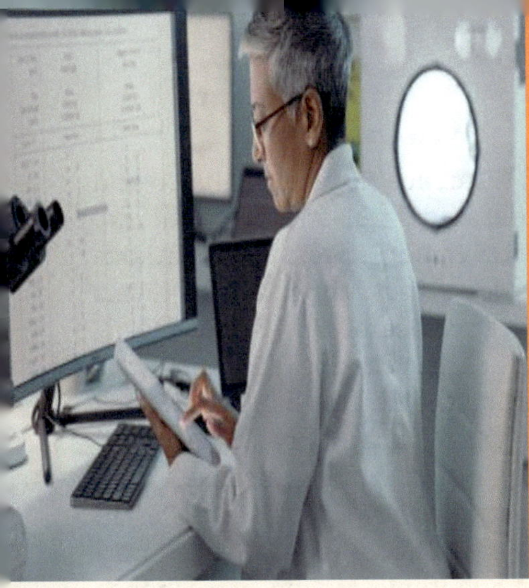

Chapter 15

PREVENTION AND PUBLIC HEALTH STRATEGIES

Contents

Introduction....483
15.1. Historical Context of Public Health....487
15.2. Epidemiology and Disease Prevention....492
15.3. Health Education and Promotion....496
15.4. Vaccination Programs....500
15.5. Policy and Legislation....504
15.6. Global Health Initiatives....508
Summary....514
References....516

Introduction

Public health intervention is the key to preventing infectious disease transmission and maximizing health benefits throughout the globe. Public health interventions are complex and entail various strategies that range from education and health promotion to technology development. The overall aim is to broaden general knowledge about health risks and confirm changes in behavior to accommodate preventive measures. As was evident during the COVID-19 pandemic, health surveillance technologies became advanced technologies to track disease transmission and support public health interventions. Such technologies present potential interventions but bring ethical and legal concerns that must be addressed carefully to build public trust and adherence (Befus et al., 2021). This early development character of health strategy highlights that the efficacy as well as implications of such measures should be evaluated in the context of broad public health objectives. Moreover, response to specific health issues demands application of targeted communication strategies. Tuberculosis (TB) is a suitable case illustrating how public health communications could influence drug compliance and disease awareness. Mass media interventions have been identified as central strategies for the provision of information promoting informed health-seeking behavior among affected populations. Nonetheless, their effectiveness is doubtful, making systematic reviews very important in terms of explaining their impact on public opinion and use of services in the case of TB (Bekker et al., 2014). These results are essential in maximizing preventive health interventions and achieving maximum efficiency in resource allocation for the purpose of obtaining the utmost benefit through public health campaigns. The relevance of effective communication and community involvement is essential in the success of any prevention program, especially in preventing diseases with multifactorial social determinants. In conclusion, the bringing together of different strategies in public health prevention plots a comprehensive framework that involves addressing contemporary health challenges. The challenge of infectious diseases demands adaptable means of response to fit changing socio-economic and health contexts. As public health institutions embrace new technologies and modes of communication, meticulous analysis is needed to regularly assess the consequences of the strategies through rigorous research, criticism, and appraisal. This dual focus on technology and message targeting not only encourages enhanced health literacy but enables community participation in disease prevention as well. A complete understanding of the forces operating in these initiatives will ultimately work to safeguard public health interests and inform future efforts aimed at creating healthier communities (Bekker et al., 2014; Befus et al., 2021) (Figure 15.1).

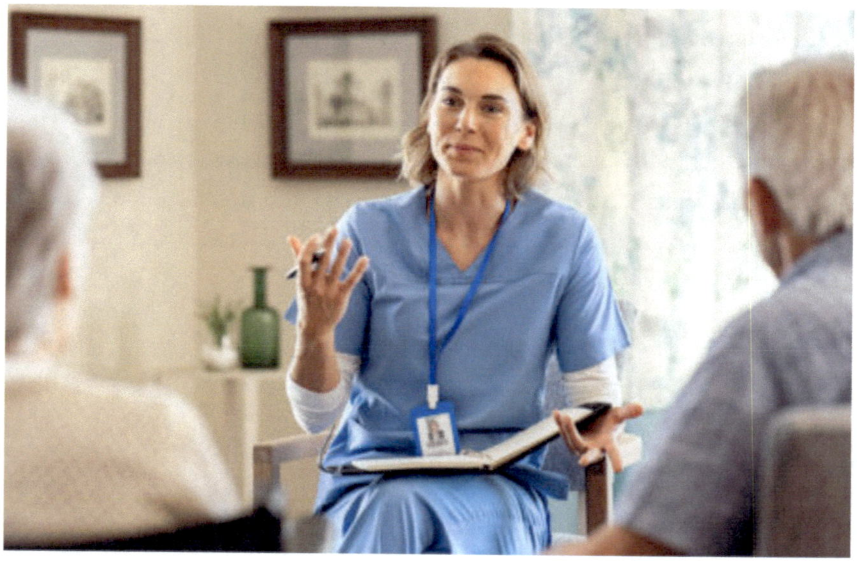

Figure 15.1. A healthcare professional providing nutrition and lifestyle counseling to older adults.

Source: https://s3.eu-north-1.amazonaws.com/cdn-site.mediaplanet.com/app/uploads/sites/42/2024/09/04095512/AdobeStock_434943694-460x295.jpg.

Definition of Public Health

The definition of public health is very extensive and encompasses many approaches for protecting and promoting the health of populations. Public health not just deals with the health of individuals but also with community health, determinants which influence health inequalities , such as environmental, economic, and social factors. This integrative style acknowledges that health outcomes are the result of a complex interaction among such determinants of health as education, income, and access to healthcare services. Effective public health initiatives emphasize prevention and health promotion, avoiding communicable diseases, chronic diseases, and environmental dangers. By designing a healthy environment and promoting informed health choices, public health practitioners can significantly enhance the quality of people's and communities' lives. To further illustrate public health's real-world applications, consider the mixed response to the COVID-19 pandemic across the globe. Arctic countries employed disparate health directives and transmission prevention protocols to stem the spread of the virus, which is evidence of the ability of public health to respond to crises. For example, state government policies included travel restrictions and communication measures with particular attention to local populations, which were pivotal in maintaining case rates low at the initial stages of the outbreak. The convergence of official guidelines and local efforts in such regions underscores that public health is not merely the domain of government but is equally, though more subtly, the art of involving local communities in health decisions. These coordinated actions provide an example for how public health collaborative activities can be most effectively addressed to emerging health issues, particularly in cases of crisis (Peterson et al., 2023). Besides, recognition of the involvement of the community in public health interventions plays a significant role in addressing individual health problems, for instance, addiction in local settings. Market community research in South Belfast demonstrates how public health interventions can be informed by resident knowledge. The collaboration between Queens Communities and Place and the Market Development Association shows the benefit of accessing community knowledge to identify gaps in services and develop targeted educational programming. These community-based approaches have the potential to enable residents to bring public health challenges to their solution through solutions tailored to their needs, increasing involvement and improving health outcomes. This model illustrates how public health strategies flourish through collaborative power between communities and researchers, which in turn directs more optimal intervention towards meeting the complex requirements of specific groups (Brannan et al., 2019).

Importance of Prevention in Health

Public health values the preventive role above all, as it is a major tool for reducing the incidence of disease while maintaining well-being. Preventive measures , such as vaccination, lifestyle modification, and routine screening are essential elements in decreasing the burden of infectious and chronic illnesses. For instance, access to comprehensive eye care can prevent illnesses that cause blindness and visual impairment, which already afflict hundreds of millions of individuals around the globe, most of whom belong to low- and middle-income countries. Given the understanding that vision impairment cases that exceed 90% can be avoided, investment in preventive eye health is bound to translate into quality of life and economic benefit in terms of greater productivity as well as foregone health care costs (Burton et al., 2021). Preventive health interventions are, thus, not merely about mitigating pain but are essential for ensuring sustainability and fostering development at the societal level. Aside from that, preventive health interventions must be outlined in the frame of equitable access among patients within the different populations to rectify structural inequities in health status. Disparities persist in health access; wherein vulnerable groups are disproportionately impacted by avoidable illnesses. The COVID-19 pandemic highlighted the need for effective public health interventions with a focus on prevention, given that the most at-risk have been disproportionately impacted by related health outcomes. For instance, front-line healthcare workers and nurses experience important stress and ethical dilemmas while struggling to provide care to those already badly affected by the virus, as evidenced by their own reported despair and exhaustion (Maben and Bridges, 2020). Redressing these inequalities through preventative health programs ensures that vulnerable populations not only receive access to the preventative interventions they require but also contribute to a sense of trust in the healthcare system overall, leading to better health outcomes for everyone. Public health policy with prevention also requires an interdisciplinary approach, involving education, community involvement, and coordination of services. Promoting health literacy is critical in empowering people to make informed choices about their health, thus enhancing compliance with preventive measures. Furthermore, community interventions involving local leaders can ensure culturally sensitive interventions that target risky groups. Such interventions can eliminate barriers to access and empower people in their healthcare through screening programs, promotion of health, and support systems. An integrated approach that encompasses prevention and education does not just enhance individual health but also aids in overall public health goals, like the Sustainable Development Goals, where the improvement of vision health further adds to social and economic benefits (Burton et al., 2021). So, prioritizing prevention sets the stage for more sustainable healthcare systems that can handle current and future burdens in health (Figure 15.2).

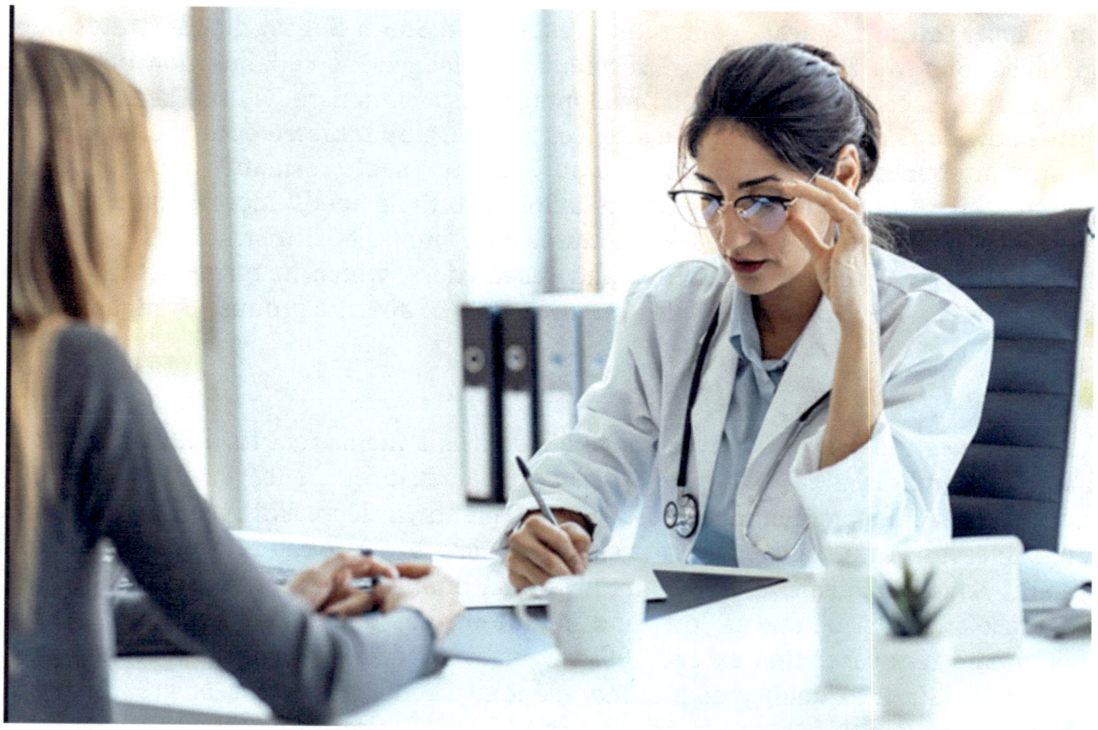

Figure 15.2. Doctor providing health advice to support public health awareness.

Source: https://cdn.prod.website-files.com/5f691b0fe3052600d45359de/64dc392ee3175bfdb74dca00_Arcadia_Gather%20Voices_4%20Steps%20to%20Effectively%20Spread%20Public%20Health%20Awareness.jpg.

Overview of Public Health Strategies

Public health interventions are also very important in the preservation of health and prevention of illness among populations. There are a wide variety of interventions aimed at various determinants of health, including environmental, behavioral, and policy determinants. The improvement of healthcare workers' knowledge and skills through education is an effective measure. For instance, the Moving Healthcare Professionals program (MHPP) is an example of an organized model of education aimed at incorporating prevention and promotion of physical activity into practice. Through combining content across the continuum of medical education from undergraduate to continuing professional development, the MHPP is trying to instill a culture of health throughout the clinical environment. This approach equips clinicians as well as enhances patient involvement, ultimately leading to healthier communities sustained by enlightened healthcare practice (Brannan et al., 2019). Socioecological framework (SEF) is also an imperative of public health, one that promotes a comprehensive understanding of health-related issues, , such as sport-related concussions. Under this framework, athletic trainers can develop targeted prevention and education plans because they recognize that various interacting determinants shape health outcomes. Education by itself might not be enough to alter behaviors; thus, factoring in the different layers of society involved is crucial. With the use of SEF, athletic trainers are able to build robust concussion management policies that echo the sophistication of individual and community interactions. This multi-faceted approach supports convergence between various settings to enhance the effectiveness of public health initiatives towards injury control, like concussions and finally a safer sporting culture (Register-Mihalik et al., 2017). Apart from education and policy change, public health initiatives must address community engagement to achieve maximum outcomes. Community members' participation in health promotional activities can lead to greater awareness and advocacy for public health initiatives. For example, physical activity or nutrition education programs can sustain themselves with local partnerships that spur participation and sustain long-term change. In addition, programs can enable crossings between healthcare providers and target populations that establish trusting relationships for preventive care. When communities are involved in public health strategy development, the likelihood of long-term behavioral change and increased health benefits is greater. Hence, a community-based, cooperative system is one of the main cornerstones of any effective model of public health for prevention and general health improvement.

15.1. Historical Context of Public Health

The development of public health practice is largely shaped by historical occurrences that have shaped population reactions to health emergencies. The recognition of contagious diseases and the need for ordered interventions became prominent in the 19th century when urbanization and industrialization accelerated disease transmission , such as cholera and typhoid. These epidemics pushed early public health reformers to advocate for improved sanitation, vaccination, and the creation of public health departments. These early efforts laid the foundation for the public health movement of today, which emphasizes that health cannot be separated from social and environmental conditions. Since such relationships were viewed by communities, preventive action became increasingly evident, and there was a more concerted effort in public health with a focus on protection and health promotion on a broader scale. The historical context under which viral diseases have afflicted populations, ranging from HIV/AIDS to hepatitis, shows the vital role that efforts in public health have played in addressing the widespread nature of health afflictions. For instance, the HIV/AIDS epidemic, which was recognized in the 1980s, highlighted the pressing need for effective testing and treatment methods. As outlined in the authoritative review of HIV testing in Uganda, the country witnessed some of the highest rates of prevalence in East Africa, prompting health authorities to implement targeted response plans that included enhanced access to testing and new diagnostic technologies. At the same time, the response of public health to hepatitis B and C has also been altered, which directly impacts rates of liver cancer, or hepatocellular carcinoma (HCC).

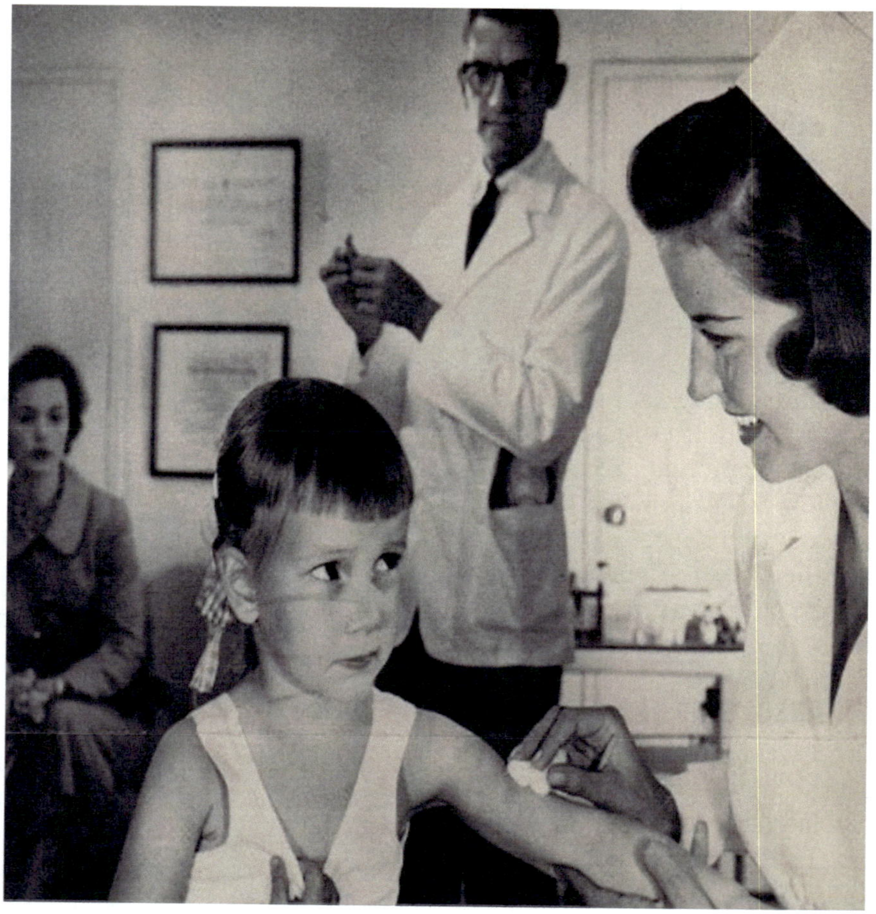

Figure 15.3. Historic scene of childhood vaccination in early public health care.

Source: https://s3.amazonaws.com/libapps/accounts/8921/images/new-vaccines.jpg.

Awareness of the previous trends among these viral diseases informs prevention strategies as well as policies that aim to reduce their impact on affected populations, thus enhancing the effectiveness of public health interventions (Moses, 2024). Moreover, the study of the history of public health illustrates the complex relationship between socio-economic determinants and health outcomes. Disparities in access to healthcare, usually influenced by wealth and geography, have been a significant obstacle to successful disease control and prevention. For instance, as highlighted in the history of hepatitis viruses, differences between industrialized and developing nations with respect to vaccine coverage and access to antiviral medication remain a major concern. This lopsided distribution of resources is also an indicator of the necessity to have global health approaches that bridge these gaps and enhance equity in access to prevention interventions. With continued development in public health, learning from history is important to developing comprehensively integrated approaches that tackle biological as well as social determinants of health to reduce health inequities and improve resilience in communities to new health risks (Stroffolini and Stroffolini, 2023) (Figure 15.3).

15.1.1. Evolution of Public Health Practices

Growth in public health practice has been significantly influenced by the emergence of novel infectious diseases and evolving population health trends. Previous pandemics, , such as 19th-century cholera, were landmark moments that helped shape public health response and evidence. The control of cholera, which was characterized by its swift emergence, necessitated innovative practices like the development and use of oral cholera vaccines (OCVs). These vaccines evolved through a collaborative network model of innovation, which sustained their development for decades. This development is used to show how stakeholder relations, knowledge management, and global access strategies have been crucial to promoting vaccine use in cholera control. The learning points from this experience are achievable to inform current public health policies with a perspective of adaptive interventions that vary as emerging health problems occur to enhance population health on a global scale (Large et al., 2025). Secondly, public health interventions can also be viewed through the lens of dealing with chronic diseases as well as non-communicable diseases. The transition from the sole focus on infectious diseases to an all-encompassing one encompassing chronic diseases is a broadening of the determinants of health understanding. Strategies , such as health education, lifestyle modification, and early detection have been pivotal in curbing the rising incidence of chronic diseases. The evolution of HIV testing practice in Uganda, for example, can be used as an illustrative case. Beginning from voluntary counseling and testing, the approaches have evolved to include provider-initiated testing and emerging self-testing technologies. This process was not free from danger, including stigma and discriminatory service delivery. Nonetheless, the continuous efforts of organizations like the Uganda AIDS Commission have encouraged uptake of testing and follow-up HIV treatment programs, pointing to the need for public health interventions that address both infectious and chronic conditions to optimize total health outcomes (Moses, 2024). The future cannot emphasize enough the need to integrate technological innovations into public health interventions. New diagnostic technologies, data analysis, and communication can unlock health service delivery. For instance, the expansion of telemedicine and mobile health applications has reached new horizons for accessibility and participation, particularly in disadvantaged communities. Furthermore, utilizing data on determinants and trends in health allows for more targeted intervention and adaptation based on population needs. Such ongoing improvement in public health practice should also involve the incorporation of inclusive policies that bridge gaps in access to healthcare, particularly in the arena of global disparities highlighted by recent health emergencies. Through the development of an innovative-supportive environment and, simultaneously, inequality reduction, an achievable future of public health is both efficient and equitable and can provide advantages to all segments of the population (Large et al., 2025; Moses, 2024).

15.1.2. Significant Public Health Achievements

Public health development is defined by some significant milestones that reflect the revolutionary developments in health strategies over the years. One of the significant milestones was the introduction of vaccination programs, which turned out to be a turning point towards the eradication of smallpox and the dramatic decline in polio. The success of such immunization campaigns is not only a measure of scientific advancement, however, but also a demonstration of the value of the community's role and education as part of public health initiatives. The role of community health workers in educating and vaccinating, for instance, is an excellent illustration of the crucial intersection between healthcare provision and targeted public health intervention. As observed with the ongoing need for vaccination across various groups, these early interventions open the door for subsequent work focusing on preventive health measures and disease burden reduction in public populations. Another milestone of public health is the establishment of integrated policies for health, focusing on rectifying social determinants of health.

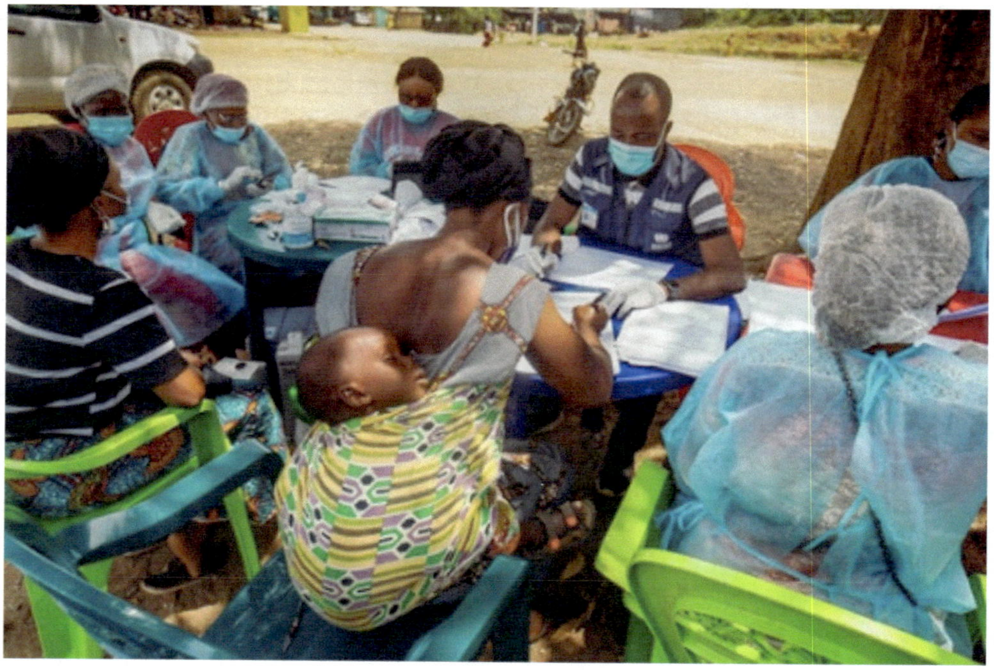

Figure 15.4. Health workers providing community care during Ebola response efforts.

Source: https://cdn.who.int/media/images/default-source/who-campaigns/who75/public-health-milestones/2016_ebola.tmb-549v.jpg?Status=Master&sfvrsn=6fbc5de5_14.

The integration of health-focused approaches into larger socioeconomic frameworks, such as the solutions presented in Brown et al. (2015), is a holistic approach to reducing health disparities. Public health officials and policymakers have realized that the provision of healthcare alone is insufficient without considering determinants like poverty, education, and housing stability. *For example*, recent policy briefs emphasize the importance of developing implementable plans, which incorporate such determinants, in order to achieve ideal results in health. With the promise of an integrated approach, public health interventions can be more effective in delivering long-term benefits, hence reducing inequalities among susceptible populations and ensuring equitable access to healthcare services. Initiation of public health campaigns to address specific health crises is another milestone for public health. Campaigned initiatives, particularly those tackling contagious diseases , such as HIV/AIDS and tuberculosis, have mobilized resources and support systems from communities. Assessment of the accomplishment during sessions, such as the 6th Annual Joint Health Sector Review showed both achievement and still developing care needs, as highlighted in Smithson et al. (2005). In addition, such campaigns tend to use public-private partnerships to promote better resource utilization and expertise exchange, thus bolstering the healthcare infrastructure. The combined resolve seen between stakeholders, including government bodies and NGOs, is a perfect example of the necessity for partnership in public health. By constantly having to modify strategies in response to new health issues, public health milestones become key points of inflection that inform future health interventions in an ever-dynamic societal context (Figure 15.4).

15.1.3. Impact of Historical Pandemics on Health Strategies

Pandemics throughout history have greatly impacted public health policy, and health organizations and governments have been forced to re-strategize in terms of prevention and response. Pandemic experiences , such as the 1918 influenza pandemic and the COVID-19 pandemic, have highlighted the importance of preparedness and adaptability. The pandemics put vulnerabilities in healthcare systems to test, , such as being unprepared and having policies that were not specifically tailored for high-risk groups, i.e., children. Specifically, a specific analysis points out that readiness in the U.S. to treat children in the case of a potential pandemic flu outbreak was substandard, which was an indication of a lack of clearly defined actions taking into account appropriate vaccine dosage and treatment administration management for this group (6th Annual Joint Health Sector Review). With the ongoing development of the health situation globally, such factors become imperative in designing comprehensive measures that focus on equal treatment accessibility and resource allocation during future pandemics. The response to previous pandemics also emphasizes the value of knowledge-informed decision-making and scenario planning within public health. The 2009 influenza A(H1N1) pandemic was utilized as a case study to illustrate how years of preparatory work, in anticipation of avian influenza, had an impact on the response to an emerging virus. By analyzing current pandemic plans, researchers constructed various potential scenarios on the basis of a number of crucial parameters , such as clinical attack rates and case fatality rates. This shift in methodology to create adaptable response frameworks helped health authorities react swiftly to new threats (Barral et al., 2015). Hence, the implementation of sophisticated analytics and simulation models has emerged as a norm of modern public health practice, allowing for risk reduction and outcome improvement during outbreaks of infectious disease. Beyond improving readiness, previous pandemics have resulted in a reassessment of the role of communication and community mobilization in health policy. During crises, public understanding of health information is essential to maintain health advisory compliance as well as avert misinformation. History indicates that open and transparent communication can go a long way in gaining the trust and cooperation of the public and resulting in improved health outcomes overall. Further, engaging communities in decision-making creates resilience since committed communities that are engaged in making decisions regarding health will adhere to prevention measures. As emerging lessons come from ongoing pandemics challenges, there is a need for public health strategies to include robust communication frameworks prioritizing inclusivity and stakeholder involvement. A forward-looking approach is critical to fostering public trust and successful health interventions against future pandemics.

15.2. Epidemiology and Disease Prevention

The application of epidemiology is critical to guiding public health policy to prevent disease. By examining the distribution and determinants of health states within populations, epidemiologists are able to identify risk factors for health conditions. This scientific basis allows for the formulation of evidence-based interventions that can adequately reduce disease burden. For instance, identification of lifestyle-related risk factors , such as obesity, smoking, and physical inactivity, has provided opportunities for preventive interventions promoting healthier lifestyles. Furthermore, epidemiological research informs policymakers about the effectiveness of interventions , such as vaccination campaigns or campaigns for health education, with foundations for evidence-based decision-making at public health and ultimately at the community level of well-being. Effective disease prevention is essential to minimizing health inequities and maximizing population health outcomes.

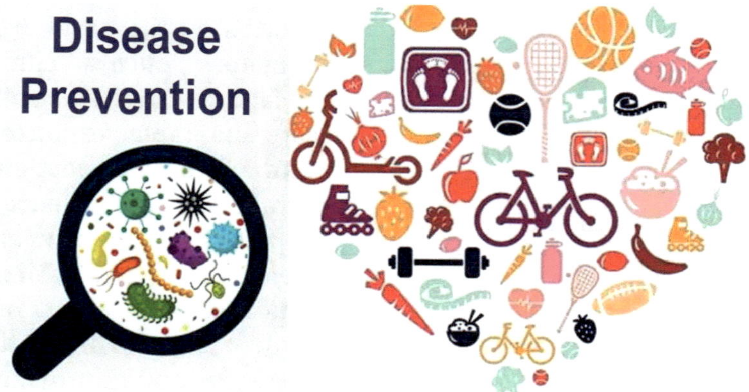

Figure 15.5. A healthy diet and active lifestyle support disease prevention.

Source: https://microbenotes.com/wp-content/uploads/2021/12/Disease-Prevention-Levels-Approaches-Key-Components.webp.

Use of preventive interventions, particularly among vulnerable populations, has been shown to improve long-term health indicators. For example, public health programs that emphasize the need for regular health check-ups and immunizations have been shown to reduce the incidence of infectious diseases, , such as measles or influenza, and also of chronic conditions , such as diabetes and hypertension. Additionally, the use of community-based interventions ensures that interventions are culturally relevant and accessible, thus promoting enhanced community engagement and compliance. These interventions aim not only at the immediate health requirements of populations but also at the socioeconomic factors that tend to bring about health inequalities, creating a more long-term model for public health. Prevention of chronic illnesses, which are now more prevalent amongst vulnerable groups, is one area that is prioritized by public health programs. Early identification and management of risk factors , such as obesity, hypertension, and diabetes will lay the ground for the prevention of conditions , such as CKD and heart disease. Certain public health interventions to promote healthy lifestyles and reduce exposure to risk factors are essential to this process. Development of multisectoral policies favoring environments conducive to health is also important in leading to long-term success. For example, investments in wholesome access to food and recreational spaces that are not harmful can reduce the prevalence of lifestyle diseases among various populations. Ultimately, through collective action in solving the multifaceted issues posed by chronic diseases, public health interventions can significantly influence community resilience and health equity towards the achievement of a healthier future for all (Bello et al., 2020) (Figure 15.5).

15.2.1. Role of Epidemiology in Public Health

Epidemiology forms the basis of public health policy through the generation of critical knowledge pertaining to the epidemiology of disease transmission and health outcome determinants. Risk factors and patterns that direct preventive interventions are identified by epidemiologists by conducting a systematic investigation of the distribution and determinants of states related to health among specified populations. This scientific discipline not only estimates the incidence and prevalence of disease, but also the socio-economic and environmental determinants for health inequity. To give an example, knowing the way in which certain pathogens, including antibiotic-resistant Staphylococcus aureus strains, are being transmitted between populations enables public health administrations to design targeted interventions to stop outbreaks. By ensuring the collection and review of data under strict scrutiny, epidemiology constructs evidence-based models to address public health problems with the ultimate goal of reducing disease burden and improving community health status in the long term. Additionally, the use of epidemiological evidence is central to the design of public health policy and guidelines. By analyzing disease surveillance and epidemiology data, health authorities are able to take prevention measures against high-risk groups. The increasing rates of infection with antibiotic-resistant organisms, particularly MRSA, partly underscore the requirement for having stringent surveillance systems and antibiotic stewardship programs. In most countries in Europe, for example, there is a high rate of *S. aureus* infection caused by MRSA strains, which consequently places the imperative of active public health interventions (Jorge, 2012). Such epidemiological data help to inform health campaigns that seek to raise awareness of proper use of antibiotics, hygiene practices, and the necessity of vaccination, thereby facilitating the reduction in rates of transmission as well as the overall health setting. Finally, the inclusion of epidemiology in public health also emphasizes the relevance of cross-disciplinary collaboration. Epidemiologists must work with healthcare providers, policymakers, microbiologists, and community organizations to create an integrated plan for disease prevention and health promotion. HVISA development poses not only clinical treatment challenges but also a multilevel challenge that requires education, research, and investment (Goglio and Stefani, 2010). Collaborative action facilitates the development of creative, person-centered solutions addressing both short-term pressures of infectious disease epidemics and longer-term social determinants driving health inequities. Through synergies between epidemiological data and interdisciplinary capability, public health interventions can be refined to address the intermixed array of factors influencing population health effectively, ultimately producing a more resilient health system.

15.2.2. Disease Surveillance and Monitoring

Surveillance and monitoring of disease occupy a pivotal role in setting effective public health interventions that are fundamental to prevention work. Through the systematic acquisition, analysis, and interpretation of health-related data, these surveillance systems enable the detection of outbreaks of disease and the identification of trends over time by health authorities. For instance, the Registration and Monitoring of Hypertensive Diabetics System of Brazil (HIPERDIA Program) provides crucial data on the prevalence and control of hypertension among the elderly. Information obtained through such data not only has an impact on healthcare policy but also facilitates targeted intervention for improving health outcomes, pointing towards the importance of surveillance integration in public health measures for the facilitation of well-being among a population (Medeiros et al., 2015). Effective disease surveillance requires a unified collaborative approach that engages various stakeholders at the local, regional, and national levels. Multi-disease surveillance strategies, particularly in resource-limited settings, have the potential to promote early detection of communicable diseases, which are leading causes of morbidity and mortality. WHO has encouraged such strategies for promotion in Africa, where communicable diseases represent vast health risks. Through linking national health systems, health facilities, and community health workers, these strategies enable health staff to make evidence-based decisions based on reliable epidemiological data. This comprehensive and systematic monitoring system ultimately leads to effective deployment of resources and intervention implementation, hence advancing public health goals (World Health Organization Regional Office for Africa. Division of Communicable Disease Prevention and Control, 2014).). In addition, the impact of inadequate disease surveillance can be disastrous, resulting in preventable outbreaks and increased health costs.

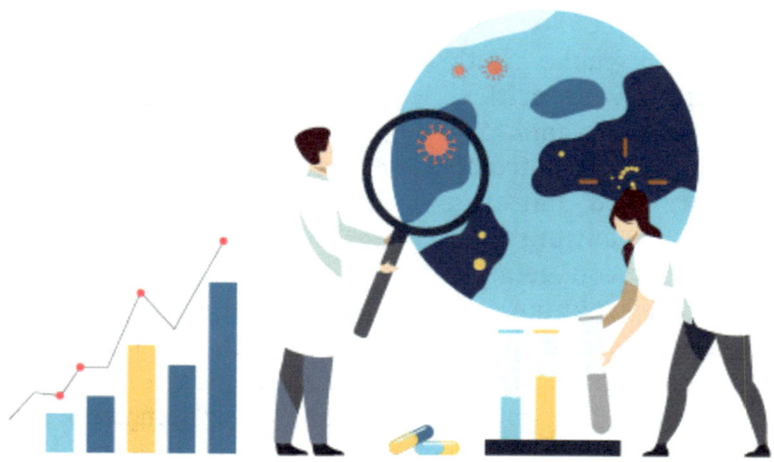

Figure 15.6. Global epidemiological surveillance through research and data analysis.

Source: https://www.epiconcept.fr/wp-content/uploads/SURMESURE-surveillance-epidemio.svg.

Most of the time, the unavailability of timely and accurate information is the barrier to health authorities' efforts to implement required public health intervention. To prevent these problems, there is a need to build local capacities for disease monitoring and reporting. Training health professionals to gather and analyze surveillance data effectively can allow them to react to health emergencies successfully. According to various epidemiological studies, , such as vaccine-preventable disease monitoring programs, increased surveillance allows programs to quantify success in prevention programs and to adjust strategy accordingly. Lastly, robust disease surveillance systems are central to developing public health infrastructure and maintaining healthy populations at risk (World Health Organization Regional Office for Africa. Division of Communicable Disease Prevention and Control, 2014; Medeiros et al., 2015) (Figure 15.6).

15.2.3. Strategies for Outbreak Control

Managing outbreaks has to be approached by a multi-component approach, with vaccination as the anchor for effective prevention and response. Not only does it protect the individual, but it is also in attaining herd immunity, which is needed in managing diseases having high transmission rates. Various vaccines, , such as injectable Vi polysaccharide vaccine (ViPS) and oral Ty21a vaccine, have been utilized in endemic regions to pre-emptively prevent anticipated outbreaks or reactively control outbreaks once they occur. The evidence indicates that these vaccination strategies are largely viable and acceptable among affected populations, and they bring great effectiveness in reducing the prevalence of disease among targeted groups. However, as promising as they are, the underuse of typhoid vaccines helps to highlight the need for directed public health interventions encouraging use and addressing obstacles in high-incidence environments World Health Organization Regional Office for Africa. Division of Communicable Disease Prevention and Control, 2014). An eventual course of action will have to emphasize measures that maximize the performance of immunization programs in endemic and outbreak contexts. In addition to vaccination, robust disease surveillance systems play a fundamental role in the early control of outbreaks. By leveraging advanced data collection and distribution systems, public health officials can identify imminent threats and respond in a timely manner. Lessons learned from previous health crises, , such as the COVID-19 pandemic and Ebola virus outbreaks, indicate the importance of timely intervention strategies that are guided by up-to-date information. The existence of effective channels of communication ensures that stakeholders ranging from health workers to the general public are well informed and engaged in the exercise of containment. Targeted interventions , such as contact tracing and community outreach, also consolidate these surveillance exercises, enabling more capacity for rapid and efficient response to outbreaks. In the mpox epidemic, for instance, linking learning from past responses has played a central role in strengthening surveillance capabilities and overall readiness (Ahmed et al., 2024). Lastly, combating misinformation and winning public trust are central features of outbreak control efforts. Communication is not merely about presenting facts; it is also about community relationship-building in a way that the message gets received and implemented. Public health efforts must actively dispel myths and provide transparent information to dispel myths about vaccine safety and transmission of disease. Encouraging community engagement and leveraging influencers at the community level has a high probability of following public health recommendations. Consistent messaging and evidence of effectiveness for health interventions can also boost trust in health authorities. Thus, whenever communities trust their health care systems and believe that the prevention interventions are owned, they will be more likely to contribute to vaccination drives and abide by public health advice, thereby increasing overall efficiency of outbreak control interventions (Ahmed et al., 2024).

15.3. Health Education and Promotion

Health education and promotion are the dominant aspects of effective public health policy. Primed to target individuals and communities, health education programs aim to improve knowledge regarding health status, behavior, and resource availability that can contribute to improved health. Whole-school sexuality education, for example, addresses central topics like consent, protected practices, and reproductive health, enabling young people to make life-affecting decisions. This kind of requirement has become increasingly urgent, particularly in regions like Argentina, where rates of sexually transmitted disease (STI) infection and unwanted pregnancy indicate the true cost of poor education. Education targeted at these issues can actually reduce health inequities and support healthier lifestyles among high-risk groups, therefore playing a critical role in the overall prevention and public health intervention strategy (Arduzzi et al., 2025).

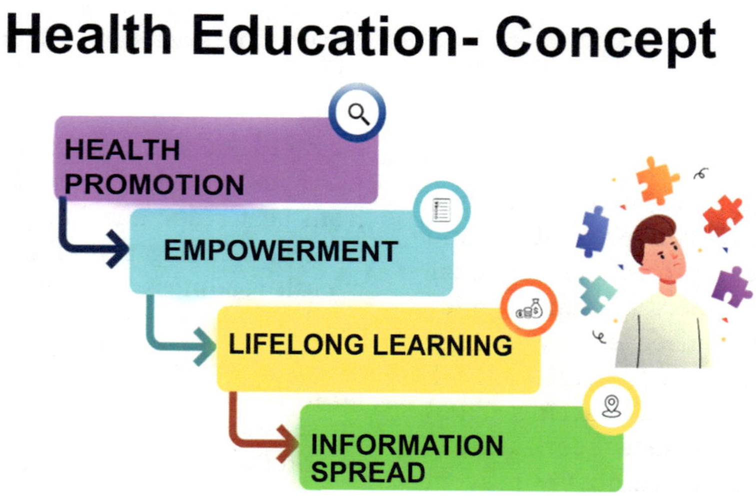

Figure 15.7. Core components of health education: promotion, empowerment, lifelong learning, and spread information.

Source: https://prepwithharshita.com/wp-content/uploads/2023/11/Champagne-and-Colorfull-Step-by-Step-Buid-Your-Business-Graph.png.

The integration of Primary Health Care (PHC) and community nursing further enhances the efficiency of health education and promotion interventions. PHC emphasizes the importance of accessible and evidence-based care with a bias towards preventive and educational strategies that enhance health awareness among communities. Community nursing is an important bridge between health care systems and populations, and thus, tailored health promotion interventions become easily feasible. Nurses perform outreach, allocation of resources, and advocacy, thereby fulfilling their important role in the efficient provision of health education. With this integrated framework, PHC and community nursing address the unique health needs of individuals, thus effectively improving health literacy and enabling citizens to adopt healthier living styles. Such connections are vital in coming up with a responsive healthcare environment that centers on prevention and community-based health strategies (Arduzzi et al., 2025). Strategic public-private partnerships have been shown to optimize resources and fortify health promotion efforts in marginalized environments. Collaborative efforts, , such as those fostered by the Pan American Health Organization (PAHO), emphasize transparent accountability and interinstitutional cooperation to solve key health concerns. For instance, in Ecuador, the Ministry of Public Health (MSP) promotes decentralized networks that ensure equal provision of health services to marginalized groups. Statistics collected from outreach programs paint a picture of high health care demand, particularly among women and patients suffering from chronic illnesses. Outcomes of such endeavors highlight the imperative of creating integral strategies that prioritize health education, preventive services, and inter-institutional coordination to fill voids in community health systems and improve quality of life (Figure 15.7).

15.3.1. Importance of Health Literacy

Health literacy is a foundation of effective public health interventions, defining the way individuals search, read, and use health information. A high health-literate population will be more capable of making informed decisions regarding preventive services, thereby relieving the burden on healthcare systems. For instance, individuals who can comply with medical counsel have a better likelihood of following prescribed medications and practicing preventive health measures. This knowledge becomes more indispensable in the era of new health risks, especially infectious diseases, which require timely and effective information for community responsiveness. Hence, enhancing health literacy needs to be a topmost concern in public health initiatives, developing a morally sustainable society to efficiently manage current and emerging health complications, as evidenced in recent research into new communication methods in health care settings, , such as graphic medicine and culturally tailored educational promotions (Pavarina et al., 2025). Besides individual benefits, health literacy is crucial for maximizing community-wide health outcomes. Public health campaigns founded on effective communication can bridge the understanding gap among heterogeneous populations, particularly in rural and underprivileged populations. For example, targeted educational programs employing local languages and culturally relevant materials may cross the socioeconomic status as well as literacy level barriers. The success of such programs has been widely reported in the instance of Mpox-type diseases, where the application of grassroots movements has shown promising results in terms of awareness as well as preventive behavior. With active involvement of the population in public health education, health programs will likely respond positively and have a long-lasting impact. Greater health literacy enables citizens to take ownership of their health, thus creating an empowered culture of wellbeing that cascades into the wider community (Afzal et al., 2025). In addition, the adoption of public health interventions via health literacy fills long-standing gaps in access to healthcare and treatment. Low health-literate populations are found to have higher proportions of chronic disease and poorer health outcomes because of an inability to understand the preventions and treatments available. Utilizing large-scale training of local health workers and partnership with the community, public health programs can make health information both available and understandable. Techniques , such as mobile health units and community outreach programs, aim at offering individualized education, particularly where typical healthcare facilities fail to exist. While issues continue to emerge in accomplishing this, the prospects of increased health literacy in creating change are significant, presenting avenues to equalizing health outcomes and raising resistance to public health catastrophes (Afzal et al., 2025; Pavarina et al., 2025).

15.3.2. Community Outreach and Engagement

Effective public health interventions for preventing disease and promoting health depend greatly on effective community outreach and engagement. By these means, collaboration among health workers and citizens is achieved, generating synergy that increases sensitivity and enables interventions to be facilitated with greater ease. Engaging local residents in decision-making processes ensures that health programs are culturally relevant and tailored to the specific needs of individual communities. As evident in recent campaigns for Mpox awareness in underprivileged populations, local tastes and knowledge-informed strategies yield more effective results. Community focus not only increases the dissemination of information but also yields trust, ultimately increasing participation levels in health programs for disease prevention.

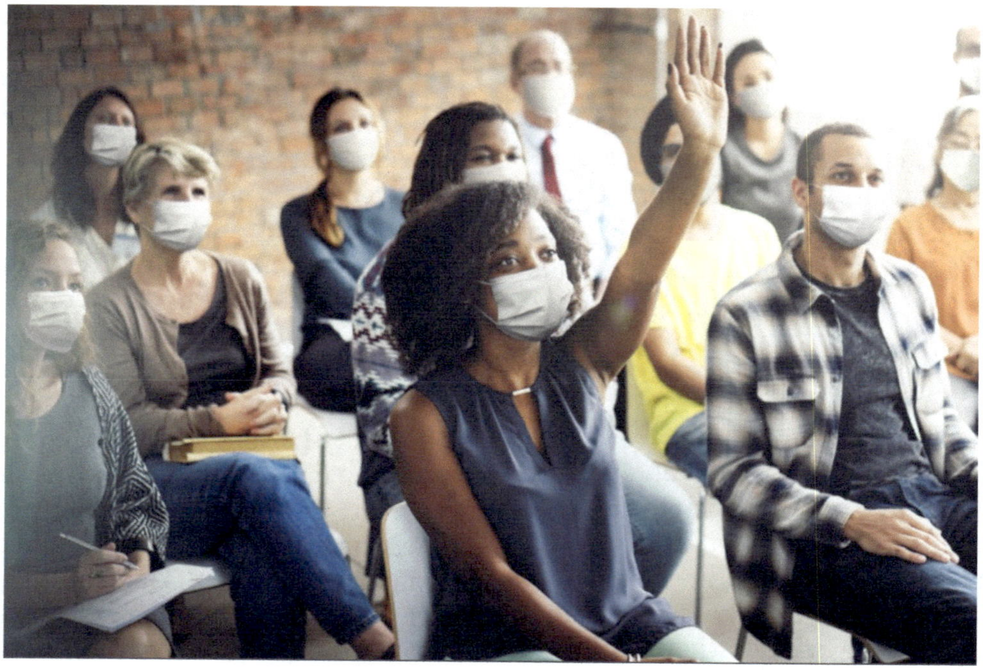

Figure 15.8. Masked community members participate in an interactive public health education session.

Source: https://icma.org/sites/default/files/2021-04/AdobeStock_406571643.jpg.

Thus, successful public health interventions must address the development of genuine partnerships with communities to achieve health outcomes in the long term (Afzal et al., 2025). New, creative education materials are the foundation of community outreach by framing difficult health problems in terms that individuals can relate to. Efforts , such as the Cancer School, illustrate the worth of employing interactive materials , such as booklets and games, to convey essential information about cancer prevention and biology in a context applicable to different populations. By adapting established pedagogy to online media and social media, efforts can reach and impact many more individuals. Cancer School project, owing to its interactive approach and active online engagement, has successfully facilitated community participation by making it possible for followers to engage, ask questions, and participate in health education. Active learning, in addition to enhancing public awareness, also makes it possible for individuals to own their own health decisions, ultimately resulting in better community health outcomes (Souza et al., 2025). Community outreach challenges must be resolved as well to provide fair access to information and health resources. Socioeconomic disparities, linguistic diversity, and misinformation may compromise the effectiveness of outreach. Prevention efforts against Mpox in India underscore the need for culturally and linguistically tailored communication strategies that resonate with various populations. By identifying and resolving such barriers, public health campaigns can build an inclusive platform that invites the participation of marginalized populations. Furthermore, building alliances with local institutions can allow bridging of infrastructure and resource gaps, enabling more effective outreach. Lastly, prevention and public health interventions are effective based on the readiness to advance community voices and act accordingly to address particular challenges during outreach activities, hence establishing a healthier society for all (Afzal et al., 2025) (Figure 15.8).

15.3.3. Use of Social Media in Health Promotion

The creation of social media has unquestionably revolutionized the health promotion scene with new avenues to disseminate information and engage diverse populations. Social media platforms allow real-time messaging, which allows health organizations to message necessary health information and campaigns to mass audiences almost in real time. By employing participatory content materials, , such as video, infographics, and interactive posts, public health programs can incite public concern and encourage healthier behaviors. Besides, the interactive nature of social media enables users to share their own health stories and challenges, which fosters a culture of shared responsibility and community. Such living engagement not only creates awareness but also encourages individuals to adopt healthier lifestyles, hence making public health interventions intended for prevention and disease control effective. Integration of social media into health promotion efforts continues to be among the most valuable strategies in managing contemporary health challenges. Social media has also shown effectiveness in reaching groups that may otherwise be underunderserved through other forms of health communication. In particular, successive generations have increasingly looked at online spaces for health information, and therefore, outreach through these channels is a necessary endeavor for public health practitioners. Social media influencers play a critical role in disseminating health messages to their followers, hence expanding their visibility and credibility to influence healthier choices. Personalized advertising and messaging tailored around a person's own interests and habits can also achieve the highest impact of health interventions. As recent studies have pointed out, content optimization for target populations guarantees that key health messages ring true with the target audience and bridge gaps in accessibility and knowledge. No greater promise is held by social media in making health promotion efforts wider-reaching, since it creates well-informed and health-oriented communities with remarkable effectiveness. The ethical implications of social media use in health promotion also need to be strictly analyzed to guide responsible use. As useful as these platforms are, there is a risk of misinformation and abuse of the vulnerable. Use of culturally sensitive messaging and tackling the psychological susceptibilities of online content are also essential for achieving the maximum positive effects of health promotion interventions. As discussed under the challenges and recommendations for mobilizing minority groups, there is a requirement to integrate tailored interventions that factor in communications styles as well as cultural diversity. By doing so, public health interventions can establish trust and credibility and address skepticism as well as misconceptions inherent in internet discourse. A balanced framework prioritizing ethical practice and community engagement will ultimately optimize the effectiveness of social media as a health promotion strategy in alignment with the broader goals of public health and prevention efforts (George et al., 2024; Gore et al., 2024).

15.4. Vaccination Programs

Vaccination campaigns are a bulwark against communicable diseases and play a fundamental role in prevention and public health efforts. These campaigns usually change according to the individual epidemiological situation of an area, using different vaccines to contain both endemic and epidemic diseases. For instance, the strategic use of injectable Vi polysaccharide vaccine (ViPS) and oral Ty21a vaccine has been appreciated in regions like Asia, where typhoid fever infection is rampant. Vaccination policies may be split between proactive measures of endemic control or reactive interventions in the occurrence of outbreaks to ensure a tailored approach to disease prevention.

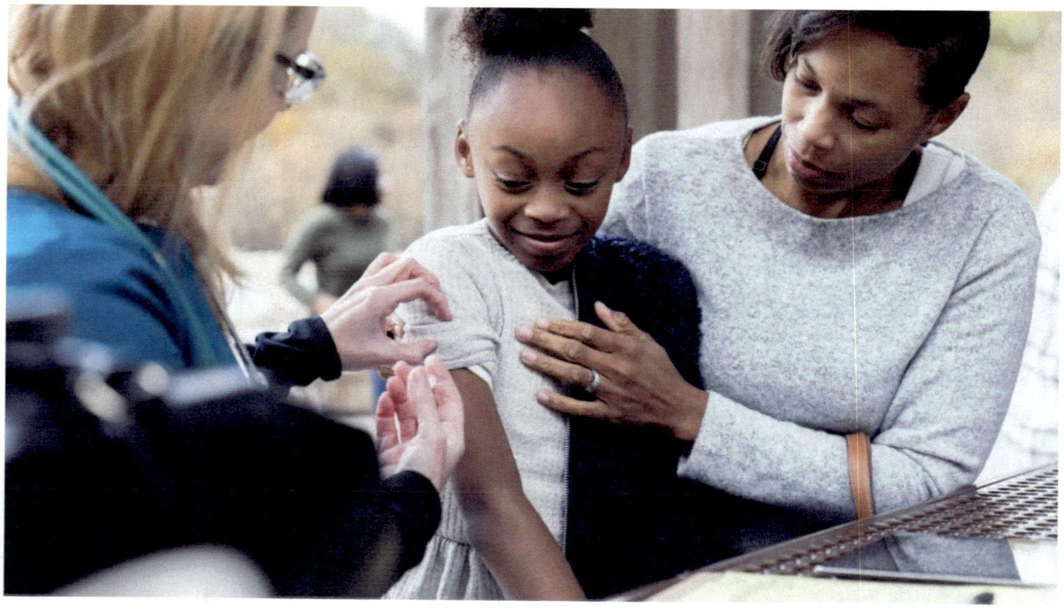

Figure 15.9. Child receiving vaccination with parental support to promote immunization and public health.

Source: https://www.merck.com/wp-content/uploads/sites/124/2024/02/Girl_Vaccination_Doctor.jpg?resize=1188,672.

Despite proven effectiveness and acceptability of such vaccination programs, some remain underutilized, primarily due to poor implementation frameworks and support for health authorities (N/A). Expansion with new vaccines, including the typhoid conjugate vaccines (TCVs), offers the potential to improve existing programs significantly. Although TCVs are presently undergoing World Health Organization (WHO) prequalification assessment, their projected benefits—extended duration of protection and incorporation within infant immunization programs—render them essential tools in developing public health programs. Observations from current vaccination programs can be applied when developing these new programs in such a manner that they are not merely effective but also pragmatic and affordable in high-incidence settings. As has been observed from numerous other nations, in which vaccination programs have had impressive public health payback, incorporating sound operations research and local evaluation in program planning is a vital necessity (N/A). As the trend of global disease indicates, the potential application of vaccines to combat other pathogens, , such as HIV, highlights the difficulty of implementing new vaccine programs. Research indicates that an arguably effective HIV-1 vaccine would have dramatic impacts in regions like southern India, saving millions of lives. But their implementation involves meticulous planning, , such as target group designation and creation of sustainable delivery systems. In addition, maintaining vaccine coverage in the long term involves constant investments in health education as well as more extensive prevention efforts. As underscored by studies, effective vaccination is not a standalone activity; it is optimally effective as part of a comprehensive public health initiative that incorporates addressing behavior, surveillance, and mobilization at the community level (Figure 15.9).

15.4.1. Overview of Vaccination Strategies

Vaccine strategies are key components of public health to avert infectious disease, particularly in populations at risk. The success of these strategies is largely founded upon knowledge of the epidemiology of the diseases to be targeted and the context in which vaccination is to be implemented. One famous case in point is the use of the Vi polysaccharide vaccine (ViPS) against typhoid fever, which is notable for its application in both endemic and outbreak contexts. Various approaches , such as community-based routine immunization, school-based activity, and focused mass vaccination campaigns, have been tested in terms of acceptability and performance. Evidence indicates that the approaches are not just feasible but also exert a substantial health impact in high-burden settings. However, despite their high effectiveness, typhoid vaccines are not being taken up adequately, suggesting an acute shortcoming in global vaccination strategy, warranting the development and deployment of optimum vaccination strategies (Gostin &Berkman, 2007). For HIV-1 prevention, vaccine strategies must consider public health infrastructure and selected population dynamics. As demonstrated in the study, an imperfect vaccine is still going to have a great effect on disease burden, particularly where there is such a high disease burden as is observed in southern India. There is a need to consider integrated delivery strategies targeting vulnerable populations based on the cost implications of mass vaccination initiatives. Covering the political and social dimensions, including vaccine acceptance, is necessary to enhance overall vaccination coverage. Among the planning elements are enhanced health surveillance structures, innovative outreach tactics, and continuous engagement with communities to foster trust. Making sure vaccination programs fit within other prevention activities will yield a unified effort towards public health concerns around HIV/AIDS, thereby illustrating the complexity and gravity of multi-component vaccine approaches (Jha et al., 2025). For maximum returns on vaccination investment, there is always a necessity to measure the program and community levels of effectiveness. Adapting vaccination programs to respond to the local epidemiological needs, cost-effectiveness, and logistical conditions has tremendous potential to maximize program success. For typhoid vaccines, experience has shown that integrating vaccines into routine health services can facilitate the process of improving acceptance and coverage. Further, the development of new vaccines, , such as the typhoid conjugate vaccine (TCV), is based on an estimate of their potential advantage over existing vaccines. Similarly, in HIV, sustained investment in large-scale prevention efforts alongside vaccination is needed to sustain health gains. Addressing infrastructure problems, guaranteeing the delivery of vaccines to the most at-risk populations, is a keystone of quality public health interventions and spurring success in disease prevention programs (N/A).

15.4.2. Impact of Vaccines on Public Health

Vaccine development has revolutionized public health, and it has had a significant role in curbing infectious diseases. Traditionally, the introduction of vaccinations has led to a sudden decline in morbidity and mortality rates caused by diseases , such as measles, polio, and smallpox. Such declines highlight the very basis that not only does immunization protect an individual, but also herd immunity is assured, thus protecting populations at large. Resource investment in immunization programs is a good strategic investment in public health infrastructure and an integral part of disease control interventions.

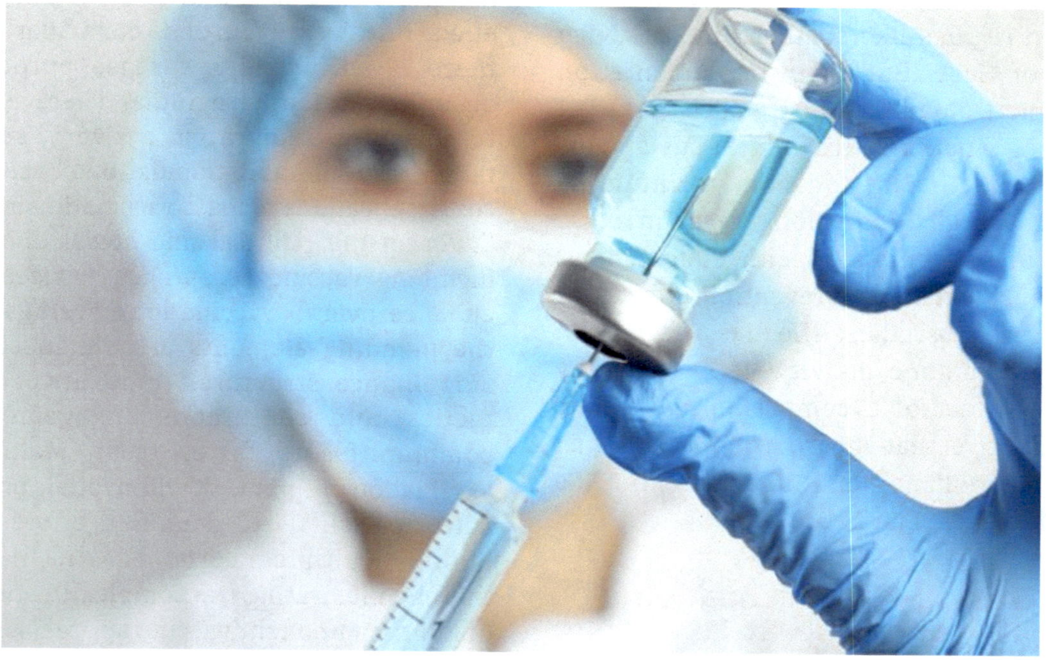

Figure 15.10. Close-up of vaccine preparation by a masked healthcare worker, emphasizing immunization safety.

Source: https://www.ihi.europa.eu/sites/default/files/styles/news_block_sticky_image/public/events/shutterstock_1730302936_Doctor%20filling%20syringe%20with%20medication%2C%20closeup.%20Vaccination%20and%20immunization.jpg?itok=dE6mA3Kt.

End-to-end immunization programs demonstrate vaccines' potential to prevent outbreaks and save healthcare costs, with implications for society at large. Such strategies are consistent with best evidence-based practice and emphasize prevention rather than reaction, thus proving the efficacy of vaccines in enhancing general public health outcomes. Response to rapidly emerging infectious diseases also demonstrates the agility of vaccination strategies under the public health umbrella. In particular, rapid vaccine development against viruses , such as SARS-CoV-2 proves the potential of new immunization technologies in addressing public health crises. These new vaccines are an expedited research effort required to facilitate timely intervention against threats to global health, highlighted by advances in vaccine research methods favoring efficiency and access (Gostin &Berkman, 2007). The overall implications of these developments extend beyond the short-term management of outbreaks; they are to reestablish the public's faith in immunization as a fundamental defense mechanism. By enabling widespread vaccination coverage by means of public health outreach and education efforts, public health officials can effectively mobilize communities as active agents in infectious disease control, thereby slowing the spread and increasing population resilience. As much as vaccines have taken their place firmly in public health orthodoxy, their introduction cannot be without ethical dilemma. Vaccine distribution and specifically pandemics present complex problems of access and distribution of resources. Ethical models must balance how the population's needs are balanced against individual rights and guarantee interventions do not undermine the freedom of individuals in the pursuit of maximum health gains (Gostin &Berkman, 2007). Public health policy must thus balance the risk of social division and resistance to vaccination programs. Engaging in open discussion about the worth of immunization, as well as directly responding to concerns over autonomy and privacy, can help to create trust between the public. Thus, the success of vaccine programs is not strictly a function of scientific efficacy but also of ethical integrity, and vaccines become an essential linchpin in the overall strategy to avoid disease and ensure public health (Figure 15.10).

15.4.3. Challenges in Vaccine Distribution and Acceptance

The problems that come with vaccine coverage and use are complex and very embedded with socio-political as well as cultural contexts. One significant problem is the differential state-level policies that tend to suppress universal vaccine coverage. For instance, states that are likely to be conservative politically or have very high levels of religiosity have lower completion rates for vaccines , such as the human papillomavirus (HPV) vaccine. These factors create an environment where misinformation can thrive, discouraging individuals from seeking vaccination. Consequently, comprehensive strategies must be developed that not only address individual concerns but also engage communities effectively, leveraging local health education initiatives to foster an understanding of vaccine benefits. This emphasizes the need for well-fitted public health interventions that consider the individual sociopolitical and cultural contexts of specific regions to enhance vaccination rates and overcome resistance according to contextual determinants (Brownson et al., 2019). Apart from sociopolitical determinants, logistical factors significantly complicate the vaccination delivery process. In the majority of regions, particularly rural and disadvantaged ones, there is a glaring disparity in the availability of healthcare resources, including centers for vaccination. Limited transportation access and disinformation regarding vaccine availability or safety can contribute further to these groups' difficulties. Mass marketing methods of recruitment for immunization programs are generally inadequate. There is evidence suggesting that focused outreach, , such as direct community approach and grass-roots effort, can significantly increase acceptance of vaccines among diverse populations, representing a paradigm shift in public health practice. By targeting local networks and known community influencers to disseminate information, public health officials can combat misinformation and gain trust. Lastly, understanding public attitudes toward vaccination is essential in overcoming acceptance concerns. Vaccine hesitancy is usually born out of a lapse in confidence in healthcare systems, fueled partially by historical injustices perpetrated on marginalized populations. This legacy can generate mistrust of vaccine campaigns, particularly when outreach is not conducted with multiple viewpoints or when communities do not feel they are represented equitably in clinical trials. For instance, having racially and ethnically diverse subjects participate in vaccine trials is significant so that vaccines are deemed safe and effective in various populations. Recent data indicate white participants were overrepresented in trials where high interest was seen among various populations, reflecting systemic recruitment strategy hurdles (Edupuganti et al., 2013). To spur broader acceptance, public health initiatives must ensure that inclusiveness and transparency are their top concern, highlighting an effort to undo the imbalances while ensuring equal access to vaccines.

15.5. Policy and Legislation

The convergence of law and policy is central to the reality of public health interventions that aim at disease prevention and health promotion.

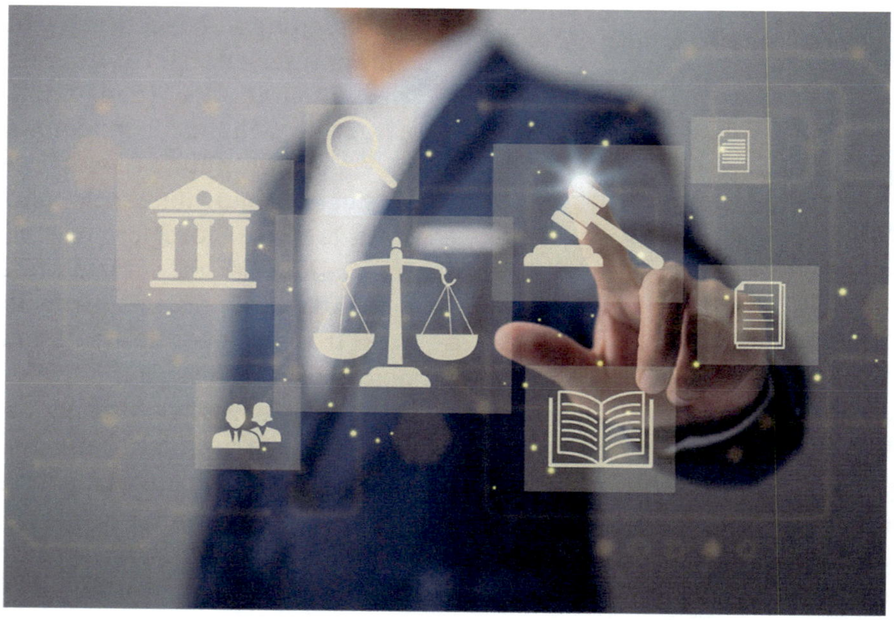

Figure 15.11. Digital interface illustrates legal policies and regulatory frameworks.

Source: https://www.indeson.net/wp-content/uploads/2022/12/policy-legaislation-services.jpg.

Political and administrative government agencies particularly set up frameworks for how public health programs are developed, funded, and administered. Effective policies blend evidence, stakeholder engagement, and interdisciplinarity in order to make the public health interventions salient and effective. For example, public health-primary care integration in states , such as Oregon and North Carolina has been led by collaborative policy structures that focus on common purpose and resource maximization. Such efforts promote cohesive health systems that can address the needs of the community and enhance the responsiveness of public health infrastructure to evolving health issues, a principle underlying all of the discussions that are in process to enhance public health outcomes through facilitative legislation and pioneering partnerships (Baum et al., 2024). Law has a pivotal function to play in regulating activities that impact public health, and the level of its regulation is also evidently reflected in the context of drug use policies.

The legalization of cannabis for non-medical use in Canada in 2018 is a useful example where the aims of public health were particularly embedded in legislative actions. Youth access to cannabis was one of the key targets while promoting public education on its dangers simultaneously. With the prevalence of young people who use cannabis increasing, the law is able to make a significant impact on patterns of use and related health effects. Integrated public health policies, in the Cannabis Act, reflect evolving knowledge about the ways that policy is able to act upon underlying health disparities and foster community health in a manner that translates to global discussions of the intersection of substance use and public health control (Kourgiantakis et al., 2024). Moreover, successful public health policies are often informed by their adaptability and responsiveness to emerging evidence and shifting societal needs. Through the ability to modify policies in accordance with emerging research developments, public health interventions may always stay relevant and effective. For instance, states identified crucial approaches of relationship building and communication towards promoting beneficial collaboration with the integration of primary care and public health systems. By adopting the use of coordinated bodies to justify interactions between stakeholders, such policies demonstrate proactive governance aimed at enhancing public health capacity. Moreover, the emphasis on prevention via education and population mobilization is a hallmark of an inherent shift towards an integrated response in problem-solving public health issues, hence cementing the position of policy and legislation in fostering healthier communities (Baum et al., 2024) (Figure 15.11).

15.5.1. Role of Government in Public Health

The role of the government in public health is critical, particularly in developing and drafting prevention strategies that protect and enhance public health. All levels of government should promulgate policies and programs that will act against health risks and address public health crises. During the COVID-19 pandemic, for instance, governments had put in place Community Activity Restrictions (PPKM) to facilitate total health measures, including compulsory mask use, social distancing, and vaccination campaigns designed to reduce the infection rate. The measures underpinned the necessity for strong government action to guide public behavior, thereby entrenching the importance of organized frameworks for health management. Moreover, the success of these interventions relied significantly on compliance and uptake by the communities, indicating the collective intervention between government agencies and citizens in ensuring health despite adversity, as evidenced through the study results in the guise of sustained public commitment to health regulations during the pandemic (Munir and Puspitasari, 2023). Outside of emergency response, governments play an important part in the resolution of long-term public health issues, , such as obesity, through policy and the legal system that promotes healthy living. CDC's legal preparedness framework explains how laws and legal authority can inform obesity prevention through settings like nutrition and healthy places. For example, local and state government agencies can use food marketing regulations and zoning ordinances to create spaces that promote physical activity and consumption of healthy food. Innovative approaches , such as taxing and subsidizing food can also be used to promote healthier eating habits among the population. This integrated model shows how the influence of the power of governments can shape social behavior and environments that support long-term health benefits, thereby securing the government's pivotal role in public health interventions (Gostin et al., 2009). Further, effective public health policies depend not only on legislative action but also on interagency collaboration and coalition building at the community level. Governments must mobilize different stakeholders, like healthcare providers, schools, and local civil society groups, to bring forth an integrated approach for public health. Through active community involvement in health programs, governments can develop more trust and cooperation, which are vital to successful prevention programs. For instance, volunteer efforts during health crises like immunization and disease prevention awareness campaigns can complement government efforts significantly and touch a large number of people. Lastly, the governmental role of establishing policy, supplying resources, and forming collaborations at the community level positions it as a groundwork for effective public health policy and optimizing health outcomes for all citizens (Munir and Puspitasari, 2023).

15.5.2. Key Public Health Policies and Legislation

Effective public health policy and regulation are imperative in advancing health outcomes and disease prevention among populations. By adopting frameworks that target key health determinants, such policies are capable of mitigating established risks of many public health hazards. For instance, effective hospital wastewater (HWW) management is highly crucial, especially in low- and middle-income economies (LMICs), where untreated effluents can lead to significant environmental and health risks, including the spread of antibiotic-resistant bacteria (ARB) and genes (ARGs). Implementation of strict regulations demanding treatment of HWW can greatly reduce these pathogens in the environment, hence protecting public health. Also, through the implementation of efficient monitoring mechanisms, such treatment systems do not lose their efficiency, hence indirectly addressing the call to global action against antimicrobial resistance (AMR) and reasserting the role of comprehensive public health policy in the avoidance of health risks from wastewater disposal (Hounmanou et al., 2025). But still another critical area of public health policy is that of acting to address gambling as a health issue, where calling out its potential harm must be followed by enactments. While gambling has been legalized in the majority of the world, with over 80% of countries permitting it, public health is typically secondary to economic interests, including but not limited to generating revenue. Current estimates indicate that prevention interventions nearly wholly depend on individual responsibility, rather than the overall societal determinants of gambling harms. Failure to encompass a balanced policy response not only defeats public health objectives but also limits the potential for effective harm reduction that may be able to address the political, economic, and commercial determinants of gambling. While the public health stakeholders advocate for an integrated approach, the challenge is to ensure wellbeing and health take precedence in gambling legislation, which, to date, has shown limited consonance with public health objectives (Feldens et al., 2023). There needs to be a dialogue between policy within public health and regulation methods to enhance healthier environments and communities. For example, the introduction of strict smoking prohibitions and tobacco sale-specific legislation has evidently reduced the prevalence of smoking and related morbidity. Similarly, addressing hazardous waste in healthcare settings, particularly in

LMICs, requires efficient regulatory regimes to protect the environment and public health. By imposing tighter regulations on hazardous waste disposal and promoting environmentally friendly practices, public health authorities can preempt future occurrences of health complications from environmental degradation. Besides, these regulations must be supported by education and resource allocation to enable communities to implement efficient prevention policies. Ultimately, an active and comprehensive public health policy framework can lead the way for creative regulation that protects the public's health and enables sustainable development in the face of new health challenges (Feldens et al., 2023; Hounmanou et al., 2025) (Figure 15.12).

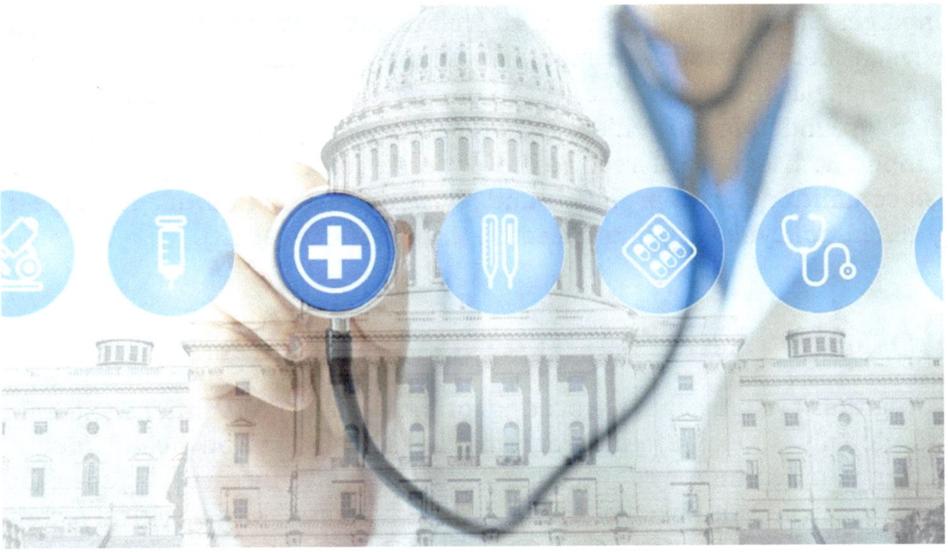

Figure 15.12. Symbolic representation of healthcare policy and governmental reform initiatives.

Source: https://www.publichealth.columbia.edu/sites/default/files/styles/cola_media_1280_16_9/public/media/images/2022-01/healthcare-reform-banner.jpg?itok=9HnELq-q.

15.5.3. Advocacy for Health-Related Legislation

Successful advocacy for legislation that addresses health issues is a central factor in the formulation of public health policies that respond to pressing community demands. Advocacy for legislation encompasses a broad range of stakeholders, including public health organizations, legislators, and community advocates, who collaborate to build an impact on health. The outreach most commonly involves increasing awareness about specific health issues, , such as mental health provider burnout, which has increased across the board, particularly in burgeoning regions like Charlotte, North Carolina. Self-care and burnout prevention advocacy not only addresses the existing issues faced by mental health professionals but can also potentially serve to improve patient care and overall community health outcomes. When health practitioners articulate their needs and network around common goals, they contribute to a more informed and responsive legislative setting that focuses on health-oriented activities (Marcy, 2023). The achievement of health legislations by advocacy coalitions attests to the importance of collaborative action among various groups focused on public health. The California menu labeling law case highlights how state policy can be effectively influenced by public health coalitions that make concerted efforts and communicate effectively to push for legislative action. The public health coalition in this case mobilized various resources, , such as public opinion polls and media relations, to build support for well-informed consumer choice. This demonstrates the efficacy of advocacy coalitions not only in placing policies on the agenda but in communicating effectively with legislative panels to enact necessary change. Through their collective expertise and standing together as a united wall, these coalitions can be instrumental in public health legislation, ensuring it adheres to community needs and the most current evidence regarding health promotion (Cousineau et al., 2017). Moreover, good lobbying for health legislation often entails a multi-faceted approach, both addressing the symptoms of public health issues as well as their causes. This entails lobbying to help mental health practitioners through education campaigns and financial support, as well as attempts at influencing systemic shifts in healthcare delivery. Methods , such as mobilizing money to finance mental health interventions, are useful in the fight against causative forces of provider burnout. As the campaigns go along, they must remain grounded in the evidence of prevention and public health interventions, merging stakeholders' input with empirical realities to endorse solutions. Lastly, effective advocacy is a bridge between committed health problems and legislative action in order to shape a better world through enlightened policymaking and collective effort (Marcy, 2023).

15.6. Global Health Initiatives

Global health programs are crucial in advocating for preventive interventions and enhancing public health systems globally. Global health programs focus on narrowed health inequalities among disadvantaged communities, thereby advocating for health equity. By executing specialized programs, they aim to narrow down health obstacles to health care accessibility, a critical factor in successful disease prevention. For example, maternal and child health initiatives have registered significant progress toward health gains through the provision of vital services and education to high-risk populations. Moreover, government-nongovernmental organization-international institutional joint efforts maximize their impact, unveiling a collective action against major global health risks. Increasing not only the health systems but also allowing societies to deal with emerging health risks more capable is the secondary gain from this collective action. The evaluation of global health programs proves the importance of evidence-based interventions in guiding public health policy. Based on the application of information from various health interventions, such programs can identify successful interventions and those that require modification. For instance, a comparison of the outcome of vaccination programs may guide public acceptability as well as logistics. Such an evidence-based approach enables policymakers to make informed choices, with the confidence that they are utilizing resources effectively and efficiently. Furthermore, continuous monitoring and assessment are central to strategy modification in countering changing health environments. Such adaptability is critical in countering unforeseen events, , such as epidemics, and learning from each initiative and then applying those lessons to future efforts is paramount. Thus, careful knowledge of past global health initiatives informs future preventive and public health policy direction. Tackling the social determinants of health continues to be at the heart of work in global health since these conditions immensely affect health outcomes. Interventions that integrate education, socioeconomic development, and environmental factors in public health initiatives yield more sustainable improvements in health. One such example is interventions on the built environment, like access to improved water and sanitation, which can make a huge impact on community health. Through understanding the complex interplay of these determinants, programs for health can best guide their interventions. Community participation is also at the core of ensuring programs are appropriate for those they aim to assist, in order to foster ownership and accountability. The findings and recommendations from global health programs, as demonstrated in Birnbaum et al. (2011), point towards the need for an integrated plan that addresses long-standing social issues alongside using preventive health measures. It is such a comprehensive strategy that is needed for effective long-term public health achievements (Figure 15.13).

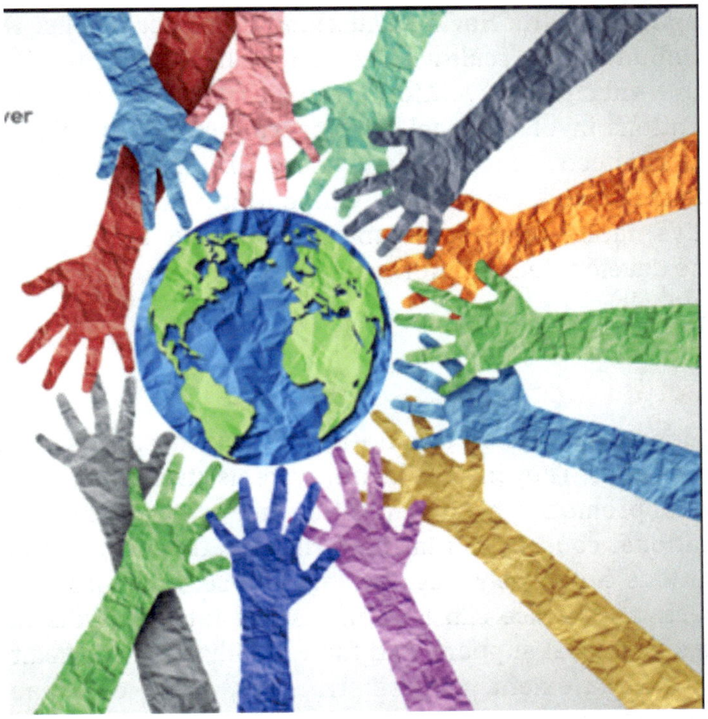

Figure 15.13. Hands of diverse colors encircling the globe, symbolizing global cooperation and equity in health.

Source: https://aidspan.org/wp-content/uploads/2023/10/Reimagining-the-future-of-GHIs.png.

15.6.1. International Organizations and Their Roles

International bodies play a key role in guiding prevention and public health policy, particularly in attending to complex issues of global health. Institutions , such as the World Health Organization (WHO) and the United Nations Children's Fund (UNICEF) are at the core of mobilizing global action on health crises and also advocating for policy reform. Their objective is to join hands in marshaling research, provision of sharing knowledge, and employing best practices among member nations. This cooperative structure allows nations to more effectively act upon swift public health concerns, , such as pandemics and maternal mortality, allowing for a more cohesive global strategy. Furthermore, these agencies fund individual programs that directly contribute to improving outcomes in health, exhibiting their central function within the overall body of public health prevention methods. The role of including men and boys in public health programs has been underscored in numerous strategies submitted by global bodies. For example, programs to prevent sexual violence highlight the requirement for men to be included in order to help refute negative gender norms and push for good behavior. Organizations like Oak Foundation, in their report commissioned, have applied broad-based analysis to establish effective intervention strategies in engaging men in preventing child sexual abuse (N/A, 2012). Focus on the engagement of men not only enhances preventive measures for vulnerable groups but also encourages a culture of responsibility. By encouraging awareness and utilization of educational programs, global agencies can effectively reduce the rate of violence and assist in improving general community health. In addition, gender-based violence is crucial to be addressed with an integrated strategy by global agencies committed to public health. Having understood violence against women as a ubiquitous issue entwined with profound social realities, institutions like the United Nations have introduced detailed examinations of effective prevention strategies (Bott et al., 2025). These institutions aim to evaluate interventions involving legal reforms, community mobilization, and health sector responses. By recognizing effective methods and those that need further research, international organizations can expand their efforts towards eliminating intimate partner violence and sexual assault. The collaborative nature of these organizations allows for the sharing of resources and expertise, facilitating the development of informed policies and programs that ultimately contribute to healthier societies globally.

15.6.2. Global Strategies for Disease Prevention

Global disease control measures involve a multi-faceted approach of a series of interventions at global, national, and local levels. They involve health systems strengthening, enhancing surveillance and response systems, and promoting health education and behavior change. WHO places emphasis on the need for international cooperation in the form of nations coming together to address the challenges that their nations collectively face, including those that emanate from globalization and climate change. A collective response can help in disease infectious disease prevention through sharing of best practices, technical support, and fund mobilization for health programs. Universal health coverage is also a key element in these strategies, giving everyone accesses to essential health services without resulting in financial hardship. Public health programs play a significant role in disease prevention through eco-friendly measures, particularly in urban settings. Design and use of public space can bring healthy behavior in neighborhoods. For instance, public space development not only provides recreational areas but can also promote physical activity, thereby reducing the incidence of noncommunicable diseases , such as diabetes and obesity. Evidence shows that effective public space initiatives can be coordinated with the development of population health, thereby ensuring a just healthy environment. These strategies, though, overall, would, when integrated with community engagement, lead to sustainable and healthier outcomes. After the need for systemic review of public space projects in African cities, evidence a greater recognition of the effect of environmental factors on health and wellbeing. This is in alignment with international strategies of prevention via health promotion and community-level empowerment (Brannan et al., 2019). Research and technology investment play a crucial role in augmenting disease prevention strategies around the globe. With data analytics and digital health technologies, it is easier to monitor outbreaks of diseases as well as track risk factors affecting various populations. Technology also facilitates telemedicine and remote consultations that can increase accessibility to healthcare, especially for rural populations. The promotion of vaccine research and provision also points to a significant aspect of global health policies aimed at disease avoidance. Through the extension of equal access to vaccines in the developing world, the global community can progress toward the control and elimination of diseases that disproportionately affect vulnerable populations.

Also, promoting collaborations between governments, non-profit sectors, and private agencies can lead to significant development in public health programs, thereby fostering the comprehensive frameworks required for effective global disease prevention (Brannan et al., 2019) (Figure 15.14).

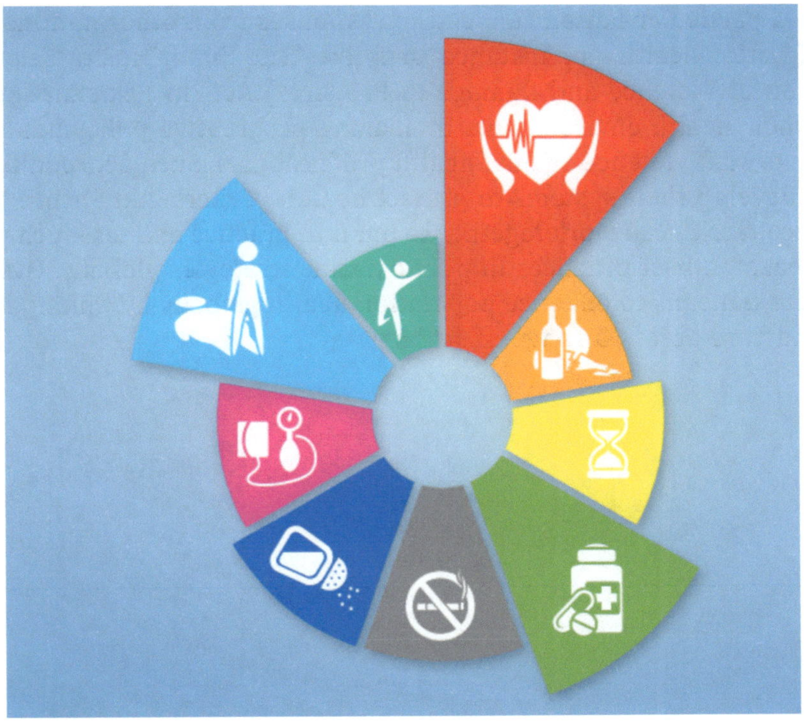

Figure 15.14. Key components of NCD prevention depicted through lifestyle and health management icons.

Source: https://ncdalliance.org/sites/default/files/news/WHO%20graphic.png.

15.6.3. Collaboration Between Countries for Health Improvement

Coordination between countries is essential to enhancing health outcomes and developing effective prevention strategies during an age of globalization. Coordination is typically attained through international conventions, organizations, and joint efforts for dealing with pressing issues in health , such as pandemics, drug dependency, and workplace violence. Through resource aggregation, data, and technical expertise, countries are able to significantly elevate the profile of their work in public health. For instance, integrated surveillance systems help nations monitor and respond to epidemics better, and collaborative research can assist in yielding innovative solutions unique to an individual health emergency. Ultimately, all this works towards standardizing procedures and fostering a culture of mutual responsibility in health development efforts. Along with that, the exchange of best practices and educational materials between countries makes it easier to get to know various health systems and their vulnerabilities. As was evidently demonstrated by the global drug abuse epidemic, pharmacists are increasingly acclaimed for their indispensable contribution to public health work outside the borders. Their involvement in outreach work, educational campaigns, and community engagement places them above other drug prevention activities since they work in cooperation with several healthcare providers. Additionally, countries have lessons to learn from others' successes and failures of strategies, modeling their efforts to fit local contexts while maintaining a commitment to enhancing global health. Such collaborative learning is instrumental in solving complex health issues that span state lines and must be addressed collectively. Legislative initiatives taken by a particular nation can lead to responses from other nations such that there is a cascade effect of better health. For instance, acts like "The Sindh Health Service Providers and Facilities (Prevention of Violence and Damage to Property) Act" in Pakistan show how countries are able to shape their health environments by making progressive policymaking, with a view to addressing issues like staff violence against health professionals. Such acts could possibly motivate other countries to develop their systems to protect health workers and ensure the quality of care provided. Different countries can work together to put into practice and test such policies, producing a strong evidence base on best practices in public health strategies globally. Overall, international cooperation provides a means to enhance population health globally by linking forces to maximize both prevention and care across a range of settings.

CLOSER LOOK

PUBLIC HEALTH

Public health is a multidisciplinary field focused on improving the health and well-being of populations through prevention, education, policy-making, and organized efforts to reduce health disparities. Unlike clinical medicine, which centers on treating individuals, public health works at the community and societal level, aiming to prevent diseases before they occur. It encompasses a wide range of activities, from promoting healthy lifestyles and improving sanitation to controlling infectious disease outbreaks and shaping health policies. One of the core goals of public health is to create conditions in which people can be healthy, regardless of their socioeconomic status, geographic location, or background. This includes addressing social determinants of health—such as education, income, housing, and access to healthcare—which significantly impact health outcomes. Public health has played a critical role in some of the most important health advancements in history, including vaccination programs, tobacco control, improved maternal and child health, and the development of clean water systems. However, the field faces growing challenges in the modern world. Emerging infectious diseases like COVID-19 have highlighted both the strengths and limitations of global public health systems. Meanwhile, non-communicable diseases (NCDs) such as obesity, heart disease, and diabetes continue to rise due to lifestyle factors, urbanization, and aging populations. Climate change also poses new threats, increasing the frequency of heatwaves, natural disasters, and vector-borne diseases. Mental health, long overlooked in public health discussions, is now gaining attention as a vital component of overall well-being. The importance of effective communication, health education, and community engagement has become more apparent than ever in light of recent global health crises. At the same time, public health professionals must navigate misinformation, political resistance, and resource limitations while advocating for science-based interventions. Technology and data analytics are now playing a growing role in public health, offering tools for disease surveillance, health trend analysis, and targeted interventions. Ultimately, the success of public health depends on collaboration across sectors—including governments, healthcare providers, educators, and communities—to develop sustainable solutions that promote equity and long-term health. As we look to the future, public health must continue to evolve, addressing both traditional and emerging challenges with innovation, resilience, and a strong commitment to the collective good.

SUMMARY

Effective public health responses should embed a multi-dimensional approach to address the dynamics of health crises , such as the COVID-19 pandemic. This embedding is premised on balancing individual confidentiality and public good outcomes in health, since the release of information will significantly affect prevention outcomes. The empirical findings reveal that the inherent contradiction between privacy demands and the demand for information disclosure may be balanced by leading internet users to conduct expectations for public health while ensuring personal data security. In this way, awareness campaigns and incentives serve a major role in remaking user conduct in order to develop community resistance to health threats (Xiao et al., 2021). Further, pandemic social media discourse illuminates the public's mixed emotional responses to health news. These emotions, ranging from hope to fear, are directly translated into the community's perception and response to epidemic advancement. Since the findings have been demonstrated, a majority of the population is engaging in arguments on critical matters , such as sources of transmission and prevention measures, which reflect that the population is actually searching for information and enlightenment. This attests to the necessity for health officials to release factual and timely information to control the mood of the masses, consequently developing an enlightened and responsive public sphere for health programs (Zhong, 2020). Finally, the integration of privacy concerns and sound communication policies can increase the overall efficiency of public health interventions. With solutions to both the issue of misinformation as well as emotional instability, health authorities can make individuals contribute meaningfully towards the collective efforts of health. Policies that center on open communication, along with guarantees through emotions, can minimize public fear and facilitate compliance with health policies. Lastly, the lessons from the COVID-19 pandemic demonstrate the necessity of developing robust frameworks that prioritize the rights of individuals and the well-being of the population as a whole, paving the way for improved-resilient public health responses in the future (Xiao et al., 2021).

With regard to effective prevention and public health, it is important to account for the severity of health matters, particularly in regions of high disease prevalence like HIV. Poverty and gender inequality, for instance, are foremost socioeconomic determinants in South Africa, which more specifically exacerbate the HIV spread and disproportionately affect the 15–24-year-olds. It has been proven through studies that countries with good antiretroviral therapy (ART) programs, , such as Botswana, have recorded impressive gains in the reduction of new infections. However, stigma and poor healthcare accessibility still pose challenges, necessitating increased public health interventions. The findings echo the need for community-based interventions in developing resilience as well as breaking down the barriers posed by the affected groups to effectively battle the chronic HIV epidemic (Khupe et al., 2025). An added effective method in public health involves community participation and empowerment, or in the context of substance use issues. A good example of this method is the alliance between the Market Development Association (MDA) and Queens Communities and Place (QCAP). In encouraging community participation in dialogue regarding substance use as well as in mapping out service gaps, the MDA and QCAP were able to find out more about the particular concerns and needs of the community. The thematic analysis revealed the high levels of community knowledge and change optimism, where the emphasis was on the promise of effective interventions. This reflects the potential of leveraging community wisdom to inform public health interventions and impact service delivery, demonstrating that inclusive strategies lead to effective prevention programs (Brannan et al., 2019). Lastly, long-term investment in prevention cannot be overstated. As reflected in ongoing efforts to develop education initiatives and enhance support services within the Market area, forward-thinking planning would best have long-term community health objectives as its first priority. Initiatives to educate parents about drug use, develop youth tools, and implement health navigator position are all steps toward supporting informed decision-making and improving service access. Furthermore, establishing bridges between local health professionals and the community can also enhance service delivery and reduce access barriers to care. Public health interventions are ultimately effective depending on thorough knowledge of the needs of the community, which necessitates both short-term and long-term efforts toward the establishment of a healthier future (Brannan et al., 2019).

References

1. Ahmed, A., Dzinamarira, T., Gahamanyi, N., Gashema, P., et al. (2024). Mpox in East Africa: Learning from COVID-19 and Ebola to strengthen public health responses. https://core.ac.uk/download/621338081.pdf (accessed on 13th June 2025).
2. Ali, S. T., Muffadil, T., Yasir, M., Otho, M. S., & Siddiqui, M. B. (2024). Assessing the needs of healthcare providers to comply with the Sindh Health Service Providers and Facilities Act (2021) on violence prevention in Karachi, Pakistan. *International Journal of Endorsing Health Science Research*. https://www.semanticscholar.org/paper/ea95894cd6d82943717d2c55294403724e7330c6 (accessed on 13th June 2025).
3. Barral, M., Beresniak, A., Bonnevay, S., Bounekkar, A., et al. (2015). Assessment of human influenza pandemic scenarios in Europe. https://core.ac.uk/download/54524838.pdf (accessed on 13th June 2025).
4. Baum, N. M., Iovan, S., & Udow-Phillips, M. (2024). Strengthening public health through primary care and public health collaboration: Innovative state approaches. *Journal of Public Health Management and Practice, 30*, E47–E53. https://www.semanticscholar.org/paper/aec6d86131a6e4f71d32d035d6d1d5040fc0a6c4 (accessed on 13th June 2025).
5. Befus, D., Burkell, J., Comer, L., Cooke, S., et al. (2021). Digital technology and disease surveillance in the COVID-19 pandemic: A scoping review protocol. https://core.ac.uk/download/534388148.pdf (accessed on 13th June 2025).
6. Bekker, L. G., Nglazi, M. D., Shey, M. S., Uthman, O. A., et al. (2014). The impact of mass media interventions on tuberculosis awareness, health-seeking behavior and health service utilization: A systematic review protocol. https://core.ac.uk/download/19553650.pdf (accessed on 13th June 2025).
7. Bello, A. K., Cherney, D. Z. I., & Luyckx, V. A. (2020). Preventing CKD in developed countries. https://www.zora.uzh.ch/id/eprint/186565/1/PIIS2468024919315864.pdf (accessed on 13th June 2025).
8. Gostin, Lawrence O. and Berkman, Benjamin E., "Pandemic Influenza: Ethics, Law, and the Public's Health" (2007). *Georgetown Law Faculty Publications and Other Works*. 449. https://scholarship.law.georgetown.edu/facpub/449(accessed on 13th June 2025).
9. Birnbaum, N., Masterson, E., & Schoomaker, H. (2011). *State of Health Equity Movement, 2011 Update Part B: Catalog of Activities* (DRA Project Report No. 11-02). https://core.ac.uk/download/pdf/18491811.pdf (accessed on 13th June 2025).
10. Birnbaum, N., Masterson, E., & Schoomaker, H. (2011). *State of Health Equity Movement, 2011 Update Part C: Compendium of Recommendations* (DRA Project Report No. 11-03). https://core.ac.uk/download/pdf/18491812.pdf (accessed on 13th June 2025).
11. Bott, S., Ellsberg, M., & Morrison, A. (2025). Preventing and responding to gender-based violence in middle and low-income countries: A global review and analysis. https://core.ac.uk/download/pdf/6645361.pdf (accessed on 13th June 2025).
12. Brannan, M., Bernardotto, M., Clarke, N., & Varney, J. (2019). Moving healthcare professionals–A whole system approach to embed physical activity in clinical practice. *BMC Medical Education, 19*. https://doi.org/10.1186/s12909-019-1517-y (accessed on 13th June 2025).

13. Brown, L., Philpart, M., & Masoud, S. (2015). *Building Place-Based Initiatives for Boys and Men of Color and Vulnerable Populations: A Community Planning Guide.* https://core.ac.uk/download/75782836.pdf (accessed on 13th June 2025).

14. Brownson, R. C., Franco, M., Mazzucca, S., Padek, M., et al. (2019). Going beyond the individual: How state-level characteristics relate to HPV vaccine rates in the United States. https://core.ac.uk/download/223009500.pdf (accessed on 13th June 2025).

15. Cousineau, M. R., Lewis, L. B., Nichol, M. B., Payán, C., et al. (2017). Advocacy coalitions involved in California's menu labeling policy debate: Exploring coalition structure, policy beliefs, resources, and strategies. https://core.ac.uk/download/323063874.pdf (accessed on 13th June 2025).

16. Feldens, E., Ukhova, V. D., University of Helsinki, & Promotion and Prevention. (2023). Embracing public health approaches to gambling? A review of global legislative and regulatory trends. *The European Journal of Public Health, 33.* https://www.semanticscholar.org/paper/c57e0330d925e2a7344ea7dbaab4b80759f33df6 (accessed on 13th June 2025).

17. George, B., & Ravola, M. (2024). Fighting fire with fire: Reclaiming social media to promote healthy eating behaviors among children. https://core.ac.uk/download/634253112.pdf (accessed on 13th June 2025).

18. Goglio, A., & Stefani, S. (2010). Methicillin-resistant *Staphylococcus aureus*: Related infections and antibiotic resistance. https://core.ac.uk/download/572837588.pdf (accessed on 13th June 2025).

19. Gore, M., Patil, R., & Tiwari, R. (2024). Understanding health communication processes and challenges: Cultural insights from Katari tribal in western Maharashtra, India. https://core.ac.uk/download/630038246.pdf (accessed on 13th June 2025).

20. Gostin, L. O., Gottfried, R. N., Jacobson, P. D., Pomeranz, J. L., et al. (2009). Assessing laws and legal authorities for obesity prevention and control. https://core.ac.uk/download/70374065.pdf (accessed on 13th June 2025).

21. Jha, P., Seshadri, S. R., & Subramaniyam, P. (2025). The potential demand for and strategic use of an HIV-1 vaccine in Southern India. https://core.ac.uk/download/pdf/6644967.pdf (accessed on 13th June 2025).

22. Jorge, A. M. (2012). Insights into cell wall synthesis and cell division in *Staphylococcus aureus.* https://core.ac.uk/download/157625622.pdf (accessed on 13th June 2025).

23. Khupe, S., Salibi, G., & Tzenios, N. (2025). HIV prevalence in Southern African countries, complete with summaries and important points for each part. *Special Journal of the Medical Academy and Other Life Sciences.* https://www.semanticscholar.org/paper/cf0d4cd6fb52e2ef2b3ed94d674215d006151300 (accessed on 13th June 2025).

24. Maben, J., & Bridges, J. (2020). COVID-19: Supporting nurses' psychological and mental health. *Journal of Clinical Nursing, 29*, 2742–2750. https://doi.org/10.1111/jocn.15307 (accessed on 13th June 2025).

25. Marcy, R. (2023). Preventing burnout among mental health professionals in Charlotte, NC. https://core.ac.uk/download/580004978.pdf (accessed on 13th June 2025).

26. Medeiros, A. C. T. de, Medeiros, F. de A. L., Nóbrega, M. M. L. da, Oliveira, L. M. M., et al. (2015). Characterization of older hypertensive registered in the state of SISHIPERDIA Paraíba: Allowance for health surveillance. https://www.ssoar.info/ssoar/bitstream/document/53967/1/ssoar-revpesquisa-2015-Supl.-oliveira_et_al-Characterization_of_older_hipertensive_registered.pdf (accessed on 13th June 2025).
27. Munir, Z., & Puspitasari, M. (2023). Volunteer health service in COVID-19 prevention at Exit Toll Laces Probolinggo. https://core.ac.uk/download/591386592.pdf (accessed on 13th June 2025).
28. Stroffolini, T., & Stroffolini, G. (2023). A historical overview on the role of hepatitis B and C viruses as etiological factors for hepatocellular carcinoma. *Cancers, 15*. https://www.semanticscholar.org/paper/8258e812336c28e63582edea9ea0b069d54f22ba (accessed on 13th June 2025).
29. World Health Organization Regional Office for Africa. Division of Communicable Disease Prevention and Control. (2014). *Integrated Disease Surveillance and Response in the African region*. https://core.ac.uk/download/144179434.pdf (accessed on 13th June 2025).
30. Xiao, Y., Xu, W., Zeng, S., & Peng, Q. (2021). Online user information sharing and government pandemic prevention and control strategies—Based on evolutionary game model. *Frontiers in Public Health, 9*. https://www.semanticscholar.org/paper/378b722038f464030772ac3b2cf081747d7307dc (accessed on 13th June 2025).

INDEX

A

Abnormal bone 243, 250
Academic growth 157
Acceptable Macronutrient Distribution Range (AMDR) 40
Adequate nutrition 146, 147, 148, 158, 159
Adiposity 282, 284, 311
Adolescents 348, 349, 352, 353, 362, 363, 365, 370, 372, 373, 380
Amino acidopathies 314
Amino acids 40, 43, 44, 45, 46, 48, 49, 50, 53, 54, 57, 61
Anorexia Nervosa 352, 367
Anthropometric assessment 113
Anthropometric measurements 107, 108, 112, 113, 114, 119, 120, 133
Anthropometry 111
Antimicrobial resistance 2, 34, 37, 384, 411
Antiretroviral therapy (ART) 514
Artificial Intelligence (AI) 115
Assimilation 1
Asymptomatic 244, 245, 250
Asymptomatic patients 244
Atypical presentations 314
Autism Spectrum Disorder (ASD) 422
Autosomal Recessive 323
Average nutrient requirement (ANR) 114

B

Balance mental health 348
Bariatric surgery 252, 254, 255
Behavioral therapy 278
Behavior change 510
Beta-Oxidation 58
Bile production 383, 388
Binge Eating 354, 363
Binge Eating Disorder (BED) 354
Bioavailability 74, 78, 80, 81, 82, 83, 84, 85, 87, 88, 90, 94, 95, 96, 105
Biochemical assessment 107, 112
Biological pathways 248
Biological tissues 111
Bisphosphonates 244, 248, 251, 262, 263
Blood glucose control 212, 230, 233
Body mass index (BMI) 111, 113, 119, 122, 124, 137
Bone biology 248
Bone structure 244, 245, 247, 252, 258, 266, 267
Brain-derived neurotrophic factor (BDNF) 171
Broader system 176
Bulimia Nervosa 353, 354, 367

C

Calcium 93, 96, 245, 246, 247, 248, 249, 251, 252, 255, 256, 258, 262, 263, 264, 266, 267, 271
Carbohydrate 318

Carbohydrates 39, 40, 41, 43, 44, 45, 46, 47, 49, 50, 51, 52, 55, 57, 58, 60, 62, 63, 64, 66, 68
Cardiometabolic disease 280
Cardiovascular disease 2, 3, 10, 11, 19, 22, 23, 37, 175, 176, 178, 184, 185, 186, 201
Causing physical sickness 422
Cellular energy 40, 56
Cellular integrity 74
Chemotherapy-induced nausea and vomiting (CINV) 151
Chronic illnesses 485, 492, 497
Chronic kidney disease (CKD) 159, 422
Chronic pain disease 282
Chronic poverty 153
Circumstances 148, 154
Cirrhosis 383, 385, 395, 396, 397, 398, 400, 402, 404, 408, 413
Climatic change 161
Coeliac disease 420
Coenzymes 91
Cognitive Behavioral Therapy (CBT) 367
Colorectal cancer (CRC) 74
Combined Nutritional and Environmental Life Cycle Assessment (CONE-LCA) 110
Community health 179, 197
Community intervention 178, 194
Community involvement 484, 486, 506
Community-oriented approach 2
Community public 210
Complexities 109, 128
Complexity 180, 193, 199
Complexity of nutrition 422
Comprehensive management programs 385
Concurrent assessment 314
Critical information 109
Critical thinking 175
Cultural transformation 175
Cystic fibrosis 420

D

Data analysis 489, 494
Deficiency 246, 247, 251, 252, 253, 262, 264, 273, 274
Deficiency-related health 74
Dermatologic presentations 155
Detoxifying process 383
Developmental Origins of Health and Disease (DOHaD) 74
Diabetes 209, 210, 211, 212, 213, 214, 215, 216, 217, 218, 219, 220, 221, 222, 223, 224, 225, 226, 227, 228, 229, 230, 231, 232, 233, 234, 235, 236, 237, 238, 239, 240, 241, 242
Diabetes mellitus 210, 216, 222, 224, 238, 241
Diagnosis 161, 163
Dietary absorption 422
Dietary alterations 209
Dietary intake 145, 148, 149
Dietary Management 330
Dietary patterns 39, 69
Dietary questioning 107
Dietary sources 143
Diet behavior 419
Dietitians 385, 393, 403, 406
Diet transition 383
Digestion 387, 388, 389, 390, 403, 409
Digital health technologies 510
Disability-adjusted life years (DALYs) 155
Disastrous complications 210
Disease 73, 74, 76, 77, 79, 85, 88, 92, 94, 96, 98, 99, 100, 101
Disease expression 390
Disease management 108, 217, 233, 315
Disease mechanisms 73
Disease risk reduction 449
Disproportionately 485, 486, 510, 514
Disrupt food availability 147
Diversity 383
Dual-energy X-ray absorptiometry (DEXA) 112, 248, 258, 260
Dysfunctions 154
Dysregulation 390, 391

E

Eating Disorders 347, 348, 350, 351, 355, 363, 379, 380, 381
Economic instability 161

Economic status 110, 115, 128
Efficient assessment 110
Elaborate metabolic 315
Emotional eating 179, 184
Emotional instability 514
Emotional pain 347
Endocannabinoid system (ECS) 390, 406
Energy consumption 143, 151
Energy formation 39
Enzymatic defects 4
Enzyme phenylalanine hydroxylase 314, 319, 334
Ethnic populations 417
Etiology 244, 245, 252, 253, 260, 262, 273, 275

F

Fatty liver 145
Fecal microbiota transplantation (FMT) 215
Fluid accumulation 155
Food certification 114
Food choice behaviors 422
Food consumption 150, 151, 166
Food insecurity 150, 153
Food intake data 111, 112
Food service 157
Functional heartburn (FH) 393

G

Galactosemia 314, 317, 323, 326, 336, 337
Gastroesophageal reflux disease (GERD) 384, 387, 391, 394, 402, 405
Gastrointestinal disease 384, 385, 386, 387, 389, 393, 402, 403, 407, 408, 409, 411, 412
Gastrointestinal (GI) 390
Gastrointestinal illnesses 384
Gastrointestinal system 384, 385, 388, 389, 390, 399, 409
Gastrointestinal tract 383, 384, 386, 389, 390, 391, 399, 401, 403, 406, 409, 413, 414
Gene expression 74
Gene-nutrient interactions 454
Genetic diversity 450, 475, 476
Genetic population 450
Genetic susceptibility 278, 286, 301, 450, 459, 466
Genotypes 254, 316, 323
Gestational diabetes mellitus (GDM) 176, 183, 192, 213, 216
Global disease control 510
Global health 143, 145, 146, 161
Global healthcare system 178
Global Leadership Initiative on Malnutrition (GLIM) 161
Global population 215, 248
Glucagon 61, 63
Glucose 51
Glucose metabolism 73, 75, 101
Glycemic control 211, 214, 217, 218, 222, 225, 226, 229, 230, 231, 234, 235, 238, 239, 242
Glycogen Storage Diseases (GSDs) 318
Glycolysis 56
Gut-brain interactions 391, 394
Gut health grows 387
Gut microbiota 40, 42, 46, 47, 48, 49, 52, 53, 54, 55, 61, 62, 65, 68, 69, 70

H

Healthcare 108, 110, 113, 120, 124, 125, 126, 127, 128, 132, 133, 134, 137, 138, 383, 384, 387, 393, 399, 412
Healthcare decisions 108
Healthcare infrastructure 491
Healthcare policy 212
Healthcare professionals 244, 252
Healthcare systems 486, 491, 497, 504
Healthcare systems worldwide 383
Health consequences 243
Health disorders 108, 124
Health disparities 490, 505
Health landscape 175
Health literacy 422, 424
Health professionals 107, 109, 123, 124, 132, 133, 419, 421, 428, 430, 432
Health-related quality 108
Healthy food 418, 422, 424, 437
Hepatitis 383, 385, 388, 395, 396, 397, 398, 402, 404
Heterogeneity 214, 222

Holistic approach 175, 196, 202
Homeostasis 39, 40, 42, 43, 44, 45, 48, 52, 54, 57, 59, 60, 61, 62, 63, 66
Hormonal 245, 246, 248, 253, 254, 264, 271, 272
Human beings 383, 391
Hybrid models 348
Hyper-caloric 176
Hyper-consumption 176
Hyperglycemia 209, 210, 211, 214, 220, 222, 223, 224, 230, 238
Hyperlipidemia 282, 283

I

Immune defense 389
Immune function 73, 74, 79, 92, 100, 101, 153
Immune system 384, 386, 389, 391, 397
Immunity 426, 427
Immunization 490, 495, 500, 501, 502, 503, 506
Immunological health 389
Immunosuppressive 392, 397
Inadequate intake 147
Inadequate management 384
Inadequate mineralization 245
Inborn errors of metabolism (IEMs) 313, 315, 316, 321, 324, 325, 332, 333, 343
induced pluripotent stem cells (iPSCs) 316
Infant feeding behavior 147
Infection resistance 75
Inflammation 215
Inflammatory 383, 384, 387, 389, 390, 393, 394, 396, 399, 400, 401, 402, 404, 405, 406, 407, 411, 415
Inflammatory bowel disease (IBD) 150
Inherited causes 315
Insulin 42, 59, 60, 64
Insulin pumps 214
Insulin resistance 213, 214, 215, 216, 220, 221, 230, 234, 238
Insulin secretion 210, 213, 231, 238
Integrated approach 210, 216
Intersection 111, 132
Iron 88
Iron deficiency 419
Irritable bowel syndrome 384, 389, 391, 402, 405, 406, 408, 409, 414
Irritable bowel syndrome (IBS) 384, 391, 402, 405, 406, 408, 409

L

Lifestyle diseases 451, 457
Lipid imbalance 280, 282
Lipid metabolism 277, 278, 280, 281, 290, 302
Lipid metabolism enzymes 277, 285, 292
Lipolysis 45
Lipoproteins 54
Liver disease 383, 384, 385, 386, 387, 388, 389, 390, 391, 395, 396, 397, 398, 399, 400, 402, 403, 404, 405, 406, 407, 408, 409, 411, 412, 415
Liver injury 215
Low-density lipoprotein (LDL) 280, 281, 282, 298

M

Macronutrient metabolism 39, 55, 62
Macronutrients 1, 11, 39, 40, 41, 42, 43, 44, 45, 46, 47, 48, 50, 55, 56, 57, 58, 59, 60, 63, 65, 66, 68, 69
Malabsorption 420
Malabsorption syndromes 420
Malnutrition 2, 6, 107, 108, 109, 110, 111, 113, 114, 116, 117, 119, 127, 128, 129, 137, 138, 140
Malnutrition Inflammation Score (MIS) 161
Malnutrition-poverty cycles 143
Maple Syrup Urine Disease (MSUD) 335
Marasmus 144, 145, 151, 152, 153
Market Development Association (MDA) 514
Medical professionals 255, 261, 348, 360, 374
Medicine modalities 212
Mental health 419, 433, 434, 435, 438, 447
Metabolic 178
Metabolic activity 151
Metabolic bone diseases 243, 244, 245, 246, 248, 249, 251, 252, 253, 254, 256, 257, 258, 259, 260, 262, 264, 265, 266, 269, 271, 272
Metabolic bone disorders 243, 244, 245, 248, 251, 252, 253, 254, 255, 256, 258, 259, 261, 262, 264, 266, 267, 268, 271
Metabolic disease 176, 204, 207

Metabolic diseases 2, 4, 8, 15, 16, 22, 24, 28, 34, 35, 37
Metabolic disorders 1, 2, 3, 4, 5, 8, 9, 10, 13, 15, 17, 18, 19, 20, 21, 23, 25, 26, 27, 28, 29, 31, 32, 34, 35, 37, 313, 314, 315, 316, 317, 319, 322, 323, 324, 326, 327, 328, 329, 331, 333, 336, 339, 343, 344, 346
Metabolic disturbances 314, 326, 330, 334
Metabolic dysfunction 246
Metabolic efficiency 41, 51, 66
Metabolic functions 73, 74, 79, 80, 87, 92, 97
Metabolic health 40, 41, 42, 44, 48, 51, 53, 57, 58, 61, 62, 63, 64, 65, 66, 68, 69, 74, 77, 79, 83, 92, 103
Metabolic illnesses 2
Metabolic medicine 316
Metabolic regulation 383, 388, 395
Metabolic responses 449, 460, 462, 464
Metabolic syndrome 213, 215, 216
Metabolism 1, 4, 5, 10, 11, 12, 14, 18, 19, 20, 23, 25, 29, 30, 34, 35, 37
Metabolite analysis 314
Methodology 315
Microbial regulation 278
Microbiota 385, 386, 389, 391, 392, 394, 395, 397, 399, 411, 414, 415
Microbiota-gut-brain 278, 310
Micronutrient 152, 153
Micronutrient deficiencies 427, 436
Micronutrient-insecure 73
Micronutrient intake 73, 76, 80, 85, 99, 103
Micronutrient metabolism 73, 74, 75, 77, 78, 79, 80, 81, 82, 83, 84, 85, 87, 88, 89, 90, 91, 92, 94, 95, 96, 98, 103, 104
Micronutrients 73, 74, 75, 76, 77, 78, 79, 80, 81, 82, 83, 84, 85, 86, 87, 88, 89, 90, 91, 92, 93, 96, 97, 98, 99, 100, 101, 103, 104, 105
Mid-upper arm circumference (MUAC) 113
Mineral homeostasis 450
Mineralization processes 243
Mineral metabolism 245, 251, 271
Mini Nutritional Assessment (MNA) 108, 113, 164
Mobile health 216, 240
Morbidity 145, 150, 164
Morphology 246
Mortality 144, 145, 146, 158, 160, 164, 165, 174
Mortality worldwide 383
Moving Healthcare Professionals program (MHPP) 487
Multi-faceted approach 487, 508, 510
Multiple acyl-coenzyme A dehydrogenase deficiency (MADD) 283
Muscles 144, 153, 155
Mycoprotein 152
Myriad of disorders 40

N

Neonatal complications 177
Neonatal health 183
Neoplastic liver diseases 386
Neurodegenerative effects 278
Neurological abnormalities 314
Neurological health 282
Neurologic training 314
Non-alcoholic fatty liver disease (NAFLD) 179, 215
Non-communicable diseases (NCDs) 184
Nutrient absorption 148, 150, 154, 157, 164, 165
Nutrient uptake 383, 389, 409
Nutrigenomics 449, 450, 451, 452, 453, 454, 455, 457, 458, 459, 460, 461, 462, 463, 464, 465, 466, 467, 468, 469, 470, 471, 472, 473, 474, 475, 476, 478, 479, 480, 481, 482
Nutrition 108, 109, 110, 111, 112, 113, 114, 115, 116, 118, 122, 123, 124, 125, 126, 127, 128, 129, 130, 131, 132, 133, 134, 135, 137, 138, 141
Nutritional assessment 107, 108, 109, 110, 111, 112, 113, 114, 115, 116, 117, 118, 119, 120, 122, 123, 125, 126, 127, 129, 130, 131, 132, 133, 135, 138
Nutritional deficiencies 146, 157, 159, 166
Nutritional deficiency 110, 148, 158
Nutritional disorders 2, 417, 418, 419, 420, 421, 422, 424, 425, 427, 428, 429, 430, 432, 433, 436, 437, 438, 439, 440, 441, 442, 443, 445
nutritional issues 150
Nutritional Rehabilitation 369
Nutritional science 39, 42, 449, 457, 458

Nutrition counseling 3
Nutritionists 348, 375

O

Obesity 2, 3, 4, 6, 8, 10, 12, 14, 15, 17, 18, 19, 20, 21, 22, 23, 27, 28, 29, 30, 31, 34, 37
obesity epidemic 176, 180, 182, 183, 188, 205
Oral cholera vaccines (OCVs) 489
Organic acidemias 314
Osteodystrophy 251
Osteomalacia 244, 245, 246, 247, 248, 249, 251, 257, 259, 263, 274
Osteomalaciaoarthritis 248
Osteoporosis 243, 245, 246, 248, 249, 251, 252, 253, 254, 256, 257, 258, 259, 262, 263, 266, 267, 268, 269, 427, 434
Other specified foods or eating disorders (OSFED) 348
Overnutrition 18, 19
Oxygen transport 74, 78, 79

P

Paget's disease 243, 245, 247, 248, 250, 258
Parathyroid hormone (PTH) 253
Pathogenesis 277, 282, 286, 309
Pathophysiological 383, 393, 411
Pathophysiology 247, 249, 250, 260, 272
Pathophysiology of Paget's disease 247
Patient education 384, 385, 395, 411
Patient health 244
Perpetuate stigma 347
Pharmacogenomics 384
Pharmacologic 248
Pharmacologic drugs 282
Pharmacologic regimens 210
Pharmacologic treatment 245, 262
Phenylalanine 314, 319, 324, 329, 330, 334
Phenylketonuria (PKU) 314, 319, 328, 329, 330, 334, 339
Phosphorus 245, 248, 251, 258, 267, 271
Physical health 420, 432
Physical inactivity 383
Physiological functions 39, 43, 45, 50
Physiological variables 348
Policy determinants 487
Polycystic ovary syndrome (PCOS) 253
polyphyletic collection 277
Poor health globally 450
Population health 177, 192, 198
Post-traumatic stress disorder (PTSD) 377
Potential nutritional 108, 133
Produce blood cells 246
Productivity 384
Professional organizations 387
Promote better resource 491
Promote nutritional 160
Promoting health literacy 486
Protein 143, 144, 145, 147, 150, 151, 152, 153, 154, 155, 158, 159, 160, 161, 162, 163, 164, 165, 166, 167, 171, 173, 174
Protein-energy malnutrition 161
Protein-energy malnutrition (PEM) 143, 151
Proteins 39, 40, 41, 43, 44, 45, 46, 48, 49, 50, 51, 53, 54, 55, 57, 58, 60, 61, 62, 63, 64, 66, 68
Psychiatric 278
Psychological 347, 348, 350, 351, 352, 353, 354, 355, 356, 357, 358, 360, 361, 362, 363, 364, 365, 366, 367, 369, 370, 372, 374, 377, 378, 379, 380, 381
Psychological development 143
Psychologists 348, 350
Psychosocial 418, 419, 425, 436, 440
Psychosocial aspects 391
Psychosocial dysfunction 419
Psychosocial influences 217
Psychotherapy 393
Public health 2, 3, 4, 5, 6, 7, 10, 13, 14, 15, 19, 21, 22, 23, 24, 34, 35, 109, 110, 111, 113, 115, 116, 117, 118, 119, 120, 125, 129, 130, 131, 132, 134, 137, 138, 383, 384, 387, 396, 397, 411, 412
Public health communications 484
Public health intervention 483
Public health policy 252
Public health programs 450, 453, 466
Public policy 175, 190

Q

Queens Communities and Place (QCAP) 514

R

Residential aged care (RAC) 157

S

Short-chain fatty acids (SCFAs) 40, 46, 52, 62, 65, 68
Single-nucleotide polymorphisms (SNPs) 449, 453
Skeletal health 245, 247, 254, 263
Skeletal integrity 251, 267
Social media's idealization 347
Social pressure 347, 348
society 2, 5, 15, 34
Sociocultural 347, 348, 355, 356, 357, 377, 378
Socioecological framework (SEF) 487
Socio-economic 145, 146, 147, 149, 150, 151, 152, 161, 168, 171
Socioeconomic frameworks 490
Socioeconomic progress 146
Socioeconomics 143, 171
Sodium 2
Special populations 417, 418, 419, 420, 423, 424, 427, 434, 435, 436, 438, 439, 440, 441, 442, 443, 445, 446, 447
Spectacular cognitive 144
Spectrum 1, 5, 13
Stem cell technologies 316
Stereotypes 417
Subjective Global Assessment (SGA) 164
Sustainable Development Goals 486

T

Therapeutic modalities 419
Therapeutic treatments 278
Triggers hypertension 2
Triglycerides 54, 55
Tuberculosis 483
Type 1 diabetes mellitus (T1DM) 212, 214, 238
Type 2 diabetes mellitus (T2DM) 213

U

Undernutrition 6
Urea cycle disorders (UCD) 316

V

Vitamin A 90
Vitamin C 78
Vitamin D 78, 92, 100
Vitamin D deficiency 245, 246, 247, 248, 271, 273
Vitamins 7, 73, 74, 75, 76, 77, 78, 79, 80, 81, 82, 85, 86, 87, 89, 90, 91, 92, 95, 98, 99, 103, 105, 106
Vulnerable populations 486, 492, 501, 510

W

World Health Organization 145, 146, 159, 161, 169
World Health Organization (WHO) 210

Z

Zinc 100, 101